D1611897

CARDIOVASCULAR CARE
HANDBOOK

Springhouse Corporation
Springhouse, Pennsylvania

Editor Regina Daley Ford
Clinical Editor Susan Marks Weiner, RN, BSN
Assistant Editor Jo Lennon
Designer Lorraine Lostracco Carbo
Production Coordinator Susan Powell-Mishler
Copy Supervisor David Moreau
Art Production Manager Robert J. Perry III
Director, Typography/Editorial Computer Services David C. Kosten
Production Manager/Books Wilbur D. Davidson

The clinical procedures described and recommended in this publication are based on research and consultation with nursing, medical, and legal authorities. To the best of our knowledge, these procedures reflect currently accepted practice; nevertheless, they can't be considered absolute and universal recommendations. For individual application, all recommendations must be considered in light of the patient's clinical condition and, before administration of new or infrequently used drugs, in light of latest package-insert information. The authors and the publisher disclaim responsibility for any adverse effects resulting directly or indirectly from the suggested procedures, from any undetected errors, or from the reader's misunderstanding of the text.

Material in this book was adapted from Nurse's Reference Library® and Nurse's Clinical Library™.

Library of Congress Cataloging-in-Publication Data
Main entry under title:
Cardiovascular care handbook.

"Material in this book was adapted from Nurse's reference library and Nurse's clinical library"—T.p. verso.
 Includes bibliographies and index.
 1. Cardiovascular disease nursing—Handbooks, manuals, etc.   I. Springhouse Corporation. II. Nurse's reference library.   III. Nurse's clinical library. [DNLM: 1. Cardiovascular Diseases—nursing. WY 152.5 C26743] RC674.C358 1986 610.73'691 85-17376
ISBN 0-916730-98-0

TABLE OF CONTENTS

ADVISORY BOARD, CONTRIBUTORS, AND CLINICAL CONSULTANTS

ADVISORY BOARD

Lillian S. Brunner, RN, MSN, ScD, FAAN, Nurse/Author, Brunner Associates, Inc., Berwyn, Pa.

Donald C. Cannon, MD, PhD, Resident in Internal Medicine, University of Kansas, School of Medicine, Wichita

Luther Christman, RN, PhD, Dean, Rush College of Nursing; Vice-President, Nursing Affairs. Rush-Presbyterian-St. Luke's Medical Center, Chicago

Kathleen A. Dracup, RN, DNSc, FAAN, Associate Professor, School of Nursing, University of California at Los Angeles

Stanley J. Dudrick, MD, FACS, Professor, Department of Surgery, and Director, Nutritional Support Services, University of Texas Medical School at Houston; St. Luke's Episcopal Hospital, Houston

Halbert E. Fillinger, MD, Assistant Medical Examiner, Philadelphia County

M. Josephine Flaherty, RN, PhD, Principal Nursing Officer, Department of National Health and Welfare, Ottawa, Ont.

Joyce LeFever Kee, RN, MSN, Associate Professor, College of Nursing, University of Delaware, Newark

Dennis E. Leavelle, MD, Associate Professor, Mayo Medical Laboratories, Mayo Clinic, Rochester, Minn.

Roger M. Morrell, MD, PhD, FACP, Professor, Neurology and Immunology/Microbiology, Wayne State University, School of Medicine, Detroit; Chief Neurology Service, Veterans Administration Medical Center, Allen Park, Mich.; Diplomate, American Board of Psychiatry and Neurology

Ara G. Paul, PhD, Dean, College of Pharmacy, University of Michigan, Ann Arbor

Rose Pinneo, RN, MS, Associate Professor of Nursing and Clinician II, University of Rochester, N.Y.

Thomas E. Rubbert, BSL, LLB, JD, Attorney-at-Law, Pasadena, Calif.

Maryanne Schreiber, RN, BA, Product Manager, Patient Monitoring, Hewlett-Packard Co., Waltham (Mass.) Division

Frances J. Storlie, RN, PhD, ANP, Director, Personal Health Services, Southwest Washington Health District, Vancouver

Claire L. Watson, RN, Clinical Documentation Associate, IVAC Corporation, San Diego

CONTRIBUTORS

Edward Averill, RN, BSN, CEN, Staff Nurse, Portland (Ore.) V.A. Hospital

Katherine G. Baker, RN, MN, Clinical Specialist, UCLA Center for the Health Sciences, Los Angeles

Carol K. Barker, RN, MSN, MEd, Associate Professor, Bergen Community College, Paramus, N.J.

Patricia L. Baum, RN, BSN, Consultant in Peripheral Vascular Nursing, Boston

Frank Lowell Brown, UT, Chief Urology Technician, Maricopa Medical Center, Phoenix, Ariz.

CONTRIBUTORS *(continued)*

Marie Scott Brown, RN, PNP, PhD, Professor of Nursing, Oregon Health Science University, Portland

Judith Byrne, BS, MT(ASCP), Consultant and Author, Norristown, Pa.

Catherine R. Davis, RN, MSN, Assistant Professor of Nursing, Hahnemann University, Philadelphia

Charlotte M. Dienhart, PhD, Assistant Professor of Anatomy and Associate Professor of Community Health, Emory University School of Medicine, Atlanta

Gail D'Onofrio, RN, MS, Student, Boston University School of Medicine

Jeanne E. Doyle, RN, BS, Nurse Consultant/Peripheral Vascular Surgery, University Hospital, Boston

Kathleen Dracup, RN, DNSc, CCRN, Associate Professor, UCLA School of Nursing, Los Angeles

Diane Dressler, RN, MSN, CCRN, Clinical Nurse Specialist, Midwest Heart Surgery Institute, Milwaukee

Barbara Boyd Egoville, RN, MSN, West Chester, Pa.

John J. Fenton, PhD, DABCC, Associate Professor of Clinical Chemistry, West Chester (Pa.) University; Director of Chemistry, Crozer-Chester Medical Center, Chester, Pa.

Regina Daley Ford, RN, BSN, MA, Editor, Springhouse Corporation, Springhouse, Pa.

Richard K. Gibson, RN, MN, JD, CCRN, Staff Nurse, Critical Care, Kaiser Foundation Hospital, San Diego

Barbara A. Gleeson, RN, MSN, CCRN, Cardiac Rehabilitation Nurse Specialist, Albert Einstein Medical Center, Mount Sinai/Daroff Division, Philadelphia

Rebecca G. Hathaway, RN, MSN, Executive Assistant Director of Nursing Service; Assistant Clinical Professor of Nursing, UCLA Medical Center, Los Angeles

Patrice M. Harman, RN, Staff Builders, Ventura, Calif.

Annette Remington Harmon, RN, MSN, Director of Nursing, Memorial Hospital, San Leandro, Calif.

Sr. Mary Brian Kelber, DNSc, Associate Professor, University of San Francisco

Catherine E. Kirby, RN, MSN, Clinical Instructor, Nursing Department, Lehigh Valley Hospital Center, Allentown, Pa.

Diane Monkowski Magnuson, RN, BSN, Staff Nurse, Doylestown (Pa.) Hospital

Elizabeth Anne Mallon, MS, MT(ASCP), Transplant Coordinator, Thomas Jefferson University Hospital, Philadelphia

Carolyn G. Smith Marker, RN, MSN, CNA, Consultant/Instructor, Resource Applications, Baltimore

Nancy L. Mauldin, RN, Cardiovascular Nurse/Technician, Saint Mary's Hospital, Galveston, Tex.

Marylou K. McHugh, RN, MSN, Academic Counselor, Department of Nursing, LaSalle University, Philadelphia

Patricia Gonce Miller, RN, MS, Instructor, University of Maryland School of Nursing, Baltimore

Terri Murrell, RN, MSN, Cardiovascular Clinical Nurse Specialist, Scripps Clinic, La Jolla, Calif.

Lynda Palmer, RN, BA(HS), Head Nurse, The Toronto Western Hospital

Phyllis Pietz, RN, MSN, Staff Nurse, Surgical ICU, Veterans Administration Regional Medical Center, Wilmington, Del.

Katherine S. Puls, RN, MS, CNM, Certified Nurse Midwife, Women's Alternative Health Care of Barrington (Ill.), Ltd.

Patricia A. Simpson, RN, BSN, Clinical Instructor, Cardiac Intensive Care, Duke University Medical Center, Durham, N.C.

Suzanne Marr Skinner, RN, MS, Consultant, University of Maryland School of Nursing, UMBC Expansion, Baltimore

Janis Blocdel Smith, RN, MSN, Nurse Consultant, Wilmington, Del.

Arlene Strong, RN, MN, ANP, Cardiac Clinical Specialist, Adult Nurse Practitioner, Portland (Ore.) V.A. Hospital

CONTRIBUTORS *(continued)*

CPT (P) Marie Rose Taubman, RN, MSN, CCRN, Clinical Coordinator, Progressive Cardiology Unit, Walter Reed Army Medical Center, Washington, D.C.

Paula Brammer Vetter, RN, BSN, CCRN, Nursing Instructor, Lorain County Community College, Elyria, Ohio

Peggy L. Wagner, RN, MSN, CCRN, Cardiovascular Clinical Nurse Specialist, Saint Michael Hospital, Milwaukee

Elaine Gilligan Whelan, RNC, MA, MSN, Associate Professor of Nursing, Bergan Community College, Paramus, N.J.

Nancy Wiedemer, RN, MSN, Staff Nurse, Intensive Care Unit, Medical College of Pennsylvania, Philadelphia

CLINICAL CONSULTANTS

Linda K. Menzel, RN, MSN, Staff Nurse, Medical/Cardiac Intensive Care Unit, Medical Center Hospital of Vermont, Burlington

Patricia A. Rivest, RN, CNT, Cardiac Rehabilitation Coordinator, Grand View Hospital, Sellersville, Pa.

FOREWORD

New knowledge and new procedures for detecting and treating various cardiovascular disorders have profoundly changed cardiovascular nursing. When it applies to acute illness, cardiovascular nursing now takes place almost exclusively in highly specialized cardiac care and surgical intensive care units.

But that's just part of it. The new emphasis on holistic and preventive care has expanded nursing involvement during early prodromal stages of cardiovascular illness and during chronic maintenance as well. Such involvement often takes place at sites away from the hospital, where nurses must practice more independently than ever before. For example, nurses have become coordinators of cardiac rehabilitation programs. In this role, they work with exercise physiologists, cardiologists, and nutritionists. They define patient entrance criteria, set exercise protocols, and establish patient education programs. Similarly, nurses have entered collaborative practices with cardiac surgeons and cardiologists in outpatient clinics—notably those for patients with hypertension or pacemakers—in which they manage patient care under standardized protocols and conduct independent and collaborative research in cardiac care settings. In the emergency department and all other hospital departments, nurses must be ready to handle sudden dysrhythmia, shock, or cardiac arrest, knowing which situations are likely to provoke cardiovascular complications or emergencies and how to handle them correctly.

To meet these challenging new responsibilities, nurses need to continuously expand and update their understanding of the cardiovascular system and its normal function, and the devastating effects of its dysfunction on interlocking vital systems. *Cardiovascular Care Handbook* will help you meet these new challenges. The first three chapters profile the cardiovascular patient, review the anatomy and physiology of the cardiovascular system, and explain how to do a comprehensive nursing assessment of the cardiovascular patient. The latter section includes pediatric, geriatric, and emergency assessment.

Chapters 4 through 11 contain specific information pertaining to disorders of cardiac musculature, electroconduction, pump failure, and circulation. Each disorder comprises five major sections: causes, diagnosis, treatment, signs and symptoms, and nursing management. Each chapter includes a discussion of nursing diagnoses, a summary of patient care goals, and suggested nursing interventions needed to achieve them. The remaining chapters of the book focus on treatment and monitoring procedures, cardiovascular emergencies, drug therapy, and rehabilitation.

Throughout this volume, scores of useful anatomic drawings, illustrations, charts, and diagrams clarify and augment the text. Three appendices provide supplementary information on cardiovascular conditions, dysrhythmias, and cardiovascular drugs.

Given nursing's expanding role in health care, nurses have a special need to keep their knowledge of cardiovascular disorders current and accurate. This volume—which offers such knowledge in both theoretical and practical forms—will be an excellent reference for nurses at all professional levels.

KATHLEEN A. DRACUP, RN, DNS, CCRN, FAAN
Associate Professor, School of Nursing
University of California, Los Angeles

1

CARDIOVASCULAR PATIENT PROFILE

Artificial hearts—for all their drama—are not the most important advancement in the treatment of cardiovascular disease (CVD). Less sensational, but more widespread in impact, are improvements in prevention, diagnosis, and treatment of CVD. Especially during the last 10 years, these improvements have lowered cardiovascular mortality, so that, today, more people with various types of CVD are living longer.

As a result, nurses have to deal with CVD more often—no matter where they practice.

The American Heart Association statistics on CVD and hypertension are startling:
• CVD is the leading cause of death in the United States.
• Roughly 42 million Americans suffer from CVD, many from more than one disorder.
• Each year, CVD claims almost as many lives as the other four leading causes of death (cancer, accidents, chronic obstructive pulmonary disease, and pneumonia) combined.
• The most common cardiovascular diseases are hypertensive heart disease (37 million patients), coronary heart disease (4.5 million), rheumatic heart disease (2 million), and cerebrovascular accident (1.8 million).
• Congestive heart failure (CHF) is becoming more common as more patients survive cardiac damage or live long enough to develop cardiac weakness. Patients with CHF account for 10% to 15% of all hospital admissions.

• According to current estimates, 60 million people need clinical support and instruction in an active antihypertensive program.

While anyone can develop primary hypertension or CVD, some people are more at risk than others. Risk factors include a family history of heart disease; obesity; smoking; a high-fat, high-carbohydrate diet; a sedentary life-style; a psychologically stressful life; diabetes; hypercholesterolemia; or hereditary hyperlipoproteinemia. Of course, many of these risk factors are controllable, so with proper education and attitude people can lessen their chances of CVD.

Demographics also play a part in determining CVD risk. People between ages 35 and 55 are particularly prone to hypertension, especially if one or both parents had high blood pressure or heart disease. Race and sex are factors, too—risk increases significantly if the person is black or male.

In coronary artery disease (CAD), which is near epidemic in the Western world, more men than women and more whites than blacks are affected. CAD is also more prevalent in industrial areas and affects more affluent people than poor people. Characteristic atherosclerotic changes may occur as early as age 10, but they usually occur after age 30. Most patients do not have angina until the lumen of the artery is narrowed by 70% to 75%.

These are grim statistics—but the picture is changing. Health professionals have launched an all-out effort to educate the public about CVD and hypertension, and today, the number of Americans dying from CVD is decreasing.

As a result of the concerted effort to educate the public about CVD, you will be expected to play a larger role in promoting good health, in preventing and controlling disease, and in developing and implementing community health education programs. You will also be challenged to develop new teaching methods to reach the *healthy* population. Finally, as more sophisticated technologies and treatments emerge, you will need expanded assessment and therapeutic management skills.

CVD is controllable—perhaps even avoidable. Helping to prevent, diagnose, and treat it could be your biggest challenge.

2

ANATOMY AND PHYSIOLOGY REVIEW

CARDIOVASCULAR COMPONENTS

The cardiac system

Basic functions of the cardiovascular system

The two basic functions of the cardiovascular system are to deliver oxygenated blood to the body tissues and to remove waste substances through the action of the heart. Specialized pacemaker cells and conduction fibers innervate the heart and initiate and propagate its beat. The heart of an average person beats 60 to 100 times/minute, pumping 4 to 6 qt (4 to 6 liters) of blood in this time—and on the average, it does this for more than 70 years.

Controlled by the autonomic nervous system, the heart pumps blood through the entire body. The vascular network that carries blood through all body systems consists of high-pressure arteries that deliver the blood and low-pressure veins that return it to the heart. This complex network keeps the pumping heart filled with blood and maintains blood pressure. (See *The Cardiovascular System,* page 4.)

Pericardium

The pericardium is a closed, invaginated, serous sac that surrounds the heart and roots of the great vessels. It has two contiguous layers: an inner (visceral) layer that forms the epicardium and an outer (parietal) layer that is continuous with the covering of the great vessels. A potential slitlike space, the pericardial cavity, lies between the two layers and contains 10 to 50 ml of serous fluid. Fibrous connective tissue (fibrous pericardium) strengthens the parietal layer, anchoring the sac to the diaphragm, the sternum, and the great vessels. The posterior surface of the pericardium contacts the esophagus, thoracic aorta, and bronchi. Its lateral surfaces lie against the mediastinal pleurae, with only the phrenic nerves and blood vessels intervening.

Location and form

The heart is a hollow, muscular, four-chambered organ, enveloped by the pericardium. Roughly cone-shaped, the heart lies obliquely in the chest, with two thirds located to the left of the midline. The average male adult heart weighs about 300 g; the average female heart, about 250 g. (See *The Heart: Anterior and Posterior Views,* page 5.)

The heart varies in shape and position, depending on the age of the person, his body build, and the changing position of the body. Its axis is more vertical in a tall, slender person and more transverse in a person who is broad and stocky. Respiration also alters the position of the axis of the heart. During inspiration, the axis becomes more vertical as the diaphragm descends; during expiration, as the diaphragm rises, it becomes more transverse.

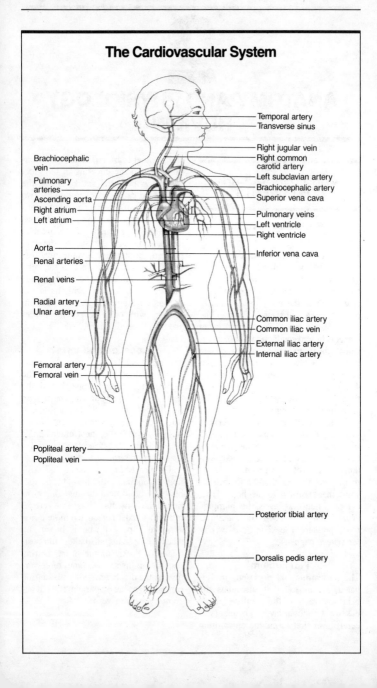

The Cardiovascular System

Temporal artery
Transverse sinus

Right jugular vein
Right common carotid artery
Left subclavian artery
Brachiocephalic artery
Superior vena cava

Brachiocephalic vein

Pulmonary arteries
Ascending aorta
Right atrium
Left atrium

Pulmonary veins
Left ventricle
Right ventricle

Aorta
Renal arteries
Renal veins

Inferior vena cava

Radial artery
Ulnar artery

Common iliac artery
Common iliac vein
External iliac artery
Internal iliac artery

Femoral artery
Femoral vein

Popliteal artery
Popliteal vein

Posterior tibial artery

Dorsalis pedis artery

The Heart: Anterior and Posterior Views

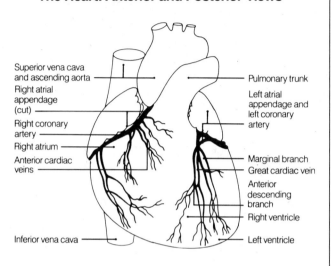

Superior vena cava and ascending aorta
Right atrial appendage (cut)
Right coronary artery
Right atrium
Anterior cardiac veins
Inferior vena cava

Pulmonary trunk
Left atrial appendage and left coronary artery
Marginal branch
Great cardiac vein
Anterior descending branch
Right ventricle
Left ventricle

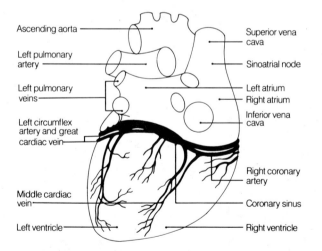

Ascending aorta
Left pulmonary artery
Left pulmonary veins
Left circumflex artery and great cardiac vein
Middle cardiac vein
Left ventricle

Superior vena cava
Sinoatrial node
Left atrium
Right atrium
Inferior vena cava
Right coronary artery
Coronary sinus
Right ventricle

These illustrations show the arterial and venous blood supply of the heart and the position of its four chambers. The heart rests in the mediastinum, the space between the lungs. It slants forward, with its narrowest part, the apex, being forwardmost. The heart is not precisely centered in the thoracic cavity—about two thirds of it lies to the left of the midsternal line.

Cardiac Depolarization-Repolarization

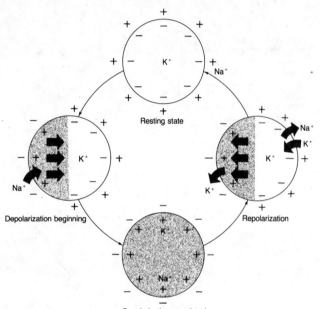

Resting state

Depolarization beginning

Repolarization

Depolarization completed

Heart muscle cells are arranged so that they act together as a single network. Alternating waves of electrical activity—depolarization and repolarization involving exchange of sodium (Na^+) and potassium (K^+) ions across the cell membrane—flow through this network. During depolarization, the cells are stimulated and the muscle contracts; during repolarization, the muscle relaxes. The diagram above shows what goes on at the cellular level of the myocardium.

During the resting (polarized) state, the number of positive charges outside the cell membrane equals the number of negative ones inside it. The concentration of sodium ions is greater outside the cell than inside it, while potassium concentration is greater inside than outside. A stimulus from the SA node briefly reverses this ionic status and causes depolarization. Sodium ions move from outside to inside the cell until the charges on the inner and outer surfaces are reversed and the membrane is fully depolarized. Immediately after the cell is fully depolarized, potassium ions begin to flow from inside to outside the cell, and the cell repolarizes. It returns to its resting state through the action of an ion-transport mechanism called the sodium-potassium pump, which is fueled by energy from adenosine triphosphate as it is changed to adenosine diphosphate by the enzyme adenosinetriphosphatase.

Cross Section of the Heart

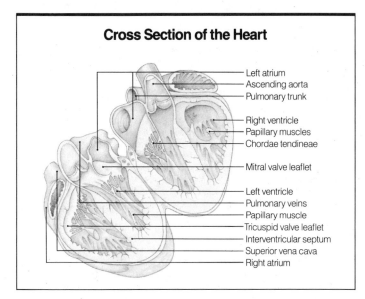

- Left atrium
- Ascending aorta
- Pulmonary trunk
- Right ventricle
- Papillary muscles
- Chordae tendineae
- Mitral valve leaflet
- Left ventricle
- Pulmonary veins
- Papillary muscle
- Tricuspid valve leaflet
- Interventricular septum
- Superior vena cava
- Right atrium

Internal structure

The *endocardium,* an endothelial layer continuous with the lining of the vascular system, forms the smooth inner layer of the heart. The cardiac muscle (called the *myocardium*) makes up the bulk of the heart wall. Heart muscle cells are arranged so that they act together as a single network. Alternating waves of electrical activity—depolarization and repolarization involving exchange of sodium (Na^+) and potassium (K^+) ions across the cell membrane—flow through the network. During depolarization, the cells are stimulated and the muscle contracts; during repolarization, the muscle relaxes. (See *Cardiac Depolarization-Repolarization.*) Externally, the visceral layer of the pericardium comprises the *epicardium.* The interior heart has 4 chambers (2 atria and 2 ventricles), 11 openings, and 4 valves.

The right atrium receives venous blood from the superior and the inferior venae cavae; the blood then passes through the tricuspid valve into the right ventricle. The right ventricular myocardium is thicker than that of either atrium but only one third as thick as that of the left ventricle. The right ventricle receives blood from the right atrium and expels it through the pulmonic valve into the pulmonary artery.

Smaller than the right atrium but with slightly thicker walls, the left atrium receives blood from the lungs via four pulmonary veins and delivers it to the left ventricle through the mitral valve. The posterior surface of the left atrium constitutes most of the base of the heart.

Longer and more conical than the right ventricle, the left ventricle forms the apex of the heart and most of its left border and diaphragmatic surface. The interventricular septum is mostly muscle with an oval-shaped, upper membranous part attached to the fibrous rings surrounding the atrioventricular (AV) and arterial openings. The left ventricular myocardium is about three times as thick as the right ventricular myocardium and produces about three times the pressure. The left ventricle receives blood from the left atrium and expels it through the aortic valve into the ascending aorta.

The Conduction System

The conduction system of the heart contains specialized muscle fibers that generate and conduct their own electrical impulses. The SA node—located in the right atrium, beneath the orifice of the superior vena cava—normally controls heart rate and is called the "pacemaker." It sends an impulse through the internodal pathways and atrial muscle to the AV node in the lower posterior part of the right atrium, near the lumen of the coronary sinus. As an impulse passes through the atrial muscles, the atria contract. After a short delay in the AV node, the impulse continues down the His bundle—which divides into right and left bundle branches—and finally, into the subendothelial Purkinje fibers, which transmit the impulse into the ventricular myocardium, causing it to contract.

After this contraction, the myocardium repolarizes, while the ventricles relax and begin to fill with blood in preparation for the next impulse from the SA node. Evidence of this conduction of electric currents through the heart may be picked up on the skin surface and graphically recorded by the electrocardiogram (EKG).

The SA node discharges 60 to 100 impulses/minute. If it fails to generate the expected impulses, the AV node can also discharge, but at a slower rate of 40 to 60 impulses/minute. If both nodes fail to discharge the Purkinje fibers can discharge at a rate of 15 to 40 impulses/minute. The ability of the heart to spontaneously generate and maintain its own impulse rate is known as *automaticity.* When any part of the heart other than the SA node takes over to pace the heart, this part is known as an ectopic pacemaker. If the electrical impulse is too weak, it will not excite the muscle fiber at all; if it is strong enough to cause the fiber to reach its electrical threshold potential, excitation occurs. The current then spreads to neighboring fibers by virtue of the low resistance of their cell walls, and the entire muscle mass reacts as a unit. This response is called the "all-or-nothing" principle.

Functional valves guard four openings in the heart. The cusps of the two atrioventricular valves (the tricuspid, which normally has three leaflets, and the mitral, which normally has two) are connected to fibrous rings around the openings, part of the skeleton of the heart. Their free margins are attached by the thin but strong chordae tendineae to the ventricular papillary muscles. When blood passes through the opening, it pushes the cusps aside. During ventricular contraction, the papillary muscles contract, pulling on the cords and preventing the cusps from prolapsing into the atria. (See *Cross Section of the Heart,* page 7.)

The two semilunar valves guard the orifices of the pulmonary artery and the aorta. Each contains three crescent-shaped cusps (right, left, and anterior for the pulmonic valve and right, left, and posterior for the aortic valve) that appear concave when viewed from above. The aortic valve cusps are thicker, larger, and stronger than the pulmonic valve cusps. Blood expelled from the ventricles pushes the cusps into the orifices of the vessels. On ventricular relaxation, arterial pressure forces the blood back toward the heart, and the cusps meet, closing the orifices and preventing backflow into the ventricles.

Blood supply to the heart

Two arteries supply blood to the heart; seven major veins drain blood from it. The two main coronary arteries encircle the heart like crowns. They arise from the right and left aortic sinuses at the root of the aorta. During left ventricular contraction, blood is ejected into the aorta, and the coronary ostia fill. During diastole, the ventricular muscle relaxes, allowing the coronary arteries to open and passively fill.

Ordinarily, the right coronary artery supplies the right atrium and the right ventricle (including the sinoatrial and atrioventricular nodes of the conduction system, and the atrioventricular bundle). It also supplies variable amounts of blood to the left atrium and left ventricle. The left coronary artery, which splits into the left anterior descending (interventricular) and circumflex arteries, supplies both ventricles, the interventricular septum, and the left atrium.

Although anastomoses between the two coronary arteries are small or absent at birth, multiple anastomoses between *arterioles* develop with age. Nevertheless, sudden occlusion of a major branch usually leads to necrosis of the affected cardiac muscle region, with subsequent infarction and scar tissue replacement.

The major veins, which lie superficial to the arteries, drain venous blood from the myocardium. These veins do not encircle the heart as the arteries do. They are called *cardiac,* rather than *coronary,* veins. The largest vein, the coronary sinus, lies in the posterior part of the coronary sulcus and opens into the right atrium. The coronary sinus is the terminus for most of the major cardiac veins except for the two or three anterior cardiac veins, which empty directly into the right atrium.

Cardiac innervation

The *intrinsic nerve supply* or *conduction system* for the heart includes the sinoatrial (SA) and AV nodes, the AV bundle of His and its branches, and the Purkinje system. Specialized cardiac muscle fibers initiate the heartbeat and coordinate chamber contraction. All these specialized fibers can initiate the contraction, but the SA node usually paces the heart because it has the greatest degree of self-excitation among the

Preload and Afterload

Preload—a key factor in the increased contractility of the heart—is a passive stretching force exerted on the ventricular muscle at end-diastole.

Afterload refers to the pressure the ventricular muscles must generate to overcome the higher pressure in the aorta. Normally, end-diastolic pressure in the left ventricle is 5 to 10 mm Hg; but in the aorta, it is 70 to 80 mm Hg. This difference means that the ventricle must develop enough pressure to force open the aortic valve. Drugs may sometimes be used to gradually reduce afterload, which increases stroke volume and cardiac output.

elements of the conduction system. (See *The Conduction System.*)

The *extrinsic nerve supply* consists of cardiac nerves of the autonomic nervous system that control the conduction system and the contractility of the heart. Thus, the heart can respond to the changing physiologic needs of the body by altering the rate and force of its contractions.

Stimulation of the sympathetic fibers that supply the SA and AV nodes and all four chambers increases the heart's rate, force, and relaxation phase. Stimulation of the vagal (parasympathetic) fibers that supply the SA node and the atria decreases the rate. Dilatation of the coronary arteries results from stimulation of sympathetic fibers that supply the coronary arteries.

Visceral afferent pain fibers from the coronary arteries enter the first and second thoracic spinal cord segments. These segments also receive afferent pain fibers from the upper left extremity's ulnar aspect, which is the reason angina pectoris attacks may cause referred pain in this area.

The Cardiac Cycle

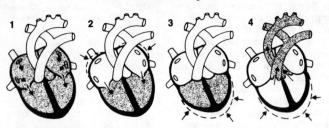

These schematic drawings show events during a single cardiac cycle.
Period of rapid ventricular filling (1): Unoxygenated blood returning from the tissues enters the right atrium at the same time that oxygenated blood from the lungs enters the left atrium. The atria and ventricles are passively filled.
Atrial kick (2): About 70% of incoming blood flows through the atria directly into the ventricles before the atria contract; when they do, they force an additional 30% of blood into the ventricles—the atrial kick.
Period of isovolumic contraction (3): The ventricles begin contracting before emptying.
Period of ejection (4): The ventricles contract, pushing unoxygenated blood into the pulmonary arteries and oxygenated blood into the aorta.

Adapted with permission from M. Jackle and M. Halligan, *Cardiovascular Problems: A Critical Care Nursing Focus* (Bowie, Md.: Robert J. Brady Co.), 1980.

Cardiac cycle

The cardiac cycle (one complete heartbeat) consists of two phases: contraction (systole) and relaxation (diastole). When the heart rate is 72 beats/minute, one cardiac cycle occurs every 0.8 second—0.3 second for ventricular systole and 0.5 second for ventricular diastole. Remember, the duration of the cardiac cycle varies with the heart rate. As the rate increases, systolic and diastolic phases shorten.

As ventricular systole begins, pressure builds in the ventricles, closing the AV valves and preventing the backflow of blood into the atria. When the ventricle contracts, ventricular pressure rises sharply—to about 120 mm Hg in the left ventricle and 26 mm Hg in the right ventricle. When this pressure becomes greater than aortic and pulmonary arterial pressures, the semilunar valves open. Blood is then ejected into the aorta and pulmonary artery—most of it during the first third of ventricular systole.

After ejection, ventricular diastole begins. The ventricles relax and pressure begins to drop. When it falls below the pressures in the aorta and pulmonary artery, the semilunar valves snap shut, preventing backflow into the ventricles.

Meanwhile, the pulmonary veins and venae cavae have filled the atria with blood, and atrial pressure starts to rise toward the end of ventricular systole. As ventricular pressure drops below atrial pressure, the AV valves open and the ventricles rapidly fill with blood. Seventy percent of the blood flow from the great veins goes directly through the atria into the ventricles before the atria contract. Atrial systole then completes ventricular filling. (See *The Cardiac Cycle*.)

Adequate circulation or tissue perfusion depends on cardiac output and peripheral vascular resistance. *Cardiac output* is the quantity of blood pumped

Stroke Volume and Starling's Law

Total ventricular volume in each cardiac cycle reaches 120 to 130 ml during diastolic filling (end-diastolic volume) and falls to 50 to 60 ml as the ventricles empty during contraction; this 70-ml difference represents the *stroke volume*. The stroke volume multiplied by heart rate/minute equals *cardiac output*, or the volume of blood pumped in 1 minute. Normally, the cardiac output for a resting person is about 5 liters, but this amount varies with body size, heart rate, and stroke volume.

The remarkable ability of the heart to deliver equal volumes of blood each minute, even when the right and left ventricles deliver very different volumes of blood per stroke, is explained by *Starling's law:* the force of contraction of each heartbeat depends on the length of the muscle fibers of the walls of the heart. Thus, if right ventricular output exceeds left ventricular output, the fibers of the left ventricle lengthen at end-diastole to increase the force of contraction. In the diagram, at (A), normal diastolic filling during diastole causes normal fiber stretch, contractile force, and stroke volume. At (B), increased filling during diastole increases fiber stretch, force of contraction, and stroke volume.

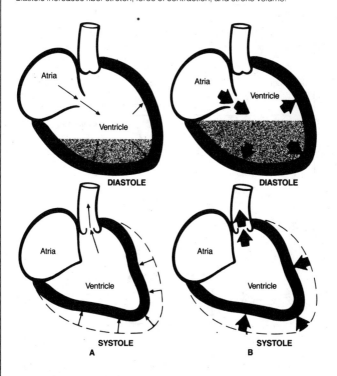

Adapted with permission from S.A. Price and L.M. Wilson, *Pathophysiology: Clinical Concepts of Disease Processes* (New York: McGraw-Hill Book Co.), 1978.

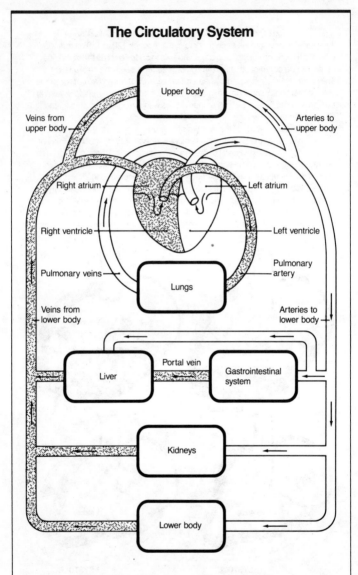

The Circulatory System

Upper body

Veins from upper body

Arteries to upper body

Right atrium

Left atrium

Right ventricle

Left ventricle

Pulmonary veins

Pulmonary artery

Veins from lower body

Lungs

Arteries to lower body

Portal vein

Liver

Gastrointestinal system

Kidneys

Lower body

This schematic representation shows how arteries transport blood from the heart and distribute it throughout the body and how veins transport blood back to the heart. Note the pattern of distribution, to better understand how blood circulation works.

Blood Vessels: A Closer Look

The thick muscle layer of the artery helps it withstand high pressure. Because a vein withstands less pressure than an artery, its walls are thinner and more compliant. In the illustration above, note the valve of the vein, which prevents blood backflow.

by the left ventricle into the aorta each minute; it is calculated by multiplying the *stroke volume* (the amount of blood the left ventricle ejects during systole) by *heart rate* (strokes/minute). Through an increase in either stroke volume or heart rate, cardiac output increases to meet cellular demand. Stroke volume depends on the volume of blood (or pressure exerted by the volume) in the ventricle at the end of diastole (preload), resistance to ejection (afterload), and the contractile strength of the myocardium. Changes in preload, afterload, and con-

The Highs and Lows of Blood Flow

How much do varying size and structure of blood vessels dictate the speed and pressure at which blood flows through the circulatory system? Blood flows easily through the aorta, at an almost constant mean arterial pressure of 100 mm Hg. But pressure begins to drop as soon as blood enters the arteries, and by the time it reaches the arterioles, mean blood pressure decreases to about 85 mm Hg.

As blood continues on its way to smaller arterioles and capillaries, blood pressure drops further, to about 35 mm Hg. Such low pressure in capillary beds allows the blood to deposit optimum amounts of oxygen and other nutrients in body tissues in exchange for carbon dioxide and other wastes.

By the time blood begins its return trip through the veins to the heart, blood pressure is only about 15 mm Hg. Pressure continues to decrease steadily as the blood flows through ever-widening veins and venules.

tractile strength can alter the volume of blood ejected (stroke volume). In turn, the volume of blood ejected alters preload, afterload, and contractile strength. (See *Preload and Afterload*, page 9, and *Stroke Volume and Starling's Law*, page 11.)

Heart sounds

Heart sounds are thought to result from vibrations associated with the sudden closure of heart valves and the acceleration and deceleration of adjacent blood flow. These vibrations are transmitted to the body surface and are heard as heart sounds. The contribution of atrial and ventricular muscle contractions to audible heart sounds is uncertain.

Usually heard at the apex, the first heart sound (S_1) is associated with tricuspid and mitral valve closures. Because the mitral valve usually closes before the tricuspid, the sound splits into two components.

The second heart sound (S_2) is associated with aortic and pulmonic valve closures. Physiologic splitting of S_2 results when the pulmonic valve closes later than the aortic during inspiration. The aortic component is normally much louder than the pulmonic component. Two events cause this split. First, during inspiration, blood rushes into the thorax through large veins and increases venous return to the right heart, prolonging right ventricular filling and ejection and delaying pulmonic valve closure. Second, during inspiration, increased pulmonary capacity slightly reduces left ventricular blood volume, and the aortic valve closes slightly earlier than the pulmonic valve.

Although frequently heard in children, the physiologic third heart sound (S_3) is not normally audible in adults. A low-pitched sound that occurs during rapid ventricular inflow, shortly after S_2 in early diastole, S_3 probably results from vibrations caused by abrupt ventricular distention or increased compliance.

The fourth sound (S_4) is almost always inaudible in the normal individual and probably results from vibrations initiated by sudden, forceful ejection of atrial blood into already distended ventricles. *Murmurs* are sounds resulting from turbulent blood flow in the heart.

The vascular system

The vascular system comprises the arteries, arterioles, capillaries, venules, and veins. Both arteries and veins have three layers: a *tunica intima* (inner coat) of endothelial, connective, and elastic tissues; a *tunica media* (middle coat) of smooth muscle fibers and elastic and collagenous tissue; and a *tunica adventitia* (external coat) of connective, smooth muscle and elastic tissue. Cap-

How Blood Vessel Size Affects Pressure

To some degree, differences in vessel-wall thickness and structure account for blood pressure changes as blood courses through the body. Arteries, thick-walled and muscular, can withstand high pressure; veins, thinner-walled and wider, accommodate lower pressure.

As the graph below illustrates, blood leaves the left ventricle of the heart under very high pressure. Pressure drops rapidly as blood travels through increasingly smaller arterial vessels, then more gradually as it returns through the venous system to the venae cavae, then back to the right atrium.

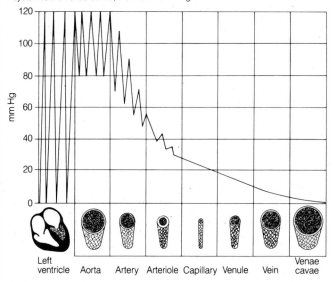

illaries consist of endothelial tissues one cell thick, while venules and arterioles have a variable composition, depending on their size.

Arteries, which contain 15% of circulating blood volume, carry blood away from the heart. Normally, the aorta (the largest artery) and its branches can withstand large changes in cardiac pressure that distend them during ventricular contraction. These pressure changes are detectable as a palpable wave (pulse) in certain arteries near the skin. The aorta and other large arteries add little to total peripheral vascular resistance since they do not ordinarily impede blood flow. The arterioles largely control the degree

of total peripheral resistance and, consequently, the amount of blood flow to and in the tissues by their ability to dilate and contract.

The veins carry blood toward the heart and contain 50% of total circulating blood volume. The superior and inferior venae cavae, which empty into the right atrium, are the largest veins in the body. In the venous system, pressure changes only slightly with vessel dilation or constriction. However, total circulating blood volume, heart and lung function, venomotor tone, and the condition of the one-way venous valves in the limbs may affect the capacitance and the pressure of the venous system. (See

The Pulmonary Blood Supply

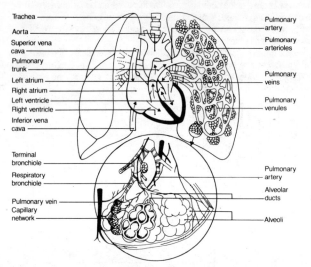

The respiratory and circulatory systems work closely together to transport gases to and from the lungs. To understand this relationship, follow the arrows in this illustration.

The right and left pulmonary arteries take unoxygenated blood from the right side of the heart to the lungs. These arteries divide into distal branches, called arterioles, that terminate as a concentrated capillary network in the alveoli and alveolar sacs. Here, gas exchange occurs. The pulmonary veins also divide into branches. The venules collect the oxygenated blood from the capillaries and pass it along to larger vessels, which carry it back to the heart. The pulmonary veins terminate at the left side of the heart, where they deliver oxygenated blood to be distributed throughout the body.

The Circulatory System, page 12.)

In coronary circulation, blood flow occurs during diastole and depends directly on the *perfusion pressure* (the pressure gradient between the coronary arteries and the right atrium). Coronary blood flow may diminish if aortic pressure decreases or right heart pressure increases. It may also be influenced by tachycardias, which reduce diastolic flow time, and by conditions that reduce diastolic perfusion pressure, such as hypotension.

Coronary circulation constitutes 5% of total cardiac output in the resting heart. It uses 70% of the arterial oxygen. Increased oxygen demand requires increased coronary blood flow, since the heart extracts virtually all oxygen from the blood, even at rest.

Blood vessels and peripheral pulses

Arteries are thick-walled vessels that carry blood from the heart and distribute it through the systemic and pulmonary circuits to all parts of the body.

They serve as low-resistance lines, conducting blood to the organs, and as a pressure reservoir, sending blood through the tissues.

The largest artery, the *aorta,* is the trunk of the systemic circuit. The aorta and its branches are called *elastic arteries* because their middle layers contain many elastic fibers. The distributing arteries, which carry blood to the organs, have more smooth muscle in their middle layers and are called *muscular arteries.* The pulmonary artery and its branches constitute a low-pressure system that transports blood to the lungs for reoxygenation.

Veins have thinner walls but larger diameters than arteries, and return blood to the heart through the venae cavae and pulmonary veins. The venous system consists of *deep veins,* which accompany companion arteries, and *superficial veins,* which lie in the superficial fascia under the skin. The veins are low-resistance lines that carry blood from the tissues to the heart and can adjust their own capacity to compensate for blood volume variations. (See *Blood Vessels: A Closer Look,* page 13.)

Capillaries are high-resistance, thin-walled tubes composed of one endothelial layer. They connect the smallest arteries (*arterioles*) with the smallest veins (*venules*). About 5% of the total circulating blood is always flowing through the capillary beds. The work of the capillaries is the ultimate function of the entire cardiovascular system: to exchange nutrients and metabolic end products. The rest of the system functions solely to bring blood into and out of the capillaries.

Maximum blood pressure (*systolic pressure*) occurs during peak ventricular ejection; minimum pressure (*diastolic pressure*) occurs just before ventricular contraction. The pulse that can be felt in any artery results from the difference between systolic and diastolic pressures (called *pulse pressure*). The easiest arteries to palpate are the radial, carotid, femoral, popliteal, posterior tibial, dorsalis pedis, ulnar, and superficial tem-

Mechanics of Respiration

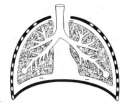

At rest
- Inspiratory muscles relax
- Atmospheric pressure present in tracheobronchial tree
- No air movement

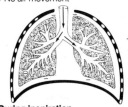

During inspiration
- Inspiratory muscles contract
- Chest expands
- Diaphragm descends
- Negative alveolar pressure present
- Air moves into lungs

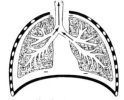

During expiration
- Inspiratory muscles relax, causing lung recoil
- Diaphragm ascends
- Positive alveolar pressure present
- Air moves out of lungs

KEY:
− = negative intrapleural pressure
⊖ = negative alveolar pressure
⊕ = positive alveolar pressure

poral. (See *The Highs and Lows of Blood Flow*, page 14, and *How Blood Vessel Size Affects Pressure*, page 15.)

RESPIRATORY COMPONENTS

The cardiopulmonary system

Thoracic cage, lungs, and pleurae

The anterior boundary of the thoracic cage, which contains the lungs and pleurae, is the sternum. Its posterior boundary is formed by the thoracic vertebrae; its inferior boundary, by the costal margins, xiphoid process, and diaphragm.

The right lung has three lobes and is larger than the left, which has two. The medial inferior surface of the left lung curves slightly around and under the heart and forms a tonguelike structure called the *lingula pulmonis sinistri*. The inferior surfaces of both lower lobes are separated from the abdominal viscera by the diaphragm. The apices of the two upper lobes are slightly above the first rib, about 1" (2.5 cm) above the clavicles. The lateral boundary of both lungs is the chest wall.

The *visceral pleura*, a serous membrane adhering closely to the lung parenchyma, envelops each lung and separates it from the mediastinal structures—the heart and its great vessels, the trachea, the esophagus, and the bronchi. The parietal pleura, which lines the thoracic cavity from the hilum, covers all areas that contact the lungs. The visceral pleura meets the parietal pleura at the hilum, forming a narrow fold called the *pulmonary ligament*. These membranes consist of connective and epithelial tissue and a single layer of secreting epithelium. As they rub together during respiration, secretions minimize friction. The area between the two membranes is only a potential space and cannot be seen unless air or excess fluid occupies it. Normally, pleural fluid maintains the surface tension forces.

Mechanics of respiration

Voluntary and intercostal muscles, working with the diaphragm, produce normal inspiratory and expiratory movement of the lungs and chest wall. The tendency of the lungs to recoil inward, balanced by the tendency of the chest wall to spring outward, creates a subatmospheric pressure in the closed pleural cavity. This pressure, which is about -5 mm Hg below atmospheric pressure, makes lung ventilation (gas volume movement) possible. (See *Mechanics of Respiration*, page 17.)

Pulmonary blood supply

Oxygen-deficient blood is pumped from the right ventricle of the heart to the pulmonary trunk. This trunk then branches laterally into the right and the left pulmonary arteries, which further divide into smaller arteries that closely follow the bronchial tree airways throughout the lungs. Eventually, pulmonary arterioles enter the lung lobules, where arterioles and venules form the capillary beds around the alveoli. This is where gas exchange occurs. The venous system then returns oxygenated blood to the left atrium of the heart to be pumped throughout the body. The tissues of the airways and pleura receive blood from the bronchial arteries, which arise from the aorta and its branches. (See *The Pulmonary Blood Supply*, page 16.)

3

NURSING ASSESSMENT OF THE CARDIOVASCULAR SYSTEM

No matter where you practice nursing, the overwhelming prevalence of cardiovascular disease ensures that cardiovascular assessment will be one of your regular responsibilities. Some routine cardiovascular assessment techniques, such as recording pulse rates and blood pressures, are easy to perform. But a complete assessment, including evaluation of the heart and peripheral vascular system, is complex, requiring special skills and knowledge.

This chapter will help you sharpen your cardiovascular assessment skills and understand the delicate balance between cardiac and other bodily functions.

ADULT ASSESSMENT

Subjective data

To interpret your examination results, you will need the subjective data that only the patient can provide. Conduct the patient interview as a conversation, starting with biographical information.

First, record the patient's age, sex, and race. Then ask what caused him to seek medical help (his chief complaint). The most common complaints in cardiovascular disorders are *chest pain* or *discomfort, dyspnea* (particularly paroxysmal nocturnal dyspnea and orthopnea), *fatigue* and *weakness, irregular heartbeat,* and *peripheral changes* (especially weight change with edema, dry skin,

and extremity pain). Record the chief complaint in the patient's own words.

History of present illness
Depending on the complaint, explore the history of his present illness by asking the following types of questions:
• **Chest pain.** *How would you characterize the pain? Does it burn or produce a squeezing sensation? Where in your chest do you feel the pain? Does it radiate?* Ischemic pain usually affects a large chest area, and the patient has difficulty localizing it. If he can circumscribe the painful area, the pain probably is not ischemic. *How long have you been having this pain? How long does an attack last?* The patient's answers will help identify the origin and severity of his cardiovascular disorder. (See *Assessing Chest Pain,* pages 20 to 23.)
• **Dyspnea.** *When do you experience shortness of breath?* This symptom may indicate transient congestive heart failure or left ventricular failure. If the dyspnea occurs with exertion, ask how much activity is required to cause it. Dyspnea at rest suggests advanced disease; increasing dyspnea with less exertion may indicate progressive pathology and failing compensatory mechanisms.
• **Paroxysmal nocturnal dyspnea (PND),** a classic symptom of left ventricular failure, occurs at night when the patient is sleeping. He awakens with a feeling of suffocation. Maneuvers that cause gravity to drain fluid from the lungs to the feet—for example, sitting on the edge of the bed or walking to the window for fresh air—relieve PND. The

Assessing Chest Pain

CONDITION	LOCATION AND RADIATION	CHARACTER
Myocardial ischemia (angina pectoris)	• Substernal or retrosternal pain spreading across chest • May radiate to inside of either or both arms, the neck, or jaw	• Squeezing, heavy pressure, aching, or burning discomfort
Myocardial infarction	• Substernal or over precordium • May radiate throughout chest and arms to jaw	• Crushing, viselike, steady pain
Pericardial chest pain	• Substernal or left of sternum • May radiate to neck, arms, back, or epigastrium	• Sharp, intermittent pain (accentuated by swallowing, coughing, deep inspiration, or lying supine)
Pulmonary embolism	• Inferior portion of the pleura • May radiate to costal margins or upper abdomen	• Stabbing, knifelike pain (accentuated by respirations)
Spontaneous pneumothorax	• Lateral thorax • Does not radiate	• Tearing, pleuritic pain
Infectious or inflammatory processes (pleurisy)	• Pleural • May be widespread or only over affected area	• Moderate, sharp, raw, burning pain
Aortic aneurysm (dissecting)	• Anterior chest • May radiate to thoracic portion of back	• Excruciating, knifelike pain

ONSET AND DURATION	PRECIPITATING EVENTS	ASSOCIATED FINDINGS
• Sudden onset • Usually subsides within 5 minutes	• Mental or physical exertion; intense emotion • Hot, humid weather • Heavy food intake; especially in extreme temperatures or high humidity	• Feeling of uneasiness or impending doom
• Sudden onset • More severe and prolonged than anginal pain	• Occurs spontaneously, with exertion, stress, or at rest	• Dyspnea • Profuse perspiration • Nausea and vomiting • Dizziness, weakness • Feeling of uneasiness or impending doom
• Severe, sudden onset • Usually relieved by bending forward • May occur intermittently over several days	• Upper respiratory tract infection • Myocardial infarction • Rheumatic fever • Pericarditis	• Distended neck veins • Tachycardia • Paradoxical pulse possible with constrictive pericarditis • Pericardial friction rub
• Sudden onset • May last a few days	• Anxiety (associated with coughing)	• Dyspnea; tachypnea • Tachycardia • Cough with hemoptysis
• Sudden onset • Relieved by aspiration of air	• Trauma • Ruptured emphysematous bleb • Anxiety	• Dyspnea; tachypnea • Mediastinal shift • Decreased or absent breath sounds over involved lung
• Occurs on inspiration • Relief usually occurs several days after effective treatment	• Underlying disease of lung, such as pneumonia	• Fever • Cough with sputum production
• Sudden onset • Unrelieved by medication or comfort measures • May last for hours	• Hypertension	• Lower blood pressure in one arm than in other • Possible paralysis • Possible murmur of aortic insufficiency or pulsus paradoxus • Hypotension and shock

(continued)

Assessing Chest Pain (continued)

CONDITION	LOCATION AND RADIATION	CHARACTER
Esophageal pain	• Substernal • May radiate around chest to shoulders	• Burning, knotlike pain (simulating angina)
Chest wall pain	• Costochondral or sternocostal junctions • Does not radiate	• Aching pain or soreness

attack usually subsides in a few minutes.

• **Orthopnea.** *How many pillows do you use to make breathing easier? Do you use more now than you used to?* An increase in the number of pillows indicates developing orthopnea. The number of pillows the patient uses helps determine the degree of left ventricular failure. Record the patient's response as *two-pillow orthopnea, three-pillow orthopnea,* and so on.

• **Unexplained weakness and fatigue.** *Do you tire easily? What activities cause you to feel tired? How long can you perform these activities before becoming tired? When did you first notice weakness and fatigue? Is it getting worse? Is it relieved by rest?* Fatigue and weakness on mild exertion, especially if relieved by rest, may be a sign of heart disease. The heart of such a patient cannot provide sufficient blood to meet the slightly increased metabolic needs of the cells. These symptoms are often the hallmark of early progressive heart failure.

• **Irregular heartbeat.** *Does your heart pound or beat too fast?* Palpitations usually reflect dysrhythmias, especially tachyarrhythmias. *Does your heart ever skip a beat or seem to jump?* Skipped beats often indicate premature ventric-

ular contractions. *Do you ever faint or feel dizzy? When?* These symptoms may be related to transient dysrhythmias, often caused by coffee, tea, or cola.

• **Weight change with edema.** *Does your weight fluctuate, or have you gained weight recently?* Weight changes are common in cardiovascular disease, especially weight gain from sodium and water retention secondary to congestive heart failure and hypertension. *Are your ankles or feet swollen? Do your shoes feel tight or uncomfortable at the end of the day? Is the swelling relieved by elevating your feet or lying down?* Edema associated with cardiovascular disease is readily mobilized.

• **Dry skin.** *Have you noticed any skin dryness or scaliness, especially on your legs?* Dry skin may be associated with peripheral vascular disease.

• **Extremity pain.** *Have you experienced any pain or discomfort in your arms or legs?* Ischemia from peripheral vascular disease can cause aches or cramps when the patient moves the affected arm or leg. *Do you feel pain or cramps in your legs when you walk? Is the pain relieved by rest? Does elevating the leg cause pain that is relieved by dangling or low-*

ONSET AND DURATION	PRECIPITATING EVENTS	ASSOCIATED FINDINGS
• Sudden onset • Relieved by diet or position change, antacids or belching • Usually brief duration	• May occur spontaneously • Eating	• Regurgitation
• Often begins as dull ache, increasing in intensity over a few days • Usually long lasting	• Chest wall movement	• Symptoms and physical findings vary with specific musculoskeletal disorder

ering the leg? Intermittent claudication results from advanced atherosclerosis of the femoral arteries. *How many stairs or city blocks can you walk before the symptoms begin? Is the pain associated with walking over any particular kind of terrain, in certain temperatures, or at a particular pace?* These factors affect the intensity of exertion. *Does the pain increase with prolonged standing or sitting?* Pain that is most severe during prolonged standing or sitting indicates venous insufficiency. Venous pain located in the calf and lower leg, usually described as an aching, tired, or full feeling, is commonly accompanied by leg edema and obvious varicosities.

Ask about previous conditions, and explore the following relevant areas:

• **Hypertension.** *Have you ever had your blood pressure taken? Can you recall what it was? Have you ever been told you had high blood pressure? Have you ever taken medication for blood pressure?* Pressure above 160/90 correlates positively with ischemic heart disease, renal failure, cerebrovascular accident (CVA), and an accelerated rate of coronary artery disease (CAD).

• **Hyperlipoproteinemia.** *Have you ever been told by your doctor that you have high cholesterol or triglyceride levels?* Elevated serum levels of cholesterol, triglycerides, and free fatty acids probably correlate directly with a higher incidence of CAD. The two most common hyperlipoproteinemia patterns in patients with premature atherosclerosis are Type II—elevated cholesterol with normal or slightly elevated triglycerides—and Type IV—elevated triglycerides with normal or slightly elevated cholesterol.

• **Diabetes mellitus.** *Have you ever been told you had sugar in your urine? Have you ever had a test for blood sugar? Was it normal?* The relationship between diabetes mellitus and CAD is still controversial, but patients with the most common types of hyperlipoproteinemia usually show abnormal carbohydrate metabolism. Patients with CAD also have a high incidence of diabetes mellitus, and patients with diabetes seem to have a tendency toward atheroma formation. Such atherosclerosis occurs not only in the coronary artery system, but also in the arteries of the systemic circulation, particularly in the aorta and in the femoral and carotid arteries.

Reviewing Cardiac Physiology by Systems

SYSTEM	SYMPTOMS	POSSIBLE CONDITIONS
General	• Weakness • Chronic fatigue • Significant weight changes • Poor tolerance for exercise	• Decreased cardiac output • Congestive heart failure • Infectious endocarditis
Integumentary (skin)	• Ulcers or sores • Loss of body hair	• Vascular insufficiency (arterial or venous)
Ears, eyes, nose, and throat	• Frequent headaches • Impaired vision • Pain behind eyes • Nosebleeds • Occasional dizziness or syncope	• Stress • Retinal hemorrhage or arteriosclerosis • Diabetes • Blood dyscrasia • Cardiac dysrhythmia
Respiratory	• Labored breathing when active • Labored breathing when upright • Sudden labored breathing during sleep • Hacking cough with sputum production	• CHF • Pulmonary edema
Cardiovascular	• Chest pain • Palpitations • Ankle swelling • Pain in buttocks while walking	• Angina pectoris • Myocardial infarction • Cardiac dysrhythmia • CHF • Aortic aneurysm
Genitourinary	• Increased amount of urine • Concentrated urine • Diminished amount of urine • Nocturia	• Vascular changes in kidney (from hypertension, CHF, or diabetes) • CHF
Musculoskeletal	• Muscle aches • Fatigue • Ankle edema	• Arterial insufficiency • Decreased cardiac output • CHF
Gastrointestinal	• Nausea and vomiting	• Myocardial infarction

• *Rheumatic fever. Did you ever have rheumatic fever? Were you ever told you had a heart murmur?* Many people have so-called innocent or functional heart murmurs unrelated to rheumatic fever or structural congenital heart disease. But rheumatic fever or repeated streptococcal infections can permanently damage heart valves—especially the mitral and aortic—leaving them *insufficient* (unable to close) or *stenosed* (scarred, rigid, and unable to open fully). Knowing whether the patient has had these conditions will help you interpret heart murmurs common in patients with post–rheumatic fever heart disease.

• *Medications. Have you ever taken diuretics? Do you know why the doctor prescribed them? Have you ever taken any drugs for your heart or circulation?* Knowledge of medications the patient is taking or has taken can provide valuable information on past or present cardiovascular disorders.

Next, ask about any family history of the following conditions:

• *Cardiovascular disease.* Ask the patient about any family history of angina, acute myocardial infarction, hypertension, CVA, diabetes, or renal disease. The incidence of CAD is higher in patients with a family history of advanced plaque disease or one or more deaths from a CAD-related event.

• *Acquired behavior.* Genetic predisposition to cardiovascular disease may exist, but acquired behavior—including diet (high sodium intake, high lipid levels, obesity), personality, and lifestyle—is a significant contributing factor.

Explore the following areas in the psychosocial history of your patient:

• *Personality.* How does the patient view himself? His personality is the most significant aspect of his psychosocial history.

• *Occupation.* A person's occupation can place him under a great deal of stress, a factor that may be important in the diagnosis of cardiovascular disease. Commuting long distances can also be stressful.

• *Domestic problems.* Problems at home can be more stressful than occupational problems and may also predispose a person to cardiovascular disease.

Examine the following aspects of the daily life of your patient for patterns that may predispose him to cardiovascular problems:

• *Physical activity.* A healthy person should engage in aerobic activity at least three times a week. Exercise benefits general cardiovascular conditioning.

• *Smoking.* If the patient smokes cigarettes, determine the duration of his habit and the amount he smokes, and record this data as *pack years* (the number of years multiplied by the number of packs/day). Nicotine, a sympathetic nervous system stimulator, increases heart rate, stroke volume, cardiac output, cardiac work, and vasoconstriction. Smoking is a significant risk factor for peripheral vascular disease, and the mortality for patients with coronary artery disease is about 70% higher in middle-aged men who smoke one pack a day than in those who do not smoke. The percentage decreases for older men, and the correlation is not as clear for women. This risk does not apply to pipe and cigar smokers, probably because they generally do not inhale as much as cigarette smokers.

• *Diet.* A brief history of the eating habits of your patient, particularly his intake of carbohydrates and fats, may help determine his potential for CAD. A high-sodium diet can aggravate the development of edema and may be one of the factors associated with the development of hypertension.

Finally, ask your patient about signs and symptoms that may indicate cardiovascular dysfunction. (See *Reviewing Cardiac Physiology by Systems.*)

Objective data

After completing the interview, ensure the privacy of the patient and explain that you will now conduct a systematic

Choosing—and Using—a Stethoscope

To accurately auscultate heart sounds, you will need a stethoscope with double-barrel ear tubings, comfortable earpieces, a two-headed endpiece, and short tubing. The double-barrel ear tubings ensure good transmission of sound. Earpieces should fit comfortably to channel heart sounds directly into your ear canal. The two-headed endpiece includes a diaphragm side for detecting high-frequency sounds (normal heart sounds) and a bell side for detecting low-frequency sounds (murmurs and abnormal heart sounds). Since the diaphragm endpiece screens low-frequency sounds, it is most useful when auscultating the base of the heart, where most sounds are relatively high-pitched. Short tubing—no longer than 12″ to 15″ (30 to 38 cm)—minimizes the distance sound must travel, thereby preventing ambient noise.

To auscultate heart sounds:
• Have the patient lie on his back. If he has difficulty breathing in this position, raise the head of the bed to a 30° to 45° angle. Next, warm the endpiece of the stethoscope with your hands before applying it to the skin.
• To obtain best results from the diaphragm side, use a firm touch; to obtain best results from the bell side, use a light touch. Improve control of the bell side by placing two or three fingers of your dominant hand on the apex of the chest. Then use your other fingers to hold the bell in place. Initially, plant the bell firmly against the chest; then slowly decrease pressure. As you do, heart sounds should become louder and clearer. Next, lift the bell off the chest. The sounds should become softer.
• Slowly move the appropriate side of the endpiece across the chest from the apex to the tricuspid area. Then move upward to the pulmonic area, across to the aortic area, and return diagonally across the chest to the apex. Avoid skipping from one valve area to another, and always listen for one sound component (such as intensity) at a time.
• To hear louder sounds at the apex, have the patient lie on his left side. To hear otherwise inaudible murmurs at the left sternal border and base, have the patient sit. If breath sounds mask distant or weak heart sounds, listen while the patient holds his breath for as long as he is comfortable.
• Recognize that age and physique may affect what you hear. Auscultating the chest of a young athlete may be easier than auscultating the chest of an older or obese patient. Also, you may hear the same sounds at slightly different sites in different patients.

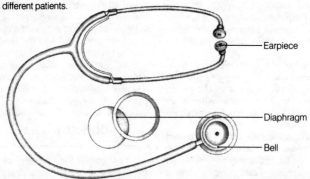

physical examination. Then ask him to lie in a supine position, with his head and thorax comfortably supported at about a 45° angle.

Gather the necessary equipment: stethoscope, blood pressure cuff, and ruler. (See *Choosing—and Using—a Stethoscope*.)

Make sure the height of the bed or examination table allows inspection of the patient in a supine, sitting, and left lateral position. Also, make sure the room is quiet enough to allow accurate auscultation of heart and lung sounds.

To enhance vision, place the light source across the areas you will inspect, not directly on them.

During the examination, stand on the right side of the patient. This allows you to reach comfortably across the precordium for palpation and auscultation and to palpate the liver area on the right side correctly.

General inspection

During your general inspection, record your initial impressions of the patient's body type, posture, gait, and movements as well as his overall health and basic hygiene. Also note observable cardiac risk factors, such as cigarette smoking, obesity, and fatty skin deposits *(xanthomas)*. Observe his facial expressions for signs of pain or anxiety. During conversation, assess his mental status, particularly the appropriateness and the clarity of his speech. Determine his apparent mood. Is he cooperative, withdrawn, fearful, or depressed?

Obtain some general information about the cardiovascular system of the patient. Assess his skin color and condition and further assess his level of consciousness, if appropriate. Skin color, especially in the face, mouth, earlobes, and fingernails, helps determine the adequacy of cardiac output. Pallor or cyanosis may indicate poor cardiac output and tissue perfusion. (Remember, a dark-skinned patient with a cardiac disorder may appear gray. Inspect his lips and nail beds for cyanosis and his conjunctivas and mucous membranes for

Recognizing Pulse Abnormalities

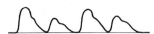

Pulsus alternans is an alteration in pulse size and intensity occurring with every other beat. The rhythm of pulsus alternans is regular, but its volume varies. If you take the blood pressure of a patient with this abnormality, you will first hear a loud Korotkoff sound and then a soft sound, continually alternating. Pulsus alternans frequently accompanies left ventricular failure and states of poor contractility.

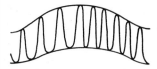

Pulsus paradoxus is an exaggerated decrease in blood pressure during inspiration resulting from an increase in negative intrathoracic pressure. A pulsus paradoxus that exceeds 10 mm Hg is considered abnormal and may result from pericardial tamponade, constrictive pericarditis, severe lung disease, or advanced heart failure.

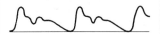

Pulsus bigeminus is a basic heart rhythm irregularity in which premature beats alternate with sinus beats. The premature beat usually has such a poor stroke volume (because of its timing in the cardiac cycle and its inadequate diastolic filling period) that it does not perfuse to the periphery. Because only the sinus beat perfuses to the periphery, the pulse may be slower than normal.

Perfecting Blood Pressure Technique

When you take blood pressure, you are measuring the lateral force that blood exerts on arterial walls as the heart contracts *(systolic pressure)* and relaxes *(diastolic pressure)*. Systolic pressure normally ranges from 110 to 140 mm Hg; diastolic pressure, from 60 to 90 mm Hg. Obtaining an accurate reading depends on how well you prepare the patient, select the equipment, and carry out the procedure, as described below.

• Before taking the blood pressure of the patient, encourage him to relax. Do not take blood pressure after meals, during or directly after exercise or an emotional upset, or just before or after urination or defecation.

• Choose a cuff of the correct size. The bladder should be 20% to 25% wider than the patient's arm circumference. Also, be sure that the cuff works properly. Do not use a cuff that inflates or deflates erratically or has faulty pressure bulb screw clamps.

• After you prepare the patient and the equipment, support the patient's arm at heart level on a table or bed. Then, center the cuff over the brachial artery, and wrap it smoothly and securely around the upper arm.

• Palpate the brachial pulse and rapidly inflate the cuff until the pulse disappears. Continue inflating the cuff until pressure rises an additional 30 mm Hg.

• Place the bell of the stethoscope lightly over the brachial artery. Then, deflate the cuff at 2 to 3 mm Hg/second. If you deflate it too slowly, venous congestion in the arm can result in a spuriously high reading. However, if you deflate it too quickly, diastolic pressure cannot be accurately assessed.

• Listen for the Korotkoff sounds as you deflate the cuff. These sounds occur in five phases: phase I—clear tapping sounds; phase II—tapping sounds with a blowing murmur or whooshing sound; phase III—louder and higher-pitched tapping sounds; phase IV—muffled sounds; and phase V—silence.

When you hear the first two consecutive tapping sounds of phase I, record the systolic pressure. For an accurate reading, keep the mercury column on a level surface and view the meniscus at eye level.

When you hear the first two consecutive muffled sounds of phase IV, record the diastolic phase IV pressure. With the onset of silence, record the diastolic phase V pressure. For example, in a reading of 120/90/80, the systolic pressure equals 120, the diastolic phase IV pressure, 90, and the diastolic phase V pressure, 80.

If you fail to hear all five phases of the Korotkoff sounds, you will have to record blood pressure somewhat differently. This often happens in children and, occasionally, in adults. For example, the muffled sounds of phase IV may continue, without fading into silence. When this happens, record one diastolic pressure— the first two muffled sounds of phase IV.

Phase IV may occasionally be absent. Silence—not muffled sounds—follows the loud tapping sounds of phase III. If this occurs, record one diastolic pressure—the onset of silence of phase V. An auscultatory gap—an interval of silence lasting 5 to 10 seconds—can also interrupt the sequence of Korotkoff sounds. This gap occurs after the tapping sounds of phase I and may take the place of phase II. If this happens, record the pressures when the silence begins and when the pulse sounds return. To prevent a false reading due to an auscultatory gap, inflate the cuff 30 mm Hg above the point at which the pulse disappears.

In the blood pressure measurement at right, the interval of silence or absence of pulse sounds known as the *auscultatory gap* is nonexistent.

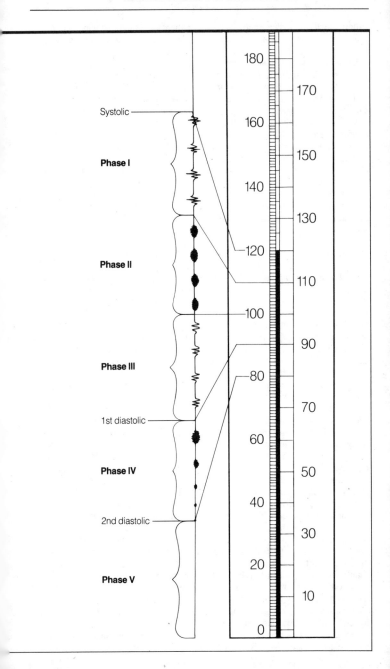

pallor, which may indicate anemia.)

Feel the patient's arm to assess its warmth and dryness. Dry, warm skin indicates adequate cardiac output and tissue perfusion. If the skin is perspiring and feels cool or cold, suspect peripheral vasoconstriction; this can be an early compensatory response in shock.

While assessing the skin, also palpate the radial artery pulse to determine if the pulse rate, quality, and volume are within normal limits. (See *Recognizing Pulse Abnormalities*, page 27.) Generally, the rate should be 60 to 100 beats/ minute, and the quality should be strong and regular. This gross determination indicates whether the cardiovascular system is stable or seriously compromised and requires immediate intervention. To complete your general inspection, record vital signs. (See *Perfecting Blood Pressure Technique*, pages 28 and 29.)

Inspecting the venous pulse

Blood from the jugular veins flows directly into the superior vena cava and the right heart. Thus, you can assess the adequacy of your patient's circulating blood volume, right heart function, and venous pressure by examining external and internal jugular vein pulsations. External jugular veins, which lie superficially, are visible above the clavicle. Internal jugular veins are larger, lie deeper along the carotid arteries, and transmit their pulsations outward to the skin covering the neck.

Normally, neck veins are visible when a person lies down and are flat when he stands up. The semi-Fowler's position is best for inspection, because at a 45° elevation, neck veins should not be prominent if right heart function is normal. Position the patient properly, and turn his head slightly away from you. Use a small pillow to support the head, but do not flex the neck sharply. Remove clothing around the neck and thorax to prevent constriction. Arrange the lighting to cast small shadows along the neck.

Learn about right heart dynamics by analyzing the venous waveform of the patient's right internal jugular vein. Use his carotid pulse or heart sounds to time the venous pulsations with the cardiac cycle.

The jugular venous pulse consists of five waves. The three ascending waves—*a, c,* and *v*—produce an undulating pulsation normally seen ⅜″ to ¾″ (1 to 2 cm) above the clavicle, just to the medial side of the sternocleidomastoid muscle, as follows:

• The *a wave* is the initial pulsation of the jugular vein, produced by right atrial contraction and retrograde transmission of the pressure pulse to the jugular veins. It occurs just before the first heart sound. Time the atrial contraction by placing your index finger on the patient's opposite carotid to feel the carotid pulse or by listening for the first heart sound at the apex. The first jugular pulsation you see just before feeling the carotid pulse or hearing S_1 is the *a* wave. Remember that this wave will not appear in dysrhythmias lacking atrial contraction, such as atrial fibrillation, atrial flutter, and junctional rhythm. Also, the *a* wave may be exaggerated in chronic obstructive pulmonary disease, pulmonary embolism, and pulmonic or tricuspid stenosis—conditions causing elevated right atrial pressure. *Cannon wave* is a giant *a* wave occurring when the atrium contracts against a closed tricuspid valve during ventricular systole. This condition results from ectopic heartbeats, especially premature ventricular contractions, atrioventricular (AV) dissociation, or complete AV block.

• The *c wave* begins shortly after the first heart sound and may result from the impact of the carotid artery on the adjacent jugular vein or pressure transmission from right ventricular contraction during ventricular systole. This wave may be hard to see.

• The *v wave* results from continued passive atrial filling during ventricular systole and peaks just after the second heart sound, when the tricuspid valve opens.

Two descending waves complete the jugular venous pulse:

Estimating Central Venous Pressure

This illustration shows how to indirectly measure central venous pressure. To begin, place the patient at a 45° angle, and identify his internal jugular vein. (Although you can use the external or the internal jugular vein, the internal is more reliable.) Observe the internal jugular to determine the highest level of visible pulsation *(meniscus)*.

Next, locate the *angle of Louis,* or sternal notch. To do this, palpate the clavicles where they join the sternum (the *suprasternal notch*). Place your first two fingers on the suprasternal notch, and then, without lifting them from the skin surface, slide them down the sternum until you feel a bony protuberance. This is the angle of Louis. The right atrium lies approximately 5 cm below the angle of Louis.

To estimate central venous pressure in centimeters, measure the vertical distance between the highest level of visible pulsation and the sternal notch. Normally, this is less than 3 cm. Add 5 cm to this figure to estimate the distance between the highest level of pulsation and the right atrium. If your estimate is more than 10 cm, consider the central venous pressure of your patient elevated and suspect right heart failure.

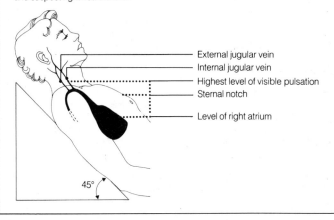

- External jugular vein
- Internal jugular vein
- Highest level of visible pulsation
- Sternal notch
- Level of right atrium

45°

- *x descent,* the descent of the *a* and *c* waves, results from right atrial diastole, as well as from the tricuspid valve's being pulled down during ventricular systole, reducing right atrial pressure.
- *y descent* is the fall in right atrial pressure from the peak of the *v* wave following tricuspid valve opening. It occurs during rapid atrial emptying into the ventricle in early diastole.

Measuring venous pressure

Obtain more information about the right side of your patient's heart by determining his venous pressure level. (*Venous*

pressure, the force exerted by the blood in the venous system, normally ranges from 6 to 8 cm of water.) Factors affecting venous pressure include circulating blood volume, vessel wall tone, vein patency, right heart function, respiratory function, and pulmonary pressures, as well as the force of gravity.

Examples of alterations in venous pressure due to respiration include Kussmaul's sign and the hepatojugular reflux. *Kussmaul's sign,* a paradoxical rise in the height of jugular pressure during inspiration, may be seen in patients with chronic constrictive pericarditis. The

Valsalva's Maneuver

Valsalva's maneuver is any forced expiratory effort against a closed airway, as when a person holds his breath and tightens his muscles in a concerted, strenuous effort to move a heavy object or to change position in bed. Most healthy people perform Valsalva's maneuver during normal daily activities without any injurious consequences, but such efforts are dangerous for many patients with cardiovascular diseases, especially if they become dehydrated, increasing the viscosity of their blood and the attendant risk of blood clotting. Constipation increases the risk of cardiovascular trauma in such patients, especially if they perform the maneuver when trying to move their bowels. Patients who may be endangered by performing the maneuver are commonly instructed to exhale instead of holding their breath when they move. The exhalation decreases the risk of cardiovascular trauma.

hepatojugular reflux is increased venous pressure from abdominal compression during normal respirations. Although compressing the abdomen increases right heart volume, venous pressure should not rise significantly. If it does (a positive hepatojugular reflux), the patient may have congestive heart failure.

You can describe jugular venous pressure by characterizing the neck veins as mildly, moderately, or severely distended and by measuring pressure levels in fingerbreadths of distention above the clavicle. Such a report might read: "The patient's neck veins are moderately distended to a level of three fingers above the clavicle, at a level of 45° from the horizontal." Generally, you should observe the veins bilaterally to confirm true venous distention. Unilateral jugular venous distention may be caused by a local obstruction. (See *Estimating Central Venous Pressure*, page 31.)

How to examine the carotid pulse

Carefully inspect and palpate the carotid arteries of your patient. This is essential because the carotid pulse correlates with central aortic pressure and reflects cardiac function more accurately than peripheral vessels. During diminished cardiac output, peripheral pulses may be difficult or impossible to feel, but the carotid pulse should be easy to palpate.

Examine the carotid pulse for rate, rhythm, equality, contour, and amplitude. Observe the carotid area for excessively large waves, indicating a hypervolemic or hyperkinetic state of the left ventricle, as in aortic regurgitation. With the patient in the semi-Fowler position and his head turned toward you, use these techniques to palpate the carotid arteries:
• To prevent possible cerebral ischemia, palpate *only one* carotid artery at a time.
• Feel the trachea and roll your fingers laterally into the groove between it and the sternocleidomastoid muscle (below and medial to the angle of the jaw).
• Do not exert too much pressure or massage the area; this may induce excessive slowing of the heart rate.

The carotid pulse correlates with S_1. To gain information about heart rate and rhythm in a patient with a regular rhythm, palpate the pulse for 30 seconds. If the rhythm is irregular, palpate for 1 to 2 minutes. Remember, you cannot determine the pattern of irregularity or the presence of an apical-radial pulse deficit until you analyze the precordium and apical pulse.

Describe the amplitude of the carotid pulse as increased (hyperkinetic) or decreased (hypokinetic). Increased pulses are large and bounding, with wide pressures. You will feel a rapid upstroke, a brief peak, and a fast downstroke. This is common during exercise and when anxious or afraid. Increased amplitude may also accompany hyperthyroidism, anemia, aortic regurgitation, complete heart block, extreme bradycardia, and hypertension. A bounding carotid pulse may indicate that the left ventricle is generating excessive pressures to accomplish adequate cardiac output.

Decreased amplitude is characterized by small, weak pulsations that show diminished pressure and by a slow, gradual, or normal velocity of upstroke, a delayed systolic peak, and a prolonged downstroke. This type of pulse results from left heart failure, severe shock, constrictive pericarditis, or aortic stenosis.

After palpating both carotid pulses, auscultate them in this fashion:

• Turn the patient's head slightly away from you to allow space for the stethoscope.

• Auscultate only one carotid artery at a time.

• Place the bell of the stethoscope on the skin overlying the carotid artery.

• Ask the patient to hold his breath. Avoid Valsalva's maneuver—forced exhalation against a closed glottis—which may initiate dysrhythmias. (See *Valsalva's Maneuver.*)

Blood flow through the arteries is silent except in a patient with occlusive arterial disease. Auscultation of the blood flow in such a patient usually produces a blowing sound called a *bruit*. (See *Auscultation for Bruits,* page 34.) Arteriovenous fistulas and various high-cardiac-output conditions, such as anemia, hyperthyroidism, and pheochromocytoma, may also cause bruits. If you hear a bruit, gently repalpate the artery with the pads of your fingers to detect the *thrill* (a vibrating sensation similar to the feel of the throat of a purring cat) that frequently accompanies it. A thrill results from turbulent blood flow caused by arterial obstruction.

Precordium inspection

Begin inspecting the precordium by identifying anatomic landmarks. The critical landmarks for cardiovascular assessment are the suprasternal notch and the xiphoid process (see *Identifying Cardiac Landmarks,* page 37). Other important landmarks include the midsternal line, the midclavicular line (MCL), and the anterior axillary, midaxillary, and posterior axillary lines.

Place the patient in a supine position, and elevate his upper trunk 30° to 45°. Remember, you can examine the precordium best by standing to the right of the patient and using lighting that casts shadows across his chest.

Inspect the entire thorax for shape, size (including thickness), symmetry, obvious pulsations, and retractions. (Certain congenital heart diseases can cause left-chest prominence.)

Next, observe the apical impulse, which is normally located in the fifth intercostal space (ICS) at about the MCL. You can see this apical beat as a pulsation produced by the thrust of the contracting left ventricle against the chest wall during systole. This apical beat is evident in about half the normal adult population. Because it occurs almost simultaneously with the carotid pulse, simultaneous palpation of a carotid pulse helps you identify it.

The apical impulse reflects cardiac size, especially left ventricular size and location. In left ventricular hypertrophy, the impulse is sustained and forceful. In left ventricular distention, the impulse is laterally displaced. You will see left ventricular hypertrophy in patients with hypertension, mitral regurgitation, aortic stenosis, and hypertrophic cardiomyopathy. A rocking motion at the apex is commonly associated with left ventricular hypertrophy.

Inspect the right and left lower sternum of the patient for excessive pulsation and any bulging, lifting, heaving, or retraction. A slight retraction of the chest wall just medial to the MCL, in the fourth ICS, is a normal finding, but retraction of the rib is abnormal and may result from pericardial disease. When the work and force of the right ventricle increase markedly, a diffuse and lifting pulse can usually be seen or felt along

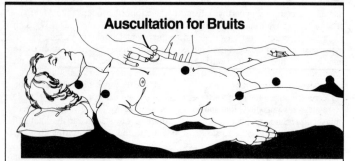

Auscultation for Bruits

Auscultation of the neck, abdomen, and limbs is essential for complete arterial assessment. Moving from head to toe, auscultate for *bruits*—swishing sounds caused by turbulent blood flow—in these areas:

• **The neck.** A narrowing or obstruction may cause bruits. A bruit that is loudest close to the jaw is significant since that is where the carotid artery divides; a bruit over the collarbone may have been transmitted up along the arteries from the heart or the aortic root—so listen over the heart, too.

• **The abdomen.** Bruits heard in the abdominal aorta should alert you to assess arterial perfusion in the legs. Absence of pulses indicates decreased blood flow (dissecting aneurysm or arterial embolus is possible).

• **The groin and inner aspect of the thigh, where the femoral artery runs.** In the lower part of the thigh, slightly above the knee, is the adductor canal, probably the most common site for hardened arteries of the legs.

• **Behind the knee.** Significant narrowing of the popliteal artery can cause bruits.

Preventing problems

Auscultation requires experience, judgment, and finesse. Keep these tips in mind:

• If you press too hard with the stethoscope where arteries are close to the skin, you may compress the artery and create a false bruit. But you do need good contact with the skin.

• It is easy to create a bruit behind the knee. To avoid this, place the patient in a supine position, put your hand behind the ankle, and lift the leg slightly so the stethoscope can be placed behind the knee without pressure.

• In an overweight person, apply moderate pressure over a big stomach or thigh. Where the vessel is far below the skin, the noise of a bruit may not be very loud, especially when bowel sounds interfere with your hearing. If you hear a bruit, decrease the pressure, but make sure the bruit does not disappear.

the left sternal border. This impulse is called a *parasternal lift* and indicates right ventricular hypertrophy.

Precordium palpation

To palpate the precordium, start at the apex and move methodically to the left sternal border and the base of the heart. (You may also palpate the epigastrium,

the right sternal border, and the clavicular and left axillary areas.) Begin by placing your right palm over the apex area—the MCL at the fifth ICS—to locate the apical impulse (the point on the anterior chest wall that the tip of the left ventricle hits during ventricular systole). Using light palpation, you should feel a tap with each heartbeat over an area the size of a nickel. The apical impulse correlates with the first heart sound and carotid pulsation. To be sure you are feeling it, use your left hand to palpate the carotid artery. If you have difficulty palpating the apical impulse, turn the patient to the left lateral decubitus position, which brings the heart closer to the left chest wall.

The apical impulse may be abnormal in size, strength, and location. Generally, a weak apical impulse indicates poor stroke volume and a weakened contractile state, such as decompensated congestive heart failure from increased lung volume. The apical impulse may be imperceptible in a patient who is muscular or obese, or whose chest wall is enlarged (as in emphysema) or deformed.

After assessing the apical impulse, palpate the apex for thrills caused by turbulent blood flow (possibly due to mitral regurgitation and stenosis):
• across a damaged valve
• through a partially obstructed vessel
• through artificial changes between arteries and veins, such as atrioventricular shunts or fistulas
• through abnormal openings between heart chambers, such as ventricular or atrial septal defects
• because of high flow rates.

Next, place your right palm on the left sternal border area of the patient. A diffuse, lifting systolic impulse indicates right ventricular hypertrophy, which occurs in fewer patients than left ventricular hypertrophy.

To continue the examination, palpate the base of the heart, located at the second left and right ICS at the sternal borders. (Keep in mind that the sternal notch, or angle of Louis, marks the exact location of the second ICS.) Normally, you will not feel any pulsations. Detection of pulsations or thrills may indicate excessive systemic or pulmonary pressures, as well as aortic or pulmonic valve disease. When your hand is over the base, the aortic valve area is under your palm and the pulmonic valve area is under your fingertips. Remember that these areas do not correspond to the exact locations of the valves, but to the sites where their sounds are normally transmitted.

Listening for heart sounds and murmurs

Listening over the precordium with a stethoscope is the most useful examination technique for learning about the heart function of your patient. While auscultating, listen selectively for each cardiac cycle component, and move the stethoscope slowly over the five main topographic areas (see *Chest Auscultation: Listening for Heart Sounds*, pages 38 to 41, and *Learning about Heart Murmurs*, pages 42 and 43). Acquiring expertise in identifying heart sounds and murmurs takes a great deal of practice, so follow the same procedure sequence every time you listen.

First, using the diaphragm of the stethoscope, listen to your patient's heart at the apex—the fifth ICS at the MCL—for the two normal heart sounds, S_1 and S_2. (S_1 is the *lub* and S_2 the *dub* of the *lub-dub* sound made by the normal heart.) You can hear S_1 best by listening as you palpate the carotid pulse, because the sound and the beat occur simultaneously. S_1 splitting is significant only if very pronounced.

S_2 immediately follows S_1. You will hear it best at the base of the heart (at the second ICS, right and left sternal borders). S_2 often splits into an aortic and a pulmonic component when the aortic valve closes slightly before the pulmonic valve during inspiration. This physiologic split is most distinct at the second ICS, left sternal border. In systemic hypertension and dilatation of the ascending aorta, the aortic component is usually loud and sharp; in severe aortic stenosis, it may be diminished or absent. In pulmonary hypertension resulting from such conditions as mitral stenosis, left ventricular failure, pulmonary emboli, or pulmonary heart disease, the pulmonic component is louder; in severe pulmonic stenosis, it is diminished. Always identify S_1 and S_2 first, because you can only recognize abnormal sounds by their relationship to diastole and systole.

Now, use the bell of the stethoscope to listen at the apex of the heart for the abnormal S_3 and S_4 sounds. (Apply the bell lightly—exerting pressure makes it work like a diaphragm.) S_3, a low-pitched sound immediately following S_2, is probably caused by abrupt limitation of left ventricular filling. Called *ventricular gallop* because of its triple sound, S_3 is an important early sign of heart failure and indicates more serious pathology than S_4. Learning to detect this extra sound takes practice and patience.' But you should develop your skill, because S_3 often appears before other significant symptoms of congestive heart failure, such as rales, dyspnea, and elevated jugular venous pressure. This means that your skill in detecting it may contribute significantly to early identification of your patient's problems. In fact, S_3 is such an important indicator of congestive heart failure that many doctors begin drug therapy as soon as it is detected. (Effective treatment for heart failure makes this sound disappear.)

S_4 occurs just before S_1 and can be more difficult to hear than S_3. Called an *atrial gallop* because of its triple sound, S_4 results from atrial contraction during diastolic ventricular filling. Normally, atrial systole is silent, but when ventricular filling pressure is high and the ventricle is stiffer than normal (as in heart disease), the atria produce an extra sound as they contract against this greater ventricular resistance. (This explains why S_4 occurs just before S_1.) Although not as specific as S_3 for congestive heart failure, S_4 is a key sign for other forms of heart disease, including hypertension, cardiomyopathies, and aortic stenosis. In adults with severe myocardial disease and tachycardia, summation (a cumulative effect) of S_3 and S_4 may occur, producing a *summation gallop*.

Pericardial friction rub is an extra cardiac sound resembling squeaking leather or a grating, scratching, or rasp-

ing sound. You can hear it best between the apex and the sternum; it may be loud enough to mask other heart sounds. Inflammation of the pericardial sac causes the parietal and visceral surfaces to rub together.

Finally, listen carefully for *heart murmurs,* which result from turbulent blood flow produced by valvular or septal wall pathology. Murmur loudness is classified in six grades, with Grade 1 the softest audible murmur and Grade 6 the loudest—audible even when the stethoscope is not touching the patient's chest. Murmurs can be classified as systolic or diastolic. Systolic murmurs occur during ventricular systole and may result from turbulent flow through a stenotic aortic or pulmonic valve, regurgitant flow through an incompetent mitral or tricuspid valve, or flow through a ventricular septal defect. Diastolic murmurs occur during ventricular diastole and may result from turbulent flow through stenotic mitral or tricuspid valves or regurgitant flow through an incompetent aortic or pulmonic valve. Listen for a pansystolic murmur during the acute stage of myocardial infarction. A murmur of this type may indicate the presence of a ventricular septal defect. (The synonymous terms *pansystolic* and *holosystolic* indicate that the murmur occurs during the entire systolic cycle; you will hear it as a whooshing sound between S_1 and S_2.)

Identifying murmurs, like identifying heart sounds, is difficult. Developing this skill may take years of study and practice. (See *Identifying Cardiac Rate, Rhythm, and Sound,* pages 46 to 49.)

Auscultation sequence

Positioning the patient properly can help you hear heart sounds better. For the apex area, begin auscultation with the patient supine. Then turn him on his left side and listen with the bell to identify low-pitched filling sounds or murmurs (as in mitral stenosis). Finally, listen to the base with the patient sitting up. To hear high-pitched diastolic murmurs (as in aortic or pulmonic insufficiency),

Identifying Cardiac Landmarks

To perform an accurate cardiovascular assessment, familiarize yourself with the landmarks illustrated here.

The *base* of the heart (the superior portion, where the ascending aorta and pulmonary trunk emerge and the superior vena cava enters) corresponds to a horizontal line at the third costal cartilages. This line begins about 1 cm from the right sternal margin and ends about 2 cm from the left sternal margin.

The *apex* of the heart (the inferior portion that points down and to the left) is normally located at the fifth left intercostal space, about 8 to 9 cm to the left of the midsternal line. The right end of the inferior surface lies under the sixth or seventh chondrosternal junction.

Determine the approximate size and shape of your patient's heart by identifying these points, marking them on his chest with a felt-tip pen, and connecting them with slightly convex lines.

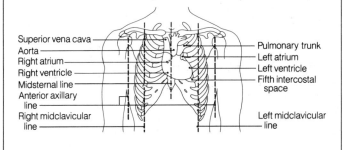

Superior vena cava — Aorta — Right atrium — Right ventricle — Midsternal line — Anterior axillary line — Right midclavicular line

Pulmonary trunk — Left atrium — Left ventricle — Fifth intercostal space — Left midclavicular line

press the diaphragm firmly against the chest wall while the patient leans slightly forward.

Use the following auscultation sequence (see *Learning Cardiac Auscultation Landmarks,* page 51.):
- With the patient in a supine or semi-Fowler position, begin auscultating with the diaphragm at the *apex* to identify rate, rhythm, S_1 (the loudest sound at this location), and S_2. Then listen for extra sounds, such as murmurs, S_3, S_4, or pericardial friction rubs.
- Turn the patient on his *left side,* and listen with the bell to identify mitral valve murmurs and the filling sounds of S_3 and S_4.
- Position the patient on his back, and inch the diaphragm up the *left sternal border* to the third ICS—Erb's point. (Murmurs caused by tricuspid valve dysfunction and pulmonic valve disor-

ders radiate to Erb's point.) Then proceed to the second ICS (pulmonic) area, where you can identify S_1 and S_2, and note the physiologic split of S_2 on inspiration. (S_2 is the more prominent sound in this base location.)
- Proceed to the second ICS at the right sternal border (aortic area), using the diaphragm. Note S_1 and S_2 (still the most prominent sounds in this area). Then ask the patient to sit forward. Press the diaphragm firmly against his chest wall and listen for the high-pitched murmurs of aortic regurgitation and, possibly, aortic stenosis.

Listening for lung sounds

To assess the flow of air through the respiratory system of the patient, auscultate his lungs and identify normal and abnormal (adventitious) breath sounds. (See *Guide to Breath Sounds,* page 52,

Chest Auscultation: Listening for Heart Sounds

SOUNDS	TIMING	PHYSIOLOGY
S_1	Beginning of systole	Mitral and tricuspid valves close almost simultaneously, producing a single sound; S_1 corresponds to the carotid pulse.
Accentuated S_1	Beginning of systole	Mitral valve is still open wide at the beginning of systole, so the valve slams shut from an open position.
Diminished S_1	Beginning of systole	Mitral valve has time to float back into an almost-closed position before ventricular contraction forces it shut, so it closes less forcefully. Softer closure may also be from an immobile, calcified valve.
Split S_1	Beginning of systole	Mitral valve closes slightly before the tricuspid valve.
S_2	End of systole	Pulmonic and aortic valves close almost simultaneously.
Physiologic split S_2 (split on inspiration but not on expiration)	End of systole	During inspiration, the pulmonic valve closes later than the aortic valve. (Pulmonic valve closure is normally delayed during inspiration, which causes decreased thoracic pressure and allows more blood into the right side of the heart, delaying pulmonic valve closure.)
Persistent wide split S_2 (split on both inspiration and expiration, but more widely split on inspiration)	End of systole	Pulmonic valve closes late or (less commonly) the aortic valve closes early.
Fixed split S_2 (equally split on inspiration and expiration)	End of systole	Pulmonic valve consistently closes later than aortic valve. Right side of heart is already ejecting a larger volume, so filling cannot be increased during inspiration. The sound remains fixed.

When auscultating the chest, listen carefully to each component of the cardiac cycle. This chart will help identify some abnormalities you may hear.

INDICATION	WHERE TO AUSCULTATE
• Normal	Apex
• During rapid heart rate • Mitral stenosis • After mitral valve disease, such as mitral prolapse	Apex
• First-degree heart block • Mitral regurgitation • Severe mitral stenosis with calcified immobile valve	Apex
• Normal in most cases • Right-bundle-branch heart block (wide splitting of S_1) • Pulmonary hypertension	Beginning at mitral area and moving toward tricuspid area
• Normal	Aortic and pulmonic areas (base); heard best at aortic area
• Normal; a physiologic S_2 split corresponds to the respiratory cycle.	Aortic and pulmonic areas; heard best at pulmonic area on inspiration
Late pulmonic valve closure: • Complete right-bundle-branch heart block, which delays right ventricular contraction. As a result, the pulmonic valve closes later. • Pulmonary stenosis, which prolongs right ventricular ejection	Pulmonic area
• Severe right ventricular failure, which prolongs right ventricular systole • Atrial septal defect, which causes blood return to the right ventricle from lungs, prolonging the ejection	Pulmonic area

(continued)

Chest Auscultation: Listening for Heart Sounds *(continued)*

SOUNDS	TIMING	PHYSIOLOGY
Paradoxical (reversed) S₂ split (widely split on expiration)	End of systole	On expiration, aortic valve closes after the pulmonic valve, from delayed or prolonged left ventricular systole. On inspiration, the normal delay of the pulmonic valve closure causes the two sounds to merge.
S₃ (ventricular gallop)	Early diastole	Ventricles fill early and rapidly, causing vibrations of the ventricular walls.
S₄ (atrial gallop)	Late diastole	Atrium makes an extra effort to fill against increased resistance.

and *Guide to Adventitious Sounds,* page 54.) Lung auscultation helps detect abnormal fluid or mucus, as well as obstructed passages. You can also determine the condition of the alveoli and surrounding pleura.

When auscultating the chest, instruct the patient to take full, slow breaths through his mouth. (Nose breathing changes the pitch of the lung sounds.) Listen for one full inspiration and expiration before moving the stethoscope. Remember, a patient may try to accommodate you by breathing quickly and deeply with every movement of the stethoscope, which can cause hyperventilation. If the patient becomes light-headed or dizzy, stop auscultating and allow him to breathe normally for a few minutes.

Using the diaphragm of the stethoscope, begin auscultating above the scapulae. Move to the area between the scapulae and the vertebral column. Then move laterally beneath the scapulae to the right and left lower lobes. Move the stethoscope's diaphragm methodically, and compare the sounds you hear on both sides of the chest before moving to the next area.

If you hear an adventitious breath sound, note its location and at which point during the respiratory process it occurs—during inspiration, for example. Then continue auscultating the patient's posterior chest.

After auscultating, instruct the patient to cough and breathe deeply. Let him rest, and listen again to the area where you heard the adventitious sound or sounds. Note any changes. Sometimes rales and rhonchi can be cleared by coughing; wheezes and friction rubs cannot be cleared this way.

In the same way you auscultated the posterior chest, auscultate the anterior and lateral chest, comparing sounds on both sides before moving to the next area. (See *Lung Auscultation Sequences,* page 53.)

Begin auscultating the anterior chest at the trachea, where you should hear bronchial (or tubular) breath sounds.

Next, listen for bronchovesicular breath sounds where the mainstem

INDICATION	WHERE TO AUSCULTATE
• Left-bundle-branch heart block (most common cause) • Aortic stenosis • Patent ductus arteriosus • Severe hypertension • Left ventricular failure, disease, or ischemia	Aortic area
• Early congestive heart failure • Ventricular aneurysm • Common in children and young adults	Mitral area and right ventricular area, using stethoscope bell, with patient on his left side
• Hypertensive cardiovascular disease • Chronic coronary artery disease • Aortic stenosis • Hypertrophic cardiomyopathy • Pulmonary artery hypertension	Apex

bronchi branch from the trachea (near the second ICS, ¾" to 1¼", or 2 to 3 cm, to either side of the sternum). Bronchial and bronchovesicular sounds are abnormal when heard over peripheral lung areas.

Now, using the standard chest landmarks, comparing right and left sides as you proceed, listen over the patient's peripheral lung fields for vesicular sounds. Be sure to auscultate his lateral chest walls. On the left side, heart sounds diminish breath sounds; on the right side, the liver diminishes them. If you hear adventitious breath sounds, describe them and note their location and timing.

Assessing the epigastric area

Assess the upper abdominal area for evidence of cardiovascular disease. A normal patient may have visible or palpable pulsations in the epigastric area (upper central abdominal region). Abnormally large aortic pulsations may result from an aneurysm of the abdominal aorta or from aortic valvular regurgitation. To distinguish right ventricular hypertrophy—which can exaggerate epigastric pulsations—from an aortic pathology, place your palm on the epigastric area, and slide your fingers under the rib cage. You will feel the aortic pulsations with your palm and the right ventricular impulses with your fingertips. Next, use the bell of the stethoscope to auscultate the vascular sounds of the abdominal aorta from the epigastric area in the abdominal midline to the umbilicus, listening for bruits, which may indicate obstruction of the aorta by plaques. (See *Locating Abdominal Sounds,* page 56.)

If you note any bruits in the abdominal aorta, assess arterial perfusion in the legs. Absence of pulses indicates decreased blood flow to the legs, so notify the doctor promptly, keep the patient quiet, and *do not* palpate his abdomen. These symptoms may reflect a dissecting aneurysm, which is a surgical emergency. The same symptoms may indicate arteriosclerosis obliterans, a chronic condition, but a doctor must make the diagnosis.

Learning about Heart Murmurs

When you listen for heart sounds, you may hear more than those identified as S_1 through S_4. You may hear a murmur, or audible vibration, when blood flow is obstructed or abnormal.

To help in identifying types of murmurs, carefully note the following indicators. Then, study the chart to learn about the different types of murmurs.

• *Timing:* Note the occurrence—is it in the systolic phase or the diastolic phase? A midsystolic murmur is also called an *ejection murmur;* a murmur heard throughout the systolic phase is called a *pansystolic,* or *holosystolic, murmur.*

• *Quality:* Describe the quality or sound of the murmur—is it blowing, harsh, musical, or rumbling?

• *Pitch:* Identify the pitch or frequency of the murmur—is it high, medium, or low?

• *Location:* Name the auscultation location where you hear the murmur best—is it aortic, pulmonic, tricuspid, or mitral?

• *Radiation:* List the bordering structures where the murmur is also heard.

• *Loudness:* Employ this rating system to describe the volume of the murmur: 1–barely heard; 2–faint but distinct; 3–moderately detectable; 4–

TIMING	QUALITY	PITCH	LOCATION	RADIATION
Midsystolic (systolic ejection)	Harsh, rough	Medium to high	Pulmonic	Toward left shoulder and neck
Midsystolic (systolic ejection)	Harsh, rough	Medium to high	Aortic and suprasternal notch	Toward carotid arteries or apex
Holosystolic	Harsh	High	Tricuspid	Precordium
Holosystolic	Blowing	High	Mitral, lower left sternal border	Toward left axilla
Holosystolic	Blowing	High	Tricuspid	Toward apex
Early diastolic	Blowing	High	Midleft sternal edge (not aortic area)	Toward sternum
Early diastolic	Blowing	High	Pulmonic	Toward sternum
Mid-to-late diastolic	Rumbling	Low	Apex	Usually none
Mid-to-late diastolic	Rumbling	Low	Tricuspid, lower sternal border	Usually none

loud; 5–very loud; 6–heard before stethoscope comes in contact with the chest.

• *Configuration:* Represents the murmur much as it would appear on a phonocardiogram. This shows the approximate relationship of the murmur to the normal heart sounds, in timing and intensity. *Crescendo* means the murmur begins softly and gets louder. *Decrescendo* means the opposite. *Crescendo-decrescendo* (diamond-shaped) is a combination of the two patterns. *Plateau* means the murmur is fairly constant, not appreciably altering in intensity.

CONDITION	CONFIGURATION
Pulmonic stenosis Aortic stenosis	S_1 S_2 **I∧I** Crescendo-decrescendo
Ventricular septal defect Mitral insufficiency Tricuspid insufficiency	S_1 S_2 **I━━I** Plateau (constant)
Aortic insufficiency Pulmonic insufficiency	S_1 S_2 S_1 **I ∖I** Decrescendo
Mitral stenosis Tricuspid stenosis	S_1 S_2 S_1 **I I∿I** Crescendo

Evaluating liver size by percussion or palpation can help determine the presence and extent of right-sided heart disease. Remember to note whether liver percussion or palpation causes the patient discomfort, because tenderness is characteristic of right heart failure resulting from excessive venous congestion.

Palpating peripheral pulses

Evaluation of the rate, rhythm, amplitude, and symmetry of peripheral pulsations, along with auscultation of the femoral pulses for bruits, reveals important information about the cardiac function and peripheral perfusion of your patient. Using your dominant hand, palpate the peripheral pulses lightly with the pads of your index, middle, and (when appropriate) ring fingers. Use three fingers where space permits and two fingers when the area you are palpating is small or angled (for example, the femoral pulses).

To determine *rate,* count all pulses for at least 30 seconds (60 seconds when recording vital signs). The normal rate is between 60 and 100 beats/minute. If you detect an irregular radial pulse, use the technique for apical-radial pulses.

To estimate pulse *volume* or *amplitude,* palpate the blood vessel during ventricular systole. Pulse amplitude reflects the adequacy of the circulating volume, the vessel tone, the strength of left ventricular contraction, and the elasticity and distensibility of the arterial walls. Normal arteries are soft and pliable. Sclerotic vessels are more resistant to occlusion by external pressure; when you palpate them, they feel beaded and cordlike. Characterize the pulse volume of your patient using this scale:
• 3 + : bounding, increased
• 2 + : normal
• 1 + : weak, thready, decreased
• 0: absent.

Palpate pulses on both sides of the body simultaneously (except the carotid pulse) to determine *symmetry;* inequality is diagnostically significant. Always assess peripheral pulses methodically, moving from the head (temporal, facial) to the arms (brachial, radial, ulnar) to the legs (femoral, popliteal, posterior tibial, pedal). For the *temporal pulse,* feel the ear immediately in front of the tragus, where the artery passes over the root of the zygomatic process of the temporal bone. Then palpate the *facial pulse* where the artery passes over the lower border of the mandible, at the anterior border of the masseter muscle.

Feel the *brachial pulse* medial to the biceps tendon. Palpate the *radial pulses* on the palmar surface of the patient's relaxed, slightly flexed wrist, medial to the radial styloid process. (The radial pulse is the most frequently used indicator of pulsation rate and rhythm.) Feel the *ulnar artery* by pressing it against the ulna on the palmar surface of the wrist. Be sure to note rate, amplitude, and symmetry for both arms.

To assess the *femoral pulses,* use the pads of your fingers to deep-palpate the area below the inguinal ligament, midway between the anterior superior iliac spine and the symphysis pubis. Then, auscultate the pulsation sites on both sides of the body for bruits, which indicate arteriosclerotic changes.

To locate the patient's *popliteal* arteries, which are relatively deep in the soft tissues behind the knee, flex his knee slightly while he is supine or in the semi-Fowler position. Use both hands to deep-palpate the pulsation. You may locate the pulse more easily by placing both thumbs on his knee and palpating behind it with the first two fingers of both hands.

Assess the *pedal pulses* by using the pads of your fingers to palpate the dorsum of the foot. To prevent excessive traction on the artery, dorsiflex the foot, preferably to 90°, and palpate where the vessel passes over the dorsum. To locate the pulsation, place your palm on the dorsum until you feel the dorsalis pedis pulse point. (The pedal pulse is a superficial pulse that can be obscured by heavy palpation.) Keeping the foot of the patient in the dorsiflexed position, use the pads of your fingers to locate the

posterior tibial pulsation on the posterior or inferior medial malleolus of the ankle.

Assessment tip: Always check the pedal pulse in patients with intermittent claudication or gangrene.

Remember that in some patients the dorsalis pedis may occupy a different position or be difficult to palpate; failure to find the pulse does not necessarily indicate arterial disease.

Assessing perfusion to arms and legs

Inspect the skin color of the patient's hands and feet. Describe skin color as *normal, cyanotic, mottled,* or *excessively pale.* Note if the patient has any petechial hemorrhages, *Osler's nodes* (tender, reddish or purplish subcutaneous nodules seen in subacute bacterial endocarditis) in his fingers, palms, or toes, or *Janeway spots* (small hemorrhagic macules diagnostic of subacute bacterial endocarditis) on his palms.

To assess arterial flow adequacy, have the patient lie down and raise his legs or arms 12″ (30 cm) above heart level; then ask him to move his feet or hands up and down briskly for 60 seconds. Next, tell him to sit up and dangle his legs or arms—which should show mild pallor, with the original color returning in about 10 seconds and the veins refilling in about 15 seconds. Significant arterial insufficiency may be present if one or both of his feet or hands show marked pallor, delayed color return ending with a mottled appearance, or delayed venous filling—or if you note marked redness of his arms or legs. (See *Performing the Allen's Test,* page 55.)

Next, assess the adequacy of the patient's venous system by inspecting and palpating his legs for superficial veins. When the legs are in a dependent position, venous distention, nodular bulges at venous valves (bifurcations of veins), and collapsing veins are normal. Evidence of *venous insufficiency* (dilated, tortuous veins with poorly functioning valves) includes peripheral cyanosis, peripheral edema that pits with pressure, unusual ankle pigmentation, skin thickening, and ulceration—especially around the ankles.

To test capillary refill, squeeze a small area of the foot or toe between your fingers to cause blanching, then release the pressure and observe how rapidly normal color returns. Immediate return indicates good arterial supply.

Test the arms and legs of the patient for normal sensations to both light and deep palpation. Also note symmetry, areas of tenderness, and increased warmth or coolness.

Examine the fingernails and toenails for quantitative changes, including decreased or increased thickness and such qualitative changes as color, contour, consistency, and adherence to the nail bed. Also check for clubbed nails, which are associated with lung and heart disease. (See *Clubbing of the Fingers*, page 57.) In patients with long-standing heart disease, nail changes may result from hypoxemia. In these patients, you will note chronic nail thickening and enlargement, as well as bulbous enlargement of the ends of fingers or toes. Inspection also reveals exaggerated curves in the nails, with obscuring of the obtuse angle between the distal portion of the finger or toe and the nail. The end root feels spongy or soft.

Now, inspect and palpate the skin of the patient for texture and hair patterns. In a patient with chronic poor circulation, the skin appears thick, waxy, fragile, and shiny; normal body hair on the arms and legs is absent.

Inspect the arms, hands, legs, feet, and ankles for edema caused by increased hydrostatic pressure and vascular fluid exudation into the tissue interspaces. (If the patient has been confined to bed, also check for edema in his buttocks and sacral areas, because it occurs in the most dependent body parts.) Palpate for edema against a bony prominence and describe its characteristics:
• type (pitting or nonpitting)
• extent and location (ankle-foot area, foot-knee area, hands, or fingers)
• degree of pitting (described in terms of depth): 0″ to ¼″ is mild (1 +); ¼″ to ½″, moderate (2 +); and ½″ to 1″, severe (3 +)
• symmetry (unilateral or symmetrical).

Inspect and palpate for evidence of deep vein inflammation or clot formation. Determine the presence of pain, tenderness, or a sense of fullness in the calf, which may be aggravated when the patient stands or walks. Next, assess for local redness, foot edema, or cyanosis of the foot, especially when it is dependent. Gently press the calf muscle with your palm; pain indicates possible thrombophlebitis. To test for Homans' sign, firmly and abruptly dorsiflex the foot while supporting the entire leg, which must be extended or slightly bent (deep calf pain indicates thrombophlebitis); then palpate the foot.

PEDIATRIC AND GERIATRIC ASSESSMENT

Pediatric considerations

Children's cardiovascular problems stem from congenital heart disease or from rheumatic fever. Congenital heart disease is the leading cause of serious illness and death in newborns and infants; rheumatic fever, the second largest cause of cardiac problems in children over age five. Even if you don't specialize in the care of children, you should know how to recognize children with these potentially fatal problems.

Developmental anatomy
The fetal heart has two extra openings: the *foramen ovale* (located between the two atria) and the *ductus arteriosus* (located between the aorta and the pulmonary artery). The foramen ovale, which normally fuses at birth, can function as an atrial septal defect. The ductus arteriosus, which normally closes soon after birth, may remain open for some time, resulting in a continuous murmur.

Identifying Cardiac Rate, Rhythm, and Sound

To identify a cardiac rhythm on an EKG, you will need to know the conduction sequence, as shown here.

When you observe these patterns, also be aware of *when* the appropriate heart sounds (S_1 and S_2, for example) occur in the sequence. Sequence frequency is important as well.

CLASSIFICATION	RATE	RHYTHM
Normal sinus rhythm	*Atrial:* 60 to 100 *Ventricular:* 60 to 100	Regular
Sinus bradycardia	*Atrial:* less than 60 *Ventricular:* less than 60	Regular
Sinus tachycardia	*Atrial:* 100 to 180 *Ventricular:* 100 to 180	Regular
Sinus arrhythmia	*Atrial:* 60 to 100 *Ventricular:* 60 to 100 Quickens on inspiration, slows on expiration	Irregular
Premature atrial contraction (PAC)	*Atrial:* 60 to 100 *Ventricular:* 60 to 100 Rate varies, depending on number of PACs	Irregular
Paroxysmal atrial tachycardia	*Atrial:* 150 to 200 *Ventricular:* 150 to 200	Regular, except at onset and termination
Atrial fibrillation	*Atrial:* 400 to 600 (controlled *and* uncontrolled) *Ventricular:* under 100 (with controlled atrial fibrillation) *Ventricular:* over 100 (with uncontrolled atrial fibrillation)	Very irregular

*Note: All rhythms are in Lead II of the EKG.

When you examine the patient, you may hear abnormal heart sounds and differences in cardiac rate and rhythm, like those occurring with a cardiac dysrhythmia. Accurate interpretation of these variations will help you identify the cardiac abnormality.

Use the chart below to identify cardiac rates, rhythms, and sounds. *Document your findings.

SOUND	
Normal (S_1 is of constant intensity; normal S_2 splitting)	
Normal	
Normal	
Normal, although S_1 and S_2 intensities may vary	
Normal, although S_1 and S_2 intensities may vary	
Normal but rapid	
S_1 intensity varies; normal S_2 splitting	

(continued)

Identifying Cardiac Rate, Rhythm, and Sound

(continued)

CLASSIFICATION	RATE	RHYTHM
Nodal rhythm	*Atrial:* 40 to 60 *Ventricular:* 40 to 60 (Atrial dysrhythmia may also exist *or* atria may be captured retrogradely)	Fairly regular
Premature ventricular contraction (PVC)	*Atrial:* 60 to 100 *Ventricular:* 60 to 100 (Rates vary depending on the number of PVCs)	Irregular
Ventricular tachycardia	*Atrial:* variable *Ventricular:* 100 to 270	Fairly regular
Ventricular fibrillation	*Atrial:* cannot be determined *Ventricular:* 400 to 600	Irregular
First-degree heart block	*Atrial:* 60 to 100 *Ventricular:* 60 to 100	Regular
Type I second-degree heart block	*Atrial:* 60 to 100 *Ventricular:* 30 to 100 (Atrial rate greater than ventricular)	Regular, although ventricular may be irregular, contraction not occurring with every atrial contraction.
Type II second-degree heart block	*Atrial:* 60 to 100 *Ventricular:* 30 to 100 (Atrial rate twice that of ventricular rate)	Regular, although ventricular may be irregular
Complete atrioventricular block	*Atrial:* 60 to 100 *Ventricular:* less than 40	Regular

SOUND

S_1 intensity varies; normal S_2 splitting

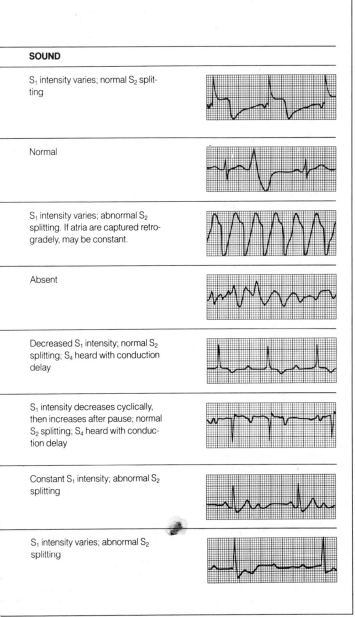

Normal

S_1 intensity varies; abnormal S_2 splitting. If atria are captured retrogradely, may be constant.

Absent

Decreased S_1 intensity; normal S_2 splitting; S_4 heard with conduction delay

S_1 intensity decreases cyclically, then increases after pause; normal S_2 splitting; S_4 heard with conduction delay

Constant S_1 intensity; abnormal S_2 splitting

S_1 intensity varies; abnormal S_2 splitting

In children under age 8, the heart is proportionally smaller. The tip of the apex (and the apical pulse) is at the fourth, not the fifth, ICS. Located 2″ to 2¼″ (5 to 6 cm) left of the sternum, the apex does not reach the MCL.

Pediatric history questions

Ask if the child has frequent upper respiratory tract infections. Then determine if he experiences shortness of breath. For an infant, ask the parents if the child has ever turned blue or had a bluish cast to his skin—especially on his face and around his mouth. Determine if the infant has trouble finishing a bottle without gasping or drinks only about 2 to 4 oz (60 to 120 ml) of milk at a time. Ask if other symptoms—such as increased breathing, rapid heartbeat, dyspnea, and diaphoresis—occur during feeding. Does the infant seem to tire easily? Also determine if his breathing is greatly labored during bowel movements. Is loss of appetite, profuse sweating, or vomiting a problem?

Ask an older child if he can keep up physically with children his age. Next, determine if the child experiences cyanosis on exertion or has dyspnea or orthopnea. Ask the parents if he constantly assumes a squatting position or sleeps in the knee-chest position; either sign may indicate tetralogy of Fallot or other cyanotic heart disease. Finally, find out if he bleeds excessively when cut.

Check the family history for indications of possible congenital heart defects. If the child is old enough, talk with him to obtain a profile of his lifestyle and daily activities. What he tells you can provide important information about his symptoms, including whether they have affected his activities. (See *Taking a Pediatric History,* pages 58 and 59.)

Inspecting the child

Examine the child for retarded growth or development. This condition may indicate significant chronic congestive heart failure or complex cyanotic heart disease. Then inspect his skin. Pallor can indicate a serious cardiac problem in an infant or anemia in an older child; in an infant or child, cyanosis may be an early sign of a cardiac condition. Cyanosis of the extremities *(acrocyanosis)* is a common and usually normal finding in neonates, but you should evaluate it when present. Acrocyanosis decreases when the infant is warm and active; cyanosis from decreased tissue oxygenation increases when the infant is crying and active.

Check for clubbed fingers, a sign of cardiac dysfunction. (Clubbing does not ordinarily occur before age 2.) Also, remember that dependent edema (a late sign of congestive heart failure in children) appears in the legs only if the child can walk; in infants, it appears in the eyelids. If the child is bedridden, also check his sacrum and buttocks.

Although it is difficult, you must measure blood pressure in children and infants because it provides important diagnostic information—for instance, it can help confirm coarctation of the aorta. First, select an appropriate cuff size. It should not be more than two thirds or less than one half of the upper arm length, and it should be about 20% wider than the diameter of the arm. Pediatric cuff sizes are 2½″, 5″, 8″, and 12″. Blood pressure may be inaudible in children under age 2. A Doppler stethoscope provides a more accurate measurement of blood pressure in children under age 2 than a regular stethoscope.

Before beginning, allow the child to handle the cuff and stethoscope to allay any fears. When you take his blood pressure, have him seated with his arm at heart level. Take the blood pressure of an infant when he is supine. Also take his thigh blood pressure, because diastolic readings lower in the legs than in the arms may indicate a coarctation of the aorta.

For children under age 1, the systolic thigh reading should equal the systolic arm reading. For older children, it may be 10 to 40 mm Hg higher, but the diastolic thigh value should equal the

Learning Cardiac Auscultation Landmarks

To perform cardiac auscultation, know the locations of the five areas shown here.

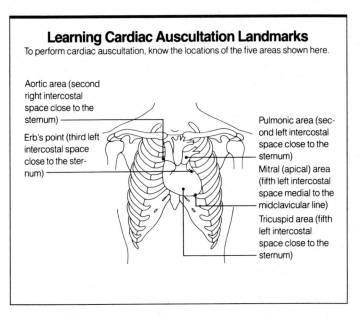

Aortic area (second right intercostal space close to the sternum)

Erb's point (third left intercostal space close to the sternum)

Pulmonic area (second left intercostal space close to the sternum)

Mitral (apical) area (fifth left intercostal space medial to the midclavicular line)

Tricuspid area (fifth left intercostal space close to the sternum)

diastolic arm value. If thigh readings are below normal, suspect coarctation.

Next, simultaneously palpate the radial and femoral pulses. If you feel the radial pulse before the femoral, suspect coarctation. (See *Pediatric Pulse Rate and Blood Pressure*, page 61.)

Palpation, percussion, and auscultation

In judging cardiac enlargement, remember that in children under age 8 the heart is proportionately smaller and the apical impulse is higher. Palpate or percuss the liver for enlargement, such as occurs in right ventricular failure, or for systolic pulsations, such as in tricuspid regurgitation.

Assessment tip: For infants, use a smaller bell on the stethoscope. If your stethoscope does not have interchangeable bells, remove the bell and use the base.

An S_3 sound is more common in a child and also more likely to be a normal finding. *Sinus arrhythmia* (a variation in which the heart accelerates on inspira-

tion and decelerates on expiration) is also more common in children and is normal. To confirm this variation in an older child, tell him to hold his breath; a true sinus arrhythmia will disappear.

Split sounds are significant in children. Carefully evaluate an S_2 split, which is easier to hear in a child than in an adult. Heard over the pulmonic area, this split occurs when the aortic valve closes slightly before the pulmonic valve. The difference in timing between the valve closures results in the S_2 split, which should increase during inspiration and decrease during expiration. A split that does not change during respiration or that changes paradoxically is abnormal.

So-called *innocent murmurs* (functional murmurs) are those which do not reflect underlying pathology. Usually such a murmur is Grade I or Grade II early systolic, without transmission, and heard at the pulmonic area. Some organic murmurs have the same characteristics as innocent ones, so until you have considerable experience, refer ev-

Guide to Breath Sounds

This chart tells what you will hear when you listen to the breath sounds of your patient, where you should and should not hear certain breath sounds, and what these findings indicate.

TYPE AND DESCRIPTION	POSITION IN RESPIRATORY CYCLE	NORMALLY HEARD OVER	ABNORMALLY HEARD OVER
Vesicular High-pitched and loud on inspiration; low-pitched and soft on expiration	More prominent during inspiration than during expiration	Peripheral lung fields	Peripheral lung fields in decreased volume; possibly indicating emphysema or pleural effusion
Bronchial or tracheal High-pitched, loud, harsh, hollow	Less prominent during inspiration than during expiration	Trachea and anterior of mainstem bronchi	Peripheral lung fields, possibly indicating consolidation, as in pneumonia
Bronchovesicular Moderate pitch and loudness	Equally prominent during inspiration and expiration	Major bronchi, upper anterior chest, and posteriorly between scapulae	Peripheral lung fields, possibly an early indication of respiratory disease

ery child with a murmur to a doctor for further evaluation. (See *Assessing the Pediatric Patient,* page 62.)

Childhood heart problems

The two primary cardiac conditions of childhood are congenital heart problems and rheumatic fever. Of every 1,000 full-term infants, 5 to 8 experience congenital heart problems, and this rate increases two to three times in premature infants. Neonates suffer the highest morbidity and mortality from congenital conditions—most deaths occur during the first week of life. Early detection and surgery could prevent at least 50% of these deaths.

The most common congenital cardiac conditions include atrial and ventricular septal defects, patent ductus arteriosus,

tetralogy of Fallot, coarctation of the aorta, aortic stenosis, pulmonic stenosis, and transposition of the great vessels. Rheumatic fever (a complication of Group A streptococcal infection), unlike these conditions, most commonly strikes children between ages 5 and 15. Children in this age-group should always be given a thorough cardiac examination 2 weeks after a streptococcal infection.

Geriatric considerations

The aging process involves changes in physical appearance, diminished sensory function, decreased body system function, and an increased vulnerability to disease. As a nurse, you must be aware of these changes when doing an assessment of an elderly patient.

Cardiovascular changes in the elderly

As a person ages, his heart usually becomes smaller. Exceptions to this rule are persons suffering from hypertension or heart disease. By age 70, cardiac output at rest has often decreased by about 35%. Fibrotic and sclerotic changes thicken heart valves and reduce their flexibility, sometimes causing a heart murmur. The elderly may also develop obstructive coronary disease and fibrosis of the cardiac skeleton. The ability of the heart to respond to physical and emotional stress may decrease markedly with age. Usually, aging also contributes to arterial and venous insufficiency as the strength and elasticity of blood vessels decrease. All these factors contribute to an increased incidence of cardiovascular disease in the elderly; coronary disease is most common.

Geriatric history questions

As you begin the interview, assess the *level of consciousness* of your patient, noting confusion or slowed mental status—occasionally, these are early signs of inadequate cardiac output. Remember that poor memory and generalized cerebral atherosclerosis may make it difficult for a patient to understand and respond to your questions.

Ask the patient about *chest pain,* which could be interpreted as angina pectoris. Remember, however, that his chief complaint may be dyspnea or palpitations rather than chest pain, because although aging contributes to coronary artery plaque development, it also promotes collateral circulation to areas deprived of perfusion. Also keep in mind that these signs and symptoms in the elderly may indicate pathology in many systems other than cardiovascular, including the urinary, endocrine, musculoskeletal, and respiratory systems.

Ask your patient about his *activities of daily living,* any signs or symptoms associated with these activities, and his

Lung Auscultation Sequences

Follow the auscultation sequences shown here to help identify lung abnormalities.

Remember to compare sound variations from one side to the other as you proceed. Document any abnormal sounds you hear and describe them carefully, including their location.

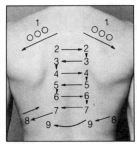

Posterior

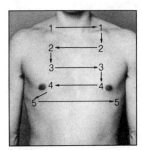

Anterior

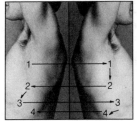

Left lateral   Right lateral

Guide to Adventitious Sounds

TYPE AND DESCRIPTION	POSITION IN RESPIRATORY CYCLE	POSSIBLE CAUSE	POSSIBLE INDICATION
Fine rales High-pitched, crackling, and popping (like rubbing hairs between your fingers)	End of inspiration	Fluid in the smallest airways	Pneumonia or congestive heart failure
Medium rales Lower-pitched, louder, and wetter (like freshly opened bottle of carbonated soda)	Mid-to-late inspiration or expiration	Fluid in the bronchioles	CHF, pneumonia, pulmonary edema, bronchitis, or emphysema
Coarse rales Lower-pitched and loud (like crushing cellophane between your fingers)	Inspiration and expiration	Fluid in the bronchi and trachea	Severe pulmonary edema
Sibilant rhonchi High-pitched, musical, and squeaky (like whistling)	Predominant in expiration	Air passing through swollen small airways	Asthma or emphysema
Sonorous rhonchi Lower-pitched and moaning (like snoring)	Throughout respiratory cycle, though predominantly heard during expiration. May clear with coughing.	Air passing through swollen large airways	Bronchitis, tracheobronchitis
Pleural rub Coarse, grating, and low-pitched (like squeaking leather)	Throughout respiratory cycle, though loudest between inspiration and expiration	Inflamed surfaces of pleurae rubbing together	Pleurisy, tuberculosis, pulmonary infection, pneumonia, or cancer

Performing the Allen's Test

The Allen's test checks the patency of the ulnar and radial arteries. If you cannot palpate a pulse in one or both of these arteries, follow these guidelines:

Instruct the patient to rest his right arm on a table. Support the wrist with a rolled washcloth, as shown here. Place your thumb over the radial artery and ask him to clench his fist tightly. Compress the artery firmly. Then ask him to relax his hand. Observe the color of his palms. If his hand flushes, the artery is patent. If it remains blanched, suspect ulnar artery occlusion. (Note: Slow blood return may also be caused by poor cardiac output or, in a patient in shock, poor capillary refill.) Continue the test, occluding the ulnar artery. Then repeat the test on the left arm and document your findings.

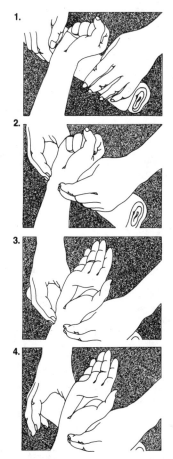

Follow these steps:

1. Have the patient rest his arm on the bedside table. Support his wrist with a rolled towel. Ask him to clench his fist.

2. Use your index and middle fingers to exert pressure over both the radial and the ulnar arteries.

3. Without removing your fingers, ask the patient to unclench his fist. His palm will be blanched because you have impaired the normal blood flow with your fingers.

Nursing tip: If the patient is unconscious or unable to clench his fist, encourage his palm to blanch by occluding both arteries, elevating his hand, and massaging his palm.

4. Release the pressure on the ulnar artery, and ask the patient to open his hand. If the ulnar artery is functioning well, his palm will turn pink in about 5 seconds, even though the radial artery is still occluded. But if blood return is slow and his fingers begin to contract, blood supply from the radial artery may not be adequate. In that case, try the Allen's test on his other wrist—you may get better results.

Note: Slow blood return does not always indicate arterial occlusion. It may mean poor cardiac output or poor capillary refill resulting from shock.

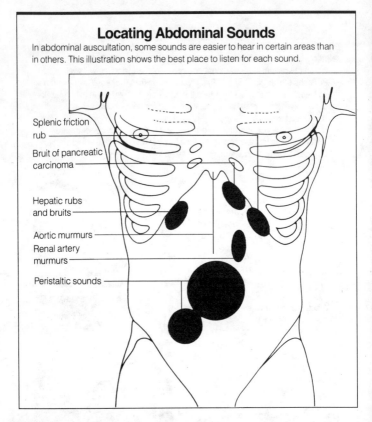

Locating Abdominal Sounds

In abdominal auscultation, some sounds are easier to hear in certain areas than in others. This illustration shows the best place to listen for each sound.

Splenic friction rub

Bruit of pancreatic carcinoma

Hepatic rubs and bruits

Aortic murmurs

Renal artery murmurs

Peristaltic sounds

response to physical and emotional exertion. Reduced cardiac reserve limits the ability to respond to such conditions as infection, blood loss, hypoxia-induced dysrhythmias, and electrolyte imbalance.

Determine if the patient has a history of smoking, frequent coughing, wheezing, or dyspnea, which may indicate *chronic lung disease*. Pulmonary hypertension resulting from pulmonary disease is a chief cause of right-sided heart failure.

Ask, too, about *medication side effects*. Weakness, bradycardia, hypotension, and confusion may indicate elevated potassium levels; weakness, fatigue, muscle cramps, and palpitations

may indicate inadequate levels of potassium. Anorexia, nausea, vomiting, diarrhea, headache, rash, vision disturbances, and mental confusion may indicate an overdose of digitalis or antiarrhythmic medications.

Physical examination guidelines
In an elderly patient who may have *chronic lung disease,* check for evidence of cor pulmonale and advanced right-sided congestive heart failure: large, distended neck veins, hepatomegaly with tenderness, hepatojugular reflux, and peripheral dependent edema. Check, too, for evidence of chronic obstructive pulmonary disease.

Carefully assess the patient for signs and symptoms associated with *cerebral hypoperfusion*—such as dizziness, syncope, confusion or loss of consciousness, unilateral weakness or numbness, aphasia, and occasionally slight clonic, jerking movements. Cerebral hypoperfusion may result in transient ischemic attacks caused by cerebrovascular spasm, carotid stenosis, microembolic phenomena, or transient bradyarrhythmias resulting from degenerative disease of the heart's conduction system (Stokes-Adams attack). Check the carotid artery or femoral pulse when these signs and symptoms occur to help you differentiate between transient ischemic attacks and Stokes-Adams attack. An extremely slow or absent pulse followed by rapid return of consciousness and a slightly increased or normal heart rate may indicate Stokes-Adams attack.

Record baseline blood pressures bilaterally and use them carefully to determine if systolic pressures are consistently above 150 mm Hg. Because aging causes arterial walls to thicken and lose elasticity, readings—especially systolic readings—may be higher than normal.

Measure the heart rate of the patient for 60 seconds, apically and radially. (Remember: As a person ages, increased vagal tone slows the heartbeat.) If the apical rate is below 50 beats/minute in a hospitalized patient, monitor his vital signs frequently. Determine if the patient has palpitations or symptoms of inadequate cardiac output.

When palpating the carotid pulse, be alert for hyperkinetic pulses and bruits over the carotids, which are common in older patients with advanced arteriosclerosis.

Kyphosis and scoliosis, also common in the elderly, distort the chest walls and may displace the heart slightly. Thus, the apical impulse and heart sounds of your patient may be slightly displaced. According to some authorities, S_4 sound is common in the elderly and results from decreased left ventricular compliance. Diastolic murmurs indicate pathology; soft, early systolic murmurs

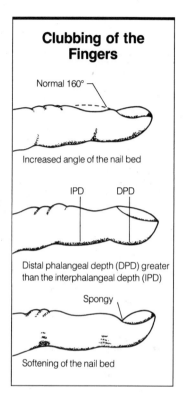

Clubbing of the Fingers

Normal 160°

Increased angle of the nail bed

IPD   DPD

Distal phalangeal depth (DPD) greater than the interphalangeal depth (IPD)

Spongy

Softening of the nail bed

may be associated with normal aortic lengthening, tortuosity, or sclerotic changes and may not indicate serious pathology. Check for signs of peripheral arterial insufficiency (See *CV Changes in the Elderly,* page 63.)

EMERGENCY ASSESSMENT

Adult patients

Cardiac emergencies can arise from chest trauma or from preexisting disorders, such as coronary artery disease or hypertension. These emergencies must be assessed quickly because they disrupt your patient's basic life processes.

Taking a Pediatric History

Chances are, the doctor's office, clinic, or hospital where you work has an interview form to follow when you document a patient's history. Be sure it covers these major points:

Identity: Document the name, age, address, religion, and sex of the child. Also document the interview date and the name and relationship of others who have provided information.

Chief complaint: What is the reason for this visit? Does the child have a specific problem, or is this a routine checkup? If he *has* a health problem, describe it thoroughly, including its duration, its signs and symptoms, whether any treatment makes the symptoms better or worse, and whether the parents have been treating the problem with medications. (Do not forget to document home remedies and over-the-counter medications, as well as any prescribed by a doctor.) Ask the child to describe his symptoms, and document his exact words or gestures.

Medical history: Include prenatal and birth complications, postnatal problems, and early feeding difficulties. These facts can provide clues to current problems. Also document all illnesses the child has had, and ask the parents to estimate how often he gets minor colds. Note any accidents (including burns and poisoning), surgeries, or hospitalizations. Of course, also document any chronic problems, such as a heart defect or diabetes. Finally, document all vaccinations. *Note:* Confirm this information with the child's medical records, if available. If the family is new to the community, stress the importance of having copies of their medical records transferred.

Medications and allergies: Is the child taking medication? If so, document its name, dosage, and the reason he needs it. Then, find out if he has any chronic allergies, including hay fever and asthma, and if he has ever had any allergic reactions to medication (particularly penicillin), food (including milk and fruit juices),

Primary assessment

Your primary emergency assessment may identify life-threatening problems involving your patient's airway, breathing, or circulation. (See *CV Emergency Assessment Checklist,* page 64.)

Airway

Begin by checking airway patency. Look and listen for such signs and symptoms as gurgling, stridor, wheezing, noisy breathing, circumoral or nail-bed cyanosis, obvious neck trauma, deviated trachea, and decreased level of consciousness. If the patient is *unconscious,* place your ear close to his nose and mouth—you should *hear* his breathing and *feel* his breath on your cheek.

If his airway is patent, you can move on to assess his breathing. If it isn't, you need to take *immediate* steps to open it.

If a conscious patient clutches his throat and starts to cough, you know that he is choking. Ask him if he can speak. If he can, encourage him to expel the obstruction himself by coughing. However, if he cannot speak or cough, or if he begins to make crowing noises, assume his airway is obstructed and intervene immediately.

If a patient is not choking, but you still do not hear or feel air movement, position him on his back and use the *head-tilt/chin-lift* method or the *head-tilt/neck-lift* method to try to open his airway. Use the *jaw-thrust without head-tilt* method if you have *any* reason to suspect cervical spine injury. Use the

insect stings, or anything else. (If necessary, describe signs of possible allergic reaction to the parents.) Document allergies on your interview form, and document medication allergies in red on the child's Kardex and chart cover. If the parents are unaware of any allergies, write "No allergies known" on your interview form.

Habits: Find out about the eating, sleeping, and elimination patterns of the child. Does he have specific eating or bedtime routines? Does he have frequent nightmares? Does he wet his bed? If the answers you get reveal anything abnormal (for example, chronic constipation), ask for more information about his eating and drinking habits. Also, inquire about play habits and the relationship of the child with his peers.

Systems review: Working from head to toe, ask about any problems. Use open-ended questions, unless you repeatedly receive negative answers. In that case, ask more specific questions. For example, if the parents insist that the child is always healthy, ask whether he ever has a runny nose.

Use the responses of the parents to guide you when you conduct a physical examination.

Family history: Does anyone in the family have a chronic illness, such as diabetes, hypertension, or asthma, or a birth defect, a severe or unusual allergy, heart or kidney disease, or cancer? Are any members of the immediate family dead? (If so, document the cause of death.) Note any major illnesses of the siblings. (Consider using a genotype or pedigree chart to document this information.)

Developmental history: Document the growth and development of the child. When did he first roll over, sit alone, stand up, and walk? When did he begin talking? When did his first tooth erupt? Pay particular attention to his interactions with you and his family. Note whether he seems older or younger than his age.

Other considerations: Briefly describe your overall impression of the child, including any physical, emotional, or developmental problems you have noticed or suspect.

"*sniff*" position if your patient is an infant. Then, use a finger sweep to clear any foreign body from the oral cavity, and suction the patient if necessary. Check again for air flow from his nose and mouth. Using the appropriate head position may open his airway and restore his breathing—especially if his tongue caused the obstruction.

Breathing

Once you have established that your patient has an open airway (or you have intervened as necessary to open it), check his breathing. If he is breathing, quickly assess the rate, depth, and quality of his respirations, noting if they are unusually fast or slow, shallow or deep, or irregular. Observe him for chest-wall expansion, abnormal chest-wall motion, and accessory muscle use.

Provide supplemental oxygen by nasal cannula or mask if he is breathing but short of breath, or if he has:
• chest pain
• signs and symptoms of poor cardiac output (decreased pulse and blood pressure)
• signs and symptoms of hypoxemia (such as confusion, anxiety, or restlessness)
• profuse bleeding
• nausea.

Remember, never give oxygen by mask at a flow rate less than 5 liters/minute. If you do, the patient will rebreathe carbon dioxide, decreasing the effectiveness of oxygen therapy.

If he is breathing adequately, move on to assess his *circulation*. If he *is not*, ventilate him immediately. (See *The ABCs of CPR*, pages 342 to 344.)

Circulation

Assess the circulatory status of your patient by first checking his pulses, starting with the carotid. If they are strong and regular, check his blood pressure. If it is stable, quickly check his *mental status* and *general appearance*—the last steps in your primary assessment. Intervene *immediately*, however, if you note any of these problems:

• *no pulse*, indicating cardiac arrest
• *irregular or abnormal pulse*, possibly indicating dysrhythmias
• *weak, rapid, thready pulse* and *decreased blood pressure*, possibly indicating shock.

If the patient has *no pulse*, he is in cardiac arrest; begin CPR *immediately* (see "Cardiopulmonary Resuscitation," pages 340 to 346), and have someone call for help or call a code. Open the patient's airway and ventilate him. Be sure he is placed on a cardiac arrest board or some other firm surface.

If the patient has an *irregular or abnormal pulse*, he may be experiencing cardiac dysrhythmias.

If the patient has *weak, rapid, thready pulses and decreased blood pressure*, he is probably in shock. Look for these signs and symptoms:

• restlessness
• dizziness or syncope
• thirst
• pallor
• diaphoresis.

General appearance and mental status

If one or more of the patient's vital functions is compromised, his general appearance will be poor and his mental status will be altered. But even if the vital functions are stable, take a few seconds to assess the patient for obvious wounds and deformities, abnormal breath or body odors, altered skin color, diaphoresis, tremors, and facial expressions indicating distress or anxiety. Determine his level of consciousness in response to verbal communication, touch, or painful stimuli.

Secondary assessment

When the airway, breathing, and circulation of the patient have been stabilized, identify his most serious problems. Your assessment will include:

• *subjective factors* (the information the patient provides about himself, including answers to history questions)
• *objective factors* (the information you uncover with inspection, palpation, percussion, and auscultation in the course of your physical examination).

When you perform an actual emergency assessment, you will combine these factors to save time, using the chief complaints of the patient to focus your physical examination.

Pediatric patients

Both your primary and secondary emergency assessments will be different if your patient is a child, because his developing body predisposes him to special problems that threaten his airway, breathing, and circulation. Also, his anxiety and (if he is very young) inability to communicate make secondary assessment more difficult.

Primary assessment

Airway obstruction and breathing difficulties, especially in infants and young children, are most often the result of viral infection. But remember, children commonly aspirate food, such as candy or peanuts, or small objects, such as toys or buttons. The tongue of a young child, proportionately larger than that of an adult, is more likely to block his airway if he is unconscious or has a seizure. And swelling or mucus—for example, in a child with croup or epiglottitis—may easily occlude his narrow airway. Be alert for signs of respiratory distress in any child with an emergency. These signs include:

Pediatric Pulse Rate and Blood Pressure

AVERAGE RESTING PULSE RATE

Age	Normal Range		Average	
Newborn	70 to 170		120	
1 to 11 months	80 to 160		120	
2 years	80 to 130		110	
4 years	80 to 120		100	
6 years	75 to 115		100	
8 years	70 to 110		90	
10 years	70 to 110		90	
	Female	Male	Female	Male
12 years	70 to 110	65 to 105	90	85
14 years	65 to 105	60 to 100	85	80
16 years	60 to 100	55 to 95	80	75
18 years	55 to 95	50 to 90	75	70

AVERAGE RESTING BLOOD PRESSURE

Age	Female	Male
4 years	98/60	98/55
6 years	105/65	105/60
8 years	108/67	105/60
10 years	112/64	110/65
12 years	115/65	110/65
14 years	112/65	114/65

- tachypnea (probably the first sign)
- intracostal, subcostal, or suprasternal retractions
- expiratory grunts
- nasal flaring
- wheezing
- cyanosis
- paradoxical breathing.

If the airway is occluded, use the head-tilt/neck-lift technique or the sniff position to try to open it.

Infants are obligate nose-breathers. So if an infant has a cold that is congesting or obstructing his nostrils, he will have to breathe through his mouth, which can create breathing difficulties. Assess his respiratory rate, remembering that in infants and young children, breathing is primarily diaphragmatic, and thoracic excursion is minimal. You may find a respiratory rate easier to obtain if you observe *abdominal* rather than *thoracic* excursion. Assess the rate for more than the usual 30 to 60 seconds to obtain an accurate count, because infants may have periodic breathing with variable rates, changing every 15 to 30 seconds. Also, a child's respiratory rate is more responsive than an adult's to illness, emotion, and exercise—it may double if he is stressed.

When you assess the circulation of a pediatric patient, remember that you can feel a carotid pulse in an older child, but you may *not* be able to feel it in an infant. Auscultate his apical pulse, or palpate his brachial pulse, because these are easier to assess. Note any increase, decrease, or irregularity, remembering that heart rate in infants and children is labile and more sensitive to stressful events. Keep in mind that many children normally have sinus arrhythmia, in which heart rate increases with inspira-

Assessing the Pediatric Patient

To assess a pediatric patient physically, use the same method you use on an adult. But observe the following variations:

• **Blood pressure reading:** The diastolic sound in an infant or child will not be as distinct as in an adult.

If you cannot hear either the diastolic or systolic sounds, which frequently happens with patients under age one, use the flush technique instead. To do this, elevate the infant's arm or thigh (arm and thigh pressure in those under age one are equal), and wait until the skin blanches. Apply the proper size cuff and inflate it to about 75 mm Hg. Then, lower the limb and begin deflating the cuff. Note the pressure reading when the entire limb flushes with color—this approximate reading is the *infant's mean blood pressure.*

Pulse pressure (the difference between systolic and diastolic readings) is 20 to 50 mm Hg throughout childhood. If it is less than 20 mm Hg, the patient may have aortic stenosis. If it is more than 50 mm Hg—and you used the proper size pressure cuff—the patient may have patent ductus arteriosis or aortic regurgitation.

• **Arterial palpation:** You may not be able to locate your patient's popliteal, post-tibial, or dorsalis pedis pulses. For pulses that can be palpated, the rate fluctuates rapidly.

Important: When you palpate radial and femoral pulses, expect them to beat synchronously. If they do not, suspect coarctation of the aorta.

• **Chest inspection:** The normal infant and young child exhibit diaphragmatic breathing and show minimal thoracic activity. So, assess the pattern of their breathing by observing their abdomens, not their chests. This pattern changes with aging. Assess the breathing patterns of older children the same way you assess adults'—by observing the chest.

• **Chest percussion:** Percuss the pediatric patient very lightly. If you hear hyperresonance over the left side of the chest, do not automatically assume this indicates a pneumothorax—it may simply be air bubbles in the stomach.

• **Chest auscultation:** Do not be discouraged if you cannot immediately differentiate between heart sounds S_1 and S_2. At first, you may also have trouble identifying heart sounds and lung sounds because your area for auscultation is so small. However, both skills can be acquired with practice.

You may hear coarse sounds in the patient's chest. Do not be alarmed. Such sounds may simply indicate mucus in his trachea. If you hear a sinus arrhythmia in a child, instruct him to hold his breath—the dysrhythmia should disappear. If you hear a sinus arrhythmia in an infant, observe his respirations as you listen to his heart. The dysrhythmia will speed up with inspiration and slow down with expiration.

tion and decreases with expiration. If your patient is able to, ask him to hold his breath for a few seconds—his heart rate will become regular if he has sinus dysrhythmia but will continue to be irregular if he has a true dysrhythmia.

Secondary assessment

Take the temperature of your patient as soon as you have stabilized his airway, breathing, and circulation. Remember that this vital sign is more labile in infants and young children than in older children and adults.

Pay attention to the mental status of the child—a sick infant may be extremely irritable or listless, whereas a young child may sulk or scream. An older child who is sick may be tearful, withdrawn, or irritable.

Geriatric patients

When you assess an elderly patient in an emergency, use the same techniques you would for any other adult. However, take into account the physiologic and biological changes that are a normal part of the aging process. Decreased respiratory and cardiovascular function may make your patient more susceptible to airway, breathing, and circulation difficulties; decreased function in other body systems may compound the effects of an emergency condition. Your elderly patient may also have one or more chronic diseases that complicate his management and care.

Primary assessment

When you assess the airway, remember that the patient may have a diminished gag reflex and be more likely than a younger adult to aspirate stomach contents if his level of consciousness decreases.

Other factors that affect the breathing of a geriatric patient include:
- decreased maximum breathing capacity
- decreased inspiratory reserve volume
- decreased vital capacity
- decreased forced expiratory volume
- increased residual volume.

Advanced age affects circulation, too. Your patient probably has:
- decreased cardiac output (by as much as 35% in many patients older than age 70)
- decreased arterial wall elasticity
- arterial and venous insufficiency.

So he is more likely than a younger adult to have chronic heart disease, hypertension, and atherosclerosis—all posing additional risks for him in an emergency. Expect him to have a slower heart

---

CV Changes in the Elderly

Typical changes
- Increased systolic pressure
- More pronounced arterial pulses because of decreased adjacent connective tissue
- Possible slight decrease in heart rate
- Orthostatic hypotension
- Irregular cardiac rhythms, including ectopic beats or dysrhythmia from degeneration of conduction system
- Soft systolic ejection murmur (S_4) heard at base of heart early in systole, from sclerotic changes in aortic valve; not a problem in absence of other signs and symptoms
- Decreased cardiac output
- EKG changes such as lengthening of PR and QT intervals and shift of the QRS axis to the left
- Myocardial hypertrophy, including thickened left ventricular wall
- Stiffened, thickened heart valves
- Varicosities, which may be painful
- Reduced cardiac pain sensation
- Increased vasovagal response

Possible problems
- Increase in *both* systolic and diastolic blood pressure. Usually, systolic pressure rises higher, creating wider pulse pressure. Patient with systolic pressure over 160 mm Hg and diastolic pressure over 95 mm Hg may require blood pressure treatment
- Clubbing of fingers or cyanosis, indicating circulatory impairment
- Fatigue
- Shortness of breath
- Angina
- Myocardial infarction
- Congestive heart failure
- CVA
- Pulmonary embolism
- Stokes-Adams syndrome
- Vertigo or syncope
- Ulcerated, inflamed, or cordlike varicosities

CV Emergency Assessment Checklist

BODY SYSTEM	WHAT TO ASSESS
Vital signs 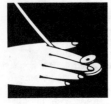	• Auscultate or palpate the patient's blood pressure. • Note the rate, depth, pattern, and symmetry of his respirations. • Palpate his radial pulse and note its rate, rhythm, and strength. • Take his temperature.
Cardiovascular 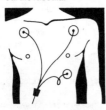	• Palpate the patient's peripheral pulses—especially of each affected body part—for rate, rhythm, quality, and symmetry. • Inspect him for jugular vein distention. • Inspect and palpate his extremities for edema, mottling and cyanosis, and temperature change. • Auscultate his heart sounds for timing, intensity, pitch, and quality, and note the presence of murmurs, rubs, or extra sounds. • Auscultate blood pressure in both arms.
Respiratory 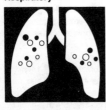	• Observe the patient for use of accessory muscles, paradoxical chest movements, and respiratory distress. • Inspect his chest for contour, symmetry, deformities, or trauma. • Auscultate his lungs for adventitious sounds and increased or decreased breath sounds. • Palpate his chest for tenderness, pain, and crepitation.

rate because of his increased vagal tone; if he has a sclerosed aorta, he may also have elevated systolic blood pressure with normal diastolic pressure.

Take his blood pressure in both arms. Peripheral pulses may *normally* be decreased if he has chronic venous and arterial insufficiency, so weak or absent peripheral pulses do not necessarily indicate shock or circulatory impairment.

Secondary assessment

Data collection for your *secondary assessment* may be difficult if the patient has decreased mental function because:
• he may have syncope or be confused from cerebral hypoperfusion.
• neuron degeneration may decrease sensory function and mentation.

The EKG of an elderly patient is normally somewhat different from that of a young adult; expect such changes as increased PR, QRS, and QT intervals and a decreased QRS complex amplitude.

4

MATERNAL-INFANT HEART DISORDERS

Pregnant women and infants with cardiovascular disease pose a special nursing challenge. Cardiovascular disease ranks fourth (after infection, toxemia, and hemorrhage) among the leading causes of maternal death. The physiologic stress of pregnancy and delivery is often more than a compromised heart can tolerate.

Infants with cardiovascular disease also have a high mortality. For every infant born with a malformed heart who survives, there is another infant who dies. But at least half of those dying from congenital heart defects may be candidates for corrective surgery if their defects are detected early enough.

THE PREGNANT PATIENT

Cardiovascular disease in pregnancy

Approximately 1% to 2% of pregnant females have cardiac disease, but the incidence is rising because medical treatment today allows more females with rheumatic heart disease and congenital defects to reach childbearing age. The prognosis for the pregnant patient with cardiovascular disease is good, with careful management. *Decompensation* (failure of the heart to maintain adequate circulation) is the leading cause of maternal death. Infant mortality increases with decompensation, since uterine congestion, insufficient oxygen-

ation, and the elevated carbon dioxide content of the blood not only compromise the fetus, but frequently cause premature labor and delivery.

Causes
Rheumatic heart disease is present in more than 80% of patients who develop cardiovascular complications. In the rest, these complications stem from congenital defects (10% to 15%) and coronary artery disease (2%).

The diseased heart is sometimes unable to meet the normal demands of pregnancy: 25% increase in cardiac output, 40% to 50% increase in plasma volume, increased oxygen requirements, retention of salt and water, weight gain, and alterations in hemodynamics during delivery. This physiologic stress often leads to decompensation. The degree of decompensation depends on the age of the patient, the duration of cardiac disease, and the functional capacity of the heart at the outset of pregnancy.

Signs and symptoms
Typical clinical features of cardiovascular disease during pregnancy include distended neck veins, diastolic murmurs, moist basilar pulmonary rales, cardiac enlargement (discernible on percussion or as a cardiac shadow on chest X-ray), and cardiac dysrhythmias (other than sinus or paroxysmal atrial tachycardia). Other characteristic abnormalities include cyanosis, pericardial friction rub, pulse delay, and pulsus alternans.

Decompensation may develop suddenly or gradually, with persistent rales at the lung bases. As it progresses, edema, increasing dyspnea on exertion, palpitations, a smothering sensation, and hemoptysis may occur.

Diagnosis

A diastolic murmur, cardiac enlargement, a systolic murmur of grade 3/6 intensity, and severe dysrhythmia suggest cardiovascular disease. Determination of the extent and cause of the disease may necessitate the following tests: electrocardiography, echocardiography (for valvular disorders, such as rheumatic heart disease), or phonocardiography. X-rays show cardiac enlargement and pulmonary congestion. Cardiac catheterization should be postponed until after delivery, unless surgery is necessary.

Treatment

The goal of antepartum management is to prevent complications and minimize the strain on the heart of the mother, primarily through rest. This may require periodic hospitalization for patients with moderate cardiac dysfunction or with symptoms of decompensation, toxemia, or infection. Older women or those with previous decompensation may require hospitalization and bed rest throughout the pregnancy.

Drug therapy is often necessary and should always include the safest possible drug in the lowest possible dosage to minimize harmful effects to the fetus. Diuretics and drugs that increase blood pressure, blood volume, or cardiac output should be used with extreme caution. If an anticoagulant is needed, heparin is the drug of choice. Digitalis and common antiarrhythmics, such as quinidine and procainamide, are often required. The prophylactic use of antibiotics is reserved for patients who are susceptible to endocarditis.

A therapeutic abortion may be considered for patients with severe cardiac dysfunction, especially if decompensation occurs during the first trimester.

Patients hospitalized with heart failure usually follow a regimen of digitalis, oxygen, rest, sedation, diuretics, and restricted intake of sodium and fluids. Patients whose symptoms do not improve after treatment with bed rest and digitalis may require cardiac surgery, such as valvotomy and commissurotomy. During labor, the patient may require oxygen and an analgesic, such as meperidine or morphine, for relief of pain and apprehension without undue depression of the fetus or herself. Depending on which procedure promises to be less stressful for the heart, delivery may be vaginal or by cesarean section.

Bed rest and medications already instituted should continue for at least 1 week after delivery because of the high incidence of decompensation, cardiovascular collapse, and maternal death during the early puerperal period. These complications may result from the sudden release of intra-abdominal pressure at delivery and the mobilization of extracellular fluid for excretion, which increase the strain on the heart, especially if excessive interstitial fluid has accumulated. Breast-feeding is undesirable for patients with severely compromised cardiac dysfunction, because it increases fluid and metabolic demands on the heart.

Nursing management

• During pregnancy, stress the importance of rest and weight control to decrease the strain on the heart. Suggest a limited fluid and sodium intake to prevent vascular congestion. Encourage the patient to take supplementary folic acid and iron to prevent anemia.

• During labor, watch for signs of decompensation, such as dyspnea and palpitations. Monitor pulse rate, respirations, and blood pressure. Auscultate for rales every 30 minutes during the first phase of labor and every 10 minutes during the active and transition phases. Check carefully for edema and cyanosis, and assess intake and output. Administer oxygen for respiratory difficulty.

• Use electronic fetal monitoring to watch for the earliest signs of fetal distress.

• Keep the patient in a semirecumbent position. Limit her efforts to bear down during labor, which significantly raise blood pressure and stress the heart.

• After delivery, provide reassurance, and encourage the patient to adhere to her treatment program. Emphasize the need to rest during her hospital stay.

Nursing diagnoses

After collecting subjective data and doing a cardiac assessment, you are ready to formulate nursing diagnoses, set goals, and plan interventions. Some typical diagnoses might be:
Alteration in cardiac output related to cardiovascular disease and decompensation. Alteration in comfort related to cardiovascular disease and pregnancy. Potential for noncompliance related to knowledge deficit of presenting condition.

Your goals are to prevent complications and help minimize strain on the heart. To achieve this, monitor vital signs often, and watch for signs and symptoms of fluid retention and cardiac decompensation.

You should also teach the patient about her condition so she will cooperate with treatment.

THE NEONATE

Ventricular septal defect

In ventricular septal defect (VSD), the most common congenital heart disorder, an opening in the septum between the ventricles allows blood to shunt between the left and right ventricles. VSD accounts for up to 30% of all congenital heart defects. The prognosis is good for defects that close spontaneously or are correctable surgically, but poor for untreated defects, which are sometimes fatal by age 1, usually from secondary complications.

Causes
In infants with VSD, the ventricular septum fails to close completely as it would normally by the eighth week of gestation. VSD occurs in some infants with fetal alcohol syndrome, but a causal relationship has not been established. Maternal ingestion of teratogens and maternal rubella during the first trimester of pregnancy have also been linked to VSD. Although most children with congenital heart defects are otherwise normal, in some, VSD coexists with additional birth defects, especially Down's syndrome and other autosomal trisomies, renal anomalies, and cardiac defects such as patent ductus arteriosus and coarctation of the aorta. VSDs are located in the membranous or muscular portion of the ventricular septum and vary in size. Some defects close spontaneously; in some defects, the entire septum is absent, creating a single ventricle.

VSD is not readily apparent at birth because right and left ventricular pressures are approximately equal, so blood does not shunt through the defect. As the pulmonary vasculature gradually relaxes, between 4 and 8 weeks after birth, right ventricular pressure decreases, allowing blood to shunt from the left to the right ventricle.

Signs and symptoms
Clinical features of VSD vary with the size of the defect, the effect of the shunting on the pulmonary vasculature, and the age of the infant. In a small VSD, shunting is minimal, and pulmonary artery pressure and heart size remain normal. Such defects may eventually close spontaneously without ever causing symptoms.

Initially, large VSD shunts cause left atrial and left ventricular hypertrophy; right ventricular hypertrophy develops later in life in uncorrected VSD because of increasing pulmonary vascular resistance. Eventually, biventricular congestive heart failure and cyanosis (from reversal of shunt direction) occur. Resulting cardiac hypertrophy may make the anterior chest wall prominent. A large VSD also increases the risk of pneumonia.

Infants with large VSDs are thin, small for their age, and gain weight slowly. They may develop congestive heart failure, with dusky skin; liver, heart, and spleen enlargement because of systemic venous congestion; diaphoresis; feeding difficulties; rapid, grunting respirations; and increased heart rate. They may also develop severe pulmonary hypertension. However, irreversible or fixed pulmonary hypertension with a right-to-left shunt (Eisenmenger's complex), causing cya-nosis and clubbing of the nail beds, does not occur until considerably later in life. The typical murmur associated with a VSD is blowing or rumbling, and its frequency varies from one beat to the next. In the newborn, a moderately loud early systolic murmur may be heard along the lower left sternal border. About the second or third day after birth, the murmur may become louder and longer. In infants, the murmur may be loudest near the base of the heart and may suggest pulmonary stenosis. A small VSD may produce a functional murmur or a characteristic loud, harsh systolic murmur. Moderate-sized and large VSDs produce audible murmurs (at least a grade 3 pansystolic), loudest

Surgical Repair of Transposition of the Great Vessels (Mustard Procedure)

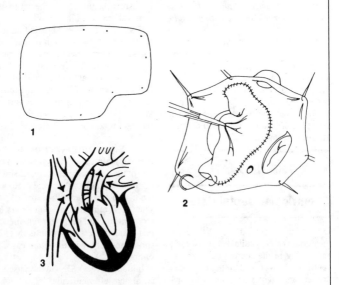

A Dacron patch (fig. 1) is sutured in the excised atrial septum (fig. 2) to divert pulmonary venous return to the tricuspid valve and systemic venous return to the mitral valve (fig. 3).

at the fourth intercostal space, usually accompanied by a thrill. In addition, the pulmonic component of S_2 is loud and widely split. Palpation reveals displacement of the point of maximal impulse to the left. When fixed pulmonary hypertension is present, a diastolic murmur may be audible on auscultation, the systolic murmur becomes quieter, and S_2 is accentuated greatly.

Diagnosis

Diagnostic tests include the following:

• *Chest X-ray* is normal in small defects; in large VSDs, it shows cardiomegaly, left atrial and left ventricular enlargement, and prominent pulmonary vascular markings.

• *Electrocardiogram (EKG)* is normal in children with small VSDs; in large VSDs, it shows left and right ventricular hypertrophy, suggesting pulmonary hypertension.

• *Echocardiography* may detect a large VSD and its location in the septum, estimate the size of a left-to-right shunt, and suggest pulmonary hypertension and is also more useful in identifying associated lesions and complications.

• *Cardiac catheterization* determines the size of the VSD and its location in the septum, and calculates the degree of shunting through a comparison of blood oxygen saturation in each ventricle. Catheterization also determines the extent of pulmonary hypertension and detects associated defects.

Treatment

Large defects usually require early surgical correction, before irreversible pulmonary vascular disease develops. Surgery consists of simple suture closure of small defects or insertion of a patch graft for moderate-to-large defects, using cardiopulmonary bypass. If the child has other defects and will benefit from delaying surgery, pulmonary artery banding normalizes pressures and flow distal to the band and prevents pulmonary vascular disease, allowing postponement of surgical correction. (Pulmonary artery banding is necessary

only when the child has other complications.) A rare complication of VSD repair is complete heart block from interference with the bundle of His during surgery. (Heart block may necessitate temporary or permanent pacemaker implantation.)

Before surgery, treatment consists of:

• digoxin, sodium restriction, and diuretics to prevent congestive heart failure

• careful monitoring by physical examination, X-ray, and EKG to detect increasing pulmonary hypertension, which, if it develops, indicates an early need for surgery

• measures to prevent infection (specifically, prophylactic antibiotics to prevent infective endocarditis).

Postoperative treatment generally includes a brief period of mechanical ventilation. Also, analgesics must be provided, and diuretics may be needed to increase urine output. Occasionally, continuous infusions of nitroprusside, adrenergic agents, or both may be necessary to regulate blood pressure and cardiac output. Rarely, a temporary pacemaker may be required.

Nursing management

Although the parents of an infant with VSD often suspect something is wrong before diagnosis, they need psychological support to help them accept the reality of a serious cardiac disorder. All physical examinations and diagnostic studies should be thoroughly explained. Because surgery, if needed, is generally scheduled some months after diagnosis, your care should emphasize parent teaching to prevent complications until the child is scheduled for surgery or the defect closes.

• Instruct the parents to watch for signs of congestive heart failure, such as poor feeding, sweating, heavy breathing, and fatigue.

• If the child is receiving digoxin or other medications, teach the parents how to administer the drugs and how to observe for side effects. Caution parents to keep medications out of the reach of all

children.
• Teach the parents to recognize and report early signs of infection and to avoid exposing the child to persons with obvious infections.
• Encourage parents to allow their child to continue normal activities without restriction.
• Teach parents the importance of endocarditis prophylaxis.

After surgery to correct VSD:
• Monitor vital signs and intake and output. Maintain the body temperature of the infant with an overbed warmer. Give catecholamines, nitroprusside, and diuretics, as ordered, and give analgesics, as needed.
• Monitor central venous pressure, intraarterial blood pressure, and left atrial or pulmonary artery pressure readings closely. Assess heart rate and rhythm for signs of conduction block.
• Check oxygenation, particularly in a child who requires mechanical ventilation. Suction, as needed, to maintain a patent airway and to prevent atelectasis and pneumonia.
• Monitor pacemaker effectiveness, if a pacemaker is needed. Watch for signs of pacemaker failure, such as bradycardia and hypotension.
• Reassure the parents, and allow them to participate in the care of their child as much as possible.
• Assist parents in encouraging their child to regain strength and resume activity.
• Tell parents that antibiotic prophylaxis to prevent endocarditis must continue.

Atrial septal defect

In an atrial septal defect (ASD), an opening between the left and right atria allows shunting of blood between the chambers. *Ostium secundum* defect (most common) occurs in the region of the fossa ovalis and occasionally extends inferiorly, close to the vena cava. *Sinus venosus* defect occurs in the superior-posterior portion of the atrial septum, sometimes extending into the vena cava, and is almost always associated with abnormal drainage of pulmonary veins into the right atrium. *Ostium primum,* a defect of the primitive septum, occurs in the inferior portion of the septum primum and is usually associated with atrioventricular valve abnormalities (cleft mitral valve) and conduction defects. ASD accounts for about 10% of congenital heart defects and appears almost twice as often in females as in males, with a strong familial tendency. Although ASD is usually a benign defect during infancy and childhood, delayed development of symptoms and complications makes it one of the most common congenital heart defects diagnosed in adults. Prognosis is excellent in asymptomatic persons but poor in those with cyanosis, due to large, untreated defects.

Causes

The cause of ASD is unknown, although factors such as rubella during the first trimester of pregnancy may lead to its development. In this condition, blood shunts from left to right because left atrial pressure normally is slightly higher than right atrial pressure. This pressure difference is sufficient to force large amounts of blood through a defect. The left-to-right shunt results in right heart volume overload, affecting the right atrium, right ventricle, and pulmonary arteries. Eventually, the right atrium enlarges, and the right ventricle dilates to accommodate the increased blood volume. If pulmonary artery hypertension develops as a consequence of the shunt (rare in children), increased pulmonary vascular resistance and right ventricular hypertrophy will follow. In some adult patients, irreversible (fixed) pulmonary artery hypertension causes reversal of the direction of the shunt, which results in unoxygenated blood entering the systemic circulation, causing cyanosis.

Signs and symptoms

ASD often goes undetected in preschoolers. Such children may complain exertion and may have frequent respiratory tract infections but otherwise appear normal and healthy. However, they may show growth retardation if they have large shunts. Children with ASD rarely develop congestive heart failure, pulmonary hypertension, infective endocarditis, or other complications. However, as adults, they usually manifest pronounced symptoms, such as fatigability and dyspnea on exertion, frequently to the point of severe limitation of activity (especially after age 40).

In children, auscultation reveals an early-to-midsystolic ejection murmur, superficial in quality, heard best at the second or third left intercostal space. In patients with large shunts—as a result of increased tricuspid valve flow—a low-pitched diastolic murmur is heard at the lower left sternal border, which becomes more pronounced on inspiration. Although the intensity of the murmur is a rough indicator of the size of the left-to-right shunt, its low pitch sometimes makes it difficult to hear. While S_1 is normal in children with ASD, S_2 is fixed and widely split because of delayed closure of the pulmonic valve. Mitral valve prolapse is occasionally seen in older children with ASD, indicated by a systolic click or a late systolic murmur at the apex.

In older patients with large, uncorrected defects and severe pulmonary artery hypertension, auscultation reveals an accentuated S_2. A pulmonary ejection click and an audible S_4 may also be present. Clubbing of the fingers and cyanosis are evident; syncope and hemoptysis may occur with severe pulmonary vascular disease.

Diagnosis

A history of increasing fatigue and characteristic physical features suggest ASD. The following findings confirm this diagnosis:

• *Chest X-ray* shows an enlarged right atrium and right ventricle, a prominent pulmonary artery, and increased pulmonary vascular markings.

• *EKG* may be normal but often shows right axis deviation, prolonged PR interval, varying degrees of right bundle branch block, right ventricular hypertrophy, atrial fibrillation (particularly in severe cases after the third decade of life), and left axis deviation in ostium primum defects.

• *Echocardiography* measures the extent of right ventricular enlargement and may locate the defect. (Other causes of right ventricular enlargement—for example, tricuspid insufficiency—must be ruled out.)

• *Cardiac catheterization* confirms ASD by demonstrating that right atrial blood is more oxygenated than superior vena cava blood—indicating a left-to-right shunt—and determines the degree of shunting and pulmonary vascular disease. Dye injection permits visualization of the size and the location of the ASD, the location of pulmonary venous drainage, and the competency of the AV valves.

Treatment

Since ASD seldom produces complications in infants and young children, surgical repair can be delayed until they reach preschool or early school age. If the defect is large, immediate surgical closure with sutures or a patch graft may be necessary. For a small ASD, an experimental procedure that inserts an umbrellalike patch using a cardiac catheter is an alternative to open heart surgery in some centers.

Nursing management

• Before cardiac catheterization, explain pre- and post-test procedures to the child and parents. If the child is old enough, use drawings or other visual aids to help with the explanation. Teach the child and family about other diagnostic procedures.

• Children with ASD and mitral valve prolapse and adults with untreated ASD require antibiotic prophylaxis to prevent infective endocarditis. Instruct them accordingly.

• If surgery is scheduled, teach the child and parents about the intensive care unit (ICU), and introduce them to the staff. Show parents where they can wait during the operation. Explain postoperative procedures, tubes, dressings, and monitoring equipment.

• Have parents tape-record a message to the child to be played in the recovery room. This way he will wake up to familiar voices.

• After surgery, closely monitor vital signs, central venous and intra-arterial pressures, and intake and output. Watch for atrial dysrhythmias, since surgical correction of ASD is only about 50% successful in eliminating them.

Coarctation of the aorta

Coarctation is a narrowing of the aorta, usually just below the left subclavian artery, near the site where the ligamentum arteriosum (the remnant of the ductus arteriosus, a fetal blood vessel) joins the pulmonary artery to the aorta. Coarctation may be associated with aortic valve stenosis (usually a bicuspid aortic valve) and, in more severe cases, with hypoplasia of the aortic arch, patent ductus arteriosus, and ventricular septal defect. Generally, prognosis for coarctation of the aorta depends on the severity of associated congenital cardiac anomalies. Prognosis for isolated coarctation is good if corrective surgery is performed before this condition induces degenerative changes in the aorta or severe systemic hypertension.

Causes and incidence

Coarctation of the aorta may develop as a result of spasm and constriction of the smooth muscle in the ductus arteriosus as it closes. Possibly, this contractile tissue extends into the aortic wall, causing narrowing. The obstructive process causes hypertension in the aortic branches above the constriction (arteries that supply the upper extremities, head, and neck) and diminished pressure in the vessels below the constriction.

Restriction of blood flow through the narrowed area of the aorta increases the pressure load on the left ventricle and causes dilation of the proximal aorta and ventricular hypertrophy. Untreated, this condition may lead to left heart failure and, rarely, to cerebral hemorrhage and aortic rupture. If VSD accompanies coarctation, blood shunts left to right, straining the right heart. This leads to pulmonary hypertension and, eventually, right heart hypertrophy and biventricular congestive heart failure.

Coarctation of the aorta accounts for about 7% of all congenital heart defects in children and is twice as common in males. When it occurs in females, it is often associated with Turner's syndrome, an absence or defect of the second sex chromosome, causing ovarian dysgenesis.

Signs and symptoms

Clinical features vary with age. During the first year of life, when aortic coarctation may cause congestive heart failure, the infant displays tachypnea, dyspnea, tachycardia, pulmonary edema, pallor, failure to thrive, cardiomegaly, and hepatomegaly. Heart sounds are generally normal in infancy, unless there are coexisting cardiac defects. However, femoral pulses are diminished or absent.

If coarctation is asymptomatic in infancy, it usually remains so throughout adolescence, as collateral circulation develops to bypass the narrowed segment. After the school-age years, this defect may produce dyspnea, claudication, headaches, epistaxis, and severe hypertension in the upper extremities despite collateral circulation. Frequently, it causes resting systolic hypertension and wide pulse pressure; high diastolic pressure readings are the same in both the arms and legs. Coarctation may also produce a visible aortic pulsation in the suprasternal notch, a continuous systolic murmur due to large collateral flow, accentuated S_2, and an S_4, caused by left ventricular failure.

Diagnosis

The cardinal signs of coarctation of the aorta are resting systolic hypertension, wide pulse pressure (high systolic readings when measured in the arms; normal or depressed readings when measured in the legs), and diminished or absent femoral pulses. The following tests confirm this diagnosis:

• *Chest X-ray* may demonstrate cardiomegaly, left ventricular hypertrophy, congestive heart failure, a dilated ascending and descending aorta, and notching of the undersurfaces of the ribs, due to extensive collateral circulation.

• *EKG* may eventually reveal left ventricular hypertrophy.

• *Echocardiography* may show increased left ventricular muscle thickness and coexisting aortic valve abnormalities at the site of the coarctation, as well as other associated cardiac defects.

• *Confirming cardiac catheterization* and *aortography* are indicated. Cardiac catheterization evaluates collateral circulation and measures pressure in the right and left ventricles and in the ascending and descending aortas (on both sides of the obstruction). Aortography locates the site and extent of coarctation. Additional cardiac defects are definitively defined and located.

Treatment

The infant with CHF due to coarctation of the aorta requires medical management with digoxin and diuretics. Surgery is recommended if medical management is unsuccessful. Older children with previous undetected coarctation may require antihypertensive therapy preoperatively. Medical management prior to surgery also includes endocarditis prophylaxis.

Surgical correction of coarctation of the aorta involves taking a flap of the left subclavian artery and using it to reconstruct an unobstructed aorta. Timing of surgery is determined by the child's symptoms, with early surgery recommended in CHF or hypertension. In the absence of these disorders, surgery is generally recommended during the preschool years.

Nursing management

• When coarctation in an infant requires rapid digitalization, monitor vital signs closely and watch for digitalis toxicity (poor feeding, EKG abnormalities).

• Balance intake and output carefully, especially if the infant is receiving diuretics with fluid restriction.

• Since the energy stores of an infant may be inadequate to maintain proper body temperature, regulate environmental temperature carefully, using an overbed warmer, if necessary.

• Monitor blood glucose levels to detect possible hypoglycemia, which may occur as glycogen stores in the liver are depleted.

• Offer the parents emotional support and an explanation of the disorder. Also explain diagnostic procedures, surgery, and drug therapy. Tell parents what to expect postoperatively.

• Closely assess blood pressure in extremities of an older child with coarctation.

• Explain any exercise restriction necessitated by significant hypertension while the child is at rest.

• Encourage endocarditis prophylaxis.

• Ensure that the parents and/or the child can administer all prescribed medications accurately and are aware of their potential side effects.

• Include all children in the explanations of diagnostic procedures or surgery whenever it is age-appropriate.

After corrective surgery:

• Monitor blood pressure closely, using an intraarterial line. Measure blood pressure in all extremities. Monitor intake and output.

• If the patient develops hypertension and requires nitroprusside or trimethaphan, administer it, as ordered, by continuous I.V. infusion, using an infusion pump. Monitor closely for severe hypotension, and regulate the dose carefully.

• Provide pain relief, and encourage a gradual increase in activity.

Six Most Common Anomalies

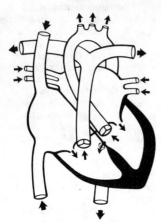

Ventricular septal defect (VSD)
One or more openings between the ventricles

CIRCULATORY
CONSIDERATIONS
Acyanotic defect. Blood flows from area of higher to area of lower pressure. This left-to-right shunt may cause pulmonary congestion and pulmonary artery hypertension.

MURMUR
Heard in lower left sternal border; may be associated with palpable thrill. Auscultatory findings depend on size of defect and amount of pulmonary vascular resistance.

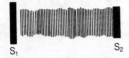

S_1 S_2

TREATMENT
Medical: Congestive heart failure regimen (sedation, rest, oxygen, digoxin, sodium restriction, diuretics)
Surgical: Simple closure or patch graft with patient on cardiopulmonary bypass

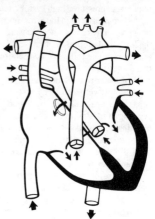

Atrial septal defect (ASD)
One or more openings between the atria. Includes ostium secundum, ostium primum, and sinus venosus

CIRCULATORY
CONSIDERATIONS
Acyanotic defect. Left-to-right shunt may cause pulmonary congestion and pulmonary artery hypertension. Atrial dysrhythmias secondary to right atrial overload and resultant interference with conduction system.

MURMUR
Systolic ejection is greatest in second and third left intercostal spaces. Fixed split S_2 on expiration heard in second, third, or fourth intercostal space.

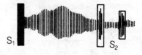

S_1 S_2

TREATMENT
Medical: Not usually necessary
Surgical: Direct closure or patch graft with patient on cardiopulmonary bypass

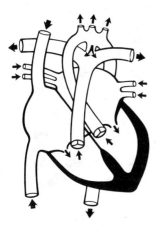

Patent ductus arteriosus (PDA)
Opening between the descending aorta and bifurcation of the pulmonary artery

CIRCULATORY CONSIDERATIONS
Acyanotic defect. Left-to-right shunt may cause pulmonary congestion and pulmonary artery hypertension. Increased incidence in premature infants. Pulse pressure may be widened; pulses, full or bounding.

MURMUR
Continuous "machinery" murmur, greatest at upper left sternal border and under clavicle.

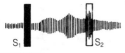

TREATMENT
Medical: Congestive heart failure regimen, indomethacin for premature infants with severe respiratory distress syndrome
Surgical: Ductal ligation in premature infants with severe respiratory distress syndrome during neonatal period; otherwise, when young children

Coarctation of the aorta
Constriction of descending aorta near the ductus arteriosus

CIRCULATORY CONSIDERATIONS
Acyanotic defect. Elevated pressures in ascending aorta and left ventricle. Insufficient mitral valve. Back pressure to lungs. Aneurysms, increased blood pressure in upper extremities, and leg cramping (may be confused with growing pains).

MURMUR
Systolic ejection click heard at base and apex of heart. Associated with systolic or continuous murmur between scapulae.

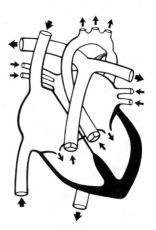

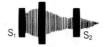

Ejection click (EJ)

TREATMENT
Medical: Congestive heart failure regimen, exercise restriction
Surgical: Resection and anastomosis, performed when patient is 6 to 12 years old

(continued)

Six Most Common Anomalies *(continued)*

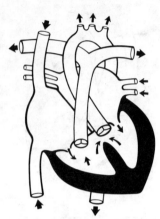

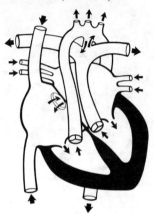

Tetralogy of Fallot
Four defects: VSD, overriding aorta, pulmonary stenosis, and right ventricular hypertrophy

CIRCULATORY
CONSIDERATIONS
Pulmonary stenosis restricts blood flow to lungs. Unoxygenated blood is shunted through the VSD. Saturated and unsaturated blood is mixed in the left ventricle and pumped out the aorta, producing cyanosis, tet spells, clubbing, and squatting.

MURMUR
Systolic murmur and single S_2 greatest in second and third intercostal spaces at left sternal border.

TREATMENT
Medical: Congestive heart failure regimen
Surgical: Palliative—Pott's, Blalock-Taussig, Waterston
Corrective—Close VSD and relieve pulmonary stenosis

Transposition of great vessels
Aorta leaves right ventricle, pulmonary artery leaves left ventricle

CIRCULATORY
CONSIDERATIONS
Unoxygenated blood flows through right atrium and ventricle and out aorta to systemic circulation again. Oxygenated blood flows from lungs to left atrium and ventricle and out pulmonary artery to lungs. Sudden severe cyanosis.

MURMUR
Loud aortic closure sound at second left intercostal space. Systolic murmur with VSD.

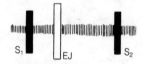

TREATMENT
Medical: Balloon septostomy, congestive heart failure regimen
Surgical: Palliative—Blalock-Hanlen
Corrective—Mustard, or Senning, procedure

- Promote adequate respiratory functioning through turning, coughing, and deep breathing.
- Observe for signs of GI and/or GU bleeding, abdominal pain, or rigidity.
- Instruct the older child with coarctation and his parents in postoperative antihypertensive therapy, if necessary.
- Explain the need for continued endocarditis prophylaxis and encourage compliance.

Patent ductus arteriosus

The ductus arteriosus is a fetal blood vessel that connects the pulmonary artery to the descending aorta. In patent ductus arteriosus (PDA), the lumen of the ductus remains open after birth. This creates a left-to-right shunt of blood from the aorta to the pulmonary artery and results in recirculation of arterial blood through the lungs. Initially, PDA may produce no clinical effects, but in time, it can precipitate pulmonary vascular disease, causing symptoms to appear by age 40. Prognosis is good if the shunt is small or surgical repair is effective. Otherwise, PDA may advance to intractable congestive heart failure, which may be fatal.

Causes and incidence

PDA affects twice as many females as males and is the most common congenital heart defect found in adults. Normally, the ductus closes within days to weeks after birth. Failure to close is most prevalent in premature infants, probably as a result of abnormalities in oxygenation (with normal lung function) or the relaxant action of prostaglandin E_1, which prevents ductal spasm and contracture necessary for closure. PDA often accompanies rubella syndrome and may be associated with other congenital defects, such as coarctation of the aorta, VSD, or pulmonary and aortic stenoses.

In PDA, the relative resistances in the pulmonary and systemic vasculature and the size of the ductus determine the amount of left-to-right shunting. The left atrium and left ventricle must accommodate the increased pulmonary venous return, in turn increasing left heart filling pressure and workload, and possibly causing congestive heart failure. In the final stages of untreated PDA, prolonged pulmonary artery hypertension because of the left-to-right shunt results in fixed, unreactive pulmonary hypertension and may cause the shunt to reverse (right to left); unoxygenated blood thus enters the systemic circulation, resulting in cyanosis.

Signs and symptoms

In infants, especially those who are premature, a large PDA usually produces respiratory distress, with signs of congestive heart failure because of the tremendous volume of blood shunted to the lungs through the patent ductus and the increased left heart workload. Other characteristic features may include heightened susceptibility to respiratory tract infections, slow motor development, and failure to thrive. Except for their cardiac examination, most children with PDA are asymptomatic, though mild symptoms of heart disease may be present (some physical underdevelopment, fatigability, increased number of respiratory infections). Adults with undetected PDA may develop pulmonary vascular disease, and by age 40 they may display fatigability and dyspnea on exertion. About 10% also develop infective endocarditis.

Auscultation reveals the classic machinery murmur (Gibson murmur): a continuous murmur (during systole and diastole) best heard at the base of the heart, at the second left intercostal space under the left clavicle in 85% of children with PDA. This murmur may obscure S_2. However, with a right-to-left shunt, such a murmur may be absent. Palpation may reveal a thrill at the left sternal border and a prominent left ventricular impulse. Peripheral arterial pulses are bounding (Corrigan's pulse), and pulse pressure is widened, due to some elevation in systolic blood pressure but a drop in diastolic pressure.

Diagnosis

• *Chest X-ray* shows increased pulmonary vascular markings, prominent pulmonary arteries, and enlargement of the left ventricle and aorta.

• *EKG* may be normal or may indicate left ventricular hypertrophy and, in advanced pulmonary vascular disease, biventricular hypertrophy.

• *Echocardiography* detects the presence and may help estimate the size of a PDA. In addition, it reveals an enlarged left atrium and left ventricle or right ventricular hypertrophy from pulmonary vascular disease. It also detects PDA.

• *Cardiac catheterization* shows pulmonary arterial oxygen content higher than right ventricular content because of the influx of aortic blood, suggesting this diagnosis. Increased pulmonary artery pressure indicates a large shunt or, if it exceeds systemic arterial pressure, severe pulmonary vascular disease. Catheterization allows calculation of blood volume crossing the ductus and can rule out associated cardiac defects. Dye injection definitively demonstrates the presence of the ductus.

Treatment

Premature infants only are given intravenous or oral indomethacin, a prostaglandin E inhibitor, to increase closure rates of PDA by inducing ductal spasm. This is done within the first 10 days of life, when it is most effective.

Asymptomatic infants with PDA require no immediate treatment. Those with congestive heart failure require fluid restriction, diuretics, and digitalis to minimize or control symptoms. If these measures do not control congestive heart failure, surgery is necessary to ligate the ductus. If symptoms are mild, surgical correction is usually delayed until age 1. Before surgery, children with PDA require antibiotics to protect against infective endocarditis.

Another form of therapy includes cardiac catheterization to deposit a plug in the ductus to stop shunting.

Nursing management

PDA necessitates careful monitoring, patient and family teaching, and emotional support.

• Watch carefully for signs of PDA in all premature infants.

• Be alert for respiratory distress symptoms resulting from congestive heart failure, which may develop rapidly in a premature infant. Frequently assess vital signs, EKG, electrolytes, and intake and output. Record response to diuretics and other therapy. Watch for signs of digitalis toxicity (feeding intolerance, poor feeding, vomiting, EKG changes).

• If the premature infant receives indomethacin to induce ductal closure, watch for possible side effects, such as diarrhea, jaundice, bleeding, or renal dysfunction.

• Explain the necessity of endocarditis prophylaxis and encourage compliance.

• Before surgery, carefully explain all treatment and diagnostic procedures to parents; include the child in your explanations, if age-appropriate. Arrange for the child and family to meet the ICU staff. Tell them about I.V. lines, monitoring equipment, and postoperative procedures. Show the parents where they can wait during surgery.

• Immediately after surgery, the child may have a central venous pressure catheter and an arterial line in place. Carefully assess vital signs, intake and output, and arterial and venous pressures. Provide pain relief, as needed.

• Before discharge, review instructions to the parents about activity restrictions that are governed by the tolerance and energy levels of the child. Advise parents not to become overprotective as tolerance for physical activity increases.

• Stress the need for regular medical follow-up examinations. Advise parents to inform any doctor who treats their child about his history of operative treatment for patent ductus arteriosus— even if he is being treated for an unrelated medical problem.

Tetralogy of Fallot

Tetralogy of Fallot is a complex of four cardiac heart defects: VSD, right ventricular outflow tract obstruction (pulmonary stenosis), right ventricular hypertrophy, and dextroposition of the aorta so that it overrides the VSD. Blood shunts right to left through the VSD, permitting unoxygenated blood to mix with oxygenated blood, resulting in cyanosis. Tetralogy of Fallot sometimes coexists with other congenital heart defects, such as patent ductus arteriosus or atrial septal defect. It accounts for about 10% of all congenital heart diseases and occurs equally in boys and girls. Before surgical advances made correction possible, approximately one third of these children died in infancy.

Causes
The cause of tetralogy of Fallot is unknown but results from embryologic hypoplasia of the outflow tract of the right ventricle and has been associated with fetal alcohol syndrome and the ingestion of thalidomide during pregnancy.

Signs and symptoms
The degree of pulmonary stenosis, interacting with the size and location of the VSD, determines the clinical and hemodynamic effects of this complex defect. The VSD usually lies in the outflow tract of the right ventricle and is generally large enough to permit equalization of right and left ventricular pressures. In addition, the ratio of systemic vascular resistance to pulmonary stenosis affects the direction and magnitude of shunt flow across the VSD. Severe obstruction of right ventricular outflow produces a right-to-left shunt, causing decreased systemic arterial oxygen saturation, cyanosis, reduced pulmonary blood flow, and hypoplasia of the entire pulmonary vasculature. Right ventricular hypertrophy develops because of increased right ventricular pressure. Milder forms of pulmonary stenosis result in either no

shunt or a left-to-right shunt, in which case cyanosis is absent and pulmonary blood flow closer to normal.

Generally, the hallmark of the disorder is cyanosis, which usually becomes evident within several months after birth but may be present at birth if the infant has severe pulmonary stenosis. Between ages 2 months and 2 years, children with tetralogy of Fallot may experience cyanotic, or "blue," spells. Such spells result from increased right-to-left shunting, possibly caused by spasm of the right ventricular outflow tract, increased systemic venous return, or decreased systemic arterial resistance.

Exercise, crying, straining, infection, or fever can precipitate blue spells. Blue spells are characterized by dyspnea, deep, sighing respirations, bradycardia, fainting, seizures, and loss of consciousness. Older children may also develop other signs of poor oxygenation, such as clubbing of fingers and toes, diminished exercise tolerance, increasing dyspnea on exertion, growth retardation, and eating difficulties. These children habitually squat when they feel short of breath; this is thought to decrease venous return of unoxygenated blood from the legs and increase systemic arterial resistance.

Children with tetralogy of Fallot are also at risk for developing cerebral abscesses, pulmonary thrombosis, venous thrombosis or cerebral embolism, and infective endocarditis.

In females with tetralogy of Fallot who live to childbearing age, the incidence of spontaneous abortion, premature births, and low birth weight rises.

Diagnosis
In a patient with tetralogy of Fallot, auscultation detects a loud systolic heart murmur (best heard along the left sternal border) that may diminish or obscure the pulmonic component of S_2. If a large patent ductus is present, the continuous murmur of the ductus may obscure the systolic murmur. Palpation often reveals a cardiac thrill at the left sternal border. In addition, the inferior sternum appears prominent and a prom-

inent right ventricular impulse can be palpated.

The results of special tests confirm the diagnosis:
• *Chest X-ray* demonstrates decreased pulmonary vascular markings, depending on the severity of the pulmonary obstruction, and a boot-shaped cardiac silhouette.
• *EKG* shows right ventricular hypertrophy, right axis deviation, and possibly right atrial hypertrophy.
• *Echocardiography* identifies septal overriding of the aorta, the VSD, and pulmonary stenosis and detects the hypertrophied walls of the right ventricle.
• *Cardiac catheterization* confirms diagnosis by visualization of the pulmonary stenosis and the VSD, as well as the overriding aorta, and by ruling out other cyanotic heart defects. This test also measures the extent of oxygen resaturation in aortic blood.
• *Laboratory findings* reveal diminished arterial oxygen saturation and polycythemia (hematocrit may be more than 60%) if the cyanosis is severe and long-standing, predisposing to thrombosis.

Treatment

Effective management of tetralogy of Fallot necessitates prevention and treatment of complications, measures to relieve cyanosis, and palliative or corrective surgery. During cyanotic spells, the knee-chest position and administration of oxygen and morphine improve oxygenation by relieving the spasm of the right ventricular outflow tract. Propranolol (a beta-adrenergic blocking agent) may control the occurrence of cyanotic spells.

Palliative surgery is performed on infants with potentially fatal hypoxic spells or rapidly increasing cyanosis and rising hematocrit. The goal of surgery is to enhance blood flow to the lungs to reduce hypoxia. This is most often accomplished by joining the subclavian artery to the pulmonary artery (Blalock-Taussig procedure). Supportive measures include prophylactic antibiotics to prevent infective endocarditis or cere-

bral abscess administered before, during, and after bowel, bladder, or any other surgery or dental treatments. Management may also include phlebotomy in children with polycythemia.

Complete corrective surgery to relieve pulmonary stenosis and close the VSD, directing left ventricular outflow to the aorta, requires cardiopulmonary bypass with hypothermia to decrease oxygen utilization during surgery, especially in young children. This may be accomplished in infants without prior palliative surgery and is generally recommended when hypoxia and polycythemia are progressive (rather than at a specific age), impairing the child's quality of life. Surgery is generally required at some point before the school-age years.

Nursing management
• Explain tetralogy of Fallot to the parents. Inform them that children with tetralogy of Fallot will set their own exercise limits and will know when to rest. Make sure they understand that the child can engage in physical activity, and encourage them not to be overprotective.
• Teach parents to recognize serious hypoxic spells (dramatically increased cyanosis, deep, sighing respirations, loss of consciousness). Tell them to place the child in the knee-chest position and to report such spells immediately. Emergency treatment may be necessary.
• To prevent infective endocarditis and other infections, warn parents to keep their child away from people with obvious infections. Urge them to encourage good dental hygiene and to watch for ear, nose, and throat infections and dental caries, all of which necessitate immediate treatment. When dental care, infections, or surgery requires prophylactic antibiotics, tell parents to make sure the child completes the prescribed regimen.
• If the child requires medical attention for an unrelated problem, advise the parents to inform the doctor immediately of the child's history of tetralogy

of Fallot, since any treatment must take this serious heart defect into consideration.

• During hospitalization, alert the staff to the condition of the child. Because of the right-to-left shunt through the VSD, treat I.V. lines like arterial lines. Remember, a clot dislodged from a catheter tip into a vein can cross the VSD and cause cerebral embolism. The same thing can happen if air enters the venous lines.

After palliative surgery:

• Monitor oxygenation and arterial blood gas values closely in the ICU.

• If the child has undergone the Blalock-Taussig procedure, do not use the arm on the operative side for measuring blood pressure, inserting I.V. lines, or drawing blood samples, since blood perfusion on this side diminishes greatly until collateral circulation develops. Note this on the child's chart and at his bedside.

After corrective surgery:

• Carefully monitor the EKG for right bundle branch block, more serious disturbances of atrioventricular conduction, and ventricular ectopic beats.

• Be alert for other postoperative complications, such as bleeding, right heart failure, and respiratory failure. Some transient congestive heart failure is not uncommon postoperatively and may require treatment with digoxin and/or diuretics.

• Monitor left atrial pressure directly. A pulmonary artery catheter may also be used to measure central venous and pulmonary artery pressures.

• Frequently assess color and vital signs. Obtain arterial blood gas measurements regularly to assess oxygenation. Suction as needed to prevent atelectasis and pneumonia. Monitor mechanical ventilation.

• Record intake and output accurately.

• If atrioventricular block develops with a low heart rate, a temporary external pacemaker may be necessary.

• If blood pressure or cardiac output is inadequate, catecholamines by continuous I.V. infusion may be ordered. To decrease left ventricular workload, administer nitroprusside, as ordered. Provide analgesics, as needed.

• Keep the parents informed about the progress of their child. After discharge, he may still require prophylactic antibiotics, digoxin, diuretics, and other drugs. Stress the importance of complying with the prescribed regimen, and make sure the parents know how and when to administer medications. Teach the parents to watch for signs of digitalis toxicity (anorexia, nausea, vomiting). Prophylactic antibiotics to prevent infective endocarditis will continue to be required. Encourage parents to avoid becoming overprotective as the child becomes more physically active.

Transposition of the Great Arteries

In this complex congenital heart defect, the great arteries are reversed: the aorta arises from the right ventricle and the pulmonary artery from the left ventricle, producing two noncommunicating circulatory systems (pulmonary and systemic). Transposition accounts for up to 5% of all congenital heart defects and often coexists with other congenital heart defects, such as ventricular septal defect, atrial septal defect, patent ductus arteriosus, and ventricular septal defect with pulmonic stenosis. It affects males two to three times more often than females.

Causes

Transposition of the great vessels results from faulty embryonic development, but the cause of such development is unknown.

In transposition, oxygenated blood returning to the left side of the heart is carried back to the lungs by a transposed pulmonary artery. Unoxygenated blood returning to the right side of the heart is carried back to the systemic circulation by a transposed aorta.

Communication between the pulmonary and systemic circulations is necessary for survival. In infants with isolated transposition, blood mixes only at the *patent foramen ovale* (an opening in the atrial septum) and at the patent ductus arteriosus, resulting in slight mixing of unoxygenated systemic blood and oxygenated pulmonary blood. In infants with concurrent cardiac defects such as ASD or VSD, greater mixing of systemic and pulmonary blood occurs, re-sulting in less cyanosis and improved chances for survival initially, but later complicating definitive surgical correction.

Signs and symptoms
Within the first few hours after birth, neonates with transposition of the great vessels but without other associated heart defects generally show cyanosis

Fetal Circulation

Note the structures involved in fetal circulation, especially the umbilical vein, ductus venosus, foramen ovale, ductus arteriosus, and umbilical arteries. Shortly after birth, the umbilical vein, ductus venosus, ductus arteriosus, and umbilical arteries functionally close to adjust pulmonary blood circulation. Within 3 months, the foramen ovale also functionally closes, adjusting to the changing blood pressure between the right and left atria.

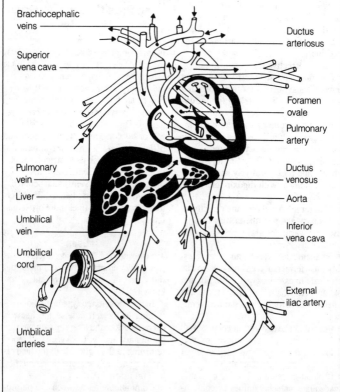

- Brachiocephalic veins
- Superior vena cava
- Pulmonary vein
- Liver
- Umbilical vein
- Umbilical cord
- Umbilical arteries
- Ductus arteriosus
- Foramen ovale
- Pulmonary artery
- Ductus venosus
- Aorta
- Inferior vena cava
- External iliac artery

vessels but without other associated heart defects generally show cyanosis and tachypnea, which worsen with crying. After several days or weeks, such infants usually develop signs of congestive heart failure (gallop rhythm, tachycardia, dyspnea, hepatomegaly, and cardiomegaly). S_2 is louder than normal, because the anteriorly transposed aorta is directly behind the sternum; often, however, no murmur can be heard during the first few days of life. Associated defects (ASD or VSD) present with their typical murmurs and allow arterial and venous blood to mix, which decreases cyanosis but causes other complications (especially severe congestive heart failure). VSD with pulmonic stenosis presents with a characteristic murmur in the infant with transposition and also results in severe cyanosis.

As infants with this defect grow older, cyanosis is their most prominent abnormality. They also develop diminished exercise tolerance, fatigability, coughing, clubbing of nail beds, and murmurs if ASD, VSD, patent ductus arteriosus, or pulmonary stenosis are present.

Diagnosis
• *Chest X-rays* are normal in the first days of life. Within days to weeks, right atrial and right ventricular enlargement cause the heart to appear oblong (resembling an egg on its side). X-rays also show increased pulmonary vascular markings, except when pulmonary stenosis accompanies transposition.
• *EKG* reveals right axis deviation and right ventricular hypertrophy but may be normal in the newborn.
• *Echocardiography* demonstrates the reversed position of the aorta and pulmonary artery and records echoes from both semilunar valves simultaneously, due to the displacement of the aortic valve. The existence of other cardiac defects is also demonstrated.
• *Cardiac catheterization* reveals decreased oxygen saturation in left ventricular blood and aortic blood; increased right atrial, right ventricular, and pulmonary artery oxygen satura-

tion; and right ventricular systolic pressure equal to systemic pressure.
• *Dye injection* reveals the transposed vessels and the presence of any other cardiac defects.
• *Arterial blood gas measurements* indicate hypoxia and secondary metabolic acidosis.

Treatment
At cardiac catheterization of an infant with transposition, emergency atrial balloon septostomy (Rashkind procedure) enlarges the patent foramen ovale and creates an ASD if there is none, thereby improving oxygenation by allowing better mixing of the pulmonary and systemic circulations. Atrial balloon septostomy requires passage of a balloon-tipped catheter through the foramen ovale and subsequent inflation and withdrawal across the atrial septum. This procedure alleviates hypoxia to some extent. Afterward, digoxin and diuretics can lessen congestive heart failure until the infant is ready to withstand corrective surgery (usually between the neonatal period and age 1).

There are three operative procedures available and currently in use to correct transposition. The Mustard procedure replaces the atrial septum with a Dacron or pericardial partition that allows systemic venous blood to be channeled to the left ventricle and pulmonary artery and oxygenated blood returning to the heart to be channeled through the pulmonary veins into the right ventricle and aorta. (See *Surgical Repair of Transposition of the Great Vessels [Mustard Procedure],* page 68.) The Senning procedure accomplishes the same result, using the right atrial wall and the atrial septum to create a partition to redirect systemic and pulmonary venous return to the appropriate ventricle. In the arterial switch, or Jantene procedure, now available for some children with transposition, the transposed arteries are surgically anastomosed to the appropriate ventricle. This procedure requires that the left ventricle be accustomed to pumping at systemic pressures, as is true in neonates or in children with transposition who have a large VSD, a large PDA, or left ventricular outflow obstruction. The patient with a coexisting VSD requires patch closure of this defect. Surgery also corrects other heart defects, such as pulmonary stenosis, ASD, or PDA.

Nursing management
• Explain cardiac catheterization and the Rashkind procedure to the parents. Offer emotional support and explain all other diagnostic procedures as well.
• Monitor vital signs, arterial blood gases, urinary output, and central venous pressure, watching for signs of congestive heart failure. Give digoxin and I.V. fluids, as ordered, being careful to avoid fluid overload.
• Teach the parents to recognize signs of congestive heart failure and digoxin toxicity (poor feeding, vomiting) and to report them immediately. Stress the importance of regular checkups to monitor cardiovascular status.
• Encourage the parents to protect their infant from exposure to individuals with infections.
• Assist parents in encouraging their infant and/or child in normal growth and development. Activity need not be restricted, as these children will set their own limits for physical activity.
• If the child is scheduled for surgery, explain the procedure to him and his parents. Show them the ICU, and introduce them to the staff. Also explain postoperative tubes, catheters, dressings, and monitoring devices.
• Preoperatively, monitor arterial blood gases, acid-base balance, intake and output, and vital signs.
  After corrective surgery:
• Monitor cardiac output by close assessment of blood pressure, skin color, heart rate, urinary output, central venous and left atrial pressures, and level of consciousness. Report any abnormalities or significant changes.
• Carefully measure arterial blood gases to evaluate adequacy of mechanical ventilation and/or respiratory function.

• For early detection of supraventricular conduction blocks and dysrhythmias, monitor the patient carefully. Watch for evidence of atrioventricular blocks, atrial dysrhythmias, and impaired sinoatrial function.
• Assess the child for the development of baffle obstruction following either the Mustard or Senning procedures. Obstruction is most common at the superior vena cava, resulting in marked facial and upper extremity edema.
• Teach the parents about the importance of antibiotic prophylaxis for infective endocarditis, if it is recommended postoperatively.
• Provide emotional support to help parents during the difficult hours and days immediately following surgery. Encourage them to assist their child in assuming new activity levels and independence. (See also *Six Most Common Anomalies*, pages 74 to 76.)

Nursing diagnoses

With infants, subjective data will have to be supplied by the parents. Your physical examination supplies the objective data. In formulating nursing diagnoses, keep in mind that because of the small size of the infant, any alteration in the cardiac status will affect his comfort and feeding. Typical nursing diagnoses might include:
Alteration in cardiac output related to PDA, VSD, transposition of great vessels, coarctation of the aorta, and so forth; potential alteration in nutrition related to shortness of breath while feeding; alteration in comfort related to inadequate gas exchange in the lungs.
  Your goals are to help the infant breathe and eat with as little stress as possible. Teach the mother appropriate feeding and positioning techniques.
  Observe the mother (or primary caretaker) for signs of noncompliance to the treatment regimen, since she will be the one responsible for it. Also help her understand the problems of the infant and what can be beneficial for him.

5

CORONARY ARTERY DISEASE AND VASCULAR DISORDERS

I f your patient suffers an acute myocardial infarction (AMI), oxygen
supply to some part of his heart has
failed to meet metabolic demands.
Normally, coronary arteries respond to
increased myocardial oxygen demand by
dilating and supplying a greater volume
of blood to cardiac tissues. But during
AMI, this compensatory mechanism is
not sufficient.

Current research indicates that coronary artery thrombosis may occur in
more than 90% of all transmural infarctions (those involving the entire heart-
wall thickness) and in 33% to 50% of all
subendocardial (nontransmural) infarctions.

Coronary artery disease

The dominant effect of coronary artery
disease (CAD) is the loss of oxygen and
nutrients to myocardial tissue because
of diminished coronary blood flow. This
disease is near-epidemic in the Western
world. CAD occurs more commonly in
men, in whites, and in the middle-aged
and elderly. In the past, this disorder
rarely affected premenopausal women,
but that is no longer the case, perhaps
because many women now take oral
contraceptives, smoke cigarettes, and
are employed in stressful jobs that used
to be held exclusively by men. (See *Atherosclerosis: Recognizing Risk Factors*,
page 86.)

Causes
Atherosclerosis is the usual cause of

CAD. In this form of arteriosclerosis,
fatty, fibrous plaques narrow the lumen
of the coronary arteries, reduce the volume of blood that can flow through
them, and lead to myocardial ischemia.
Plaque formation also predisposes to
thrombosis, which can provoke myocardial infarction.

Atherosclerosis usually develops in
high-flow, high-pressure arteries, such
as those in the heart, brain, kidneys, and
aorta, especially at bifurcation points. It
has been linked to many risk factors:
family history, hypertension, obesity,
smoking, diabetes mellitus, stress, sedentary life-style, and high serum cholesterol or triglyceride levels.

Uncommon causes of reduced coronary artery blood flow include dissecting aneurysms, infectious vasculitis,
syphilis, and congenital defects in the
coronary vascular system. Coronary artery spasms may also impede blood
flow.

Signs and symptoms
The classic symptom of CAD is angina,
the direct result of inadequate flow of
oxygen to the myocardium. It is usually
described as a burning, squeezing, or
crushing tightness in the substernal or
precordial chest that radiates to the left
arm, neck, jaw, or shoulder blade. Typically, the patient clenches his fist over
his chest or rubs his left arm when describing the pain, which is often accompanied by nausea, vomiting, fainting,
sweating, and cool extremities. Anginal
episodes most often follow physical exertion but may also follow emotional

Atherosclerosis: Recognizing Risk Factors

What causes the plaque deposits characteristic of atherosclerosis? Although no one knows all the answers, the following risk factors play a part:

• *Hyperlipidemia.* High serum levels of cholesterol and other lipids clearly contribute to the development of atherosclerosis. Although the relationship between diet and hyperlipidemia remains controversial, high dietary intake of low-density lipoproteins rich in cholesterol and saturated fats seems to contribute to plaque formation. High-density lipoproteins, on the other hand, may provide some measure of protection against plaque formation, possibly by transporting cholesterol out of arterial lesions.

• *Diabetes.* Though the reasons are unclear, atherosclerosis commonly develops in patients with diabetes mellitus—even when blood glucose levels seem well controlled.

• *Hypertension.* In conjunction with other risk factors, hypertension appears to promote the development of atherosclerosis.

• *Stress.* Studies have shown a relationship between prolonged periods of stress, either physical or emotional, and the formation of atherosclerotic plaques.

• *Genetic factors.* Patients with type II familial hyperlipoproteinemia are likely to develop atherosclerosis at a relatively early age. Those with parents or siblings who have developed coronary artery disease are more prone to develop atherosclerosis than the general population.

• *Cigarette smoking.* Evidence strongly supports a relationship between smoking and coronary artery disease. Among the mechanisms postulated are: increased platelet adhesiveness, increased carbon monoxide levels, and nicotine-induced increases in myocardial oxygen demand.

• *Obesity.* In combination with other risk factors—particularly hyperlipidemia and smoking—obesity may increase the risk of coronary artery disease.

• *Sedentary life-style.* People who exercise regularly seem to be at lower risk than inactive people. Possible reasons include alterations in lipid metabolism and improved cardiac efficiency.

---

excitement, exposure to cold, or a heavy meal.

Angina has three major forms: *stable* (pain is predictable in frequency and duration and can be relieved with nitrates and rest), *unstable* (pain increases in frequency and duration and is more easily induced), or *decubitus* (anginal pain recurs even at rest). Severe and prolonged anginal pain generally suggests MI, with potentially fatal dysrhythmias and mechanical failure. (See *A Closer Look at Coronary Artery Spasm,* page 88.)

Diagnosis

Patient history—including the frequency and duration of angina and the presence of associated risk factors—is crucial in evaluating CAD. (See *Diagnostic Profile for Angina,* page 89.) Additional diagnostic measures include the following:

• *Electrocardiogram (EKG)* during angina shows ischemia and, possibly, dysrhythmias, such as premature ventricular contraction. The EKG is apt to be normal when the patient is pain-free. Dysrhythmias may occur without infarction, secondary to ischemia.

• *Treadmill or bicycle exercise test* may provoke chest pain and EKG signs of myocardial ischemia in response to physical exertion.

• *Coronary angiography* reveals coronary artery stenosis or obstruction, col-

lateral circulation, and the condition of the coronary arteries beyond the narrowing.
• *Myocardial perfusion* imaging with thallium 201 detects ischemic areas of the myocardium, which are visualized as "cold spots."

Treatment
The goal of treatment in patients with angina is either to reduce myocardial oxygen demand or increase oxygen supply. Therapy consists primarily of nitrates, such as nitroglycerin (given sublingually, by mouth, or applied topically in ointment form), isosorbide dinitrate (sublingually or by mouth), calcium antagonists (sublingually or by mouth), or propranolol (by mouth). Obstructive lesions may necessitate coronary artery bypass surgery using vein grafts or the internal mammary artery. Angioplasty, an experimental procedure, may be performed during cardiac catheterization with a balloon to compress fatty deposits and relieve occlusion in patients with no calcification and partial occlusion. This procedure carries a certain risk, but its morbidity is lower than that for surgery. Laser angioplasty is an even newer but unproved procedure.

Because CAD is so prevalent, prevention is of incalculable importance. Dietary restrictions aimed at reducing intake of calories (in obesity) and of salt, fats, and cholesterol serve to minimize the risk, especially when supplemented with regular exercise. Abstention from smoking and reduction of stress are also beneficial. Other preventive actions include control of hypertension (with sympathetic blocking agents, such as methyldopa and propranolol, and with nitrates, calcium antagonists, or diuretics, such as hydrochlorothiazide); control of elevated serum cholesterol or triglyceride levels (with antilipemics, such as clofibrate, and with sitosterols, and niacin); and measures to minimize platelet aggregation and the danger of blood clots (with aspirin or dipyridamole, which may be prescribed after MI; however, their effectiveness is controversial).

Nursing management
• Successful nursing management of a patient with CAD requires a thorough history and accurate assessment. During anginal episodes, monitor blood pressure and heart rate. Take an EKG during unstable anginal episodes and before administering nitroglycerin or other nitrates. Record duration of pain, amount of medication required to relieve it, and accompanying symptoms.
• Be aware of the patient's anxiety level, and recognize its effect on the cardiovascular system.
• Keep nitroglycerin available for immediate use. Instruct the patient to call at the first sign of chest, arm, or neck pain. Place the call bell within easy reach.
• Before cardiac catheterization, explain the procedure to the patient. Make sure he knows why it is necessary, understands the risks involved, and realizes that its results may indicate a need for surgery. Assess peripheral pulses for baseline data.
• After catheterization, review the expected course of treatment with the patient and his family. Monitor the catheter site (usually the groin or the antecubital fossa) for bleeding. Also check for distal pulses. To counter the diuretic effect of the dye, make sure the patient drinks plenty of fluids. Assess potassium levels.
• If the patient is scheduled for surgery, explain the procedure to him and his family, and answer their questions. Take them on a tour of the intensive care unit (ICU), and introduce them to the staff.
• After surgery, provide meticulous I.V., pulmonary artery catheter, and endotracheal tube care. Monitor blood pressure, intake and output, breath sounds, chest tube drainage, and EKG, watching for signs of ischemia and dysrhythmias. Also observe for and record chest pain. Push pulmonary toilet including incentive spirometry and coughing.
• Before discharge, emphasize the importance of following the prescribed

A Closer Look at Coronary Artery Spasm

The oxygen supply/demand imbalance that causes ischemia usually occurs when increased exertion creates oxygen demands that coronary arteries—made rigid by spasm—cannot expand to fill. But coronary artery spasm also causes ischemia from insufficient oxygen *supply*: a sudden smooth-muscle contraction temporarily narrows the arterial lumen, halting or drastically reducing blood flow to part of the myocardium.

Coronary artery spasm occurs in both normal and atherosclerotic arteries. Typically, spasm manifests itself through chest pain that occurs:

• while the patient is at rest
• at about the same hour of the day with each recurrence
• more intensely and for a longer time than the pain of classic exertional angina
• with no preceding rise in heart rate or blood pressure.

What causes coronary artery spasm? Researchers have not yet found a definitive answer. However, they have been able to induce coronary artery spasm with vasoconstrictive substances. The results of these studies suggest that excessive sensitivity to these substances may be one predisposing factor. Another factor involves calcium release within the cell. Because calcium release helps to initiate smooth-muscle contraction, researchers believe that it may be a precondition to coronary artery spasm. If so, controlling calcium release may provide a key to controlling coronary artery spasm.

medication regimen (antihypertensives, nitrates, antilipemics, for example), exercise program, and dietary restrictions. Encourage moderate but regular exercise. Refer patients who smoke to a self-help program.

Myocardial infarction (Heart attack)

In MI, reduced blood flow through one of the coronary arteries results in myocardial ischemia and necrosis. (See *Atherosclerosis: Plaque Progression,* page 90.) In cardiovascular disease, death usually results from the cardiac damage or complications of MI. Mortality is high when treatment is delayed, and almost half of sudden deaths due to an MI occur before hospitalization, within 1 hour of the onset of symptoms. Prognosis improves if vigorous treatment begins immediately.

Causes and incidence

Predisposing factors to CAD and MI include:

• family history of early MI or hyperlipidemias
• hypertension
• smoking
• elevated serum triglyceride and cholesterol levels
• diabetes mellitus
• obesity or excessive intake of saturated fats, simple carbohydrates, or salt
• sedentary life-style
• aging
• stress

Men are more susceptible to MI than women, although incidence is rising among women, especially those who smoke, take oral contraceptives, and are working in high stress jobs.

The site of the MI depends on the vessels involved. Occlusion of the circumflex branch of the left coronary artery causes a lateral wall infarction; occlusion of the anterior descending branch of the left coronary artery causes an anterior wall infarction. True posterior or inferior wall infarctions generally result from occlusion of the right coronary artery or one of its branches. In transmural MI, tissue damage extends through all myocardial layers; in subendocardial MI, only in the innermost layer. Right ventricular infarctions are usually due to occlusion of the right coronary artery. They can accompany inferior infarctions and may result in right-sided failure, even in the absence of left-sided failure. (See *Infarction Sites and Structural Injury*, page 91.)

Signs and symptoms

The cardinal symptom of MI is persistent, crushing substernal pain that may radiate to the left arm, jaw, neck, or shoulder blades. Such pain is often described as "heavy," "squeezing," or "crushing" and may persist for 12 hours or more. However, in some MI patients—particularly the elderly or diabetics—pain may not occur at all. In others, it may be mild and confused with indigestion. In patients with CAD, angina of increasing frequency, severity, or duration (especially when not precipitated by exertion, a heavy meal, or cold and wind) may signal an impending infarction.

Other clinical effects include a feeling of impending doom, fatigue, nausea, vomiting, and shortness of breath. The patient may experience catecholamine responses, such as coolness in extremities, perspiration, anxiety, and restlessness. Fever is unusual at the onset of an MI, but a low-grade temperature elevation may develop during the next few days. Blood pressure may vary among MI patients; hypotension or hypertension may be present.

The most common post-MI complications include recurrent or persistent chest pain, dysrhythmias, left ventricular failure (resulting in congestive heart failure [CHF] or acute pulmonary edema), and cardiogenic shock. Unusual but potentially lethal complications that may develop soon after infarction include thromboembolism; papillary muscle dysfunction or rupture, causing mitral regurgitation; rupture of the ventricular septum, causing ventricular septal defect; rupture of the myocardium; and ventricular aneurysm.

Diagnostic Profile for Angina

EKG abnormalities during and after exercise:
- Chest X-rays
- Cardiac catheterization before surgery
- Nitroglycerin shortens attack or increases exercise tolerance.

Stable angina: occurs over a long time in same pattern of onset, duration, and intensity of symptoms

Unstable angina: frequency, intensity, and duration of symptoms increase as atherosclerotic process progresses; about 50% of patients infarct within 3 to 18 months after onset

Prinzmetal's angina: chest discomfort at rest due to coronary artery spasm causing transient ST segment elevation and pain

Angina decubitus: chest discomfort that occurs in the recumbent position; relieved by sitting or standing

Nocturnal angina: occurs only at night, but not necessarily in the recumbent position

Intractable angina: chronic chest discomfort that is physically incapacitating and refractory to medical treatment

---

Within 2 weeks to several months after infarction, Dressler's syndrome may develop, characterized by pericarditis, pericardial friction rub, chest pain, fever, and possibly pleurisy or pneumonitis and leukocytosis.

Diagnosis

A history of CAD, persistent chest pain, changes in EKG, and elevated serum CPK-MB enzyme levels over a 72-hour period usually confirm an MI. Auscultation may reveal diminished heart sounds, gallops, and, in papillary dysfunction, the apical systolic murmur of mitral regurgitation over the mitral valve area.

Atherosclerosis: Plaque Progression

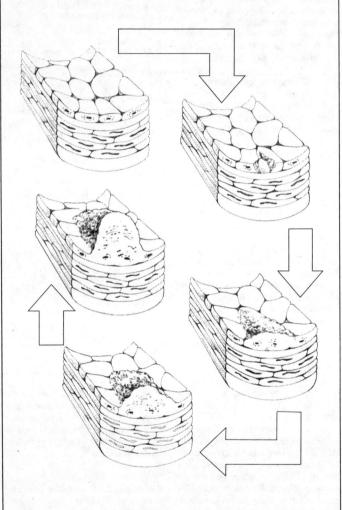

Injury to healthy arterial tissue (1) exposes the intima and leads to formation of lipid deposits. These may develop into fibrous plaques (2) that accumulate and narrow the arterial lumen (3,4). Reinjury can occur before the original lesion heals, causing additional plaque buildup, which may completely occlude the artery.

Infarction Sites and Structural Injury

What cardiac structures does an acute MI injure, and which heart functions may become impaired as a result? The answer depends on the location of the infarction and the specific coronary artery affected.

After EKGs or other diagnostic tools have identified the site of the infarction, this chart can help you anticipate complications that may result from the structural damage sustained.

Infarction sites	Blocked artery	Injured structures
Anteroseptal/ anterior	Left anterior descending	• Anterior wall of left ventricle • Anterior interventricular septum • Apex of left ventricle • Bundle of His and bundle branches • Papillary muscles
Anterolateral/ posterior, lateral	Left circumflex (LC)	• Left atrium • Lateral and posterior left ventricle • Posterior interventricular septum • Sinoatrial (SA) node* • Atrioventricular (AV) node*
Inferior/posterior	Right coronary (RC)*	• Right atrium (occasionally) • Right ventricle (occasionally) • Inferior left ventricle • SA node* • AV node* • Posterior and inferior interventricular septum • Left ventricle (rarely)

*Damage to these structures varies from one person to the next, depending on anatomic differences. In about 9 out of 10 people, the RC artery supplies the AV node; in those remaining, the LC artery supplies the AV node. The RC artery also supplies the SA node in over half of all persons; in the rest, the LC artery performs this function.

When clinical features are equivocal, assume MI until special tests rule it out. Diagnostic laboratory results include the following:

• *serial 12-lead EKG:* EKG abnormalities may be absent or inconclusive during the first few hours following an MI. When present, characteristic abnormalities show serial ST-T changes in subendocardial MI and Q waves representing transmural MI. (See *Characteristic EKGs in MI*, page 92.)

• Echocardiogram shows ventricular wall dyskinesis if the MI is transmural.

• *serial serum enzymes:* elevated CPK—especially elevated CPK-MB isoen-

Characteristic EKGs in MI

Infarctions in different sites of the heart cause EKG changes. Recognizing these changes will help you assess the patient.

• An *inferior wall MI* will show typical pattern changes—a pathologic Q wave, ST segment elevation, and T-wave inversion—in leads II, III, and aVF.

• Sometimes an inferior or posterior wall infarction will involve the lateral wall as well. *Lateral wall involvement* will cause a reduced R wave, a T-wave inversion, and, in some cases, an elevation of the S-T segment in the lateral leads V_5, V_6, aVL, and L_1.

• A *posterior wall infarction* causes a tall R wave and upright T wave in V_1.

• An *anterior MI* will produce a typical infarction pattern in leads I, aVL, and V_2 to V_6.

• An *anteroseptal infarction* will cause the typical pattern in leads V_1 to V_4.

• An *anterolateral infarction* will produce the typical pattern in leads I, V_5, and V_6.

• An infarction within the anterolateral surface of the left ventricle—a *high anterolateral infarction*—will produce

typical changes in leads aVL, L_1, and V_6.

Change for the better

These EKG patterns gradually return to normal. Recovery after an MI can be divided into four phases:

PHASE I (acute phase): Immediately after onset or within 48 hours, leads reflecting the injured area show abnormal Q waves, an elevated S-T segment, and inverted T waves. Reciprocal changes, such as S-T depression, occur in leads reflecting the uninjured area.

PHASE II: This phase covers the gradual return of the elevated S-T segment to the baseline.

PHASE III: Most T waves return to normal or near-normal configuration.

PHASE IV (stabilized phase): An abnormal Q wave may be the only sign of infarction.

These four phases may be completed in 3 days or may take as long as 10. Remember always to interpret EKGs in light of other laboratory findings and the patient's symptoms.

zyme, the cardiac muscle fraction of CPK—lactic dehydrogenase (LDH) isoenzymes—especially LDH_1 and LDH_2—serum glutamic-oxaloacetic transaminase (SGOT), and alpha-hydroxybutyric dehydrogenase

• *elevated erythrocyte sedimentation rate (ESR)* and *white blood cell count (WBC)*

• *serial chest X-rays:* normal in MI, but with development of CHF show cardiomegaly, pulmonary vascular congestion, or bilateral pleural effusion.

Scans using I.V. technetium 99 can identify acutely damaged muscle by picking up radioactive nucleotide, which appears as a "hot spot" on the film. They are useful in localizing a recent MI.

Treatment

The goals of treatment are to relieve chest pain, stabilize heart rhythm, and reduce cardiac workload. Dysrhythmias, the predominant problem during the first 48 hours after the infarction, may require antiarrhythmics, a pacemaker, and, rarely, electrocardioversion.

Therapy includes:

• lidocaine for ventricular dysrhythmias or, if lidocaine is ineffective, other drugs, such as procainamide, quinidine, bretylium, or disopyramide

• atropine I.V. or a temporary pacemaker to treat heart block or bradycardia

• nitroglycerin (sublingual, topical, or I.V.), isosorbide dinitrate (sublingual or oral), or calcium antagonists (sublingual, oral, or I.V.) to relieve pain by

COMMON DYSRHYTHMIAS

PACs

Treatment: Often none, but quinidine may be used

PAT

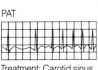

Treatment: Carotid sinus pressure, verapamil, or propranolol

AV BLOCK — SECOND-DEGREE

Treatment: Atropine, Isuprel, or pacemaker

AV BLOCK — THIRD-DEGREE

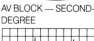

Treatment: Atropine, Isuprel, or pacemaker

PVCs

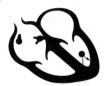

Treatment: Lidocaine, Pronestyl, or atropine, if associated with bradycardia

VENTRICULAR TACHY-CARDIA

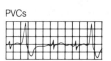

Treatment: Cardioversion (except for patients on digitalis, since digitalis toxicity may cause tachy-cardia), lidocaine, Pronestyl, or bretylium tosylate

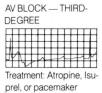
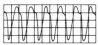

redistributing blood to ischemic areas of the myocardium, increasing cardiac output, and reducing myocardial workload

• morphine or meperidine I.V. for pain and sedation
• bed rest with bedside commode to decrease cardiac workload
• oxygen administration (by face mask or nasal cannula) at a modest flow rate for 24 to 48 hours; a lower concentration if the patient has chronic obstructive pulmonary disease
• pulmonary artery catheterization to detect left ventricular failure and to monitor response to treatment
• drugs that increase contractility or blood pressure, as needed, or an intraaortic balloon pump for cardiogenic shock
• thrombolytic therapy within 4 to 6 hours postinfarction, using I.V. streptokinase (intracoronary or systemic); experimental methods include thrombolysis by laser and intravenous tissue plasminogen activator.

Nursing management

Nursing care is directed toward detecting complications, preventing further myocardial damage, and promoting comfort, rest, and emotional well-being. Most patients with MI receive treatment in the cardiac care unit (CCU), under constant observation for complications. (See *Secondary Causes of AMI*, page 94, and *Complications of Myocardial Infarction*, page 96.)

• On admission to the CCU, monitor and record EKG, blood pressure, temperature, and heart and breath sounds.
• Assess pain, and administer analge-

Secondary Causes of AMI

Any condition that reduces coronary blood flow may contribute to the development of AMI. Shock, hemorrhage, and dehydration, for example, all decrease blood pressure and diminish cardiac output. When this happens, blood flow to myocardial tissue is decreased.

The conditions listed below can lead to AMI in patients with or without atherosclerosis:

• Carbon monoxide poisoning
• Congenital coronary artery anomalies (for example, anomalous origin of the coronary arteries)
• Coronary arteritis
• Disseminated intravascular coagulation
• Emboli to coronary arteries (for example, prosthetic valve emboli)
• Hypercoagulability
• Luminal narrowing by mechanisms other than atherosclerosis (for example, dissection of a coronary artery)
• Myocardial contusion
• Polycythemia vera
• Prolonged hypotension
• Trauma to coronary arteries (for example, myocardial laceration).

sics as ordered. Always record the severity and duration of pain. Avoid giving I.M. injections, since absorption of I.M. injections from the muscle is unpredictable as a result of low cardiac output and diminished peripheral perfusion.
• Check blood pressure after giving nitroglycerine, especially the first dose, for hypotension.
• Frequently monitor EKG to detect rate changes or dysrhythmias. Place rhythm strips in the patient's chart periodically for evaluation.
• During episodes of chest pain, obtain EKG, blood pressure, and pulmonary artery catheter measurements to determine changes.

• Watch for signs of fluid retention (rales, cough, tachypnea, edema), which may indicate impending heart failure. Monitor daily weight, intake and output, respirations, serum enzyme levels, and blood pressure. Listen for adventitious breath sounds (patients on bed rest frequently have atelectatic rales, which may disappear after coughing) and for S_3 or S_4 gallops.
• Plan patient care to maximize uninterrupted rest.
• Ask the dietary department to provide a clear liquid for the patient diet until nausea subsides. A low-cholesterol, low-sodium diet, without caffeine-containing beverages, may be ordered.
• Provide a stool softener to prevent straining during defecation, which causes vagal stimulation and may slow heart rate. Allow the patient to use a bedside commode, and provide as much privacy as possible.
• Assist with passive range-of-motion exercises. If the patient is completely immobilized by a severe MI, turn him often. Antiembolism stockings and subcutaneous heparin help prevent venostasis and thrombophlebitis.
• Provide emotional support, and help reduce stress and anxiety; administer tranquilizers, as needed. Explain procedures and answer questions. An explanation of the CCU environment and routine can lessen the patient's anxiety. Involve the family as much as possible in the patient's care.

Carefully prepare the MI patient for discharge:
• To promote compliance with drug regimen and other treatment measures, thoroughly explain dosages and therapy. Warn about drug side effects, and advise the patient to watch for and report signs of toxicity (for example, anorexia, nausea, vomiting, and yellow or double vision if he is receiving digitalis).
• Review dietary restrictions. If the patient must follow a low-sodium or low-fat and low-cholesterol diet, provide a list of undesirable foods. It may be helpful to have the dietitian speak to the

patient and family.
• Counsel the patient about resuming sexual and other activities gradually but progressively.
• Advise him about appropriate responses to new or recurrent symptoms.
• Advise the patient to report to the doctor typical or atypical chest pain. Postinfarction syndrome may develop, producing chest pain that must be differentiated from recurrent MI, pulmonary infarct, or CHF. (See *Compensating for Ischemia,* page 98.)
• If the patient has a Holter monitor in place, explain its purpose and how to use it.
• Emphasize the need to stop smoking. If necessary, refer the patient to a self-help group.
• Refer the patient to a stress reduction program.
• Counsel the patient that postinfarction depression is common but self-limiting as activity increases.

Nursing diagnoses

After collecting subjective data from the patient interview and objective data from the cardiovascular assessment, formulate nursing diagnoses. They should clearly explain the patient's problems, allowing you to plan appropriate goals and interventions. They should also reflect the physiologic and psychological consequences of angina and acute MI and the need for patient teaching about drug and surgical treatments during hospitalization and after discharge.

Typical diagnoses for angina might include:

Alteration in comfort (chest pain) related to oxygen embarrassment to cardiac muscle

Potential alteration in sleep-rest pattern related to chest pain of coronary disease

Potential disruption of activity resulting from chest pain of CAD.

Your goals are to prevent MI, restore the balance between myocardial oxygen supply and demand, and relieve pain.

Typical diagnoses for MI might include:

Alteration in cardiac output related to acute MI and an altered hemodynamic status of the body.

This diagnosis suggests the potential for sudden death, lethal dysrhythmias, and other life-threatening complications. Your goals are to provide constant patient monitoring, promptly detect changes in the patient's condition, prevent sudden death and complications, and limit the size of the infarction.

Potential alteration in comfort related to severe chest pain from an AMI. Your goals are to relieve chest pain and promote rest. To achieve them, assess, document, and report to the doctor the location, radiation, and duration of pain and any factors that affect it. Also report the effect of chest pain on perfusion to the heart, brain, kidneys, and skin.

Anxiety and fear of death resulting from an AMI.

Your goals are to reduce anxiety and fear in the patient and his family, help prevent extension of the infarction, encourage expression of feelings, and promote effective coping mechanisms.

Aneurysm

Thoracic aneurysm is an abnormal widening of the ascending, transverse, or descending portion of the aorta. The aneurysm may be dissecting, a hemorrhagic separation in the aortic wall, usually within the medial layer; saccular, an outpouching of the arterial wall, with a narrow neck; or fusiform, a spindle-shaped enlargement encompassing the entire aortic circumference. Some aneurysms may progress to serious and, eventually, lethal complications, such as rupture of untreated thoracic dissecting aneurysm into the pericardium, with resulting tamponade.

Abdominal aneurysm, an abnormal dilation in the arterial wall, generally occurs in the aorta between the renal arteries and iliac branches. Such aneurysms are four times more common in men than in women and are most prevalent in whites aged 50 to 80. More than

Complications of Myocardial Infarction

COMPLICATION	DIAGNOSIS	TREATMENT
Dysrhythmias	• In inferior wall MI, EKG shows bradycardia and junctional rhythms or AV block; in anterior wall MI, tachycardia or heart block; in all MIs, premature ventricular contractions, ventricular tachycardia, or ventricular fibrillation.	• Antiarrhythmics, atropine, cardioversion, and pacemaker
Congestive heart failure	In left heart failure, chest X-rays show venous congestion and cardiomegaly. Catheterization shows increased pulmonary artery, pulmonary capillary wedge, and central venous pressures.	• Diuretics, vasodilators, inotropes, cardiac glycosides
Cardiogenic shock	• Catheterization shows decreased cardiac output and increased pulmonary artery and pulmonary capillary wedge pressures. • Other signs include hypotension, tachycardia, decreased level of consciousness, decreased urinary output, neck vein distention, and cool, pale, moist skin.	• I.V. fluids, vasodilators, cardiotonics, cardiac glycosides, intraaortic balloon pump (IABP), and beta-adrenergic stimulants
Mitral regurgitation	• Auscultation reveals crackles and apical holosystolic murmur. • Catheterization shows increased pulmonary artery and pulmonary capillary wedge pressures with prominent V waves. • Dyspnea is prominent. • Echocardiogram shows valve dysfunctions.	• Nitroglycerine, nitroprusside, IABP, and surgical replacement of the mitral valve and concomitant myocardial revascularization

50% of all people with untreated abdominal aneurysms die, primarily from aneurysmal rupture, within 2 years of diagnosis; over 85% die within 5 years.

Causes and incidence
Commonly, an aneurysm results from atherosclerosis, which weakens the aortic wall and gradually distends the lumen at the weakened area. The initiating factor in dissecting aneurysm (in about 60% of patients) is an intimal tear in the ascending aorta. Other causes include:
• infection (mycotic aneurysms) of the aortic arch and descending segments
• congenital disorders, such as coarctation of the aorta and Marfan's syndrome (often associated with dissecting aneurysm)
• trauma, usually of the descending

COMPLICA-TION	DIAGNOSIS	TREATMENT
Ventricular septal rupture	• In left-to-right shunt, auscultation reveals a harsh holosystolic murmur and thrill. • Catheterization shows increased pulmonary artery and pulmonary capillary wedge pressures. • Confirmation is by increased oxygen saturation of right ventricle and pulmonary artery.	• Surgical correction (may be postponed several weeks), IABP, nitroglycerin, or nitroprusside
Pericarditis, or Dressler's syndrome (post-myocadial infarction syndrome)	• Auscultation reveals a friction rub. • Chest pain is relieved by sitting up, intensifies by deep breathing. • Chest X-rays may show pleural effusion.	• Anti-inflammatory agents
Ventricular aneurysm	• Chest X-ray may show cardiomegaly. • EKG may show dysrhythmias and persistent ST segment elevation. • Left ventriculography shows altered left ventricular motion (akinesis) or paradoxical motion (dyskinesis). • Complications include congestive heart failure, dysrhythmias, and systemic embolization.	• Cardioversion, antiarrhythmics, vasodilators, anticoagulants, cardiac glycosides (digitalis), and diuretics; if conservative treatment fails to control complications, surgical resection is necessary
Thromboembolism	• Sudden onset of severe dyspnea and chest pain if pulmonary; neurologic changes if cerebral. • Nuclear scan shows ventilator/perfusion (V/Q) mismatch. • Angiography shows arterial blockage.	• Oxygen, heparin, endarterectomy

aorta, from an automobile accident that damages the aorta by shearing it transversely (acceleration-deceleration injuries)

• syphilis, usually of the ascending aorta (now uncommon because of effective antibiotic therapy)

• hypertension (in dissecting aneurysm)

Thoracic aneurysms are most common in men between ages 50 and 70; dissecting aneurysms, in blacks.

Abdominal aneurysms develop slowly. First, focal weakness in the muscular layer of the aorta (tunica media), due to degeneration changes, allows the inner layer (tunica intima) and outer layer (tunica adventitia) to stretch outward. Blood pressure within the aorta progressively weakens the vessel walls and enlarges the aneurysm.

Compensating for Ischemia

Ischemia does not always progress to acute MI. Even without medical intervention, the heart can defend itself, to some extent, by compensatory mechanisms. These mechanisms can help restore perfusion and prevent, or at least limit, an infarction (so successfully, in some cases, that the patient never realizes he has had a heart attack).

Let's look at how these mechanisms operate and how each may be able to help the patient.

Collateral circulation.
Many of the small terminal branches of left and right coronary arteries mingle and interconnect, forming natural bypass routes. As atherosclerosis gradually occludes an artery, this network of arterial branches provides a possible detour around the blockage. The arterial lumina along this detour respond to the increased blood flow by gradually widening and strengthening their walls.

A patient whose circulatory system has established such collateral routes may feel little effect from a small infarction, since almost as much blood as usual may reach the affected myocardium by alternate routes.

Alpha-receptor stimulation.
The sympathetic nervous system (SNS) provides another compensatory mechanism. After a few seconds of reduced cardiac output, SNS activity in tissue immediately around the infarct begins to stimulate alpha receptors. The receptors respond by causing vasoconstriction, as well as increasing heart rate and contractility, to restore some cardiac output and stroke volume and so prevent infarct enlargement.

However, this mechanism does not always have the desired effect. Increasing heart rate shortens filling time and increases myocardial oxygen consumption. If the heart does not fill sufficiently, the left ventricle ejects too little blood (reduced stroke volume) with each beat, possibly decreasing coronary artery perfusion. The result: increased oxygen demand, decreased supply, and possible infarction extension.

Limitations.
Collateral circulation and alpha stimulation may be able to balance the effect of a small infarction. But a large infarction—or many small ones—can exceed the heart's ability to compensate. In such cases, the patient needs outside intervention—drugs, oxygen, cardiopulmonary resuscitation, even surgery—to help him survive an AMI.

Signs and symptoms

The most common symptom of thoracic aneurysm is pain. In dissecting aneurysm, such pain may be sudden in onset, with a tearing or ripping sensation in the thorax or the anterior chest. It may extend to the neck, shoulders, lower back, or abdomen but rarely to the jaw and arms, which distinguishes dissecting aneurysm from MI.

Accompanying signs include syncope, pallor, sweating, shortness of breath, increased pulse rate, cyanosis, leg weakness or transient paralysis, diastolic murmur (caused by aortic regurgitation), and abrupt loss of radial and femoral pulses or wide variations in pulses or blood pressure between arms and legs. Paradoxically, although the patient appears to be in shock, systolic blood pressure is often normal or significantly elevated.

Clinical effects caused by thoracic aneurysms (saccular or fusiform) vary according to the size and location of the aneurysm and the compression, distortion, or erosion of surrounding structures, such as the lungs, trachea, larynx and recurrent laryngeal nerve, esophagus, and spinal nerves. If the aneurysm is located in the ascending aorta, it has potential for extension into the aortic root, resulting in aortic valve insufficiency. Sudden onset of a diastolic murmur will alert the nurse to this potential catastrophic event.

Characteristic associated symptoms may include a substernal ache in the shoulders, lower back, or abdomen; marked respiratory distress (dyspnea, brassy cough, wheezing); hoarseness or loss of voice; dysphagia (rare); and possibly, paresthesias or neuralgia. Such aneurysms can occasionally rupture.

Abdominal aneurysms usually do not manifest symptoms; most are evident (unless the patient is obese) as a pulsating mass in the periumbilical area, accompanied by a systolic bruit over the aorta. Some tenderness may be present on deep palpation. A large aneurysm may produce symptoms that mimic renal calculi, lumbar disk disease, and duodenal compression. Abdominal aneurysms rarely cause diminished peripheral pulses or claudication, unless embolization occurs.

Lumbar pain that radiates to the flank and groin from pressure on lumbar nerves may signify enlargement and imminent rupture. If the aneurysm ruptures into the peritoneal cavity, it causes severe, persistent abdominal and back pain, mimicking renal or ureteral colic. Signs of hemorrhage—such as weakness, sweating, tachycardia, and hypotension—may be subtle, since rupture into the retroperitoneal space produces a tamponade effect that prevents continued hemorrhage. Patients with such rupture may remain stable for hours before shock and death occur, although 20% die immediately. (See *Types of Aortic Aneurysms,* page 100.)

Diagnosis

Diagnosis relies on patient history, clinical features, and appropriate tests. In an asymptomatic patient, diagnosis often occurs accidentally, through posteroanterior and oblique chest X-rays showing widening of the aorta (most obvious when compared with a previous chest X-ray). Other tests help confirm aneurysm:

• *Aortography,* the most definitive test, shows the lumen of the aneurysm, its size and location, and the false lumen in dissecting aneurysm.

• *Computed tomography* (CT) scanning may be used to confirm the position and location of the aneurysm. CT scan can also be used to monitor the progression of the aneurysm by serial exam.

• *EKG* is not diagnostic but helps differentiate between thoracic aneurysm and MI.

• *Echocardiography* may help identify dissecting aneurysm of the aortic root.

• *Hemoglobin* may be normal or decreased as a result of frank bleeding or blood loss into the hematoma from a slow-leaking aneurysm.

• *Serial ultrasound* (sonography) is accurate and allows determination of aneurysm size, shape, and location.

• *Anteroposterior and lateral X-rays* of the abdomen can detect aortic calcification, which outlines the mass at least 75% of the time.

Treatment

Dissecting aneurysm is an extreme emergency that requires prompt surgery and stabilizing measures: antihypertensives, such as nitroprusside; negative inotropic agents that decrease the force of contractility, such as propranolol; oxygen therapy for respiratory distress; narcotics for pain; I.V. fluids; and if necessary, whole blood transfusions.

Surgery is comparable to open heart surgery and consists of resecting the aneurysm, restoring normal blood flow through a Dacron or Teflon graft replacement, and (with aortic valve insufficiency) aortic valve replacement.

Postoperative measures include careful monitoring and continuous assessment in the ICU, antibiotics to prevent infection, endotracheal and chest tubes for respiratory management, EKG monitoring for cardiac management, and pulmonary artery catheterization for hemodynamic management.

Types of Aortic Aneurysms

Saccular

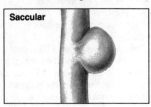

Unilateral, pouchlike bulge with a narrow neck

Fusiform

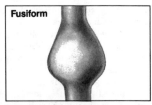

Spindle-shaped bulge encompassing the entire diameter of the vessel

Dissecting

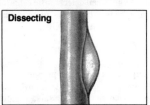

Hemorrhagic separation of the medial layer of the vessel wall, which creates a false lumen

False

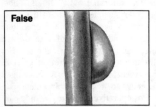

Pulsating hematoma resulting from trauma or anastomotic disruption and often mistaken for abdominal aneurysm

Nursing management

• Explain diagnostic tests. If surgery is scheduled, explain the procedure and expected postoperative care (I.V.s, endotracheal and drainage tubes, cardiac monitoring, ventilation).

• Carefully monitor blood pressure, pulmonary capillary wedge pressure, and central venous pressure. Assess pain, respirations, and carotid, radial, and femoral pulses.

• Be alert for signs of rupture, which may be immediately fatal. Watch closely for any signs of acute blood loss (decreasing blood pressure, increasing pulse and respiratory rates, cool, clammy skin, restlessness, and decreased sensorium).

• If rupture does occur, the first priority is to get the patient to surgery immediately. Medical antishock trousers may be used while transporting to surgery. Surgery allows direct compression of the aorta to control hemorrhage. Large amounts of blood may be needed during the resuscitative period to replace blood loss. In such a patient, renal failure due to ischemia is a major postoperative complication, possibly requiring hemodialysis.

• Make sure laboratory tests include a complete blood count with differential, electrolytes, type and cross match for whole blood, arterial blood gas determinations, and urinalysis.

• Insert an indwelling (Foley) catheter. Administer 5% dextrose in water or lactated Ringer's solution and antibiotics, as ordered. Carefully monitor nitroprusside I.V.; use a separate I.V. line for infusion. Adjust the dose by slowly increasing the infusion rate. Meanwhile, check blood pressure every 5 minutes until it stabilizes. With suspected bleeding from aneurysm, give whole blood transfusions, as ordered.

• In the ICU after surgery, closely monitor vital signs, intake and hourly output, neurologic status (level of consciousness, pupil size, sensation in arms and legs), and blood gases. Assess the depth, rate, and character of respirations and lung sounds at least every hour.

• After stabilization of vital signs and

respirations, encourage and assist the patient in turning, coughing, and deep breathing.

• Watch for signs of bleeding (increased pulse rate and respirations or hypotension). Check dressings for excessive bleeding or drainage. After nasogastric intubation for intestinal decompression, irrigate the tube frequently to ensure patency. Record the amount and type of drainage.

• Check respiratory function. Carefully observe and record the type and amount of chest tube drainage, and frequently assess heart and lung sounds.

• If the patient can breathe unassisted and has good lung sounds and adequate blood gases, tidal volume, and vital capacity 24 hours after surgery, he will be extubated and will require oxygen by mask. Weigh him daily to evaluate fluid balance.

• Assist with range-of-motion exercises of legs to prevent thromboembolic phenomenon due to venostasis during prolonged bed rest.

• Help the patient walk as soon as he is able.

• Monitor I.V. therapy.

• Give medications, as ordered.

• Watch for signs of infection, especially fever and excessive drainage on dressings.

• Before discharge, ensure compliance with antihypertensive therapy by explaining the need for such drugs and the expected side effects. Teach the patient how to monitor his blood pressure. Refer him to community agencies for continued support and assistance, as needed.

• Throughout hospitalization, offer the patient and his family psychological support. Answer all questions honestly, and provide reassurance. (See *Possible Nursing Diagnoses for Vascular Abnormalities,* page 102.)

Aortic arch syndrome

(Takayasu's disease, pulseless disease, brachiocephalic arteritis, panaortitis, primary arteritis of the aortic arch, ob-literative aortic disease, aortitis syndrome, and nonspecific aortoarteritis).

Aortic arch syndrome is progressive obliteration of the aorta and its branches, eventually causing bilateral loss of pulse in the arms, loss of carotid pulse, and tissue ischemia, especially of the nervous system. This rare disease occurs primarily in women in the second and third decades. It is usually fatal as a result of heart failure, hypertension, or neurologic complications.

Causes

Aortic arch syndrome may be an autoimmune response, since laboratory results in persons with this disorder show elevated alpha and gamma globulins and positive complement fixation. This disease produces a nonspecific inflammation of the arterial wall (primarily the adventitia and media) and, later, scarring and thickening of the intima, which leads to thrombus formation and occlusion of the aortic arch branches. There is some indication that aortic arch syndrome may be a hypersensitive reaction to tuberculosis.

Signs and symptoms

Early in its course, aortic arch syndrome produces nonspecific systemic symptoms similar to those of collagen vascular disease, including malaise, pallor, nausea, night sweats, arthralgias, anorexia, and weight loss. However, as the disease progresses, variable symptoms of cardiovascular dysfunction develop secondary to extensive involvement of arch vessels:

• *brachiocephalic (innominate) artery* (most common site): local pain in the neck, shoulders, and chest; bruits; and loss of radial and carotid pulses

• *carotid arteries:* diplopia, blurred vision, transient blindness, focal neurologic deficits, fainting, syncope, and dizziness due to cerebral ischemia

• *subclavian arteries:* paresthesias, intermittent claudication, loss of pulses, and decreased blood pressure in the arms. The extent of symptoms depends on the degree of involvement and the

Possible Nursing Diagnoses for Vascular Abnormalities

Most vascular abnormalities are chronic, with worsening symptoms and progressive deterioration of the patient's condition. Nursing management aims to arrest the disease.

Disorder	Nursing diagnoses	Goals
Aneurysms	• Anxiety due to knowledge deficit related to aneurysms and their complications and fear of surgery	• Reduce anxiety by providing patient teaching
	• Potential for postoperative complications of atelectasis, hemorrhage, infection, graft occlusion, and embolization, if aneurysm repair is scheduled	• Prevent complications
	• Knowledge deficit related to continuing medical regimen at home	• Provide discharge teaching
Arterial occlusive disease	• Anxiety due to knowledge deficit related to the disease	• Reduce anxiety by providing patient teaching
	• Alteration in circulation to the extremities secondary to occlusion	• Maintain circulation to the affected part
	• Alteration in comfort related to pain secondary to ischemia	• Relieve pain and promote comfort
	• Potential for injury, infection, and ulcer formation secondary to decreased circulation	• Prevent injury, infection, and ulcer formation
	• Potential for noncompliance related to knowledge deficit concerning surgery and preoperative procedures	• Provide preoperative and postoperative teaching
	• Potential for postoperative complications	• Prevent postoperative complications
	• Potential for noncompliance related to knowledge deficit concerning the medical regimen at home and steps to prevent progression of the disease	• Provide discharge teaching

Disorder	Nursing diagnoses	Goals
Polyarteritis	• Anxiety about symptoms and knowledge deficit related to the disorder and its treatment • Potential alteration in comfort related to complications of corticosteroid therapy	• Reduce anxiety by providing patient teaching • Prevent complications
Raynaud's disease	• Knowledge deficit related to the disease and its treatment • Alteration in comfort related to pain secondary to ischemia	• Provide patient teaching • Relieve pain
Aortic arch syndrome	• Knowledge deficit related to the disease and its treatment • Alteration of peripheral circulation secondary to aortic branch occlusion • Potential for postoperative complications • Potential for depression secondary to poor prognosis	• Provide preoperative and postoperative patient teaching • Maintain circulation to the affected part • Prevent complications • Help patient and family cope with the disease
Varicose veins	• Potential knowledge deficit related to diagnosis of varicose veins • Alteration in circulation secondary to venous insufficiency • Potential for complications, such as ulcer formation and postoperative infection	• Provide preoperative and postoperative patient teaching • Maintain circulation and promote venous return • Prevent complications
Deep-vein thrombosis	• Potential knowledge deficit related to diagnosis of deep-vein thrombosis • Potential for pulmonary emboli • Potential for noncompliance related to knowledge deficit concerning the continuing medical regimen at home	• Provide inpatient teaching • Prevent development of pulmonary emboli • Provide discharge teaching

development of collateral circulation.

Occasionally, aortic arch syndrome may affect the coronary arteries, generally secondary to aortic thickening, producing narrowing of the coronary arteries. This condition may lead to myocardial ischemia and infarction. Hypertension may develop secondary to the arteritis.

Diagnosis

While typical clinical findings suggest aortic arch syndrome, diagnosis requires aortography of the aortic arch to identify the affected vessels and the extent of damage. Supportive laboratory results include the following:

• elevated WBC count and ESR
• decreased hemoglobin
• positive LE cell preparation and complement fixation
• serum protein electrophoresis demonstrating increased alpha and gamma globulins.

In addition, chest X-rays may reveal cardiomegaly, rib-notching from collateral circulation, and calcification of damaged blood vessels.

Treatment

Medical treatment of aortic arch syndrome consists of corticosteroids (prednisone) if begun before irreversible organ damage occurs.

Decreasing ESR reflects the effectiveness of the steroid therapy. Digitalis and diuretics are helpful in the management of the associated heart failure, but the hypertension associated with this disease is resistant to antihypertensive agents. Antituberculosis drugs may be helpful in controlling the progression of this disease. Anticoagulants, vasodilators, and antiplatelet drugs are used but usually have not been effective.

Surgical repair of the affected arteries in a patient with aortic arch syndrome offers the best prognosis. Bypass grafting of the arteries gives symptomatic relief.

Nursing management

Patients with aortic arch syndrome require supportive preoperative and postoperative care, patient teaching, and psychological support to help them cope with this inevitably fatal disease.

• Explain necessary diagnostic procedures, such as X-rays and aortography.

• Preoperatively, provide an explanation of the surgical procedure and postoperative care, such as intensive care monitoring, I.V. therapy, and coughing, deep breathing, and leg exercises to prevent thrombus formation.

• Postoperatively, be alert for signs of arterial occlusion or thrombosis. Monitor vital signs and intake and output, and observe for signs of infection (chills, fever, excessive or foul-smelling wound drainage).

• Before starting long-term corticosteroid and anticoagulant therapy, explain its purpose, expected results, proper dosage, and side effects. Warn against stopping corticosteroids abruptly. To prevent bleeding from anticoagulant therapy, warn the patient to avoid aspirin and aspirin-containing compounds, to use a safety razor, and to avoid trauma. Stress the need for serial blood studies (prothrombin times) throughout therapy.

• If the patient has suffered a stroke due to occluded carotid arteries, assess neurologic functions carefully. If necessary, refer him to an appropriate community agency for continued rehabilitation after discharge.

• Provide psychological support and encouragement for the patient and family. (See *Possible Nursing Diagnoses for Vascular Abnormalities,* page 102.)

Thrombophlebitis

An acute condition characterized by inflammation and thrombus formation, thrombophlebitis may occur in deep (intermuscular or intramuscular) or superficial (subcutaneous) veins. Deep-vein thrombophlebitis affects small veins, such as the soleal venous sinuses, or large veins, such as the vena cava, and the femoral, iliac, and subclavian veins.

This disorder is frequently progressive, leading to pulmonary embolism, a potentially lethal complication. Superficial thrombophlebitis is usually self-limiting and rarely leads to pulmonary embolism. Thrombophlebitis often begins with localized inflammation alone (phlebitis), but such inflammation rapidly provokes thrombus formation. Rarely, venous thrombosis develops without associated inflammation of the vein (phlebothrombosis). (See *Nursing Considerations for Prevention of Deep-Vein Thrombosis,* page 106.)

Causes
A thrombus occurs when an alteration in the epithelial lining causes platelet aggregation and consequent fibrin entrapment of red blood cells, WBCs, and additional platelets. Thrombus formation is more rapid in areas where blood flow is slower because of greater contact between platelet and thrombin accumulation. The rapidly expanding thrombus initiates a chemical inflammatory process in the vessel epithelium, which leads to fibrosis. The enlarging clot may occlude the vessel lumen partially or totally, or it may detach and embolize to lodge elsewhere in the systemic circulation.

Deep-vein thrombophlebitis (DVT) may be idiopathic, but it usually results from endothelial damage, accelerated blood clotting, and reduced blood flow. Predisposing factors are prolonged bed rest, trauma, surgery, childbirth, and use of oral contraceptives such as estrogens.

Causes of superficial thrombophlebitis include trauma, infection, I.V. drug abuse, and chemical irritation due to extensive use of the I.V. route for medications and diagnostic tests. (See *Understanding Virchow's Triad,* page 108.)

Signs and symptoms
In both types of thrombophlebitis, clinical features vary with the site and length of the affected vein. Although DVT may occur asymptomatically, it may also produce severe pain, fever, chills, malaise, and swelling and cyanosis of the affected arm or leg. Superficial thrombophlebitis produces visible and palpable signs, such as heat, pain, swelling, rubor, tenderness, and induration along the length of the affected vein. Extensive vein involvement may cause lymphadenitis.

Diagnosis
Some patients with DVT may display signs of inflammation and a positive Homans' sign (pain on dorsiflexion of the foot) during physical examination; others are asymptomatic. Consequently, essential laboratory tests include:
• *Doppler ultrasonography* to identify reduced blood flow to a specific area and any obstruction to venous flow, particularly in iliofemoral deep-vein thrombophlebitis
• *plethysmography* to show decreased circulation distal to the affected area (more sensitive than ultrasound in detecting deep-vein thrombophlebitis)
• *phlebography* (usually confirms diagnosis) to show filling defects and diverted blood flow.

Diagnosis must rule out arterial occlusive disease, lymphangitis, cellulitis, and myositis.

Diagnosis of superficial thrombophlebitis is based on physical examination (redness and warmth over affected area, palpable vein, and pain during palpation or compression).

Treatment
The goals of treatment are to control thrombus development, prevent complications, and relieve pain. Symptomatic measures include bed rest, with elevation of the affected arm or leg; warm, moist soaks to the affected area; and analgesics, as ordered. After the acute episode of deep-vein thrombophlebitis subsides, the patient may begin to walk while wearing antiembolism stockings.

Treatment may also include anticoagulants (initially, heparin; later, warfarin) to prolong clotting time. The full anticoagulant dose must be discontinued during the operative period because

Nursing Considerations for Prevention of Deep-Vein Thrombosis

High-risk patients
- Patients with previous deep-vein thrombosis (DVT), pulmonary embolism, phlebitis, or varicose veins; blood disorders (especially hypercoagulation disorders, such as polycythemia vera, thrombocytosis, and antithrombin III deficiency); heart disease (especially congestive heart failure or MI); internal hemorrhage (such as from stroke); malignancy; traumatic injury (such as fractures or extensive burns); or venipuncture in leg
- Patients undergoing diagnostic procedures that may produce emboli, such as bone or tumor biopsies
- Patients undergoing surgery (especially abdominal or pelvic surgery, splenectomy, or orthopedic procedures on legs)
- Patients receiving estrogen therapy for contraceptive or therapeutic purposes (especially women more than 35 years old)
- Patients who are pregnant, obese, immobilized, or more than 60 years old.

Prophylactic drug therapy
- Studies show prophylactic heparin therapy is safe and effective in general surgical patients (even those more than 40 years old with malignancy) but not in patients undergoing prostate or hip surgery.
- In patients receiving prophylactic heparin therapy, bleeding is not a significant problem; but a slight increase (2%) in incidence of wound hematoma may occur.
- Administer prophylactic heparin, as ordered (usual dosage is 5,000 units, administered subcutaneously, every 8 to 12 hours preoperatively and postoperatively).
- Studies of effects of drugs that suppress platelet function, such as aspirin, have been inconclusive.

Leg compression
- For patients with limited activity, use below-the-knee elastic bandages or support stockings that distribute pressure uniformly.
- Intermittent pneumatic compression stockings may be ordered for long-term bedridden patients.

Activity
- Encourage early ambulation in postoperative patients. Explain its importance in preventing DVT.
- Perform passive range-of-motion exercises for bedridden patients. If patient is able, teach him how to do active range-of-motion exercises. Also instruct him to dorsiflex feet or move them in walking motion against footboard for 5 minutes every hour.
- Avoid elevating patient's knees with pillows or by adjusting bed. It can obstruct venous blood flow. If knees must be elevated, raise foot of bed.
- Instruct patient to avoid standing or sitting in one position for long time. If he must do so, teach him to exercise legs by repeatedly standing on toes or shifting weight from one foot to another, or by alternately propping one leg, then the other, on a stool.
- Instruct patient to make sure his feet are flat on floor when he sits on side of bed. This will avoid putting pressure on popliteal spaces.

Respiratory considerations
- Instruct patient to perform deep-breathing exercises postoperatively to ventilate lungs and promote venous return.
- Observe patient closely for signs and symptoms of pulmonary embolism (such as tachycardia, rales, dyspnea, hemoptysis, hypotension, pleuritic chest pain, and cyanosis).
- If patient smokes cigarettes, encour-

age him to quit.

Intravenous catheters

• Avoid inserting I.V. catheters in legs, if possible. Studies show it increases risk of infection, which predisposes patient to thrombus formation.

• Observe I.V. sites closely for inflammation.

• Change I.V. tubing every 24 to 48 hours.

• Follow instructions carefully when diluting I.V. medications.

• Stabilize I.V. catheters securely.

Miscellaneous

• Assess patient's legs and arms regularly for swelling, asymmetry in size, inflammation, pain, deep muscle or generalized tenderness, cyanosis, and venous distension.

• Perform frequent checks of circulatory, motor, and neurologic functions in arms and legs.

• Observe for low-grade fever, indicating possible thrombophlebitis.

• Maintain proper fluid balance. Both overhydration and underhydration can decrease venous return and cause venous stasis in legs. (Most patients need at least 3,000 ml of fluid every 24 hours.)

• Monitor frequency of patient's bowel movements. Patient may need stool softener to avoid straining during bowel movements. Such straining can increase venous pressure in legs.

• Use limb restraints with caution to avoid tourniquet effect.

• Pad side rails, when necessary, to avoid limb trauma.

Patient teaching

• Put instructions for taking anticoagulant *in writing.* Inform patient of purpose of medication; warn him of possible adverse reactions and interactions with other drugs. Stress importance of frequent follow-up examinations.

• Inform patient of purpose of elastic bandages and support stockings. Before discharge, teach him how to apply bandage or stocking correctly. Stress importance of applying uniform pressure, of not turning down top of bandage or stocking, and keeping bandage or stocking wrinkle-free. Instruct him to wear it until doctor tells him otherwise.

• Explain to patient that elastic bandages and support stockings can be washed with mild soap and water but will shrink if dried in clothes dryer. Tell him to replace bandage or stocking when it loses elasticity. (Patient should have at least two pairs.)

• Encourage patient to exercise regularly, if possible. Recommend walking, jogging, bicycling, and swimming. Tell him to elevate legs frequently.

• Warn patient of hazards of smoking and obesity: nicotine constricts veins, decreasing venous blood flow; and extra pounds increase pressure on leg veins. Arrange consultation with dietitian, if necessary.

• Instruct patient to discontinue use of oral contraceptives if diagnostic testing has confirmed thrombus formation. (Tell patient to use an alternate method of contraception and inform her gynecologist.)

• Advise patient to avoid restrictive clothing, such as garters, girdles, knee-high boots, and tight jeans or panty hose. Such clothing reduces venous return, increasing pressure in leg veins.

• Inform patient that if he notices swelling, pain, tenderness, or sudden dilation of superficial veins in a leg or an arm, he should notify doctor immediately.

Understanding Virchow's Triad

Unlike the arterial system, the venous system lacks an intrinsic force to propel blood through it. Venous flow depends almost entirely on the stimulating action of voluntary muscles and the competence of one-way valves. If those muscles are inactive or the valves incompetent, *stasis of venous blood*—the first of the three causes of DVT that make up Virchow's triad—occurs. In an immobilized limb, for example, venous flow will stop unless the limb is elevated above the level of the heart. Stasis of venous blood can also occur when peripheral circulation becomes sluggish from dehydration or congestive heart failure.

Intimal damage to the vein wall—the second possible cause of DVT—can result from infection, intravenous infusion of medications, trauma, or venipuncture. Damage to the intimal layer of the vein wall alters its epithelial lining, impairing the fibrinolytic activity that inhibits thrombus formation. As platelets aggregate at the site of the damage, some become trapped by fibrin, along with red blood cells and granular leukocytes, precipitating thrombus formation.

Abnormalities of the clotting mechanism make up the third possible cause of DVT. Many conditions or factors can cause blood to coagulate faster than normal—anemia (particularly sickle cell anemia), leukemia, malignancy, oral contraceptives, polycythemia vera, and trauma, for example. A deficiency of antithrombin III, a circulating anticoagulant, can also lead to increased coagulability of the blood. Normally, antithrombin III inactivates thrombin and other clotting factors. Subnormal amounts of antithrombin III, therefore, would cause thrombin and other clotting factors to proliferate, increasing the risk of thrombus formation. Possible causes of an antithrombin III deficiency include a congenital defect, liver disease, or the exhaustion of antithrombin III during the clotting process itself, as in disseminated intravascular coagulation.

---

of the risk of hemorrhage. After some types of surgery, particularly major abdominal or pelvic procedures, prophylactic doses of anticoagulant may reduce the risk of DVT and pulmonary embolism. Rarely, deep-vein thrombophlebitis may cause complete venous occlusion, which necessitates venous interruption through simple ligation to vein plication, or clipping.

Therapy for severe superficial thrombophlebitis may include an antiinflammatory, such as phenylbutazone, and antiembolism stockings.

Nursing management

Patient teaching, identification of high-risk patients, and measures to prevent venostasis can prevent deep-vein thrombophlebitis (see *Varicose Veins,* page 110.); close monitoring of anticoagulant therapy can prevent serious complications, such as internal hemorrhage.

• Enforce bed rest, as ordered, and elevate the affected arm or leg. If pillows are used for leg elevation, place them so they support the entire length of the affected leg to prevent compression of the popliteal space.
• Apply warm soaks to increase circulation to the affected area and to relieve pain and inflammation. Give analgesics to relieve pain, as ordered.
• Measure and record the circumference of the affected arm or leg daily, and compare this measurement to the opposite extremity. To ensure accuracy and consistency of serial measurements, mark the skin over the measured area.
• Administer I.V. heparin, as ordered, with an infusion monitor or pump to control the flow rate, if necessary.

• Measure partial thromboplastin time regularly for the patient on heparin therapy; measure prothrombin time for the patient on warfarin (therapeutic anticoagulation values for both are one and a half to two times control values). Watch for signs of bleeding (dark, tarry stools, coffee-ground vomitus, and ecchymoses). Suggest that the patient use an electric razor and avoid medications that contain aspirin.

• Be alert for signs and symptoms of pulmonary emboli (sudden alteration in mental status, particularly restlessness; rales; dyspnea; hemoptysis; and hypotension).

• To prevent thrombophlebitis in high-risk patients, perform range-of-motion exercises while the patient is on bed rest, use intermittent pneumatic calf massage during lengthy surgical or diagnostic procedures, apply antiembolism stockings postoperatively, and encourage early ambulation. (See *Possible Nursing Diagnoses for Vascular Abnormalities*, page 102.)

To prepare the patient for discharge:

• Emphasize the importance of follow-up blood studies to monitor anticoagulant therapy.

• If the patient is being discharged on heparin therapy, teach him or his family how to give subcutaneous injections. If he requires further assistance, arrange for a visiting nurse.

• Tell him to avoid prolonged sitting or standing to help prevent recurrence.

• Teach him how to properly use antiembolism stockings.

Arterial occlusive disease

Arterial occlusive disease is the obstruction or narrowing of the lumen of the aorta and its major branches, causing an interruption of blood flow, usually to the legs and feet. This disorder may affect the carotid, vertebral, innominate, subclavian, mesenteric, and celiac arteries. Occlusions may be acute or chronic and often cause severe ischemia, skin ulceration, and gangrene. Arterial occlusive disease is more common in males than in females. Prognosis depends on the location of the occlusion; the development of collateral circulation to counteract reduced blood flow; and, in acute disease, the time elapsed between occlusion and its removal. (See *Arterial Occlusive Disease*, page 112.)

Causes
Arterial occlusive disease is a frequent complication of atherosclerosis. The occlusive mechanism may be endogenous, due to emboli or thrombosis, or exogenous, due to trauma or fracture. Predisposing factors include smoking; aging; such conditions as hypertension, hyperlipemia, and diabetes; and a family history of vascular disorders, MI, or cerebrovascular accident (CVA).

Diagnosis
Diagnosis of arterial occlusive disease is usually indicated by patient history and physical examination. Diagnostic tests include the following:

• *Arteriography* demonstrates the type (thrombus or embolus), location, and degree of obstruction, and collateral circulation. This procedure is particularly useful in chronic disease or for evaluating candidates for reconstructive surgery.

• *Doppler ultrasonography* and *plethysmography* are noninvasive tests that show decreased blood flow in the leg distal to the occlusion.

• *Ophthalmodynamometry* helps determine the degree of obstruction in the internal carotid artery by comparing ophthalmic artery pressure to brachial artery pressure on the affected side. More than 20% difference suggests insufficiency.

• *Electroencephalogram* and *computed tomography scan* may be necessary to rule out brain lesions.

Treatment
Generally, treatment depends on the cause, location, and size of the obstruction. In mild chronic disease, treatment usually consists of supportive measures.

Varicose Veins

Varicose veins are dilated, tortuous veins, usually affecting the subcutaneous leg veins—the saphenous veins and their branches. They can result from congenital weakness of the valves or venous wall; from diseases of the venous system, such as deep-vein thrombophlebitis; from conditions that produce prolonged venostasis, such as pregnancy; or from occupations that necessitate prolonged standing.

Varicose veins may be asymptomatic or may produce mild-to-severe leg symptoms, including a feeling of heaviness; cramps at night; diffuse, dull aching after prolonged standing or walking; aching during menses; fatigability; palpable nodules; and, with deep-vein incompetency, orthostatic edema and stasis pigmentation of the calves and ankles.

In mild-to-moderate varicose veins, antiembolism stockings or elastic bandages counteract pedal and ankle swelling by supporting the veins and improving circulation. An exercise program, such as walking, promotes muscular contraction and forces blood through the veins, thereby minimizing venous pooling. Severe varicose veins may necessitate stripping and ligation, or as an alternative to surgery, injection of a sclerosing agent into small affected vein segments.

To promote comfort and minimize worsening of varicosities:
• Discourage the patient from wearing constrictive clothing.
• Advise the patient to elevate his legs above heart level whenever possible and to avoid prolonged standing or sitting.

After stripping and ligation or injection of a sclerosing agent:
• To relieve pain, administer analgesics, as ordered.
• Elevate the affected leg above heart level.
• Frequently check circulation in toes (color and temperature) and observe elastic bandages for bleeding. When ordered, rewrap bandages at least once a shift, wrapping from toe to thigh, with the leg elevated.
• Watch for signs of complications, such as sensory loss in the leg (which could indicate saphenous nerve damage), calf pain (thrombophlebitis), and fever (infection).

Risk factor modification, especially smoking cessation, control of hypertension, and continued exercise (walking) is essential. In carotid artery occlusion, antiplatelet therapy with dipyridamole and aspirin may be initiated.

Acute disease usually necessitates surgery to restore circulation to the affected area. Appropriate surgery may include:
• *embolectomy:* balloon-tipped Fogarty catheter used to remove thrombotic material from artery; used mainly for mesenteric, femoral, or popliteal occlusion
• *thromboendarterectomy:* opening of the artery and removal of the obstructing thrombus (atherosclerotic plaque) and the intimal lining of the arterial wall; usually performed after angiography; often accompanied by autogenous vein or prosthetic bypass surgery (carotid, femoral-popliteal, or aorto-femoral)
• *patch grafting:* removal of the thrombosed segment and replacement with an autogenous vein or prosthetic graft
• *bypass graft:* diversion of blood flow through an anastomosed autogenous or prosthetic graft to bypass the occluded arterial segment
• *lumbar sympathectomy:* may be an adjunct to reconstructive surgery. Rarely done.

Amputation becomes necessary with

extensive arterial occlusion precluding the possibility of bypass surgery, failure of reconstructive surgery, gangrene, uncontrollable infection, or intractable pain.

Other therapy includes heparin to prevent emboli in patients with embolic occlusion and bowel resection after restoration of blood flow in patients with occlusion of the mesenteric artery.

Nursing management

• Provide comprehensive patient teaching, such as proper foot care. Explain all diagnostic tests and procedures. Advise the patient to stop smoking and to follow the prescribed medical regimen.

Preoperatively, during an acute episode:

• Assess circulatory status by checking lower extremity pulses and inspecting skin color and temperature.

• Provide pain relief.

• If arterial embolism is suspected, administer heparin by continuous I.V. drip, as ordered. Use an infusion monitor or pump to ensure proper flow rate.

• Protect the ischemic foot from trauma and pressure by using a sheepskin pad at the foot of the bed and a footboard to keep the weight of the bed linen off of the feet. Use lamb's wool or soft cotton between the toes to prevent friction necrosis. Strictly avoid elevating or applying heat to the affected leg.

• Watch for signs of fluid and electrolyte imbalance, and monitor intake and output for signs of renal failure (urine output less than 30 ml/hour). If the patient has carotid, innominate, vertebral, or subclavian artery occlusion, check for signs of cerebrovascular ischemia (transient ischemic attacks) or CVA (numbness in an arm or leg and transient monocular blindness).

Postoperatively:

• Monitor vital signs. Continuously assess circulatory function by inspecting skin color and temperature and checking for distal pulses. In charting, compare earlier assessments and observations. Watch for signs of hemorrhage (tachycardia and hypotension), and check

dressing for excessive bleeding.

• Following carotid, innominate, vertebral, or subclavian artery surgery, assess neurologic status frequently for changes in level of consciousness and asymmetry of muscle strength or pupil size.

• Following surgery to correct mesenteric artery occlusion, connect the nasogastric tube to low intermittent suction. Monitor intake and output (low urine output may indicate damage to the renal arteries during surgery). Check bowel sounds for return of peristalsis. Increasing abdominal distention and tenderness may indicate extension of bowel ischemia with resulting necrosis, necessitating bowel resection, or may herald peritonitis. Monitor stools for the presence of blood.

• In saddle block occlusion, check distal pulses for adequate circulation. Watch for signs of renal failure and mesenteric artery occlusion (severe abdominal pain) and for cardiac dysrhythmias, which may precipitate embolus formation.

• Following bypass of aorto-iliac occlusion, check lower extremity pulses to ensure adequate circulation. Monitor cardiovascular and hemodynamic parameters carefully, as bypass patients are at risk for perioperative myocardial ischemia or dysrhythmia. If an intraabdominal surgical approach is used, pay special attention to the adequacy of respiratory function, since breathing is painful and difficult because of abdominal muscle dissection.

• In both femoral and popliteal artery bypass, carefully monitor distal pulses or Doppler ultrasound pressures of the dorsalis pedis, posterior tibial, or peroneal arteries (see *Use of the Doppler Anemometer,* page 114.) Loss of previously palpable pulses or a significant decrease in the ankle/brachial index warrants notifying the surgeon immediately. Assist with ambulation on the second or third postoperative day, limiting sitting to 20 to 30 minutes for meals and using the bathroom. Sitting with the legs dependent for an extended period worsens postoperative edema.

Arterial Occlusive Disease

SITE OF OCCLUSION	SIGNS AND SYMPTOMS
Carotid arterial system • Internal carotids • External carotids	Neurologic dysfunction: transient ischemic attacks (TIAs) due to reduced cerebral circulation produce unilateral sensory or motor dysfunction (transient monocular blindness, hemiparesis), possible aphasia or dysarthria, confusion, decreased mentation, and headache. These recurrent clinical features usually last 5 to 10 minutes but may persist up to 24 hours, and may herald a stroke. Absent or decreased pulsation with an auscultatory bruit over the affected vessels.
Vertebrobasilar system • Vertebral arteries • Basilar arteries	Neurologic dysfunction: TIAs of brain stem and cerebellum produce binocular visual disturbances, vertigo, dysarthria, and "drop attacks" (falling down without loss of consciousness). Less common than carotid TIA.
Innominate • Brachiocephalic artery	Neurologic dysfunction: signs and symptoms of vertebrobasilar occlusion. Indications of ischemia (claudication) of right arm; possible bruit over right side of neck.
Subclavian artery	Subclavian steal syndrome (characterized by backflow of blood from brain through vertebral artery on same side as the occlusion, into subclavian artery distal to occlusion); clinical effects of vertebrobasilar occlusion and exercise-induced arm claudication. Possible gangrene, usually limited to the digits.

• After amputation, check the stump carefully for drainage. If drainage occurs, record its color, the amount, and the time. Elevate the stump, as ordered, and administer adequate analgesic medication. Since phantom limb pain is common, explain this phenomenon to the patient. When the stump is adequately healed, facilitate transferring the patient to an appropriate setting for rehabilitation with a prosthesis or wheelchair.

• To prepare the patient for discharge, instruct him about foot care, circulation monitoring, actions and side effects of discharge medications, and the importance of keeping follow-up appointments. Since atherosclerotic arterial occlusive disease is a systemic process, teach him about this underlying etiology, emphasizing the need for risk factor modification, particularly smoking cessation and control of hypertension and diabetes. Be sure the patient and family know how to contact the doctor or primary care nurse, should questions or concerns arise after discharge. If necessary, coordinate home health-care services with the patient and family. (See *Possible Nursing Diagnoses for Vascular Abnormalities*, page 102.)

SITE OF OCCLUSION	SIGNS AND SYMPTOMS
Mesenteric artery • Superior (most commonly affected) • Celiac axis • Inferior	Bowel ischemia, infarct necrosis, and gangrene; sudden, acute abdominal pain; nausea and vomiting; diarrhea; leukocytosis; shock due to massive intraluminal fluid and plasma loss.
Aortic bifurcation (saddle block occlusion), medical emergency associated with cardiac embolization	Sensory and motor deficits (muscle weakness, numbness, paresthesias, paralysis) and signs of ischemia (sudden pain; cold, pale legs with decreased or absent peripheral pulses) in both legs.
Iliac artery (Leriche's syndrome)	Intermittent claudication of lower back, buttocks, and thighs, relieved by rest; absent or reduced femoral or distal pulses; possible bruit over femoral arteries. Impotence in males due to occlusive disease of the internal iliac arteries supplying blood to the pelvic organs and penis.
Femoral and popliteal artery (associated with aneurysm formation)	Intermittent claudication of calves on exertion; ischemic pain in feet; pretrophic pain (heralds necrosis and ulceration); leg pallor and coolness; blanching of feet on elevation, gangrene. Absence of palpable pulses in ankle and foot.

Raynaud's disease

Raynaud's disease is one of several primary arteriospastic disorders characterized by episodic vasospasm in the small peripheral arteries and arterioles, precipitated by exposure to cold or stress. This condition occurs bilaterally and usually affects the hands or, less often, the feet. Raynaud's disease is most prevalent in women, particularly between puberty and age 40. It is a benign condition, requiring no specific treatment and with no serious sequelae.

Raynaud's phenomenon, however, often associated with several connective tissue disorders—such as scleroderma, systemic lupus erythematosus, or polymyositis—has a progressive course, leading to ischemia, gangrene, and amputation. Distinction between the two disorders is difficult, because some patients who experience mild symptoms of Raynaud's disease for several years may later develop overt connective tissue disease—especially scleroderma.

Causes
Although the cause of Raynaud's disease is unknown, several theories have

Use of the Doppler Anemometer

The Doppler ultrasound anemometer is a diagnostic tool used to quantitate adequacy of arterial circulation in distal arteries, particularly those in vessels without palpable pulses.

Procedure: Use of the Doppler to assess distal lower extremity arterial pressures is as follows:

1. Apply a blood pressure cuff just above the ankle.
2. Using an acoustic coupling gel between the skin and Doppler probe, locate the sound of pulsatile arterial flow over the dorsalis pedis (DP) or posterior tibial (PT) artery.
3. Keeping the probe in place, inflate the blood pressure cuff until the sound of pulsatile flow is obliterated.
4. Slowly release the pressure in the cuff.
5. Record the return of audible pulsatile flow as the systolic blood pressure in the artery (diastolic pressure is not determined because of the sensitivity of the Doppler).
6. Compare the ankle artery (higher than DP or PT) pressure with the patient's brachial systolic blood pressure, and compute the ankle/brachial index (ABI).

N.B. With normal circulation the ankle systolic pressure should equal or slightly exceed brachial systolic pressure, i.e. ABI greater than or equal to 1.00 or 100%.

Example of computing ABI:

brachial artery systolic pressure	150 mm Hg
dorsalis pedis artery systolic pressure	80 mm Hg
Posterior tibial artery systolic pressure	100 mm Hg

$$\frac{\text{ankle pressure (higher of two)}}{\text{brachial pressure}} = \frac{100 \text{ mm Hg}}{150 \text{ mm Hg}} = .66 \text{ or } \frac{2}{3} \text{ or } 66\%$$

been proposed to account for the reduced digital blood flow: intrinsic vascular wall hyperactivity to cold; increased vasomotor tone due to sympathetic stimulation; and antigen-antibody immune response (the most probable theory, since abnormal immunologic test results accompany Raynaud's phenomenon).

Signs and symptoms

After exposure to cold or stress, the skin on the fingers typically blanches, then becomes cyanotic before changing to red, and from cold to normal temperature. Numbness and tingling may also occur. These symptoms are relieved by warmth.

In long-standing disease, trophic changes, such as sclerodactyly, ulcerations, or chronic paronychia, may result.

Diagnosis

Clinical criteria that establish Raynaud's disease include skin color changes induced by cold or stress; bilateral involvement; absence of gangrene or, if present, minimal cutaneous gangrene; normal arterial pulses; and patient history of clinical symptoms of longer than 2 years. Diagnosis must also rule out secondary disease processes, such as chronic arterial occlusive or connective tissue disease.

Treatment

Initially, treatment consists of avoidance of cold, mechanical, or chemical injury;

cessation of smoking; and reassurance that symptoms are benign. Drug therapy is reserved for unusually severe symptoms because of bothersome side effects. Such therapy may include phenoxybenzamine or reserpine. Sympathectomy may be helpful when conservative modalities fail to prevent ischemic ulcers and becomes necessary in less than 25% of patients.

Nursing management
• Warn against exposure to cold. Tell the patient to wear gloves in cold weather or when handling cold items.
• Advise the patient to avoid stressful situations and not to smoke.
• Instruct him to inspect his skin frequently and to seek immediate care for signs of skin breakdown or infection.
• Teach about drug use and side effects.
• Provide psychological support and reassurance to allay fear of amputation and disfigurement. (See *Possible Nursing Diagnoses for Vascular Abnormalities,* page 102.)

Buerger's disease (Thromboangiitis obliterans)

Buerger's disease—an inflammatory, nonatheromatous occlusive condition—causes segmental lesions and subsequent thrombus formation in the small and medium arteries (and sometimes the veins), resulting in decreased blood flow to the feet and legs. This disorder may produce ulceration and gangrene.

Causes
Although the cause of Buerger's disease is unknown, a definite link exists to smoking, suggesting a hypersensitivity reaction to nicotine. Incidence is highest among men of Jewish ancestry, aged 20 to 40, who smoke heavily.

Signs and symptoms
Buerger's disease typically produces intermittent claudication of the instep, which is aggravated by exercise and re-

lieved by rest. During exposure to low temperature, the feet initially become cold, cyanotic, and numb; later, they redden, become hot, and tingle. Occasionally, Buerger's disease also affects the hands, possibly resulting in painful fingertip ulcerations. Other symptoms include impaired peripheral pulses, migratory superficial thrombophlebitis, and, in later stages, ulceration, muscle atrophy, and gangrene.

Diagnosis
The patient history and physical examination strongly suggest Buerger's disease. Supportive tests include Doppler ultrasonography and plethysmography, to show diminished circulation in peripheral vessels, and arteriography to locate lesions and rule out atherosclerosis.

Treatment
The primary goals of treatment are to relieve symptoms and prevent complications. Such therapy may include an exercise program that uses gravity to fill and drain the blood vessels or, in severe disease, a lumbar sympathectomy to increase blood supply to the skin. Amputation may be necessary for nonhealing ulcers, intractable pain, or gangrene.

Nursing management
• Urge the patient not to smoke.
• Warn him to avoid precipitating factors, such as emotional stress, exposure to extreme temperatures, and trauma.
• Teach proper foot care, especially the importance of wearing well-fitting shoes and cotton or wool socks; inspecting the feet daily for cuts, abrasions, and signs of skin breakdown; and seeking medical attention immediately after any trauma.
• If the patient has ulcers and gangrene, enforce bed rest and use a bed cradle to prevent pressure from bed linens. Protect the feet with soft padding, such as cotton batting. Wash them gently with a mild soap and tepid water, rinse thoroughly, and pat dry with a soft towel. (See *Possible Nursing Diagnoses for Vascular Abnormalities,* page 102.)

6

HEART FAILURE

Congestive heart failure (CHF) and its most devastating extreme, pulmonary edema, are among the most common cardiovascular problems. Their symptoms are always distressing and often life-threatening.

Congestive heart failure

CHF is a syndrome characterized by myocardial dysfunction that leads to impaired pump performance (diminished cardiac output) or frank heart failure and abnormal circulatory congestion. Congestion of systemic venous circulation may result in peripheral edema or hepatomegaly; congestion of pulmonary circulation may cause pulmonary edema, an acute life-threatening emergency. Pump failure usually occurs in a damaged left ventricle (left heart failure) but may happen in the right ventricle (right heart failure) primarily or secondary to left heart failure. Sometimes, left and right heart failures develop simultaneously. Although CHF may be acute, as a direct result of myocardial infarction (MI), it is often a chronic disorder associated with retention of salt and water by the kidneys. Advances in diagnostic and therapeutic techniques have greatly improved the outlook for patients with CHF, but prognosis still depends on the underlying cause and its response to treatment.

Causes

CHF may result from a primary abnormality of the heart muscle—such as an infarction—inadequate myocardial perfusion due to coronary artery disease (CAD), or cardiomyopathy. Other causes include:
• mechanical disturbances in ventricular filling during diastole when there is too little blood for the ventricle to pump, as in mitral stenosis secondary to rheumatic heart disease or constrictive pericarditis and atrial fibrillation
• systolic hemodynamic disturbances, such as excessive cardiac workload due to volume overloading or pressure overload, that limit the heart's pumping ability. These disturbances can result from mitral or aortic regurgitation, which causes volume overloading, and aortic stenosis or systemic hypertension, which results in increased resistance to ventricular emptying.

Reduced cardiac output triggers three compensatory mechanisms: *ventricular dilation, hypertrophy,* and *increased sympathetic activity*. These mechanisms improve cardiac output at the expense of increased ventricular work. In *cardiac dilation,* an increase in end-diastolic ventricular volume (preload) causes increased stroke work and stroke volume during contraction, stretching cardiac muscle fibers beyond optimum limits and producing pulmonary congestion and pulmonary hypertension, which, in turn, lead to right ventricular failure.

In *ventricular hypertrophy,* an increase in muscle mass or diameter of the left ventricle allows the heart to pump

against increased resistance (impedance) to the outflow of blood but requires more oxygen. An increase in ventricular diastolic pressure necessary to
fill the enlarged ventricle may compromise diastolic coronary blood flow, limiting the oxygen supply to the ventricle,
causing ischemia and impaired muscle
contractility.

Increased sympathetic activity occurs
as a response to decreased cardiac output and blood pressure by enhancing peripheral vascular resistance, contractility, heart rate, and venous return. Signs
of increased sympathetic activity, such
as cool extremities and clamminess, may
indicate impending heart failure. Increased sympathetic activity also restricts blood flow to the kidneys, which
respond by reducing the glomerular filtration rate and increasing tubular reabsorption of salt and water, in turn expanding the circulating blood volume.
This renal mechanism, if unchecked,
can aggravate congestion and produce
overt edema.

Chronic CHF may worsen as a result
of respiratory tract infections, pulmonary embolism, added emotional stress,
increased salt or water intake, or failure
to comply with prescribed therapy. (See
Causes of Congestive Heart Failure, page
117.)

Signs and symptoms

Left heart failure produces fatigue and
dyspnea (exertional and paroxysmal
nocturnal). Right heart failure causes
engorgement of veins (when the patient
is upright, neck veins may appear distended, feel rigid, and show exaggerated
pulsations) and hepatomegaly. Many patients complain of a slight but persistent
cold and dry cough combined with
wheezing, which may be confused with
an allergic reaction.

Later symptoms include tachypnea,
palpitations, dependent edema, unexplained steady weight gain, nausea,
chest tightness, slowed mental response,
anorexia, hypotension, diaphoresis,
narrow pulse pressure, pallor, and oliguria. Auscultation reveals a gallop

---

Causes of Congestive Heart Failure

Cardiovascular causes
- Arteriosclerotic heart disease
- Myocardial infarction
- Hypertension
- Rheumatic heart disease
- Congenital heart disease
- Ischemic heart disease
- Cardiomyopathy
- Valvular diseases
- Dysrhythmias
- Noncompliance with treatment for
heart disease

Noncardiovascular causes
- Pregnancy and childbirth
- Increased environmental tempera-
ture or humidity
- Severe physical or mental stress
- Thyrotoxicosis
- Acute blood loss
- Pulmonary embolism
- Severe infection
- Chronic obstructive pulmonary
disease

---

rhythm (S_3) and bibasilar rales on inspiration. The liver may be palpable and
slightly tender.

Right heart failure often follows left
heart failure because the right heart
must pump against increased resistance
in the pulmonary system. Signs of right
heart failure vary according to the presence and extent of left heart failure but
typically include dependent edema.
Usually, such edema begins in the ankles; after 5 to 10 lb of edema accumulate, pitting occurs. Edema may progress to the severe generalized form called
anasarca.

In later stages of CHF, dullness develops over the lung bases, as well as hemoptysis and cyanosis, marked hepatomegaly, pitting ankle edema, and in
bedridden patients, edema over the sacrum.

Softened S_1 and S_2. Listen for S_1 and S_2.
These sounds may be normal or may

soften as the heart's pumping action diminishes.

Murmurs. Listen for systolic murmurs that soften. Consider any murmur of grade IV to VI intensity that softens to a grade II as a sign of cardiovascular deterioration. Such softening occurs when blood flows over the abnormal valve with diminished force, creating less turbulence than normal.

Extra heart sounds. Auscultate for extra heart sounds produced as blood flows into a compliant ventricle. You may hear S_3 (also called ventricular gallop), one of the early signs of CHF. In left heart failure, you may hear S_3 over the apex; in right heart failure, over the left sternal border. Remember that a physiologic S_3 occurs in many children and young adults. However, physiologic S_3 disappears when the patient sits erect. Pathologic S_3 does not disappear. Sometimes in CHF, you may hear a brief, low-pitched fourth heart sound just before S_1.

Complications include pulmonary edema, venostasis with predisposition to thromboembolism (especially with prolonged bed rest), cerebral insufficiency, and renal insufficiency with severe electrolyte imbalance and scanty, dark, concentrated urine.

Diagnosis
• *Electrocardiogram (EKG)* reflects heart strain, enlargement, or ischemia. It may also reveal atrial enlargement, tachycardia, and extrasystoles suggesting CHF.
• *Chest X-ray* shows increased pulmonary vascular markings, interstitial edema, or pleural effusion and cardiomegaly.
• *Pulmonary artery monitoring* demonstrates elevated pulmonary artery and capillary wedge pressures, which reflect left ventricular end-diastolic pressure in left heart failure and elevated right atrial pressure or central venous pressure in right heart failure. (See *Classifying Congestive Heart Failure (CHF)*, page 119.)

Treatment
The aim of therapy is to improve pump function by reversing the compensatory mechanisms producing the clinical effects. CHF can be controlled quickly by:
• diuresis to reduce total blood volume and circulatory congestion
• prolonged bed rest
• inotropes to strengthen myocardial contractility
• vasodilators to increase cardiac output by reducing the impedance to ventricular outflow (afterload)
• antiembolism stockings to prevent venostasis and possible thromboembolism.

Pulmonary edema requires morphine, as a venodilator, to diminish blood return to the heart; supplemental oxygen; high Fowler's position; and, possibly, rotating tourniquets (see *Applying Rotating Tourniquets,* page 120) to abruptly limit venous return. (See *Staging Pulmonary Edema,* page 121, and *Treating Pulmonary Edema,* pages 122 and 123.)

After recovery, the patient usually must continue taking digitalis and diuretics and must remain under medical supervision. If the patient with valve dysfunction has recurrent acute CHF, surgical replacement may be necessary.

Nursing management
During the acute phase:
• Weigh the patient daily (this is the best index of fluid retention), and check for peripheral edema. Also, carefully monitor I.V. intake and urinary output (especially in the patient receiving diuretics), vital signs (for increased respiratory rate, heart rate, and narrowing pulse pressure), and mental status. Auscultate the heart for abnormal sounds (S_3 gallop) and the lungs for rales or rhonchi. Report changes immediately.
• Frequently monitor blood urea nitrogen (BUN), creatinine, and serum potassium, sodium, chloride, and magnesium levels.
• When using rotating tourniquets, check radial and pedal pulses often to ensure that the tourniquets are not too

Classifying Congestive Heart Failure (CHF)

Although CHF is usually classified by site of heart failure (left heart, right heart, or both), it may also be classified by level of cardiac output, stage, and direction. However, these varying classifications simply represent different clinical aspects of CHF, not distinct diseases.

Low- and high-output failure

Achieving a precise definition of low and high cardiac output is difficult since the normal range is wide. In some patients with low-output failure, cardiac output may be normal during periods of rest but fails to rise during exertion. In some patients with high-output failure, it may settle near the upper limit of normal.

In both low- and high-output failure, the heart is unable to deliver the precise amount of oxygenated blood to the tissues. Low-output failure occurs in CAD, hypertension, primary myocardial disease, and valvular disease. High-output failure occurs in arteriovenous fistula, hyperthyroidism, anemia, sickle cell anemia, beriberi, Paget's disease, and thyrotoxicosis.

Acute and chronic heart failure

Frequently, acute and chronic heart failure overlap. For example, a patient with chronic heart failure may experience acute heart failure from MI. Acute heart failure may also occur in valvular rupture or any condition that places stress on an already diseased heart. Chronic heart failure may occur in multivalvular heart disease, cardiomyopathy, and a healed, extensive MI.

Backward and forward heart failure

Backward and forward failure cannot be clearly separated, since both types are present in most patients with chronic heart failure. In *backward heart failure*, one ventricle fails to expel blood, causing elevated ventricular end-diastolic volume and elevated pressure and volume in the atrium and venous system behind the failing ventricle. Such elevations, along with increased renal tubular reabsorption from increased renal venous pressure, cause retention of sodium and water, thereby increasing circulating blood volume.

In *forward heart failure*, the ventricles fail to expel enough blood into the arterial system. Retention of sodium and water then results from decreased renal perfusion or increased renal tubular absorption. As in backward failure, circulating blood volume increases, making the expulsion of blood even more difficult for the weakened ventricles.

High-output failure
> 3.6 liters/minute/m^2 of body surface (can be normal in athletic heart syndrome or pregnancy)

Normal levels of cardiac output
2.6 to 3.6 liters/minute/m^2 of body surface

Low-output failure
< 2.6 liters/minute/m^2 of body surface

Applying Rotating Tourniquets

You may be asked to apply rotating tourniquets to a patient with congestive heart failure or acute pulmonary edema. Rotating tourniquets help treat these conditions by impeding venous return from the patient's arms and legs to his heart.

Although not widely used today, rotating tourniquets are still used in some hospitals. The doctor may order them in conjunction with potent diuretic or digitalis therapy or after a phlebotomy fails.

Follow this procedure for connecting and monitoring a patient on a rotating tourniquet machine:

• Explain the procedure to the patient. Tell him the tourniquets may be uncomfortable and could cause temporary limb swelling and discoloration.
• Place him in Fowler's position. Then record his blood pressure and heart, respiratory, and radial and pedal pulse rates.
• Apply the tourniquets snugly over towels and around the patient's legs and arms, about 4″ (10 cm) from his groin and armpits. (You should be able to fit two fingers between tourniquet and skin.)
• *Make sure the machine is turned off.* Connect the tourniquet hoses to their color-coded mates on the machine.
• Close the tourniquet inflation valves, then turn on the machine and set its pressure dial, as ordered. Also set the inflation timing mechanism, as ordered.
• Open the tourniquet valves. Three of the four tourniquets will inflate. About every 15 minutes, one tourniquet will deflate and one will inflate. (They never inflate at the same time.)
• Make sure the tourniquets inflate in proper clockwise order.
• Regularly assess the patient's arms and legs below the tourniquets for color, temperature, and pulse. Check heart and lung sounds, and measure blood pressure often. Notify the doctor if you detect any abnormalities.
• To stop the therapy, when ordered, remove the tourniquets one by one. (Gradually stopping the therapy prevents a sudden venous blood volume increase that could cause circulatory overload.) As each tourniquet deflates, first close its inflation valve, and then remove it until all four tourniquets have deflated. Assess the patient's limbs for changes in arterial pulse rate and character and for skin color and temperature. Monitor his vital signs during weaning.

tight. At the completion of tourniquet therapy, remove *one* tourniquet at a time to prevent a sudden upsurge in circulating volume.
• To prevent deep-vein thrombosis due to vascular congestion, assist with range-of-motion exercises. Enforce bed rest, and apply antiembolism stockings. Watch for calf pain and tenderness.

To prepare the patient for discharge:
• Advise him to avoid foods high in sodium, such as canned or commercially prepared foods and dairy products, to curb fluid overload.

• Tell the patient that potassium lost through diuretics must be replaced by taking a prescribed potassium supplement and eating high-potassium foods, such as bananas, apricots, and orange juice.
• Stress the need for regular checkups.
• Emphasize the importance of taking digitalis exactly as prescribed. Instruct the patient to watch for the following signs of toxicity: anorexia, nausea, vomiting, yellow or double vision, or

Staging Pulmonary Edema

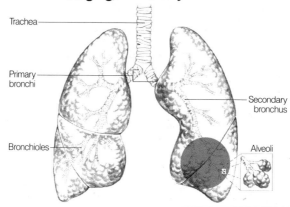

Trachea
Primary bronchi
Bronchioles
Secondary bronchus
Alveoli

STAGE	PATHOPHYSIOLOGY	SIGNS AND SYMPTOMS
Initial	Usually, left ventricular failure increases pulmonary vascular bed pressure, forcing fluid and solutes from the intravascular compartment into the interstitium of the lungs. As the interstitium overloads with fluid, fluid enters the peripheral alveoli, impairing adequate gas exchange.	Persistent cough—patient feels like he has "a cold coming on" Slight dyspnea/orthopnea Exercise intolerance Restlessness Anxiety Crepitant rales may be heard over the dependent portion of the lungs Diastolic gallop
Acute	Fluid accumulates throughout the pulmonary vasculature, causing further filling of the alveoli.	Acute shortness of breath Respirations—rapid, noisy (audible wheeze, rales) Cough more intense, producing frothy, blood-tinged sputum Cyanosis Diaphoresis, cold and clammy skin Tachycardia, dysrhythmias Hypotension
Advanced	Patient's condition rapidly deteriorates as the bronchial tree fills with fluid.	Decreased level of consciousness Ventricular dysrhythmias Shock Diminished breath sounds

Treating Pulmonary Edema

A patient is rushed to the emergency department. His skin is cold and clammy; his blood pressure is elevated and he is cyanotic. His respirations sound bubbly, with moist rales over both lungs, and he has frothy, blood-tinged secretions in the corners of his mouth. Every sign points to an advanced stage of pulmonary edema, in which fluid has accumulated in the extravascular spaces of the lung. Without immediate treatment to reduce extravascular fluid and improve gas exchange and myocardial function, the patient will die.

Here are the priorities that you should follow in this life-threatening emergency.

Relieve respiratory distress

Your first priority is to relieve respiratory difficulties. Begin by checking the patient's airway. If it is obstructed, instruct the patient to cough and expectorate. If fails to clear the obstruction, begin to suction the patient. If suctioning fails, prepare to assist the doctor with intubation, which facilitates aspiration of thick secretions and the use of intermittent positive-pressure breathing.

If the patient's airway is not obstructed, assist him to a sitting position in bed, and if possible, allow his legs to dangle over the sides to decrease venous return and relieve dyspnea. Also, give a high concentration of oxygen by mask using intermittent or continuous pressure. This method of oxygen administration overcomes the pressure barrier caused by fluid accumulation and ensures adequate blood oxygenation. To monitor oxygen administration, draw arterial blood samples for laboratory analysis.

cardiac dysrhythmias.
• Tell the patient to notify the doctor or nurse if his pulse is unusually irregular or less than 60 beats/minute; if he experiences dizziness, blurred vision, shortness of breath, a persistent dry cough, palpitations, increased fatigue, paroxysmal nocturnal dyspnea, swollen ankles, or decreased urinary output; or if weight increases 3 to 5 lb (1.36 to 2.27 kg) in a week.

Congestive cardiomyopathy

Congestive cardiomyopathy results from extensively damaged myocardial muscle fibers. This disorder interferes with myocardial metabolism and grossly dilates the ventricles without proportional compensatory hypertrophy, causing the heart to take on a globular shape and to contract poorly during systole. Congestive cardiomyopathy leads to intractable CHF, dysrhythmias, and emboli. Since this disease is usually not diagnosed until it is in the advanced stages, prognosis is generally poor.

Causes

The cause of most cardiomyopathies is unknown. Occasionally, congestive cardiomyopathies are not primary myocardial diseases but rather result from myocardial destruction by toxic, infectious, or metabolic agents, such as certain viruses, endocrine and electrolyte disorders, and nutritional deficiencies. Other causes include muscle disorders (myasthenia gravis, progressive muscular dystrophy, or myotonic dystrophy), infiltrative disorders (hemochromatosis, or amyloidosis), and sarcoidosis.

Cardiomyopathy is a possible complication of alcoholism. In such cases, cardiomyopathy may improve somewhat with abstinence from alcohol but recurs when the patient resumes drinking. How viruses may induce cardiomyopathy is still unclear, but investigation is focused

Watch for dysrhythmias

Connect the patient to a cardiac monitor. Then monitor the EKG waveforms on the oscilloscope screen, and be alert for dysrhythmias. Be sure to have resuscitation equipment ready.

Monitor response to drug administration

To remove the excess alveolar fluid, the doctor will probably order a rapid-acting I.V. diuretic, such as furosemide or ethacrynic acid. Since diuretics increase excretion of water and electrolytes, carefully monitor urinary output and serum electrolyte levels.

Along with an I.V. diuretic, the doctor will probably order morphine, unless the patient has a history of cerebrovascular accidents or chronic obstructive pulmonary disease or is in cardiogenic shock. Morphine alleviates anxiety and promotes blood flow from the pulmonary circulation to the periphery. However, because morphine can severely depress respiration, have naloxone hydrochloride and intubation equipment within easy reach.

The doctor may also order aminophylline and an inotropic agent, such as digitalis, to improve cardiac output. Aminophylline relieves severe bronchospasm and increases cardiac output, renal flow, and urinary output of sodium and water. Be sure to administer aminophylline slowly to prevent a sudden—and possibly fatal—drop in blood pressure. Also, be alert for tachydysrhythmias because aminophylline may increase heart rate. If the doctor orders digitalis, watch for signs of toxicity.

on a possible link between viral myocarditis and subsequent congestive cardiomyopathy, especially after infection with coxsackievirus B, poliovirus, and influenza virus.

Metabolic cardiomyopathies are related to endocrine and electrolyte disorders and nutritional deficiencies. Thus, congestive cardiomyopathy may develop in patients with hyperthyroidism, pheochromocytoma, beriberi (thiamine deficiency), and kwashiorkor (protein deficiency). Cardiomyopathy may also result from rheumatic fever, especially among children with myocarditis.

Antepartal or postpartal cardiomyopathy may develop during the last trimester or within months after delivery. Its cause is unknown, but it occurs most frequently in multiparous women over age 30, particularly those with malnutrition or preeclampsia. In these patients, cardiomegaly and CHF may reverse with treatment, allowing a subsequent normal pregnancy. If cardiomegaly persists despite treatment, prognosis is extremely poor.

Signs and symptoms

In congestive cardiomyopathy, the heart ejects blood less efficiently than normal. Consequently, a large volume of blood remains in the left ventricle after systole, causing signs of CHF—both left-sided (shortness of breath, orthopnea, dyspnea on exertion, paroxysmal nocturnal dyspnea, fatigue, and an irritating dry cough at night) and right-sided (edema, liver engorgement, and jugular venous distention). Congestive cardiomyopathy also produces peripheral cyanosis, narrow pulse pressure reflecting diminished stroke volume, pulses alternans, and sinus tachycardia or atrial fibrillation in some patients, secondary to low cardiac output. Auscultation reveals diffuse apical impulses, pansystolic murmur (mitral and tricuspid regurgitation secondary to cardiomegaly and weak papillary muscles), and S_3 and S_4 gallop rhythms. If tricuspid regurgitation is substantial, the patient may have a pulsatile liver and prominent regurgitant waves in the jugular venous pulse.

Diagnosis

No single test confirms congestive cardiomyopathy. Diagnosis requires elimination of other possible causes of CHF and dysrhythmias.

• *EKG* and *angiography* rule out ischemic heart disease; the EKG demonstrates nonspecific abnormalities and may also show biventricular hypertrophy, sinus tachycardia, atrial enlargement, and, in 20% of patients, atrial fibrillation.

• *Chest X-ray* demonstrates cardiomegaly—usually affecting all heart chambers—pulmonary congestion, or pleural effusion.

Treatment

In congestive cardiomyopathy, the goals are to correct the underlying causes and improve the heart's pumping ability with digitalis, diuretics, oxygen, and a restricted-sodium diet. Therapy may also include prolonged bed rest, selective use of steroids, and possibly pericardiotomy, which is still investigational. Vasodilators reduce preload and afterload, thereby decreasing congestion and increasing cardiac output. Acute heart failure necessitates vasodilation with nitroprusside I.V. or, more recently, nitroglycerin I.V. Although not yet approved for use in the United States, Salbutamol I.V. shows promise in improving cardiac status. Long-term treatment may include phenoxybenzamine, prazosin, hydralazine, isosorbide dinitrate, and, if the patient is on prolonged bed rest, anticoagulants.

When other therapeutic modalities fail, cardiac transplantation may be considered in carefully selected patients.

Nursing management

In the patient with acute failure:
• Monitor for signs of progressive failure (decreased arterial pulses, increased neck vein distention) and compromised renal perfusion (oliguria, elevated BUN and creatinine levels, and electrolyte imbalances). Weigh the patient daily.

• If he is receiving vasodilators, check blood pressure and heart rate frequently. If he becomes hypotensive, stop the infusion and place him in a supine position with legs elevated to increase venous return to the heart and ensure cerebral blood flow.

• If the patient is receiving diuretics, monitor for signs of resolving congestion (decreased rales and dyspnea) or too vigorous diuresis. Check potassium for hypokalemia, especially if therapy includes digitalis.

• Therapeutic restrictions and uncertain prognosis usually cause profound anxiety and depression, so offer support and encourage the patient to express his feelings. Be flexible with visiting hours. If hospitalization becomes prolonged, try to obtain permission for the patient to spend occasional weekends away.

• Before discharge, to help ensure continued compliance with therapy, teach the patient about his illness and its treatment. Also, emphasize the need to restrict sodium intake, watch for weight gain, and take digitalis as prescribed, watching for its toxic effects (anorexia, nausea, vomiting, and yellow vision).

• Teach the need for modest restriction of activity due to the heart's inability to increase the cardiac output commensurately.

Idiopathic hypertrophic subaortic stenosis

In this primary cardiac muscle disease, there is disproportionate and asymmetrical thickening of the interventricular septum in comparison with the remainder of the left ventricle. In idiopathic hypertrophic subaortic stenosis (IHSS), cardiac output may be low, normal, or high, depending on whether stenosis is obstructive or nonobstructive. If output is normal or high, IHSS may go undetected for years; but low cardiac output may lead to potentially fatal CHF. The course of IHSS varies—some patients demonstrate progressive deterioration, whereas others remain stable for several years.

Causes

Despite being designated as idiopathic, almost always IHSS is inherited as a non–sex-linked autosomal dominant trait. Most patients with IHSS have obstructive disease resulting from the combined effects of ventricular septum hypertrophy and the movement of the anterior mitral valve leaflet into the outflow tract during systole. Eventually, left ventricular dysfunction, due to rigidity and decreased compliance, causes pump failure.

Signs and symptoms

Generally, clinical features of IHSS do not appear until the disease is well advanced, when atrial dilation and, possibly, atrial fibrillation abruptly reduce blood flow to the left ventricle. Reduced inflow and subsequent low output may produce angina pectoris, dysrhythmias, dyspnea on exertion, syncope, orthopnea or paroxysmal nocturnal dyspnea, CHF, and sudden death. Auscultation reveals a medium-pitched systolic ejection murmur along the left sternal border and at the apex; palpation reveals a peripheral pulse with a characteristic double impulse (pulsus biferiens) and, with atrial fibrillation, an irregular pulse. (See *Idiopathic Hypertrophic Subaortic Stenosis*, page 126.)

Diagnosis

Diagnosis of IHSS depends on typical clinical findings and the following test results:
• *Echocardiography* (most useful) shows increased thickness of the interventricular septum and abnormal motion of the anterior mitral leaflet during systole, occluding left ventricular outflow in obstructive IHSS.
• *Cardiac catheterization* reveals elevated left ventricular end-diastolic pressure and, possibly, mitral insufficiency.
• *EKG* usually demonstrates left ventricular hypertrophy, ST segment and T-wave abnormalities, deep waves (due to

hypertrophy, not infarction), left anterior hemiblock, ventricular dysrhythmias, and, possibly, atrial fibrillation.
• *Phonocardiography* confirms an early systolic murmur.

Treatment

The treatment goals of IHSS are to relax the ventricle and relieve outflow tract obstruction. Propranolol, a beta-adrenergic blocking agent, slows heart rate and increases ventricular filling by relaxing the obstructing muscle, thereby reducing angina, syncope, dyspnea, and dysrhythmias. However, propranolol may aggravate symptoms of cardiac decompensation. Atrial fibrillation requires digitalis or cardioversion to treat the dysrhythmia and, because of the high risk of systemic embolism, anticoagulant therapy until fibrillation subsides. Since vasodilators such as nitroglycerin reduce venous return by permitting pooling of blood in the periphery, thereby decreasing ventricular volume and chamber size, and since they may cause further obstruction, they are contraindicated in patients with IHSS. Also contraindicated are sympathetic stimulators, such as isoproterenol, which enhance cardiac contractility and myocardial demands for oxygen, thereby intensifying the obstruction.

If drug therapy fails, surgery is indicated. Ventricular myotomy (resection of the hypertrophied septum), alone or combined with mitral valve replacement, may ease outflow tract obstruction and relieve symptoms. However, ventricular myotomy may cause complications, such as complete heart block and ventricular septal defect, and is still considered experimental.

Nursing management

• Because syncope or sudden death may follow well-tolerated exercise, warn patients against strenuous physical activity, such as running.
• Administer medication, as ordered. Caution: Avoid digitalis, nitroglycerin, and diuretics. They increase the severity of outflow obstruction by decreasing di-

Idiopathic Hypertrophic Subaortic Stenosis

IHSS carries a significant risk of sudden death, even in totally asymptomatic children and young adults. Typically, sudden death resulting from IHSS follows physical exertion.

Although the exact mechanism of sudden death in IHSS is unknown, ventricular dysrhythmias are highly suspect. Certain atrial dysrhythmias also may be implicated as a primary cause. In atrial dysrhythmias, absence of atrial systolic contraction can cause a sudden, fatal decrease in left ventricular volume and outflow. Atrial dysrhythmias also may degenerate into ventricular fibrillation, resulting in syncope and, if untreated, death.

Fortunately, IHSS does present a few diagnostic signs besides sudden death. Practically pathognomonic of this disorder is a low-pitched, apical systolic ejection murmur, heard best at the lower left sternal border and at the apex. This characteristic murmur results from turbulent blood flow through the narrowed or obstructed outflow tract. It is intensified during Valsalva's maneuver or when the patient sits upright or stands suddenly; it disappears if he squats. If CHF develops, this murmur diminishes or disappears.

Angina may also occur in the patient with IHSS. Outflow tract obstruction increases oxygen demand by increasing the left ventricular work load; the resultant disproportion between oxygen supply and demand causes angina. Because the degree of obstruction may vary without provocation or in response to changes in position or to drugs, angina may occur at rest. Syncope also may occur at rest or during exercise.

In a patient with mild-to-moderate symptoms, the course of IHSS may vary, with intervals of spontaneous improvement. But if the outflow tract obstruction is severe, CHF may gradually claim the patient's life.

astolic left ventricular volume or increasing left ventricular contractility. Warn the patient not to stop taking propranolol abruptly, since doing so may cause rebound effects resulting in MI or sudden death. To determine the patient's tolerance for an increased dosage of propranolol, take his pulse to check for bradycardia, and have him stand and walk around slowly to check for orthostatic hypotension.
• Provide psychological support. If the patient is hospitalized for a prolonged time, be flexible with visiting hours, and encourage occasional weekends away from the hospital, if possible. Refer him for psychosocial counseling to help him and his family accept the restricted lifestyle imposed by this chronic disease and cope with the poor prognosis.

• Stress antibiotic prophylaxis for dental and surgical work.
• If the patient is a child, have his parents arrange for him to continue his studies in the hospital.
• Since sudden cardiac arrest is possible, urge the family to learn cardiopulmonary resuscitation.

Restrictive cardiomyopathy

Restrictive cardiomyopathy, a disorder of the myocardial musculature, is characterized by restricted ventricular filling (the result of left ventricular hypertrophy) and endocardial fibrosis and thickening. Severe restrictive cardiomyopathy is irreversible.

Causes

An extremely rare disorder, primary restrictive cardiomyopathy is of unknown etiology. However, restrictive cardiomyopathy syndrome, a manifestation of amyloidosis, results from infiltration of amyloid into the intracellular spaces in the myocardium, endocardium, and subendocardium.

In both forms of restrictive cardiomyopathy, the myocardium becomes rigid—with poor distention during diastole, inhibiting complete ventricular filling—and fails to contract completely during systole, resulting in low cardiac output.

Signs and symptoms

Because it lowers cardiac output and leads to CHF, restrictive cardiomyopathy produces fatigue, dyspnea, orthopnea, chest pain, generalized edema, liver engorgement, peripheral cyanosis, and pallor. It also causes exercise intolerance, inspiratory increase in venous pressure (Kussmaul's sign), and S_3, or S_4 or systolic murmurs reflecting atrioventricular valvular regurgitation.

Diagnosis

• *Chest X-ray* shows advanced stages of massive cardiomegaly affecting all four chambers of the heart.
• *Echocardiography* rules out constrictive pericarditis as the cause of restricted filling by detecting increased left ventricular muscle mass and differences in end-diastolic pressures between ventricles.
• *EKG* may show low-voltage complexes, AV conduction defects, or hypertrophy.
• *Arterial pulsation* reveals blunt carotid upstroke with small volume.
• *Cardiac catheterization* demonstrates increased left ventricular end-diastolic pressure and rules out constrictive pericarditis as the cause of restricted filling.

Treatment

Although no therapy currently exists for restricted ventricular filling, digitalis, diuretics, and a restricted sodium diet benefit by easing the symptoms of CHF. Oral vasodilators—such as isosorbide dinitrate, prazosin, and hydralazine—may control intractable CHF. Anticoagulant therapy may be necessary to prevent thrombophlebitis in the patient restricted to prolonged bed rest.

Nursing management

• In the acute phase, monitor heart rate and rhythm, blood pressure, urinary output, and pulmonary artery pressure readings to help guide treatment.
• Give psychological support. Provide appropriate diversionary activities for the patient restricted to prolonged bed rest. Since the poor prognosis for severe restrictive cardiomyopathy usually causes profound anxiety and depression, be especially supportive and understanding, and encourage the patient to express his fears. Refer him for psychosocial counseling, as necessary, for help in coping with his restricted life-style. Be flexible with visiting hours whenever possible.
• Before discharge, teach the patient to watch for and report signs of digoxin toxicity (anorexia, nausea, vomiting, or yellow vision); to record and report weight gain; and, if sodium restriction is ordered, to avoid canned vegetables, pickles, smoked meats, and excessive use of table salt.

Nursing diagnoses

After collecting subjective data from the patient history and objective data from the physical examination, formulate nursing diagnoses and set goals. Typical diagnoses related to heart failure are:

Alteration in cardiac output

Such alteration causes changes in thought processes and reduces activity tolerance. With this diagnosis, your goal is to maintain hemodynamic stability. Hemodynamic monitoring—measurement of pulmonary artery end-diastolic pressure, mean pulmonary capillary wedge pressure (PCWP), and cardiac output—is a useful tool for assessing response to treatment and maintaining hemodynamic stability. PCWP is probably the most accurate indicator of impending heart failure, but measurement of cardiac output is also useful. CHF always reduces cardiac output, causing hypoperfusion.

Potential for deterioration related to inadequate gas exchange and impaired arterial and venous peripheral circulation.

With this diagnosis, your goal in planning interventions is to prevent complications: pulmonary and systemic congestion, infection, skin breakdown, thromboembolism, and cardiogenic shock.

Potential alteration in cardiac output related to electroconductive disorders of the myocardium.

With this diagnosis, your goal is to maintain electrophysiologic stability.

Anticipatory anxiety related to knowledge deficit of illness and fear of future heart failure.

The patient may experience fear of heart failure, life-style changes, powerlessness, or death; express anger and hostility as a result of his illness; or lack the knowledge necessary for full compliance. Your goal is to reduce his anxiety level. This is essential since anxiety produces vasoconstriction, increases arterial pressure and heart rate, and, according to some evidence, reduces urine output. Teach the patient relaxation techniques, and play soft music or read to him. Encourage him and his family to verbalize their fears.

7

HEART BLOCKS AND DYSRHYTHMIAS

Even if you never expect to work in a coronary-care unit, you should know how to recognize dysrhythmias and what to do about them. Dysrhythmia is one of many abnormal variations in cardiac rhythm, rate, and conduction. To deal with dysrhythmias correctly, you must distinguish the benign from the catastrophic.

Heart block

Heart block, a delay or interruption of electrical conduction, may originate in the sinoatrial (SA) node, the atrioventricular (AV) node, or elsewhere in the heart. Most patients with heart block have an AV disturbance, of which three categories exist: first degree, second degree (Type I and II), and third degree.

Causes

AV heart block may come from digitalis or quinidine toxicity, acute myocardial infarction (AMI), deteriorated myocardial conduction tissue, edema, or tissue damage from surgical manipulation. In some patients, the condition is congenital. A transient Type I AV block can be caused by rheumatic fever, vagal stimulation, or electrolyte imbalance. (See *Sick Sinus Syndrome,* page 130.)

Signs, symptoms, and diagnosis

In first-degree AV block, electrical impulses flow normally from the SA node through the atria but are delayed at the AV node. On an electrocardiogram (EKG), you will see a PR interval greater than 0.20 second (and possibly as long as 1.26 seconds). Other typical EKG features include:
- normal QRS complexes
- normal P-QRS-T sequences
- regular rhythm
- identical atrial and ventricular rates.

Second-degree AV block occurs in two forms: Type I (also called Mobitz I, or Wenckebach) and Type II (Mobitz II). (See *Types of Heart Block,* page 132.) With either type, occasionally dropped (absent) ventricular beats indicate that an impulse has been blocked at the AV node.

Type I AV block appears most commonly in patients with an inferior wall AMI or digitalis toxicity, although it may develop in patients receiving quinidine or procainamide.

In Type I AV block, diseased tissues of the AV node conduct each successive impulse earlier and earlier in the refractory period. Eventually, an impulse arrives during the absolute refractory period, when the tissue cannot conduct it. The next impulse arrives during a relative refractory period and is conducted normally. Symptoms of Type I AV heart block include:
- grouped beating
- irregular rhythm
- normal QRS complexes
- a PR interval that lengthens with each cycle until a P wave appears without a QRS complex (a dropped beat)
- a PR interval after the dropped beat that is shorter than the one preceding the dropped beat

Sick Sinus Syndrome

Sick sinus syndrome (SSS) is not a single rhythmic disturbance. Rather, it is a combination of disturbances that may include sinus bradycardia, SA exit block, sinus arrest, alternating tachycardia and bradycardia (tachy-brady syndrome), and suppression of alternate pacemakers (for example, a slower-than-normal AV junctional rhythm).

No definitive tests confirm SSS. No two cases are alike, because the individual patient's underlying heart disease dictates the form and severity of the syndrome. In some patients, SSS escapes notice—or is diagnosed as asymptomatic bradycardia. Most patients with SSS are elderly, but anyone can develop it.

Origin. What causes SSS? Any disorder that impairs the SA node's ability to initiate or conduct impulses, including ischemia, rheumatic disorders, cardiomyopathy, pericarditis, muscular dystrophy, collagen disease, and fibrosis.

SSS may also be precipitated by SA-node injury during cardiac surgery. In many patients a cause is never identified.

Common SSS types. The patient may develop *SA exit block,* a disturbance in which impulses are blocked before leaving the SA node. Early SA exit block is not evident on an EKG; but if the condition worsens, EKG tracings may periodically show dropped P waves and QRS complexes—brief periods of sinus arrest. As SA-node function deteriorates, sinus arrest may appear intermittently for two or three beats at a time.

Note: An EKG showing sinus arrest does not always mean SSS. Hyperkalemia and antiarrhythmic drugs can cause periodic sinus arrest or SA exit block.

Tachy-brady syndrome is another dysrhythmia that may result from an SA-node malfunction. The patient develops a tachycardia, which suppresses SA-node function. Known as overdrive suppression, this is a normal response. But when the tachycardia terminates, the sick SA node does not resume normal function as a healthy SA node would. As a result, the patient experiences a period of bradycardia or even asystole. To control this dangerous dysrhythmia, the doctor will insert an artificial pacemaker.

Patient care. SSS is most dangerous in patients with serious underlying conditions who are likely to have more severe signs and symptoms requiring immediate treatment. A patient without underlying disease may experience nothing worse than occasional palpitations, unexplained fatigue, sleeplessness, muscle aches, or periodic oliguria.

The doctor may order atropine or isoproterenol to treat SSS initially, but he will probably insert an artificial pacemaker as soon as possible.

● an RR interval that becomes progressively shorter
● the shortest RR interval, when double, that is longer than the longest RR interval.

Type II AV block, though not as common as Type I, is more serious—because the frequency and severity of the block are unpredictable. (See *Types of Heart Block,* page 132.)

In Type II AV block, dropped beats occur without warning because the conduction abnormality is in the bundle of His and the bundle branches.

Type II AV block generally occurs in patients with anterior AMI or severe coronary artery disease—almost never in a patient with a healthy heart. It can easily progress to third-degree heart block. Characteristic EKG tracings for

the patient with Type II AV block include:
• a normal PR interval
• a normal QRS complex (occasionally a bundle branch block may appear)
• QRS complexes periodically dropped after P waves.

In third-degree AV block (also called complete heart block), all atrial impulses are blocked at the AV junction, and the atria and ventricles beat independently. A secondary pacemaker (either junctional or ventricular) stimulates the ventricles. (See *Types of Heart Block,* page 132.)

If the secondary pacemaker is located high in the AV junction, heart rate may be nearly normal (45 to 60 beats/minute). If the secondary pacemaker is located in the ventricle itself, it produces an *idioventricular rhythm* that creates wide QRS complexes on an EKG. Heart rate may range from 20 to 40 beats/minute. (See *AV Dissociation: Not Always a Heart Block.*)

A high AV-junctional pacemaker produces a narrow QRS complex. With a block low in the AV junction and a pacemaker in the bundle of His, the QRS complex is wide. A ventricular pacemaker produces a wide, bizarre QRS complex.

Other EKG features include:
• P waves unrelated to QRS complexes
• regular RR intervals
• regular PP intervals
• slow ventricular rate (below 60 beats/minute).

Treatment
Before deciding what treatment is appropriate for the heart block, the doctor will need to determine its cause and evaluate the severity of the symptoms.

First-degree AV block rarely affects cardiac output, so the doctor may choose not to treat it. He will, however, monitor the patient closely for development of second- or third-degree AV block.

If the patient has developed Type II AV block after AMI—or if he has such symptoms as bradycardia or hypotension—he will probably have an artificial

AV Dissociation: Not Always a Heart Block
With third-degree AV block, your patient has AV dissociation: His atria and ventricles are beating independently. But not every patient with AV dissociation has third-degree AV block. AV dissociation can also result from a slowing of SA-node firing, causing a secondary pacemaker to stimulate the ventricles, and acceleration of a secondary pacemaker, as in junctional tachycardia.

pacemaker inserted to ensure adequate heart rate.

A few patients with chronic heart disease develop Type II AV block without symptoms. These patients need monitoring—but no treatment, as long as they remain stable.

If third-degree AV block develops following anterior wall injury, the patient may develop syncope or congestive heart failure (CHF). He, too, is likely to need a permanent pacemaker.

Note: Occasionally, you may encounter a patient with third-degree heart block and no symptoms except fatigue. The doctor may insert a pacemaker to ensure adequate heart rate.

Nursing management
In first-degree heart block, the patient may complain of palpitations. But unless his ventricular rate is too low to maintain normal cardiac output, he probably will not require aggressive treatment. Monitor his pulse regularly, and watch closely for signs of drug toxicity.

However, if the patient has second degree heart block, the doctor will probably transfer him to the intensive care unit. Until then, keep him connected to a cardiac monitor. As ordered, give atropine or isoproterenol I.V., and prepare for pacemaker insertion.

If a patient with third-degree AV block develops a ventricle dysrhythmia, check

Types of Heart Block

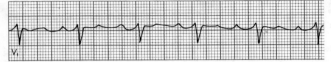

First-degree AV block

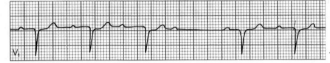

Second-degree AV block, Type I (Wenckebach)

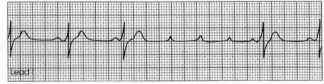

Second-degree AV block, Type II

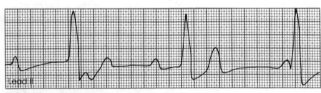

Third-degree AV block

with the doctor before giving lidocaine, procainamide, quinidine, or propranolol. These antiarrhythmic drugs could increase the block.

Cardiac dysrhythmias

In cardiac dysrhythmias, abnormal electrical conduction or automaticity changes heart rate and rhythm. Dysrhythmias vary in severity, from those that are mild, asymptomatic, and require no treatment (such as sinus arrhythmia, in which heart rate increases and decreases with respiration) to catastrophic ventricular fibrillation, which necessitates immediate resuscitation. Dysrhythmias are generally classified according to origin (ventricular or supraventricular); they can also be classified as either impulse formation disorders or impulse conduction disorders. (See *Impulse Formation Disorders*, page

134 and *Impulse Conduction Disorders,* page 135.) Their effect on cardiac output and blood pressure, partially influenced by the site of origin, determines their clinical significance.

Causes

The physiologic effects of dysrhythmia vary significantly according to cause and cardiac and vascular capacity to compensate. The normal heart adapts quickly to changes in heart rate and rhythm by compensating with coronary vasodilation, which provides sufficient oxygen to meet the demands of an increased work load. However, a diseased heart is less likely to adapt effectively. For example, the presence of coronary artery obstruction prevents adequate oxygenation; thus, dysrhythmia that increases oxygen demand can lead to progressive myocardial ischemia and, as compensatory mechanisms fail, heart failure. (See *Compensatory Mechanisms,* page 135.) In this situation, dysrhythmia may precipitate or aggravate angina or CHF. Dysrhythmias that impair AV synchrony (such as AV dissociation) also reduce cardiac output.

Dysrhythmias may be congenital or may result from myocardial anoxia, infarction, hypertrophy of muscle fiber from hypertension or valvular heart disease, toxic doses of cardioactive drugs (such as digoxin), or *sick sinus syndrome* (SSS)—degeneration of conductive tissue necessary to maintain normal heart rhythm. (See *Sick Sinus Syndrome,* page 130.)

Other causes include: electrolyte imbalances, hypoxemia, and metabolic abnormalities, such as alkalosis and acidosis. (For descriptions, causes, and treatment, see Appendix B, Cardiac Dysrhythmias.)

Signs and symptoms

No matter what the cause, reduced cardiac output results in forward heart failure, requiring vasoconstriction of the renal, mesenteric, cerebral, and musculoskeletal circulations to maintain blood pressure. Thus, the symptoms associ-

---

Impulse Conduction Disorders

Not all dysrhythmias result from impulse formation disorders. Some are caused by conduction disorders that interrupt the normal pathway of an impulse and either block or reroute it.

Conduction disorders called *exit blocks* can impede SA-node impulse transmission. As a result, a secondary pacemaker may kick in, causing an escape rhythm. A similar type of conduction disorder may cause bundle branch blocks and AV blocks.

Another conduction disorder, called *reentry,* reroutes the impulse through certain tissue segments, permitting the impulse to depolarize the same tissue more than once. Reentry, which is usually triggered by a premature beat, occurs when the following conditions are present:
• a circuit for the impulse to travel around
• slow conduction through part of the circuit
• unequal refractory periods within the circuit.

---

ated with dysrhythmia are the classic symptoms related to impaired cardiac output—pallor, cold and clammy extremities, reduced urine output, weakness, chest pain, dizziness, and (if cerebral circulation is severely impaired) syncope.

In a patient with a normal heart, dysrhythmia typically produces few symptoms. But even in a normal heart, persistently rapid or very irregular rhythms can strain the myocardium and impair cardiac output. For example, ventricular tachycardia can lead to ventricular fibrillation and sudden death. (See *Dysrhythmias and Sudden Death,* page 136.)

Diagnosis

Diagnosis of dysrhythmia is always based on patient history and symptoms

Impulse Formation Disorders

The SA node's ability to sponta-neously depolarize permits it to function as the heart's primary pacemaker. But the SA node is not the only heart tissue that can generate impulses. Other heart cells—for example, those in the atria, AV node, bundle of His, and Purkinje's fibers—also possess this property. If the SA node falters, a secondary (latent) pacemaker in one of these locations may become active. Or a secondary pacemaker may become active because of tissue irritability. An active secondary pacemaker can compete with the SA node or, if the SA node fails entirely, take over as the primary pacemaker. Either way, a dysrhythmia results.

An impulse formation disorder can cause these kinds of dysrhythmias:

• sinus tachycardia, from regular but unusually fast SA-node firing
• sinus bradycardia, from regular but unusually slow SA-node firing
• premature atrial contractions and atrial tachycardias, from the predomi-nance of a secondary atrial pace-maker
• accelerated junctional rhythms, from the predominance of a second-ary pacemaker in the AV junction or the bundle of His
• ventricular ectopic beats or rhythms, from the predominance of a ventricu-lar pacemaker.

(tachycardia, palpitations, anginal pain, extreme dyspnea, edema, or faintness) and on a detailed cardiovascular exami-nation that includes a 12-lead EKG.

Treatment

Effective medical treatment of dys-rhythmia should return pacer function to the sinus node, increase or decrease ventricular rate to normal, regain AV synchrony, and maintain normal sinus rhythm. Such treatment corrects abnor-mal rhythms through therapy with anti-arrhythmic drugs; electrical conversion with precordial shock (defibrillation and cardioversion); physical maneuvers (ca-rotid and vagal [Valsalva maneuver]); temporary or permanent placement of a pacemaker to maintain heart rate; and surgical removal or cryotherapy of an irritable ectopic focus to prevent recur-ring dysrhythmias (a new procedure, called endocardial stripping or "The Pennsylvania Peel"). Endocardial strip-ping—excision of an irritable focus (or foci) during open heart surgery—is an alternative treatment for recurrent ven-tricular tachycardia and sudden death syndrome.

Dysrhythmias often respond to treat-ment of the underlying disorder, such as correction of hypoxia. However, dys-rhythmia associated with heart disease often requires continuing and complex treatment.

Nursing management

• Assess an unmonitored patient for rhythm disturbances. If his pulse is ab-normally rapid, slow, or irregular, watch for signs of hypoperfusion, such as changes in level of consciousness, hy-potension, diminished urinary output, poor peripheral perfusion. (See *Sinus Bradycardia: Good Sign or Bad?*, page 137.)
• Document any dysrhythmias in a monitored patient, and assess for possi-ble causes and effects (See *Wolff-Parkin-son-White Syndrome*, page 138.)
• When life-threatening dysrhythmias develop, rapidly assess the level of con-sciousness, respirations, and pulse, and initiate cardiopulmonary resuscitation, as indicated.
• Evaluate for altered cardiac output re-sulting from dysrhythmias. Consider potentially progressive or ominous dys-rhythmias in determining your course of

action. Administer medications, as ordered, and prepare to assist with medical procedures, if indicated (for example, cardioversion or pacemaker insertion). (See *Carotid Sinus Massage*, page 139, and *How Carotid Massage Slows Heart Rate*, page 140.)

• Monitor for predisposing factors—such as fluid and electrolyte imbalance—and signs of drug toxicity, especially of digoxin. If you suspect drug toxicity, report such signs immediately, and withhold the next dose.

• To prevent dysrhythmias in a postoperative cardiac patient, provide adequate oxygen and reduce heart workload, while carefully maintaining metabolic, neurologic, respiratory, and hemodynamic status.

• To avoid temporary pacemaker malfunction, install a fresh battery before each insertion. Carefully secure the external catheter wires and the pacemaker box. Assess the threshold daily. Watch closely for premature contractions, a sign of myocardial irritation.

• To avert permanent pacemaker malfunction, restrict the patient's activity after insertion, as ordered. Monitor the pulse rate regularly, and watch for signs of decreased cardiac output.

• Preparation for discharge: Warn the patient about environmental hazards, as indicated by the pacemaker manufacturer, which may include microwave ovens, electrical appliances, some ham radios, and radar. Since many contemporary pacemakers are enclosed in metal containers, these hazards may not present a problem; however, in doubtful situations, 24-hour Holter monitoring may be helpful. Tell the patient to report light-headedness or syncope, and stress the importance of regular checkups.

Nursing diagnoses

When you have a clear idea of the severity and type of dysrhythmia and some idea of the cause or precipitating factors, develop nursing diagnoses, establish treatment goals, and plan care accord-

Compensatory Mechanisms

Because dysrhythmias alter heart rhythm and rate, they may affect cardiac output. Within certain limits, the heart compensates for rhythm and rate changes and maintains adequate cardiac output. Beyond these limits, however, cardiac output begins to drop and the patient experiences cardiovascular symptoms related to hemodynamic changes.

Remember that cardiac output equals heart rate times stroke volume. Consider what happens when just one element of the equation—heart rate—changes.

In bradycardia, for example, diastole lasts longer than in a normal cardiac cycle. This, in turn, increases venous return and preload. As explained by Starling's law (See Chapter 2, page 11.), an increase in preload stretches myocardial fibers more than usual, causing more forceful myocardial contractions. Thus, the heart compensates for a slow heart rate by raising stroke volume.

In contrast, tachycardia *shortens* diastole. Because ventricular filling diminishes, the amount of blood ejected with each contraction also diminishes. But up to a point, the rapid heart rate offsets this loss and maintains cardiac output.

Note: The limits beyond which the heart can compensate for bradycardia and tachycardia vary among patients and depend on the extent of MI.

ingly. For patients with dysrhythmia, your diagnoses and care plan will be similar to the following:

Potential anxiety related to knowledge deficit regarding diagnosis, possible therapy, and prognosis.

To reduce the patient's anxiety, encourage him and his family to verbalize their fears. Encourage the patient to tell

Dysrhythmias and Sudden Death

Most cases of sudden death occur before the victim reaches the hospital. In 75% of the victims of sudden death (defined as death within 1 hour of onset of symptoms), the EKGs recorded by rescue workers within minutes of collapse show ventricular fibrillation. In the remaining 25%, sudden death results from asystole, idioventricular rhythm, sinus bradycardia, and acute heart block with Stokes-Adams attacks.

These fatal dysrhythmias have multiple causes:

Cardiovascular causes —80% to 90%):
• coronary artery spasm, especially with unstable angina
• small-vessel coronary disease
• valvular aortic stenosis
• idiopathic hypertrophic subaortic stenosis
• cardiomyopathy
• pulmonary hypertension
• dissecting aortic aneurysm
• ruptured aortic aneurysm
Noncardiovascular causes:
• massive intracerebral and subarachnoid hemorrhage
• massive gastrointestinal hemorrhage
• aspiration of a food bolus.

---

electrical instability.

Your goal is to prevent the recurrence of dysrhythmia. Administer antiarrhythmic drug treatment, as ordered. If you are giving these very potent drugs intravenously, use an infusion pump or administer them by microdrip. Check every 15 minutes to ensure delivery of the correct dosage. Since antiarrhythmics are potentially lethal and dosage may need adjustment, watch carefully for symptoms of toxicity.

If the patient has received digitalis within the last 48 hours, also watch for digitalis toxicity (nausea, vomiting, diarrhea, increased ectopy, or heart block), particularly if the patient needs cardioversion. If you suspect digitalis toxicity, inform the doctor. He will postpone cardioversion. Meanwhile, make sure an I.V. line is in place and patent, and keep emergency equipment, antiarrhythmic drugs, and a pacemaker readily available. If the patient is alert, explain cardioversion to him. Continue to monitor cardiac rhythm, noting increased ectopy. Notify the doctor, as ordered.

Potential alteration in tissue perfusion related to decreased cardiac output.

Your goal is to prevent ischemic complications by maintaining adequate cardiac output. Check blood pressure every 2 hours for decreased systolic pressure and narrowed pulse pressure, showing reduced effective volume.

Watch for and immediately report any signs and symptoms of inadequate cerebral perfusion: yawning, mental confusion, dizziness, Stokes-Adams syndrome, convulsions, Cheyne-Stokes respirations. Then try to rule out other causes, such as use of antiarrhythmics or sensory deprivation. Be alert for signs and symptoms of inadequate myocardial perfusion: angina, myocardial infarction, left heart failure with pulmonary edema, and increased ectopy.

Alteration in pattern of urinary elimination related to inadequate renal perfusion.

Check urine output every 8 hours, every 1 to 2 hours if oliguria develops, and every hour if anuria develops. If

---

you about any symptoms, such as palpitations, dyspnea, or sensations of irregular beat. Maintain a quiet, calm environment, and help the patient understand dysrhythmia and its implications. Explain all scheduled tests and procedures (including pacemaker insertion and surgery). If dysrhythmia requires emergency treatment, offer the patient calm, reassuring, emotional support. If severe anxiety persists, administer a sedative, as ordered.

Potential alteration in cardiac output related to recurring dysrhythmia and

Sinus Bradycardia: Good Sign or Bad?

Bradycardia—a heart rate of less than 60 beats/minute—may stem from abnormal impulse formation, abnormal conduction, or both. Bradycardia does not always indicate a problem, however. An athlete in top condition may have asymptomatic *sinus* bradycardia.

Sinus bradycardia may have a noncardiac cause. Strong emotion or nausea and vomiting, which increase vagal tone, can suppress SA-node impulses. Pain can have the same effect, as can drugs such as propranolol and disorders such as hypothyroidism, increased intracranial pressure, and hypothermia.

For a patient with heart disease, however, sinus bradycardia can be dangerous. With a heart-rate decrease of just a few beats per minute, his cardiac output may drop enough to cause hypotension or chest pain. To compensate for the output drop, his heart may begin producing premature beats.

EKG features. Characteristics of sinus bradycardia include:
- heart rate less than 60 beats/minute
- regular rhythm
- P waves in a one-to-one relationship with QRS complexes
- a normal PR interval
- normal QRS complexes.

Patient care. Question the patient about medications he is taking, since drugs can cause bradycardia. Digitalis, morphine, and meperidine increase vagal tone and slow SA-node firing; beta blockers have the same effect by blocking sympathetic impulses.

If the patient complains of chest pain or dizziness, notify the doctor immediately. He may order atropine, which reduces vagal tone, increases SA-node conduction, and boosts heart rate. Or he may order isoproterenol, which increases heart rate by stimulating the sympathetic nervous system.

Give either drug cautiously, particularly if your patient has an AMI, because the oxygen demands caused by a faster heart rate could extend his infarction. With isoproterenol, monitor EKG closely. In addition to causing tachycardia, this drug may increase myocardial irritability and cause ventricular dysrhythmias. If these drugs do not increase the patient's heart rate, the doctor may insert a pacemaker.

Tachycardia-bradycardia syndrome (continuous strip)

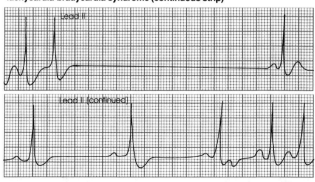

Wolff-Parkinson-White Syndrome

Wolff-Parkinson-White (WPW) syndrome commonly occurs among otherwise healthy young people. It is the most common example of *preexcitation* syndrome: any condition in which an accessory pathway bypasses some portion of the normal conduction system and provides a reentry route for electrical impulses. In WPW, impulses travel by Kent's bundle, an accessory pathway originating in an atrial wall and ending in a ventricular wall. Because impulses traveling along this pathway bypass the AV node (avoiding its delaying mechanism), they stimulate the heart prematurely.

Two dysrhythmias are associated with WPW: PSVT and atrial fibrillation with a rapid ventricular response. Either may recur frequently, possibly incapacitating the patient.

Nonsurgical treatment. Drug therapy, the first treatment for most patients, blocks premature beats that initiate reentry and delays conduction in the accessory pathway. Quinidine sulfate, which stops impulses as they pass through Kent's bundle, is effective for many patients; other drug choices include disopyramide phosphate, procainamide, propranolol hydrochloride, and amiodarone.

Mapping. If conservative measures fail, however, the doctor may sever the accessory pathway surgically. To prepare for surgery, the doctor performs an invasive mapping procedure, using an electrode catheter to locate the most likely site of the accessory pathway. Within 72 hours, he surgically severs this pathway.

---

indicated or ordered, weigh the patient daily and monitor results of laboratory tests: blood urea nitrogen, creatinine clearance, electrolyte balance (particularly potassium), and acid-base balance. Watch for changes in mental status (lethargy, confusion, anorexia, nausea, vomiting) that may indicate fluid imbalance. Know whether the drug you are administering is excreted in the urine. If it is, report altered urine output promptly.

Alteration in peripheral perfusion related to decreased coronary output.

Check all pulses for equality and quality. Assess for pallor, cooling of extremities, and claminess from peripheral arterial constriction. Report any of these signs immediately.

If necessary, assist with insertion of intraarterial lines or a pulmonary artery line (Swan-Ganz) so drugs can be given to improve peripheral perfusion. Also, position the patient to avoid compromising circulation.

Potential alteration in blood flow resulting in embolism formation related to pooling of blood from irregular myocar-

dial contraction.

To help prevent embolization, find out if the patient has a previous history of thromboembolic disease. If he does, or if his condition requires prolonged bed rest, apply antiembolism stockings and encourage range-of-motion exercises. Encourage ambulation as soon as possible. If he has chronic atrial fibrillation (a condition at higher risk for emboli) and requires cardioversion, make sure he receives anticoagulant therapy first. In any patient at high risk for emboli, watch for sudden onset of chest pain, signs and symptoms of respiratory distress, altered mental status, unexplained restlessness or anxiety, and decreased temperature, sensation, or pulses in extremities.

Potential alteration in cardiac output related to cardiac instability and possible cardiac arrest.

Be prepared to perform lifesaving resuscitation. Keep emergency equipment and drugs readily available. Keep up to date on cardiopulmonary resuscitation techniques (see "Cardiopulmonary re-

Carotid Sinus Massage

As unlikely as it may seem, a simple neck massage may halt a supraventricular tachycardia (SVT). As illustrated, carotid sinus massage results in stimulation of the vagus nerve, instantly terminating some SVTs and restoring normal sinus rhythm. It requires minimal patient cooperation—a real plus if the patient's critically ill. And it is simpler than other treatments, such as cardioversion and artificial pacing.

The doctor may also use carotid sinus massage as a diagnostic tool. Several types of dysrhythmias with similar clinical signs and EKG features can be differentiated by their responses to the maneuver. For instance, 80% to 90% of all SVTs halt abruptly after carotid sinus massage; ventricular tachycardias do not respond at all.

Minimizing risk. Before considering a patient for carotid sinus massage, the doctor will carefully evaluate both carotid arteries. If one artery is occluded, pressure applied to the other artery would reduce or eliminate the only source of cerebral blood flow.

In certain patients, carotid sinus massage can lead to prolonged asystole, life-threatening ventricular dysrhythmias, syncope, or convulsions. If the patient is over age 75 or has one of the following disorders, the doctor may decide *not* to perform carotid sinus massage or to proceed with extreme caution:

• hypertension
• coronary artery disease
• cerebrovascular disease
• diabetes
• hyperkalemia
• digitalis toxicity
• previous carotid artery surgery.

Assisting the doctor. Check hospital policy to determine if carotid sinus massage is a nursing responsibility. If it is not, assist the doctor by doing the following:

• Bring emergency resuscitation equipment to the patient's bedside.
• Position the patient on his back.
• Make sure the patient is undergoing continuous cardiac monitoring. If that is impossible, monitor cardiac rhythm by auscultating his heart and checking his pulse.

The doctor will locate the carotid sinus. With a gentle massaging motion, he will press down firmly for a few seconds.

• Monitor the patient's heart rate to see if carotid sinus massage has terminated or altered the dysrhythmia. The doctor may have to repeat the maneuver a few times to terminate the SVT.

suscitation," page 340.) Make sure you are familiar with and know how to draw up and administer emergency drugs. (See *Knowing Your Role in a Code,* page 348.) Check the defibrillator, and be prepared to defibrillate if necessary (see *How to Defibrillate,* page 350).

Self-care deficit related to lack of knowledge about pacemaker insertion.

Provide individualized teaching. Explain how the pacemaker functions and how it will correct the patient's condition. Provide written information whenever possible. Offer explanations in terms the patient understands. (See "Temporary and permanent pacemaker insertion and care," Chapter 16.)

Alteration in self-care related to lack of knowledge about home medical regimen.

Provide adequate discharge teaching. Help the patient and his family understand maintenance treatment of dysrhythmia. Explain normal heart function, dysrhythmias and the symptoms they cause, factors that might provoke them, what to do about them, and everything the patient needs to know about

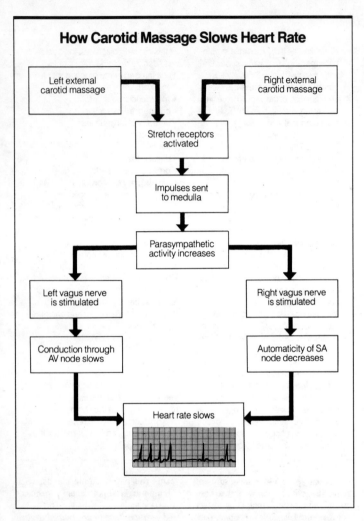

How Carotid Massage Slows Heart Rate

Left external carotid massage

Right external carotid massage

Stretch receptors activated

Impulses sent to medulla

Parasympathetic activity increases

Left vagus nerve is stimulated

Right vagus nerve is stimulated

Conduction through AV node slows

Automaticity of SA node decreases

Heart rate slows

drug therapy (purpose, dosage, timing, and side effects). If the patient has a pacemaker, explain how it works and how to care for it. Teach him when and how to take his pulse for 1 minute and when to notify his doctor of changes.

8

HYPERTENSION

I f you have ever managed hypertensive patients, you know that your biggest problem is getting them to comply with their prescribed regimens. They typically miss appointments, forget to take medications, and neglect their diets. Some sources suggest that only 13% of hypertensive patients are under good control.

Hypertension occurs as two major types: primary (essential or idiopathic), the most common, and secondary, which results from renal disease or another identifiable cause. Malignant hypertension is a severe, fulminant form of hypertension common to both types. Hypertensive crisis, which is a severely elevated blood pressure, may be fatal. (See *Glossary of Terms,* page 142.)

Primary hypertension

Hypertension is an intermittent or sustained elevation in diastolic or systolic blood pressure. It is a major cause of cerebrovascular accident, cardiac disease, and renal failure. Prognosis is good if this disorder is detected early and treatment begins before complications develop. Few conditions are as puzzling or as frustrating as primary (idiopathic or essential) hypertension. You can explain to the patient why the disease is dangerous and how it may eventually affect his body, but you cannot explain why it developed in the first place.

Causes and incidence
Hypertension affects 15% to 20% of adults in the United States. If untreated, it carries a high mortality. Risk factors for essential hypertension include family history, race (most common in blacks), stress, obesity, high dietary intake of saturated fats or sodium, use of tobacco or oral contraceptives, sedentary life-style, and aging.

Cardiac output and peripheral vascular resistance determine blood pressure. Increased blood volume, increased cardiac rate, or arteriolar vasoconstriction that increases peripheral resistance causes blood pressure to rise, but the relationship of these mechanisms to sustained hypertension is unclear. Increased blood pressure may also result from the breakdown or inappropriate response of mechanisms that intrinsically regulate it.

• The renin-angiotensin system is a neural mechanism that uses renin, a renal enzyme, to form angiotensin, a substance that directly produces vasoconstriction or indirectly stimulates the adrenal cortex to produce aldosterone, which in turn increases sodium reabsorption. Hypertonic stimulated release of antidiuretic hormone from the pituitary gland follows, increasing water reabsorption, plasma volume, cardiac output, and blood pressure. (See *How the Neuroendocrine System Responds to Blood Pressure Changes,* pages 144 and 145.)

• Changes in renal arterial pressure stimulate autoregulation of blood pressure by the kidneys. A decrease in pres-

Glossary of Terms

Hypertension is described in a variety of ways: acute or chronic (referring to blood vessel changes), benign or malignant (referring to the course of the disease), and primary or secondary (referring to the etiology of the disease). This glossary will help you understand these and other related terms.

Acute hypertension. A fluid pressure imbalance between intravascular and interstitial fluid, which increases the permeability of the arterial lining and permits fluid to shift. Edema and inflammation result.

Benign hypertension. Gradual rise in blood pressure with minimal clinical signs. The disease progresses slowly over many years, rarely causing complications until it is far advanced.

Chronic hypertension. Thickening of the medial layer of the artery from cell proliferation. Lumen narrowing restricts blood flow and reduces elasticity.

Hypertension. Sustained high blood pressure (blood pressure readings at levels associated with greater than 50% increase over expected mortality). For details on commonly accepted parameters, see the box below.

Hypertensive crisis. Acute, severe, life-threatening blood pressure rise causing rapid deterioration of brain, heart, and kidney function.

Labile hypertension. Intermittent high blood pressure.

Malignant hypertension (accelerated or necrotizing hypertension). Sudden, sustained rise in blood pressure with dramatic clinical signs. Complications appear early in the course of the disease. Fibrinoid necrosis develops in the heart, kidneys, or brain. If untreated, the disease is fatal in about 2 years.

Primary hypertension (essential or idiopathic hypertension). Sustained high blood pressure of unknown cause.

Secondary hypertension. Sustained high blood pressure caused by an identifiable disease, condition, or drug; for example, pheochromocytoma, renal artery stenosis, or oral contraceptives.

sure, for example, causes a decline in the glomerular filtration rate and increased tubular reabsorption of water, which, in turn, increase blood volume, cardiac ouput, and ultimately, blood pressure.

• Baroreceptors (pressure receptors) in the aortic arch, carotid sinus, and other large central arteries stimulate the vasomotor center to increase sympathetic stimulation of the heart by increasing epinephrine and norepinephrine levels. This increases cardiac output by strengthening the contractile force, increasing the heart rate, and augmenting peripheral resistance by vasoconstriction. Stress can also stimulate the sympathetic nervous system to increase cardiac output and peripheral vascular resistance.

• Prostaglandins, a group of at least 15 hormones derived from fatty acids, are secreted by tissue cells throughout the body. Although many of their functions are not completely understood, researchers believe that one type, prostaglandin E_2 (PGE_2), regulates blood flow through the kidneys by stimulating renal vasodilation, urinary sodium excretion, and renin release. Research indicates that PGE_2 deficiency may cause or contribute to primary hypertension.

Signs and symptoms

Hypertension usually does not produce clinical effects until vascular changes in the heart, brain, or kidneys occur. (See *Varying Stages of Hypertension*, page 146.) Severely elevated blood pressure damages the intima of small vessels, resulting in fibrin accumulation in the

vessels, development of local edema, and possibly, intravascular clotting. Symptoms produced by this process depend on the location of the damaged vessels:
- brain: cerebrovascular accident (CVA)
- retina: blindness
- heart: myocardial infarction
- kidneys: proteinuria, edema, and eventually, renal failure.

Hypertension also increases the heart's work load, leading to left ventricular hypertrophy and, eventually, to left ventricular failure, congestive heart failure, and pulmonary edema.

Diagnosis

Serial blood pressure measurements on a sphygmomanometer of more than 140/90 in persons under age 50, or 150/95 in persons over age 50 confirm hypertension. During physical examination, auscultation may reveal bruits over the abdominal aorta and the carotid, renal, and femoral arteries; ophthalmoscopy reveals arteriovenous nicking and, in hypertensive encephalopathy, papilledema. Patient history and the following additional tests may show predisposing factors and help identify an underlying cause, such as renal disease:
- *Urinalysis:* Protein, red blood cells, and white blood cells may indicate glomerulonephritis.
- *Intravenous pyelography (IVP):* Renal atrophy indicates chronic renal disease; one kidney more than ⅝" (1.5 cm) shorter than the other suggests unilateral renal disease.
- *Serum potassium:* Levels less than 3.5 mEq/liter may indicate adrenal dysfunction (primary hyperaldosteronism).
- *Blood urea nitrogen (BUN) and creatinine:* BUN normal or elevated to more than 20 mg/100 ml and creatinine normal or elevated to more than 1.5 mg/100 ml suggest renal disease.

Other tests help detect cardiovascular damage and other complications:
- *Electrocardiogram (EKG)* may show left ventricular hypertrophy or ischemia.
- *Chest X-ray* may show cardiomegaly.

Treatment

Although essential hypertension has no cure, drugs and modifications in diet and life-style can control it. Drug therapy usually begins with a diuretic alone and sympathetic blockers or vasodilators added, as needed. (See *Taking Steps to Control Hypertension,* page 147.) Life-style and dietary changes may include weight loss, relaxation techniques, regular exercise, and restriction of sodium and saturated fat intake.

Nursing management

- To encourage compliance with antihypertensive therapy, suggest the patient establish a daily routine for taking medication. Warn him that uncontrolled hypertension may cause stroke and heart attack. Tell the patient to report drug side effects. Also advise him to avoid over-the-counter cold and sinus medications, since these contain potentially harmful vasoconstrictors.
- *Assess the patient's level of understanding about hypertension:* Does he accept the fact that he has a lifelong condition requiring continuing treatment? Does he know the significance of blood pressure readings and when to report changes? Does he know how to take his blood pressure, and does he take it regularly?
- Encourage a change in dietary habits. Assist the obese patient in planning a reducing diet; stress the need to avoid foods high in sodium (pickles, potato chips, canned soups, cold cuts, processed foods) and to eliminate table salt.
- Help the patient examine and modify his life-style (such as eliminating sources of stress, exercising regularly, and decreasing or stopping smoking, as appropriate).
- Warn about alcohol intake. Explain alcohol's high caloric content and its vasodilatory and depressant effects. Check for interactions with prescribed medication and inform the patient about this verbally and in writing. The patient should be able to explain the effects of alcohol on the body and on the drugs he is taking.

How the Neuroendocrine System Responds to Blood Pressure Changes

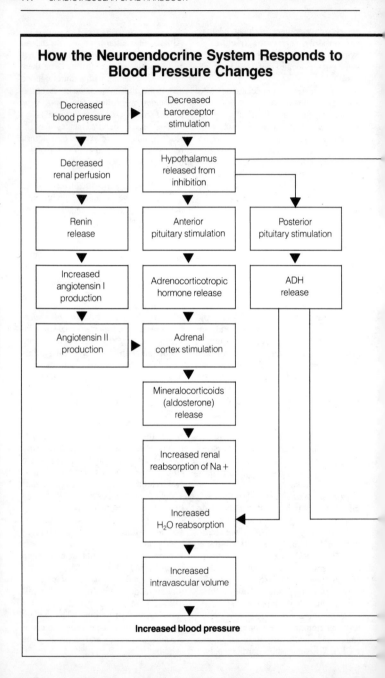

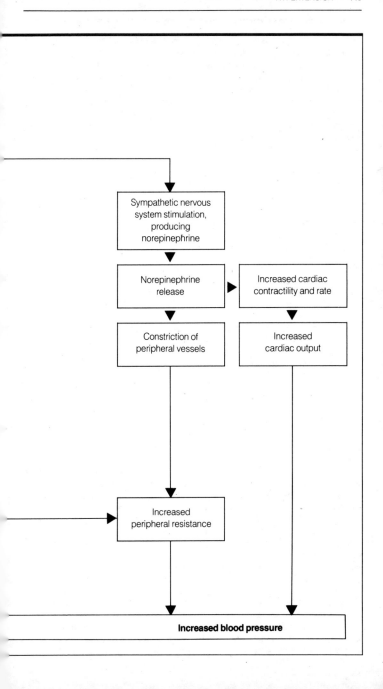

Varying Stages of Hypertension

Hypertension can be classified as primary or secondary. Primary hypertension (also called idiopathic or essential) exists in roughly 90% to 95% of patients, in whom no cause is discernible. Secondary hypertension affects the remaining 5% to 10% of those with the disease. Hypertension, whether primary or secondary, is classified as to severity based on the average of three or more diastolic blood pressure readings taken at rest, several days apart. The degrees of severity are the following:

- Class I (mild) 90 to 104 mm Hg
- Class II (moderate) 105 to 114 mm Hg
- Class III (severe) 115 mm Hg.

Common usage calls the hypertension in the first category mild. However, even at this lowest level, the risk of cardiovascular sequelae is at least twice that of normotensive persons.

Severe hypertension is further classified as either accelerated or malignant. Accelerated hypertension means blood pressure has risen to severely elevated levels in a short time. The patient with accelerated hypertension may have Grade III retinopathy (retinal exudates and hemorrhages) and a high diastolic pressure—usually above 120 mm Hg. Malignant hypertension means the patient has Grade IV retinopathy (papilledema, or swelling around the optic disk) and an even higher diastolic pressure—usually above 140 mm Hg.

The severest form of hypertension—hypertensive crisis—occurs when elevated blood pressure causes an immediate threat to the patient's life by compromising cerebral, cardiovascular, or renal function. Hypertensive crisis is not tied to a particular blood pressure level but is based on the patient's total clinical status.

You may also hear hypertension described as labile and resistant. In *labile* hypertension, blood pressure elevations occur intermittently; *resistant* hypertension is unresponsive to usual treatment.

- Teach effective stress management. Encourage the patient to verbalize his feelings. Help him identify the stressors in his own environment. Explore ways to help him cope with stress, such as taking leisurely meals or spacing activities to avoid hurrying. Help him to distinguish avoidable stressors from unavoidable ones. Teach relaxation techniques, if desired and appropriate. Recommend counseling to help him change a stressful life-style.
- Plan for chronic care. Your role in managing chronic care of hypertension has been defined by the National Task Force on the Role of Nursing in High Blood Pressure Control. This group defines the following goals of nursing care:
1. to help the patient and family recognize behaviors that promote health and so maintain stable blood pressure at the desired level with minimal target organ damage
2. to assist the patient and family in complying with the demands of therapy by supporting successful adjustments to diagnosis and therapy and by monitoring drug therapy to minimize side effects
3. to instruct, guide, and support patients in achieving and maintaining self-care so they can understand hypertension and prescribed therapy, assume responsibility for self care, and maintain stable blood pressure at the desired level.
- Explain postural hypotension. Because some patients receiving certain drugs may experience postural hypotension, explain to the patient why he may feel dizzy or faint when he stands suddenly from a lying position. Warn him to sit for a few minutes before standing up. If dizziness persists longer than 1 to

Taking Steps to Control Hypertension

For most patients with hypertension, the doctor will begin drug therapy by pre-scribing a diuretic. Before he proceeds to the next step, he will rule out poor patient compliance, excessive sodium intake or retention, use of vasoconstrict-ing drugs (such as over-the-counter cold remedies), and secondary hyperten-sion as reasons for the failure of the diuretic.

STEP 1: Diuretics

Unless contraindicated, initially give a thiazide (or thiazide-like) diuretic, as or-dered. A patient with special problems (for example, renal insufficiency) may need a loop diuretic or a potassium-sparing agent along with the thiazide di-uretic.

STEP 2: Adrenergic Inhibitors

The doctor will add a beta blocker, guanabenz acetate, clonidine hydrochloride, or methyldopa if the diuretic alone does not control blood pressure. Increase the initial dosage gradually until the drug produces the desired effect. If the dosage reaches the maximum level without producing the desired effect, or if adverse reactions appear, the doctor may add a Step 3 drug.

STEP 3: Vasodilators

The doctor will prescribe hydralazine hydrochloride or prazosin hydrochloride along with Step 1 and Step 2 drugs. Even if the doctor proceeds to a Step 3 drug because the Step 2 drug caused adverse reactions, he will continue some dosage of the adrenergic inhibitor. By doing so, he minimizes the effect of the vasodilator on the patient's heart rate.

STEP 4: Additions or Substitutions

If the patient is complying with all parts of his regimen but his blood pressure is still uncontrolled, the doctor may proceed to Step 4 of antihypertensive drug therapy. He may order a stronger adrenergic inhibitor (guanethidine sulfate) or a stronger vasodilator (minoxidil) in addition to or instead of the Step 2 or Step 3 drug. Or, he may prescribe the angiotensin-conversion inhibitor captopril.

2 minutes, the patient should sit or lie down and either decrease or omit his next scheduled drug dose; he should no-tify his doctor if dizziness continues. Encourage the patient to sleep with his head elevated; to avoid prolonged stand-ing, especially in the sun; and to avoid alcohol because of its vasodilatory ef-fects. Tell him that taking the drug at bedtime may minimize postural effects.

• Warn the patient appropriately about side effects and strongly warn against sudden discontinuation of drug treat-ment. Be sure to explain that sudden discontinuation can cause hypertensive rebound, and that drug treatment should always be stopped slowly under the doc-tor's supervision. Provide a written list of the most common side effects and what he should do about them. Recog-nize that the patient who feels fine be-fore treatment may be annoyed by side effects. Encourage him to verbalize his feelings and offer sympathy and under-standing. But emphasize that taking a drug is easier than treating complica-tions.

• Anticipate hypokalemia. Explain that certain diuretics may cause potassium deficit. To minimize potassium loss, teach the patient who must take these diuretics about the symptoms of potas-sium deficit and how to prevent it. Con-sider that he may need an adjustment of dosage or substitution of a potassium-sparing diuretic. Tell the to watch for fatigue, leg cramps, and other symp-toms of hypokalemia (provide a written list of the common ones). Also provide a list of foods high in potassium. Inform

the patient that potassium deficit needs treatment with a supplement when the potassium level in the blood drops below 3 mEq/liter or causes symptoms. Be sure to inform such a patient that replacing potassium deficit from dietary sources alone is very difficult. Instruct him how to prevent it. Instruct him to mix the prescribed potassium supplement in chilled fruit juice, preferably orange juice, to make it more palatable, and to take it after meals to minimize gastric irritation. Teach the patient that normal dietary intake of potassium should be 50 to 100 mEq/day (four glasses of orange juice or seven bananas contain 60 mEq of potassium).
• Consider sexual dysfunction. If the patient complains of sexual dysfunction after taking an antihypertensive drug, this may be a drug-related effect. However, remind the patient that such dysfunction can result from other causes, including alcohol, diabetes, stress, and marital difficulties. Initiate careful evaluation if the problem persists. It may require a change in drug therapy or referral for counseling.
• Make sure the patient understands the difference between control and cure. Inform him of what the desired blood pressure (goal) is for him. Avoid describing this goal as "normal" blood pressure. Instead, reinforce the term "well controlled" when he reaches the goal.

If a patient is hospitalized with hypertension:
• Find out if he was taking his prescribed medication. If he was not, ask why. If the patient cannot afford the medication, refer him to an appropriate social service agency. Tell him and his family to keep a record of drugs used in the past, noting especially which ones were or were not effective. Suggest that he record this information on a card so he can show it to his doctor.

When routine blood pressure screening reveals elevated pressure:
• Make sure the cuff size is appropriate for the circumference of the patient's upper arm. (See *Compensating for Improper Cuff Size*, page 149; *Korotkoff*

Sounds, page 150; and *Palpatory Systolic Pressure*, page 151.)
• Take the pressure in both arms in lying, sitting, and standing positions.
• Ask the patient if he smoked, drank a beverage containing caffeine, or was emotionally upset before the test.
• Advise the patient to return for blood pressure testing at frequent and regular intervals if his pressure is borderline.

To help identify hypertension and prevent untreated hypertension:
• Participate in public education programs dealing with hypertension and ways to reduce risk factors. Encourage public participation in blood pressure screening programs. Routinely screen all patients, especially those at risk (blacks and persons with family histories of hypertension, stroke, or heart attack).

Secondary hypertension

Unlike primary hypertension, secondary hypertension—which accounts for between 5% and 10% of all hypertension cases—has known causes. Many causes of secondary hypertension are curable.

In addition to the causes detailed below, the following conditions may lead to secondary hypertension: toxemia of pregnancy, increased intracranial pressure (for example, from a brain tumor or hematoma), and advanced collagen disease. Some drugs (such as oral contraceptives and monoamine oxidase inhibitors) may also trigger hypertension.

Causes, signs, and symptoms
• Coarctation of the aorta commonly causes systolic hypertension. Diastolic hypertension also may be present, if coarctation of the abdominal aorta is compromising renal circulation.
• This obstruction of the aorta causes hypertension in the aortic branches above the constriction—the arteries that supply blood to the arms and brain—and diminished blood pressure and pulses in vessels below the constriction. As a result, the patient's legs may be

Compensating for Improper Cuff Size

ARM CIRCUMFER-ENCE (cm)	CORRECTIONS (mm Hg)					
	REGULAR CUFF (12 x 23 cm)		LARGE CUFF (15 x 33 cm)		THIGH CUFF (18 x 36 cm)	
	Systolic	Diastolic	Systolic	Diastolic	Systolic	Diastolic
20	+11	+7	+11	+7	+11	+7
22	+9	+6	+9	+6	+11	+6
24	+7	+4	+8	+5	+10	+6
26	+5	+3	+7	+5	+9	+5
28	+3	+2	+5	+4	+8	+5
30	0	0	+4	+3	+7	+4
32	−2	−1	+3	+2	+6	+4
34	−4	−3	+2	+1	+5	+3
36	−6	−4	0	+1	+5	+3
38	−8	−6	−1	0	+4	+2
40	−10	−7	−2	−1	+3	+1
42	−12	−9	−4	−2	+2	+1
44	−14	−10	−5	−3	+1	0
46	−16	−11	−6	−3	0	0
48	−18	−13	−7	−4	−1	−1
50	−21	−14	−9	−5	−1	−1
52	−23	−16	−10	−6	−2	−2
54	−25	−17	−11	−7	−3	−2
56	−27	−19	−13	−7	−4	−3

Courtesy of *The Lancet*

poorly developed.
• Pressure in the left ventricle increases, causing dilation of the proximal aorta and ventricular hypertrophy.
• Collateral circulation above the obstruction may cause the intercostal arteries to dilate, producing rib notching (an important diagnostic sign).
• If a ventricular septal defect accompanies coarctation, blood shunts from left to right, straining the right side of the heart. This leads to pulmonary hypertension and eventually right ventricular hypertrophy and failure.

Symptoms include: headache, lower extremity claudication, leg blood pressure 20 mmHg less than arm pressure, and reduced femoral pulses.

In renovascular hypertension, causes include increased systemic blood pressure from atherosclerotic narrowing of the renal artery (most common in men aged 40 to 70) or fibroplasia of the renal artery's medial layer (most common in women age 20 to 50). Other causes include anomalies of the renal arteries, embolism, tumors and other lesions, dissecting aneurysm, or trauma. This hypertension type affects 1% to 2% of

Korotkoff Sounds

Korotkoff sounds are produced by blood movement and vessel vibration as you deflate a blood pressure cuff. As indicated below, these sounds have five phases.

You'll note systolic pressure when you hear Korotkoff phase I. But not everyone agrees on which Korotkoff phase indicates *diastolic* pressure. Some authorities specify phase IV; others, phase V. As a result, some hospitals require documentation of both phases in addition to phase I; for example, 126/70/66. Check your hospital's policy.

Phase I: Onset of a faint, clear tapping sound that gradually intensifies.

Phase II: Murmur or swishing sound.

Phase III: Crisper, louder sounds; more intensive tapping sounds.

Phase IV: Muffled tapping; softer sound that disappears.

Phase V: Silence.

all hypertensive adults.

• Stenosis or occlusion of the renal artery causes ischemia, which stimulates the affected kidney to release excessive amounts of renin and triggers the renin-angiotensin-aldosterone system. Eventually hypertension damages the unaffected kidney. When examining the patient, watch for a recent onset of accelerated hypertensive abdominal bruit on auscultation.

Acute and chronic glomerulonephritis and pylonephritis causes inflammatory changes in the kidney's interstitia and glomeruli.

• The inflammation interferes with the nephrons' excretory ability. Consequently, the kidneys lose their capacity to excrete sodium. The inflammation also interferes with blood flow, triggering the renin-angiotensin-aldosterone system.

• *Pyelonephritis*, a sudden inflammation in the interstitium, may be caused by an infection spreading from the bladder to the ureters, then to the kidneys. Vesicourethral reflux may develop. Chronic pyelonephritis is a persistent kidney infection that leads to kidney scarring and chronic renal failure.

• With *glomerulonephritis*, disease characteristics occur 10 days to 3 weeks after an infection. The kidney becomes swollen, fatty, and congested. A bloody exudate seeps from capillaries, infiltrating renal parenchyma and dimishing renal function.

As with any renal disease, the patient shows signs of dysuria, nocturia, hematuria, and recurrent urinary tract infections.

Cushing's syndrome is the excessive excretion of adrenocorticotropic hormone (ACTH), which causes hyperplasia of the adrenal cortex. Possible causes, seen in about 70% of all cases, are pituitary tumors or tumors in other tissues (sometimes called ectopic ACTH syndrome).

• In the other 30%, an adrenal tumor secretes cortisol. Cortisol, like aldosterone, promotes sodium reabsorption and potassium and hydrogen excretion.

• Patients experience persistent hyperglycemia, tissue wasting, and abnormal fat distribution along with moon face, short, thick neck, prominent abdomen, thin extremities, straie, and hirsutism.

In hyperaldosteronsim, excessive aldosterone secretion causes excessive sodium reabsorption. As the kidneys reabsorb sodium, they simultaneously excrete potassium and hydrogen. The increased sodium reabsorption not only increases intravascular fluid volume, but also causes an electrolyte imbalance from excessive potassium and hydrogen excretion (resulting in hypokalemia and metabolic alkalosis). Excessive potassium loss may lead to muscle cramps and weakness, cardiac dysrhythmias, and polyuria.

• *Primary aldosteronism* is caused by an aldosterone-producing adrenal adenoma in about 75% of all patients; most of these adenomas are benign. Another cause is bilateral adrenal hyperplasia (cell proliferation), which affects most of the remaining 25% of patients.

• *Secondary aldosteronism* is usually caused by extra-adrenal pathology that stimulates increased aldosterone production. Ovarian tumors, for example, may secrete aldosterone.

• *Pseudoaldosteronism* is caused by eating large amounts of licorice, which contains glycyrrhizic acid. This chemical is similar to aldosterone in its effects.

Pheochromocytoma affects only about 0.1% to 0.3% of all hypertensive patients. About 10% of patients with pheochromocytoma have bilateral adrenal pheochromocytoma, and about 10% have a malignant tumor.

• The tumor causes excessive secretion of the catecholamines epinephrine and norepinephrine. This may cause sustained or intermittent hypertension, thinness, headache, sweating, palpitations, elevated fasting blood sugar, orthostatic hypotension, and pallor.

Flank or renal trauma and hyperparathyroidism may also be a cause of secondary hypertension.

Diagnosis

If the doctor suspects that the patient's hypertension has a secondary cause, he will order specific laboratory tests to confirm his suspicions. Because these additional tests are expensive, he will order them only if the patient is at particular risk of secondary hypertension. Appropriate circumstances include the following:

• The patient is younger than age 20 or older than age 50.

• His hypertension has a rapid onset (especially if he has no family history of the problem).

• Routine laboratory test results suggest secondary hypertension.

• He does not respond to antihypertensive therapy.

• His hypertension suddenly worsens.

• He develops an abdominal bruit.

These tests include:

• IVP
• Renal angiography
• Rapid sequence IVP
• Plasma renin activity
• Renal vein renin concentration
• Serum aldosterone
• Urine aldosterone
• Abdominal computerized tomography
• Vanillylmandelic acid
• Urine catecholamines
• Plamsa cortisol
• Serum calcium.

Palpatory Systolic Pressure

In some patients, Korotkoff sounds temporarily vanish during one of the phases, usually phase II. Called the *auscultatory gap*, this phenomenon may mislead you into recording an erroneously low systolic pressure or, less commonly, an erroneously high diastolic pressure.

Avoid either error by determining the patient's palpatory systolic pressure *before* you take a blood pressure reading. Then, when taking the reading, inflate the cuff 20 to 30 mm Hg higher than this pressure. By doing so, you will be sure to inflate the cuff adequately for arterial occlusion.

To determine palpatory systolic pressure, follow this procedure:

• Apply the blood pressure cuff and palpate the radial pulse.

• Rapidly inflate the cuff.

• Note the pressure reading at the point when you no longer feel the radial pulse. Continue to inflate the cuff until the pressure is 20 mm Hg higher than this point.

• Release the air in the cuff at a rate of 2 mm/second. Note the point at which the radial pulse returns. This is the palpatory systolic pressure. As a rule, it is 5 to 10 mm Hg lower than auscultatory systolic pressure. (For details on Korotkoff sounds, including how to augment them when they are hard to hear, see Chapter 3, Assessment of the Cardiovascular System.)

Treatment

Unlike primary hypertension, secondary hypertension does not follow a predictable treatment regimen due to the complex nature of the causes. Treatment modalities may include a combination of drugs, surgery, diet, and palliative measures.

Nursing management

The approach used depends on the cause of the secondary hypertension.

When diagnostic tests and surgery are performed, patient teaching is extremely important. Pretest and preoperative teaching will help prepare the patient for what he will be going through and will also help to allay some of his fears. Post-test and postoperative teaching will keep him informed of his condition and prepare him for the next step in his therapy.

If the patient is being treated with medication or diet, try to educate him on all aspects of his particular regimen to improve compliance.

Hypertensive crisis

Hypertensive crisis is a severe rise in arterial blood pressure caused by a disturbance in one or more of three blood pressure-regulating mechanisms: Arterial baroreceptors, fluid volume regulation, and the renin-angiotension system.

Prolonged hypertension results in inflammation and necrosis of arterioles, narrowing blood vessels and restricting blood flow to major organs. When blood flow is severely compromised, organ damage results. Hypertensive crisis may be fatal.

Causes

The sudden, extreme, and life-threatening blood pressure elevation known as hypertensive crisis may be caused by a number of conditions. Primary hypertension can lead to crisis if it is not treated properly and an acute blood pressure increase occurs, or if an acute blood pressure increase is accompanied by a complication such as acute dissecting aortic aneurysm, leaking abdominal aortic aneurysm, or intracranial hemorrhage.

Secondary hypertension can also cause hypertensive crisis if the primary condition—for example, pheochromocytoma, acute or chronic glomerulonephritis, renovascular hypertension, or pregnancy-induced hypertension (PIH)—becomes more severe.

Antihypertensive drug withdrawal and interactions between foods and drugs are other possible causes of hypertensive crisis. If the patient is taking a monoamine oxidase inhibitor, such as pargyline hydrochloride or phenelzine sulfate (Nardil), he is at risk of crisis if he ingests anything contining tyramine—for example, avocados, Chianti wine, imported beer, chicken livers, chocolate, meats prepared with tenderizers, caviar, pickled herring, sausage meats, aged or processed cheese, or yeast extract.

Similarly, some drug interactions—for example, an interaction between guanethidine sulfate and cyclic antidepressants—can trigger hypertensive crisis.

Signs and symptoms

A patient's blood pressure reading is not the most valuable indicator of whether he is in hypertensive crisis. What is important is whether his life is in immediate danger from cerebral, cardiovascular, or renal compromise. In other words, if a patient's diastolic pressure is 140 but he is resting comfortably, then he is *not* in crisis. On the other hand, you *should* suspect crisis if a previously diagnosed hypertensive patient has some or all of the signs and symptoms listed below—even if his diastolic pressure is only moderately high.

Signs and symptoms that may accompany hypertensive crisis include:

- headache
- nausea and vomiting
- blurred vision
- drowsiness
- confusion

- limb numbness or tingling
- convulsions
- coma
- azotemia
- chest pain
- oliguria
- hemorrhagic exudates and papilledema on funduscopy
- shortness of breath.

Important: Signs and symptoms of hypertensive crisis may mimic those of other life-threatening conditions, such as CVA. Take into consideration the entire clinical picture—including the patient's history—before making a judgment. (See *How Crisis Affects Target Organs,* page 153, and *Organ Changes in Hypertensive Crisis,* page 154.)

Suspect CVA if the patient:
- shows focal or lateralizing neurologic signs, rather than generalized ones
- develops neurologic deficits suddenly, rather than progressively.

Diagnosis

Confirmation of the diagnosis is based on the patient's history and physical examination, a chest X-ray to determine the presence of cardiomegaly or left ventricular prominence, and an EKG to detect possible left ventricular hypertrophy and ischemia.

How Crisis Affects Target Organs

Four target organs are most severely affected by acute high blood pressure—the brain, eyes, heart, and kidney.

The brain. Although no one knows exactly how crisis affects the brain, two theories offer possible explanations. One is that crisis causes severe vasoconstriction. Vasoconstriction, in turn, may lead to cerebral ischemia and tissue damage.

The other possibility is that disturbances in the blood-brain barrier associated with acute hypertension allow fluid to accumulate in brain tissue. As edema builds, the patient shows signs and symptoms of hypertensive encephalopathy: severe headache, agitation or irritability, nausea and vomiting, blurred vision, drowsiness, confusion, numbness or tingling in arms or legs, convulsions, and coma.

The eye. You will see the effects of severe vasoconstriction when you examine the patient's retinal arteries. During a funduscopic exam, the retinal arteries may appear thready and one-third to one-fourth their normal size. Or, you may not be able to see them at all. If your patient suffered accelerated or malignant hypertension before the crisis occurred, you may also see grade III or IV retinopathy.

The heart. During hypertensive crisis, high blood pressure increases heart wall stress. As pressure builds, blood flow to the heart's subendocardial layer decreases. As the wall becomes ischemic, left ventricle compliance decreases, raising left ventricular end-diastolic pressure (filling pressure). Rising pressure and ischemia cause the heart to pump less efficiently. Then, as the heart begins to fail, blood backs up into the lungs, causing pulmonary edema. (Remember, the left ventricle may already be compromised by hypertrophy, a common complication of sustained hypertension.) Consequently, the hypertensive crisis patient may suffer acute shortness of breath.

The kidney. Just as hypertensive crisis causes severe cerebral vasoconstriction, crisis may cause severe vasoconstriction of the arterioles of the kidneys. Impaired renal circulation causes proteinuria, microscopic hematuria, and renal insufficiency leading to renal failure.

Note: Hypertensive crisis may also cause hemolytic anemia resulting from red blood cell damage secondary to vasoconstriction.

Organ Changes in Hypertensive Crisis

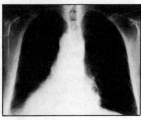

Chest X-Ray
Left ventricular hypertrophy, shown above, contributes to heart failure during hypertensive crisis.

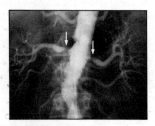

Renal Arteriogram
The X-ray shows constriction of both renal arteries (see arrows). The right renal artery is more constricted than the left.

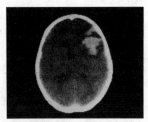

CT Scan: Head
A CT scan reveals left frontal hemorrhage (the white area) and surrounding edema (the black area).

Treatment

The first priority in hypertensive crisis treatment is to lower the patient's blood pressure. This is done by administratering antihypertensive drugs parenterally. (See Chapter 17, Cardiovascular Drug Therapy.)

A typical protocol will begin with a low drug dose. The patient's response will be carefully evaluated before proceeding.

Unless the patient responds dramatically, the doctor then gradually increases the infusion rate until the blood pressure starts dropping. Then, he will order a maintenance infusion rate. Once blood pressure stabilizes at the desired level (this may take days), the transition from I.V. to oral medication begins.

Make sure that every medication change is preceded and followed by a blood pressure reading. Watch closely for hypotension and signs of heart failure, such as tachycardia, tachypnea, dyspnea, pulmonary rales, S_3 sounds, neck vein distention, and edema.

Nursing management

Plan your interventions around the patient's condition.
• If you find severely elevated blood pressure, immediately remeasure blood pressure in both arms.
• Explain what you are doing to allay the patient's fears and gain his cooperation.
• Have him lie down in a comfortable position, away from any commotion, if possible. Report your findings to the doctor.
• Prepare to obtain a chest X-ray and EKG.
• Prepare to collect blood and urine samples for laboratory studies.
• Prepare the patient for transfer to the intensive care unit (ICU) if he is not already there.
• Establish an I.V. setup that will permit you to quickly discontinue the antihypertensive drug without sacrificing the line's patency.
• Give antihypertensive drugs, as ordered, through an infusion pump to en-

sure accuracy.
• If the patient does not have an arterial line, document his blood pressure at least every 2 minutes (or as ordered) during initial drug therapy; less frequently (but regularly) as his condition stabilizes.
• Monitor and record pulse rate, respiratory status, and fluid intake and output.
• Document any changes in physical or mental status, all medications administered, and laboratory test results.

Nursing diagnoses

Integrate the subjective data from the patient history and the objective data from your assessment to formulate nursing diagnoses.

Your diagnoses should consider the severity of hypertension, the patient's emotional state and cognitive ability to comply with treatment, and the effects of hypertention on the body systems. Keeping this in mind, you can plan appropriate goals and interventions, such as the following:

Alteration in comfort relating to pain (headache or chest pain), nausea and vomiting, shortness of breath, and so forth.

Alteration in urinary output related to the retention of fluids and edema.

Your goals are to administer medications as ordered and provide support and comfort measures. If these symptoms are side effects to antihypertensive medication, notify the doctor so he can make adjustments.

Potential noncompliance with medical regimen related to patient's perception of his own health status.

Your goal is to teach the patient as much about his condition as possible using language that is easily understood. Write important points down for him for future reference. Listen to the kinds of questions he asks to judge his level of understanding.

Disturbance in self-concept related to change in life-style.

Your goal is to help the patient readjust his daily life-style to accomodate the disease process and treatment regimen.

9

INFLAMMATORY, INFECTIOUS, AND VALVULAR DISORDERS

In the past, inflammatory, infectious, and valvular diseases of the heart were much more common and almost always fatal. But although antibiotics, cardiac catheterization, and prosthetic valve replacements have made these disorders more manageable, they still produce life-threatening changes in the heart and its structures—changes that are often difficult to recognize and treat.

Rheumatic fever and rheumatic heart disease

Acute rheumatic fever is a systemic inflammatory disease of childhood, often recurrent, that follows a Group A beta-hemolytic streptococcal infection. Rheumatic heart disease refers to the cardiac manifestations of rheumatic fever and includes pancarditis (myocarditis, pericarditis, and endocarditis) during the early acute phase and chronic valvular disease later. Long-term antibiotic therapy can minimize recurrence of rheumatic fever, reducing the risk of permanent cardiac damage and eventual valvular deformity. However, severe pancarditis occasionally produces fatal congestive heart failure (CHF) during the acute phase. Of the patients who survive this complication, about 20% die within 10 years.

Causes and incidence
Rheumatic fever appears to be a hypersensitivity reaction to a Group A beta-hemolytic streptococcal infection, in which antibodies manufactured to combat streptococci react and produce characteristic lesions at specific tissue sites, especially in the heart and joints. Since very few persons (0.3%) with streptococcal infections ever contract rheumatic fever, altered host resistance must be involved in its development or recurrence. Although rheumatic fever tends to be familial, this may merely reflect contributing environmental factors. For example, in lower socioeconomic groups, incidence is highest in children between ages 5 and 15, probably as a result of malnutrition and crowded living conditions. This disease strikes most often during cool, damp weather in the winter and early spring. In the United States, it is most common in the northern states.

Signs and symptoms
In 95% of patients, rheumatic fever characteristically follows a streptococcal infection that appeared a few days to 6 weeks earlier. A temperature of at least 100.4° F. (38° C.) occurs, and most patients complain of migratory joint pain or *polyarthritis*. Swelling, redness, and signs of effusion usually accompany such pain, which most commonly affects the knees, ankles, elbows, or hips. In 5% of patients (generally those with carditis), rheumatic fever causes skin lesions such as *erythema marginatum,* a nonpruritic, macular, transient rash that gives rise to red lesions with blanched centers. Rheumatic fever may also produce firm, movable, nontender, *subcutaneous nodules* about 3 mm to 2 cm in

diameter, usually near tendons or bony prominences of joints (especially the elbows, knuckles, wrists, and knees) and less often on the scalp and backs of the hands. These nodules persist for a few days to several weeks and, like erythema marginatum, often accompany carditis.

Later, rheumatic fever may cause transient *chorea,* which develops up to 6 months after the original streptococcal infection. Mild chorea may produce hyperirritability, a deterioration in handwriting, or inability to concentrate. Severe chorea causes purposeless, nonrepetitive, involuntary muscle spasms, poor muscle coordination, and weakness. It always resolves without residual neurologic damage.

The most destructive effect of rheumatic fever is *carditis,* which develops in up to 50% of patients and may affect the endocardium, myocardium, pericardium, or heart valves. Pericarditis causes a pericardial friction rub and, occasionally, pain and effusion. Myocarditis produces characteristic lesions called Aschoff's bodies (in the acute stages) and cellular swelling and fragmentation of interstitial collagen, leading to formation of a progressively fibrotic nodule and interstitial scars. Endocarditis causes valve leaflet swelling, erosion along the lines of leaflet closure, and blood, platelet, and fibrin deposits, which form beadlike vegetations. Endocarditis affects the mitral valve most often in women; the aortic, most often in men. In both women and men, endocarditis affects the tricuspid valves occasionally and the pulmonic only rarely. (See *Effects of Rheumatic Fever on Heart Wall.*)

Severe rheumatic carditis may cause CHF, with dyspnea, upper right quadrant pain, tachycardia, tachypnea, a hacking nonproductive cough, edema, and significant mitral and aortic murmurs. The most common of such murmurs include:
• a systolic murmur of mitral regurgitation (high-pitched, blowing, holosystolic, loudest at apex, possibly radiating to the anterior axillary line)

> # Effects of Rheumatic Fever on Heart Wall
>
> Rheumatic fever can affect one or more layers of the heart wall. If it affects all three layers, the condition is called rheumatic pancarditis.
>
> **Rheumatic myocarditis**
> Aschoff nodules usually form in the connective tissue surrounding small arteries of the myocardium. These nodules result from accumulation of leukocytes in inflamed tissues. The nodules eventually heal and become fibrotic.
>
> Rheumatic myocarditis may cause temporary loss of myocardial contractility but rarely causes permanent damage.
>
> **Rheumatic pericarditis**
> Lesions result from diffuse, nonspecific fibrinous inflammation. They may cause pericardial friction rub but usually cause no serious, long-term effects.
>
> **Rheumatic endocarditis**
> Tiny, beadlike excrescences form along the edges of valve leaflets and can cause permanent, severe valvular dysfunction.

• a midsystolic murmur due to stiffening and swelling of the mitral leaflet
• occasionally, a diastolic murmur of aortic regurgitation (low-pitched, rumbling, and almost inaudible). Valvular disease may eventually result in chronic valvular stenosis and insufficiency, including mitral stenosis and regurgitation and aortic regurgitation. In children, mitral insufficiency remains the major sequela of rheumatic heart disease.

Diagnosis
Diagnosis depends on recognition of one or more classic symptoms (carditis, polyarthritis, chorea, erythema marginatum, or subcutaneous nodules) and a detailed patient history (See *Jones Criteria (Revised) for Diagnosis of Rheu-*

Jones Criteria (Revised) for Diagnosis of Rheumatic Fever*

Major manifestations	Minor manifestations	Supporting evidence of streptococcal infection
Carditis	*Clinical*	Increased titer of antistreptococcal antibodies, ASO (antistreptolysin O), others
Polyarthritis	Previous rheumatic fever or rheumatic heart disease	
Chorea	Arthralgia	
Erythema marginatum	Fever	Positive throat culture for group A streptococcus
Subcutaneous nodules	*Laboratory*	Recent scarlet fever
	Acute phase reactants Erythrocyte sedimentation rate, C-reactive protein, leukocytosis	
	Prolonged PR interval	

*The presence of two major criteria, or of one major and two minor criteria, indicates a high probability of acute rheumatic fever, *if supported by evidence of preceding Group A streptococcal infection*.

Source: *American Heart Association, 1982.*

matic Fever). Laboratory data support the diagnosis:
• *White blood count (WBC)* and *erythrocyte sedimentation rate (ESR)* may be elevated (especially during the acute phase); blood studies show slight anemia, due to suppressed erythropoiesis during inflammation.
• *C-reactive protein* is positive (especially during acute phase).
• *Cardiac enzymes* may be increased in severe carditis.
• *Antistreptolysin O titer* is elevated in 95% of patients within 2 months of onset.
• *Electrocardiogram (EKG)* changes are not diagnostic; however, 20% of patients show a prolonged P-R interval.
• *Chest X-rays* show normal heart size (except with myocarditis, CHF, or pericardial effusion).
• *Echocardiography* helps identify valvular damage, chamber size, and ventricular function.
• *Cardiac catheterization* evaluates valvular damage and left ventricular func-

tion in severe cardiac dysfunction.

Treatment
Effective management eradicates the streptococcal infection, relieves symptoms, and prevents recurrence, reducing the chance of permanent cardiac damage. During the acute phase, treatment includes penicillin or (for patients with penicillin hypersensitivity) erythromycin. Salicylates, such as aspirin, relieve fever and minimize joint swelling and pain; if carditis is present or salicylates fail to relieve pain and inflammation, corticosteroids may be used. Supportive treatment requires strict bed rest for about 5 weeks during the acute phase with active carditis, followed by a progressive increase in physical activity, depending on clinical and laboratory findings and the response to treatment.

After the acute phase subsides, a monthly intramuscular injection of penicillin G benzathine or daily doses of oral sulfadiazine or penicillin G may be used to prevent recurrence. Such preventive treatment usually continues for at least 5 years or until age 25. CHF necessitates continued bed rest and diuretics. Severe mitral or aortic valvular dysfunction causing persistent CHF requires corrective valvular surgery, including commissurotomy (separation of the adherent, thickened leaflets of the mitral valve), valvuloplasty (repair of valve), or valve replacement (with prosthetic valve). Corrective valvular surgery is rarely necessary before late adolescence or early adulthood.

Nursing management

Because rheumatic fever and rheumatic heart disease require prolonged treatment, your care plan should include comprehensive patient teaching to promote compliance with the prescribed therapy.

• Before giving penicillin, ask the patient or his parents if has ever had a hypersensitive reaction to it. Even if the answer is no, warn that such a reaction is possible. Tell the patient or family to stop the drug and call the doctor immediately if the patient develops a rash, fever, chills, or other signs of allergy *at any time* during penicillin therapy.

• Instruct the patient and his family to watch for and report early signs of CHF such as dyspnea and a hacking, nonproductive cough.

• Stress the need for bed rest during the acute phase and suggest appropriate, physically undemanding diversions. After the acute phase, encourage family and friends to spend as much time as possible with the patient to minimize boredom. Advise parents to secure a tutor to help the child keep up with schoolwork during the long convalescence.

• Help parents overcome any guilt feelings about the child's illness. Tell them that failure to seek treatment for streptococcal infection is common, since this illness often seems no worse than a cold. Encourage parents and child to vent their frustrations during the long, tedious recovery. If the child has severe carditis, help them prepare for permanent

changes in his life-style.

• Teach the patient and family about this disease and its treatment. Warn parents to watch for and immediately report signs of recurrent streptococcal infection—sudden sore throat, diffuse throat redness and oropharyngeal exudate, swollen and tender cervical lymph glands, pain on swallowing, temperature of 101° to 104° F. (38.3° to 40° C.), headache, and nausea. Urge them to keep the child away from people with respiratory tract infections.

• Promote good dental hygiene to prevent gingival infection. Make sure the patient and family understand the importance of complying with prolonged antibiotic therapy and follow-up care and the need for additional antibiotics during dental surgery. Arrange for a visiting nurse to oversee home care, if necessary.

Myocarditis

Myocarditis is focal or diffuse inflammation of the cardiac muscle (myocardium). It may be acute or chronic and can occur at any age. Frequently, myocarditis fails to produce specific cardiovascular symptoms or EKG abnormalities, and recovery is usually spontaneous, without residual defects. Occasionally, myocarditis is complicated by CHF and, rarely, leads to cardiomyopathy.

Causes

Myocarditis results from:

• *viral infections* (most common cause in the United States): Coxsackievirus A and B strains and, possibly, poliomyelitis, influenza, rubeola, rubella, and adenoviruses and echoviruses

• *bacterial infections:* diphtheria, tuberculosis, typhoid fever, tetanus, and staphylococcal, pneumococcal, and gonococcal infections

• *hypersensitive immune reactions:* acute rheumatic fever and postcardiotomy syndrome

Causes of Inflammatory Conditions

Myocarditis
Viral infection, especially Coxsackie A and B strains
Bacterial and parasitic infection
Rheumatic fever
Toxins

Pericarditis
Viral, bacterial, or fungal infection
Rheumatic fever
Postcardiac injury
Uremia
Toxins

Endocarditis
Nonbacterial growths because of rheumatic fever, systemic lupus erythematosus, and other collagen diseases
Bacterial (streptococcal and staphylococcal) or fungal (Candida, Aspergillus, Histoplasma) infections
Infections related to I.V. drug abuse
Congenital heart disease
Prosthetic valve surgery

Rheumatic fever
Group A beta-hemolytic streptococcal infection, usually of throat or middle ear

• *radiation therapy:* large doses of radiation to the chest in treating lung or breast cancer
• *chemical poisons:* such as chronic alcoholism
• *parasitic infections:* especially South American trypanosomiasis (Chagas' disease) in infants and immunosuppressed adults; also, toxoplasmosis
• *helminthic infections:* such as trichinosis. (See *Causes of Inflammatory Conditions.*)

Signs and symptoms
Myocarditis usually causes nonspecific symptoms—such as fatigue, dyspnea, palpitations, and fever—that reflect the accompanying systemic infection. Occasionally, it may produce mild, contin-

uous pressure or soreness in the chest (unlike the recurring, stress-related pain of angina pectoris). Although myocarditis is generally uncomplicated and self-limiting, it may induce myofibril degeneration that results in right and left heart failure, with cardiomegaly, neck vein distention, dyspnea, resting or exertional tachycardia disproportionate to the degree of fever, and supraventricular and ventricular arrhythmias. Sometimes myocarditis recurs or produces chronic valvulitis (when it results from rheumatic fever), cardiomyopathy, arrhythmias, and thromboembolism.

Diagnosis
Patient history commonly reveals recent febrile upper respiratory tract infection, viral pharyngitis, or tonsillitis. Physical examination shows supraventricular and ventricular dysrhythmias, S_3 and S_4 gallops, a faint S_1, possibly a murmur of mitral regurgitation (from papillary muscle dysfunction), and if pericarditis is present, a pericardial friction rub.

Laboratory tests cannot unequivocally confirm myocarditis, but the following findings support this diagnosis:
• cardiac enzymes: elevated creatine phosphokinase (CPK), CPK isoenzyme (CPK_2), serum glutamic-oxaloacetic transaminase, and lactic dehydrogenase
• increased WBC and ESR
• elevated antibody titers (such as antistreptolysin O [ASO titer] in rheumatic fever).

EKG changes are the most reliable diagnostic aid and typically show diffuse ST segment and T wave abnormalities as in pericarditis, conduction defects (prolonged P-R interval), and other supraventricular ectopic arrhythmias.

Stool and throat cultures may identify bacteria or isolate the virus.
• Endomyocardial biopsy is used for definitive diagnosis.

Treatment
Treatment includes antibiotics for bacterial infection, modified bed rest to decrease heart work load, and careful management of complications. CHF re-

quires restriction of activity to minimize myocardial oxygen consumption, supplemental oxygen therapy, sodium restriction, diuretics to decrease fluid retention, and digitalis to increase myocardial contractility. However, digitalis necessitates cautious administration, since some patients with myocarditis may show a paradoxical sensitivity to even small doses. Dysrhythmias necessitate prompt but cautious administration of antiarrhythmics, such as quinidine or procainamide, since these drugs depress myocardial contractility. Thromboembolism requires anticoagulation therapy. Because corticosteroids may aggravate the underlying infection by suppressing systemic defense mechanisms, they are used mainly to combat life-threatening complications, such as intractable heart failure. The use of steroids and immunosuppressive therapy is controversial. Current studies have not demonstrated their efficacy.

Nursing management
• Assess cardiovascular status frequently, watching for signs of CHF (rales, dyspnea, hypotension, tachycardia, increased central venous pressure, neck vein distention, edema, weight gain, or decreased urinary output). Check carefully for changes in cardiac rhythm or conduction.
• Observe for signs of digitalis toxicity (anorexia, nausea, vomiting, blurred vision, or cardiac arrhythmias) and for complicating factors that may potentiate toxicity, such as electrolyte imbalance or hypoxia.
• Stress the importance of bed rest. Assist with bathing, as necessary. Provide a bedside commode, since this stresses the heart less than using a bedpan. Give reassurance that activity limitations are temporary. Offer diversional activities that are physically undemanding.
• During recovery, recommend that the patient resume normal activities slowly and avoid competitive sports.

Endocarditis
(Infective endocarditis, bacterial endocarditis)

Endocarditis is an infection of the endocardium, heart valves, or cardiac prosthesis, resulting from bacterial (or, in intravenous drug abusers, fungal) invasion. This invasion produces vegetative growths on the heart valves, endocardial lining of a heart chamber, or the endothelium of a blood vessel that may embolize to the spleen, kidneys, central nervous system, and lungs. Untreated endocarditis is usually fatal, but with proper treatment, 70% of patients recover. Prognosis is worst when endocarditis causes severe valvular damage, leading to insufficiency and CHF, or when it involves a prosthetic valve.

Causes
Acute infective endocarditis usually results from bacteremia that follows septic thrombophlebitis, open heart surgery involving prosthetic valves, or skin, bone, and pulmonary infections. The most common causative organisms are group A nonhemolytic streptococcus (rheumatic endocarditis), pneumococcus, staphylococcus, and rarely, gonococcus. This form of endocarditis also occurs in intravenous drug abusers, possibly from *Staphylococcus aureus,* pseudomonas, *Candida,* or usually harmless skin saprophytes.

Staphylococcus epidermis is the most common causative organism of endocarditis in patients with prosthetic heart valves.

Subacute infective endocarditis typically occurs in persons with acquired valvular or congenital cardiac lesions. It can also follow dental, genitourinary, gynecologic, and gastrointestinal procedures. The most common infecting organisms are *Streptococcus viridans,* which normally inhabits the upper respiratory tract, and *Streptococcus faecalis* (enterococcus), generally found in gastrointestinal and perineal flora.

Endocardial Vegetations

Typical vegetations on the endocardium produced by fibrin and platelet deposits on infection sites

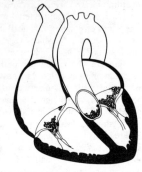

Preexisting rheumatic endocardial lesions are a common predisposing factor in bacterial endocarditis. Rheumatic endocarditis commonly affects the mitral valve; less frequently, the aortic or tricuspid valve; and rarely, the pulmonic valve.

In infective endocarditis, fibrin and platelets aggregate on the valve tissue and engulf circulating bacteria or fungi that flourish and produce friable verrucous vegetations. Such vegetations may cover the valve surfaces, causing ulceration and necrosis; they may also extend to the chordae tendineae, leading to their rupture and subsequent valvular insufficiency. Sometimes vegetations form on the endocardium, usually in areas altered by rheumatic, congenital, or syphilitic heart disease, although they may also form on normal surfaces. (See *Endocardial Vegetations*.).

Signs and symptoms

Early clinical features of endocarditis are nonspecific and include weakness, fatigue, weight loss, anorexia, arthralgia, night sweats, and in 90% of patients, intermittent fever that may recur for weeks. Endocarditis often causes a loud, regurgitant murmur typical of the underlying rheumatic or congenital heart disease. A suddenly changing murmur or the discovery of a new murmur in the presence of fever is a classic physical sign of endocarditis.

In about 30% of patients with subacute endocarditis, embolization from vegetating lesions or diseased valve tissue may produce typical features of splenic, renal, cerebral, or pulmonary infarction, or peripheral vascular occlusion:

• *splenic infarction:* pain in the upper left quadrant, radiating to the left shoulder; abdominal rigidity

• *renal infarction:* hematuria, pyuria, flank pain, decreased urinary output

• *cerebral infarction:* hemiparesis, aphasia, or other neurologic deficits. Neurologic manifestations are often the first sign of endocarditis, which appears in ≈ 30% of patients. Hemiplegia in a young adult should always suggest endocarditis.

• *pulmonary infarction* (most common in right-sided endocarditis, which often occurs among intravenous drug abusers and after cardiac surgery): cough, pleuritic pain, pleural friction rub, dyspnea, and hemoptysis

• *peripheral vascular occlusion:* numbness and tingling in an arm, leg, finger, or toe, or signs of impending peripheral gangrene. (See *Endocardial Vegetations*.)

Other symptoms include petechiae of the skin (especially common on the upper anterior trunk) and the buccal, pharyngeal, or conjunctival mucosa, and splinter hemorrhages under the nails. Rarely, endocarditis produces Osler's nodes (tender, raised, subcutaneous lesions on the fingers or toes), Roth's spots (hemorrhagic areas with white centers on the retina), and Janeway lesions (purplish macules on the palms or soles).

Diagnosis

Three or more blood cultures (possibly six for maximum yield) during a 24- to 48-hour period identify the causative organism in up to 90% of patients. The

remaining 10% may have negative blood cultures, possibly suggesting fungal infection. Other abnormal but nonspecific laboratory results include:
- elevated WBC
- abnormal histocytes (macrophages)
- elevated ESR
- normocytic, normochromic anemia (in subacute bacterial endocarditis)
- rheumatoid factor, in about half of all patients with endocarditis.

Echocardiography may identify valvular damage; EKG may show atrial fibrillation and other arrhythmias that accompany valvular disease.

Treatment

The goal of treatment is to eradicate the infecting organism. Therapy should start promptly and continue over several weeks. Antibiotic selection is based on sensitivity studies of the infecting organism—or the probable organism, if blood cultures are negative. I.V. antibiotic therapy usually lasts about 4 weeks. Bacteriocidal agents are used, sometimes in pairs, for their synergistic action with resistant strains of organisms.

Supportive treatment includes bed rest, aspirin for fever and aches, and sufficient fluid intake. Severe valvular damage, especially aortic regurgitation or infection of cardiac prosthesis, may require corrective surgery if refractory heart failure develops.

Nursing management

- Before giving antibiotics, obtain a patient history of allergies. Administer antibiotics on time to maintain consistent antibiotic blood levels. Check dilutions for compatibility with other medications the patient is receiving, and use a solution that is compatible with drug stability. (For example, add methicillin to a buffered solution.)
- Observe for signs of infiltration or inflammation at the venipuncture site, possible complications of long-term I.V. administration. To reduce the risk of these complications, rotate venous access sites.

- Watch for signs of embolization (hematuria, pleuritic chest pain, upper left quadrant pain, or paresis), a common occurrence during the first 3 months of treatment. Tell the patient to watch for and report these signs, which may indicate impending peripheral vascular occlusion or splenic, renal, cerebral, or pulmonary infarction.
- Monitor the patient's renal status (including BUN, creatinine, and urinary output) to check for signs of renal emboli or drug toxicity.
- Observe for signs of CHF, such as dyspnea, tachypnea, tachycardia, rales, neck vein distention, edema, and weight gain.
- Provide reassurance by teaching the patient and family about this disease and the need for prolonged treatment. Tell them to watch closely for fever, anorexia, and other signs of relapse about 2 weeks after treatment stops. Suggest quiet diversionary activities to prevent excessive physical exertion.
- Make sure susceptible patients understand the need for prophylactic antibiotics before, during, and after dental work, childbirth, and genitourinary, gastrointestinal, or gynecologic procedures.
- Teach patients how to recognize symptoms of endocarditis, and tell them to notify the doctor immediately if such symptoms occur.

Pericarditis

Pericarditis is an inflammation of the pericardium, the fibroserous sac that envelops, supports, and protects the heart. It occurs in both acute and chronic forms. Acute pericarditis can be fibrinous or effusive, with purulent serous or hemorrhagic exudate. Chronic constrictive pericarditis is characterized by dense fibrous pericardial thickening. Prognosis depends on the underlying cause but is generally good in acute pericarditis, unless constriction occurs.

Causes

Common causes of this disease include:

• bacterial, fungal, or viral infection (infectious pericarditis)
• neoplasms (primary, or metastases from lungs, breasts, or other organs)
• high-dose radiation to the chest
• uremia
• hypersensitivity reactions, such as acute rheumatic fever (the most common cause of pericarditis in children), and polyarteritis
• autoimmune diseases, such as systemic lupus erythematosus and rheumatoid arthritis
• acute MI
• post-MI syndrome (Dressler's syndrome)
• trauma
• postpericardiotomy syndrome
• drugs, such as hydralazine or procainamide
• idiopathic factors (most common in acute pericarditis).

Less common causes include aortic aneurysm with pericardial leakage and myxedema with cholesterol deposits in the pericardium.

Signs and symptoms

Acute pericarditis typically produces a sharp and often sudden pain that usually starts over the sternum and radiates to the neck, shoulders, back, and arms. However, unlike the pain of MI, pericardial pain is often pleuritic, increasing with deep inspiration and decreasing when the patient sits up and leans forward, pulling the heart away from the diaphragmatic pleurae of the lungs.

Pericardial effusion, the major complication of acute pericarditis, may mimic heart failure—with dyspnea, orthopnea, and tachycardia, ill-defined substernal chest pain, and a feeling of fullness in the chest. If the fluid accumulates rapidly, cardiac tamponade may occur, resulting in pallor, clammy skin, hypotension, pulsus paradoxus (a decrease in blood pressure $\geq$ 15 mm Hg during slow inspiration), neck vein distention, and eventually, cardiovascular collapse and death.

Chronic constrictive pericarditis causes a gradual increase in systemic venous pressure and produces symptoms similar to those of chronic right heart failure (fluid retention, ascites, hepatomegaly).

The most distinctive feature of pericarditis is a palpable and sometimes audible sharp pericardial "knock" occurring in early diastole when the rapidly filling ventricle encounters the nondistensible pericardium.

Diagnosis

Since pericarditis often coexists with other conditions, diagnosis of acute pericarditis depends on typical clinical features and elimination of other possible causes. A classic symptom, the pericardial friction rub, is a grating sound heard as the heart moves. It can usually be auscultated best during forced expiration, while the patient leans forward or is on his hands and knees in bed. It may have up to three components, corresponding to the timing of atrial systole, ventricular systole, and the rapid-filling phase of ventricular diastole. Occasionally, this friction rub is heard only briefly or not at all. Nevertheless, its presence, together with other characteristic features, is diagnostic of acute pericarditis. In addition, if acute pericarditis has caused very large pericardial effusions, physical examination reveals increased cardiac dullness and diminished or absent apical impulse and distant heart sounds.

In patients with chronic pericarditis, acute inflammation or effusions do not occur—only restricted cardiac filling.

Laboratory results reflect inflammation and may identify its cause:
• normal or elevated WBC, especially in infectious pericarditis
• elevated ESR
• slightly elevated cardiac enzymes with associated myocarditis
• culture of pericardial fluid obtained by open surgical drainage or cardiocentesis (sometimes identifies a causative organism in bacterial or fungal pericarditis)
• EKG shows the following changes in acute pericarditis: ST segment elevation

with preservation of normal upward concavities—evolves over a period of days, usually followed by T-wave inversions; elevation of ST segments in the standard limb leads and most precordial leads without significant changes in QRS morphology that occur with MI; atrial ectopic rhythms, such as atrial fibrillation; and in pericardial effusion, diminished QRS voltage and nonspecific ST-T wave changes.

Other laboratory data include BUN to check for uremia, antistreptolysin O titers to detect rheumatic fever, and a purified protein derivative skin test to check for tuberculosis. In pericardial effusion, echocardiography is diagnostic when it shows an echo-free space between the ventricular wall and the pericardium.

Treatment

The goal of treatment is to relieve symptoms and manage underlying systemic disease. In acute idiopathic pericarditis, post-MI pericarditis, and post-thoracotomy pericarditis, treatment consists of bed rest as long as fever and pain persist and nonsteroidal drugs, such as aspirin and indomethacin, to relieve pain and reduce inflammation. If these drugs fail to relieve symptoms, corticosteroids may be used. Although corticosteroids produce rapid and effective relief, they must be used cautiously because symptomatic episodes may recur when therapy is discontinued.

Infectious pericarditis that results from disease of the left pleural space, mediastinal abscesses, or septicemia requires antibiotics, surgical drainage, or both. If cardiac tamponade develops, the doctor may perform emergency pericardiocentesis. Signs of cardiac tamponade include pulsus paradoxus, neck vein distention, dyspnea, and shock.

Recurrent pericarditis may necessitate partial pericardectomy (surgical removal of part of the pericardium), creating a "window" that allows fluid to drain into the pleural space. In constrictive pericarditis, total pericardectomy to permit adequate filling and contraction

of the heart may be necessary. Treatment must also include management of rheumatic fever, uremia, tuberculosis, and other underlying disorders.

Nursing management

A patient with pericarditis needs complete bed rest. In addition, health care includes:

• assessing pain in relation to respiration and body position, to differentiate pericardial pain from myocardial ischemic pain

• relieving dyspnea and pain by placing the patient in an upright position and providing analgesics and oxygen, as needed

• reassuring the patient with acute pericarditis that his condition usually is temporary and responds well to treatment; explaining all diagnostic procedures to him

• monitoring the patient with pericardial effusion for decreased blood pressure and increased venous pressure—signs of cardiac compression; checking for pulsus paradoxus and reporting it and other signs of cardiac tamponade immediately; keeping a pericardiocentesis set available at all times

• explaining the surgical procedure to the patient if surgery is necessary; telling him what to expect after surgery, and showing him how to do deep breathing and coughing exercises

• giving postoperative care similar to that following cardiothoracic surgery.

Nursing diagnoses

After collecting subjective data from the patient history and objective data from the physical examination, formulate nursing diagnoses and set goals. Typical nursing diagnoses related to inflammatory heart conditions are:

Potential pericardial effusion and cardiac tamponade related to pericarditis.

Your goal is to prevent or resolve pericardial effusion or cardiac tamponade. To achieve this, monitor the patient's

Valvular Heart Diseases

DISEASE, DESCRIPTION AND CAUSES	SIGNS AND SYMPTOMS
Aortic stenosis • Stiffened valve leaflets fail to open properly, resulting in impaired blood flow from the left ventricle. • Usually caused by rheumatic fever (ages 30 to 70) or calcification of aortic valve (after age 70).	• Angina pectoris, syncope on exertion. • Left ventricular failure, indicated by signs of pulmonary congestion: dyspnea, orthopnea, paroxysmal nocturnal dyspnea.
Aortic regurgitation • Diseased aortic valve fails to close properly, causing blood backflow into left ventricle during diastole. • Usually caused by valve damage from rheumatic fever, syphilis, or endocarditis. Sometimes associated with Marfan's syndrome and rheumatoid arthritis.	• Rapidly rising and falling pulses, dysrhythmias, wide pulse pressure in severe regurgitation. Dyspnea progressing to paroxysmal nocturnal dyspnea and orthopnea, which indicates pulmonary congestion. • Severe blood backflow may cause pulmonary edema.
Mitral stenosis • Stiffened valve leaflets cannot open properly, impairing blood flow from left atrium to left ventricle. • Most commonly caused by rheumatic fever. Sometimes associated with congenital anomalies, such as tetralogy of Fallot.	• Dyspnea on exertion; fatigue; rapid, irregular pulse; palpitations; increased left atrial pressure; pulmonary hypertension; right ventricular hypertrophy and failure. • Loud S_1 or opening snap, with rumbling diastolic murmur at apex.
Mitral regurgitation • Diseased valve cannot close tightly, causing blood backflow from left ventricle to left atrium during systole. • May be caused by rheumatic fever, prolapsed valve, left ventricular dilation, papillary muscle dysfunction and, in acute regurgitation, ruptured chordae tendineae.	• Dyspnea and fatigue commonly develop late in chronic regurgitation; symptoms of pulmonary edema in acute regurgitation. Palpitations and chest pain suggest non-rheumatic disease origin. • Holosystolic murmur at apex, possible split S_2, and S_3.

TREATMENTS	NURSING INTERVENTIONS
• Drug therapy includes nitrates, digitalis, diuretics, rheumatic prophylaxis. • Valve replacement is often preferred, since symptoms generally occur late in the disease.	• Monitor vital signs (including apical pulse), lung and heart sounds, arterial blood gases (ABGs), hemodynamic status, chest X-rays, intake/output, weight. Watch for signs of drug side effects, pulmonary edema, ventricular failure. • After surgery, be alert for dysrhythmias, thrombi, hypotension, and pulmonary emboli.
• Prompt, vigorous treatment of infections and dysrhythmias. Drug therapy includes digitalis glycosides, diuretics, nitroglycerin, and for the patient with syphilitic aortitis, penicillin. • Patients symptomatic with exertion despite drug therapy require surgery.	• Monitor vital signs (including apical pulse), lung and heart sounds, ABGs, hemodynamic status, chest X-rays, intake/output, and weight. Watch for signs of ventricular failure, pulmonary edema, and drug side effects. • After surgery, be alert for dysrhythmias, thrombi, hypotension, and pulmonary emboli.
• Prophylaxis for endocarditis may be required; digitalis, quinidine, diuretics, vasodilators, sodium restriction, and activity limitation for atrial fibrillation or CHF. • Valve replacement or commissurotomy.	• Monitor vital signs (including apical pulse), lung and heart sounds, ABGs, hemodynamic status, chest X-rays, intake/output, and weight. Watch for signs of pulmonary edema, right ventricular failure, eventual left ventricular failure, and drug side effects. • After surgery, be alert for hypotension, dysrhythmias, thrombi and pulmonary emboli.
• Prophylaxis for endocarditis may be required; digitalis, quinidine, diuretics, vasodilators, sodium restriction, and limited activity for atrial fibrillation or CHF; hydralazine for reducing preload and afterload. • Valve replacement or reconstruction.	• Monitor vital signs (including apical pulse) frequently, avoid overhydration, and assess lung and heart sounds. Check for signs of decompensation, pulmonary edema, right ventricular failure, eventual left ventricular failure, and drug side effects. • After surgery, be alert for hypotension, dysrhythmias, thrombi and pulmonary emboli. *(continued)*

Valvular Heart Diseases *continued*

DISEASE, DESCRIPTION AND CAUSES	SIGNS AND SYMPTOMS
Mitral prolapse • Enlarged valve leaflets bulge backward into left atrium during ventricular systole. • Usually idiopathic and benign. Commonly inherited.	• Sharp chest pain unrelated to exercise, fatigue, palpitations, lightheadedness, syncope, dyspnea. • Mild or late systolic click followed by a late, high-pitched, musical systolic murmur at apex.
Tricuspid stenosis • Stiffened tricuspid valve leaflets cannot open properly, impairing blood flow from the right atrium to the right ventricle during diastole. • Most commonly caused by rheumatic fever; often associated with mitral stenosis; sometimes congenital.	• Increased right atrial pressure causes chamber dilatation and hypertrophy, increased pressure in the vena cava, and eventual right ventricular failure. • Blowing diastolic murmur along left sternal border. Changes on inspiration are diagnostic.
Tricuspid regurgitation • Diseased valve fails to close properly, causing blood backflow from right ventricle into right atrium during systole. • Usually occurs in right ventricular failure and, at times, in left ventricular failure and pulmonary hypertension.	• Increased right atrial pressure causes signs of right ventricular failure: distended neck veins, peripheral edema, ascites, hepatomegaly, hydrothorax, nausea, and vomiting. • Blowing holosystolic murmur at lower left sternal border, augments during inspiration.
Pulmonic stenosis • Stiffened pulmonic valve leaflets impair blood flow from the right ventricle. • Rare disorder, often caused by congenital heart defect.	• Right ventricular hypertrophy, right ventricular failure. • Systolic ejection murmur over the pulmonic area, with a widely split second sound and systolic ejection click.

TREATMENTS	NURSING INTERVENTIONS
• Nitroglycerin may relieve chest pain. Propranolol increases ventricular volume and corrects dysrhythmias. Prophylaxis for endocarditis may be required. • Valve replacement in severe symptoms.	• Reassure patient to control anxiety. Explain his condition, its treatment, and possible complications. • Watch for drug side effects; reinforce prophylactic drug therapy.
• Pulmonary and systemic congestion are treated with digitalis, diuretics, and sodium restriction. Prophylaxis for endocarditis may be required. • Valve replacement or ring annuloplasty in moderate to severe stenosis.	• Monitor vital signs (including apical pulse), ABGs, hemodynamic status, chest X-rays, intake/output, and weight. Watch for signs of ventricular failure, pulmonary edema, and drug side effects. • After surgery, be alert for hypotension, dysrhythmias, thrombi, and pulmonary emboli.
• Treatment is usually symptomatic: prophylaxis for endocarditis, digitalis, diuretics, sodium restriction, and activity limitation. • Surgery for isolated tricuspid regurgitation is seldom necessary. Valve replacement or annuloplasty may be done concurrently with mitral valve surgery.	• Monitor vital signs (including apical pulse), ABGs, hemodynamic status, chest X-rays, intake/output, and weight. Watch for signs of ventricular failure, pulmonary edema, and drug side effects. • After surgery, be alert for hypotension, dysrhythmias, thrombi, and pulmonary emboli.
• Treatment aims to correct symptoms of systemic congestion. Anticoagulants may be used if pulmonary emboli develop. • Valvotomy in severe or progressive symptoms.	• Watch for signs of ventricular failure and drug side effects. • After surgery, be alert for hypotension, dysrhythmias, thrombi, and pulmonary emboli.

(continued)

Valvular Heart Diseases *continued*

DISEASE, DESCRIPTION AND CAUSES	SIGNS AND SYMPTOMS
Pulmonic regurgitation • Diseased pulmonary valve cannot close properly, causing blood backflow into the right ventricle during diastole. • Generally caused by congenital heart disease. Often associated with other valvular or heart defects.	• Fluid overload in right ventricle leads to hypertrophy and eventual failure of ventricle. Fatigue, dyspnea, and syncope may indicate severe pulmonary hypertension. • Diastolic murmur at left sternal border increases with inspiration.
Papillary muscle dysfunction and rupture • Dysfunction: may affect mitral or tricuspid valve. Ineffective closure causes regurgitation or prolapse into atria during systole. Usually results from ischemic disease. • Rupture: usually results from infarction of the muscle in coronary artery disease.	• Dysfunction: signs of underlying heart disease. • Rupture: severe dyspnea, chest pain, syncope, hemoptysis, pulmonary edema, hyperdynamic apical pulse, tachycardia, hypotension, and signs of hypoperfusion.

hemodynamic status, observe for signs of cardiac tamponade, and if necessary, assist with pericardiocentesis. Be sure to explain all procedures to the patient and his family to help relieve their anxiety.

Potential development and migration of emboli related to endocarditis

This is most acute if the patient has endocarditis. Your goal is to promote bed rest to help prevent formation or migration of emboli. Discuss the potential for embolization, as well as its causes and treatment, with the patient to reduce anxiety.

Potential cardiac valve infection related to systemic bacterial infection

Decreased cardiac output related to cardiac valve infection (inflammation)

Your goal is to promote compliance to the medical regimen, and improve the patient's understanding of drug therapy.

Potential valvular regurgitation resulting from vegetative growths on valve leaflets

Potential alteration in coping mechanisms related to acute illness, lengthy hospitalization, and diagnostic testing procedures

Knowledge deficit about inflammation, treatment, and prevention

Your focus here is patient education. Begin by explaining the inflammatory response and its effects on the heart. Also explain the use of monitors and the purpose of diagnostic tests. Teach the patient the purpose, dosage, schedule, route of administration, and potential side effects of prescribed drugs. If appropriate, tell him that drug therapy must continue until cultures are negative for the causative organism.

TREATMENTS	NURSING INTERVENTIONS
• Without underlying disease, pulmonic regurgitation is generally well tolerated, and treatment consists of prophylactic antibiotics and continuous observation. • When pulmonic regurgitation results from other diseases, treatment is symptomatic.	• Monitor vital signs (including apical pulse), lung and heart sounds, ABGs, hemodynamic status, chest X-rays, intake/output, and weight. • Watch for signs of ventricular failure and drug side effects. • After surgery, be alert for hypotension, dysrhythmias, thrombi, and pulmonary emboli.
• Dysfunction: symptomatic (may include propranolol, nitroglycerin, digitalis, diuretics, and vasodilators). Severe mitral regurgitation and refractory heart failure may require mitral valve replacement. • Rupture: mitral valve replacement is treatment of choice. Preoperative therapy may include I.V. diuretics.	• Watch for signs of heart failure or reduced cardiac output. Auscultate for systolic murmur or S_4. • Reinforce the patient's coping mechanisms; encourage coughing and deep breathing. • After surgery, be alert for hypotension, dysrhythmias, thrombi, and pulmonary emboli.

DISORDERS OF THE VALVES

Acquired and congenital diseases of the cardiac valves have become more manageable in the last 20 years as a result of the introduction of cardiac catheterization in the 1960s, the use of prosthetic valve replacements, and modern antimicrobial and antibiotic drug therapy.

Valvular heart disease

Valvular heart disease can result from a number of disorders, including congenital defects, ischemic damage, degenerative changes, and inflammation. Rheumatic endocarditis is the most common cause. In valvular disease, two types of mechanical disruptions occur: narrowing, or stenosis, of the valve opening or failure of the valve to close completely (valvular insufficiency or incompetence). Either of these can lead to heart failure.

Valvular heart disease occurs in varying forms:
• *Mitral insufficiency:* Blood from the left ventricle flows back into the left atrium during ventricular systole, causing the atrium to enlarge to accommodate the backflow. In addition, failure of the mitral valve to close completely permits continued flow from the left atrium to the left ventricle during ventricular diastole. As a result, the left ventricle also dilates to accommodate the increased volume of blood from the atrium and to compensate for diminishing cardiac output. Ventricular hypertrophy

and increased end-diastolic pressure result in increased pulmonary artery pressure, eventually leading to both left and right ventricular failure.

• *Mitral stenosis:* Narrowing of the valve by valvular abnormalities, fibrosis, or calcification obstructs blood flow from the left atrium to the left ventricle. Consequently, left atrial volume and pressure rise and the chamber dilates. As the disease progresses, greater resistance to blood flow causes pulmonary hypertension, right ventricular hypertrophy, and, eventually, right ventricular failure.

In addition, there is inadequate filling of the left ventricle manifested by low cardiac output.

• *Aortic insufficiency:* Blood flows back into the left ventricle during diastole, causing a volume overload in the ventricle, which in turn dilates and ultimately hypertrophies. The excess volume eventually interferes with left atrium emptying, resulting in volume overload in the left atrium and, finally, in the pulmonary system. Left ventricular failure and pulmonary edema eventually result.

• *Aortic stenosis:* Increased left ventricular pressure attempts to overcome the resistance of the narrowed valvular opening. The added work load causes a greater demand for oxygen, while diminished cardiac output (caused by a decreased volume of blood ejected into the systemic circulation) causes poor coronary artery perfusion, ischemia of the left ventricle (evidenced by angina, especially on exertion), syncope, and eventually left ventricular failure.

• *Pulmonic insufficiency:* Blood ejected into the pulmonary artery during right ventricular systole flows back into the right ventricle during diastole, causing a fluid overload in the ventricle, ventricular hypertrophy, and, finally, right ventricular failure.

• *Pulmonic stenosis:* Obstructed right ventricular outflow causes right ventricular hypertrophy in an attempt to overcome resistance to the narrow valvular opening. Right ventricular failure ultimately results.

• *Tricuspid insufficiency:* Blood flows back into the right atrium during ventricular systole, decreasing blood flow to the lungs and left side of the heart. Cardiac output also lessens. Fluid overload in the right side of the heart can eventually lead to right ventricular failure.

• *Tricuspid stenosis:* Obstructed blood flow from the right atrium to the right ventricle causes the right atrium to dilate and hypertrophy. This increases pressure in the vena cava and eventually leads to right ventricular failure.

Treatment

Treatment of valvular heart disease depends on the nature and severity of associated symptoms. For example, heart failure requires digoxin, diuretics, a sodium-restricted diet, and, in acute cases, oxygen. Atrial fibrillation requires digoxin or electrical conversion, and if pulmonary edema occurs, oxygen and I.V. administration of diuretics.

If the patient has severe symptoms that cannot be managed medically, open heart surgery using cardiopulmonary bypass for valve replacement is indicated. Other appropriate measures include anticoagulant therapy to prevent thrombus formation around diseased or replaced valves and prophylactic antibiotics before and after surgery or dental care to prevent infective endocarditis.

Nursing management

• Watch closely for signs of heart failure or pulmonary edema and side effects of drug therapy.

• Teach the patient about diet restrictions, medications, symptoms that should be reported, and the importance of consistent follow-up care.

• Make sure the patient understands the necessity for anticoagulant therapy and endocarditis prophylaxis postoperatively.

• If the patient undergoes surgery, watch for hypotension, dysrhythmias, and thrombus formation. Monitor vital signs, arterial blood gases, intake and output, daily weights, blood chemistries, chest X-rays, and pulmonary artery catheter readings. (See *Valvular Heart Diseases,* pages 166 to 171.)

Nursing diagnoses

The two main nursing diagnoses related to valular disorders are:

Alteration in cardiac output related to mitral valve insufficiency, mitral steno-sis, aortic insufficiency, and so forth

Alteration in tissue perfusion related to valvular disease of the heart

Your goals are to monitor vital signs closely and watch for possible complications. If the patient is not scheduled for surgery to correct the valvular disorder, then you must teach him how to live with his disease and medication regimen.

10
UNCOMMON CAUSES OF HEART DISEASE

Cardiovascular disorders do not always follow the typical disease process. Rigorous physical training, benign cancers, or blunt trauma from an accident can also cause problems that could lead to serious complications.

Athletic heart syndrome

Athletic heart syndrome comprises a series of related cardiac changes that develop as an anatomic and physiologic response to strenuous exercise. Such changes, which do not necessarily impair heart function, include biventricular hypertrophy, intermittent systolic ejection murmur, S_3 gallop, dysrhythmias, ST-T wave abnormalities, decreased heart rate, increased stroke volume, left ventricular stroke work, and cardiac output. Because of the large number of persons currently participating in physical fitness, the incidence of athletic heart syndrome is rising.

Causes
Athletic heart syndrome is probably an adaptive physiologic response to maintain optimal cardiac performance during physical endurance training. To compensate for the sustained hemodynamic burden produced by exercise, left ventricular internal dimension (measured by left ventricular end-diastolic volumes) and cardiac wall thickness increase, enhancing contractility, improving cardiac output, and delivering more oxygen during maximum work loads.

Signs and symptoms
This syndrome usually does not produce symptoms, although it may cause chest pounding or an irregular heartbeat after strenuous activity.

Diagnosis
Athletic heart syndrome is often detected during a routine physical examination or hospitalization for an athletic injury, with the following findings:
• *History* reveals endurance training.
• *Chest X-ray* shows enlarged right and left ventricles and, occasionally, an enlarged left atrium and aortic root.
• *Echocardiography* demonstrates increased cardiac mass, including ventricular hypertrophy and, possibly, an enlarged left atrium.
• *Chest auscultation* may reveal a slow heart rate with intermittent systolic ejection murmur along the left sternal border, S_3 gallop over the mitral area (can be a normal finding in youth), and hyperdynamic ventricular impulse at point of maximum impulse.
• *Electrocardiogram (EKG)* (resting and during exercise) may show sinus bradycardia (as low as 40 beats per minute), increased QRS and T amplitude in both standard and precordial leads, elevated ST segment in precordial leads (V_2 to V_5), appearance of U wave due to abnormal repolarization or left ventricular hypertrophy, and dysrhythmias.
  Isolated findings—bradycardia, for example—may indicate primary organic heart disease or may be a normal finding.

Treatment

Athletic heart syndrome does not necessitate treatment, but underlying cardiac disease may require the athlete to discontinue training.

Nursing management

• Provide an explanation of diagnostic procedures. Inform the patient that while there is no evidence that strenuous exercise causes heart damage or increases the risk of early death from cardiac disease, the long-term effects of athletic heart syndrome are still unknown and are being studied.

• Explain that future risk of heart disease is closely linked to a family history of cardiovascular disorders. To minimize future risk, recommend regular checkups with resting and exercise EKGs.

• Advise the patient that an extensive medical evaluation may be necessary to distinguish normal variations from disease states.

Benign cardiac tumors

Benign cardiac tumors can arise from the endocardium, myocardium, and pericardium and constitute 75% of all primary lesions found in the heart. Myxomas and rhabdomyomas are the two most common benign tumors, with myxomas accounting for at least half of these. Rarer benign tumors include fibromas, lipomas, teratomas, angiomas, and hamartomas. Although histologically benign, these tumors can be fatal, and they often produce cardiac dysfunction, such as pericardial effusion and tamponade, potentially lethal dysrhythmias, refractory heart failure, and sudden death. Clinical course for this rare disorder varies with tumor type and location. With early recognition of signs and symptoms, removal of benign cardiac tumors by open heart surgery can greatly improve prognosis.

Causes and incidence

Myxomas may develop from mural thrombi or may be of neoplastic origin (true tumor). As single or multiple lesions, myxomas arise from the endocardium and occupy the left atrium three times more often than the right; however, they may be bilateral. Myxomas are most prevalent in women between ages 30 and 60. *Angiomas* and *lipomas* may also be intracavitary, occurring in the atria.

Rhabdomyomas may result from congenital tissue malformation or from a localized disorder of glycogen metabolism resulting from an enzyme defect. They may not be true tumors and, when multiple, coexist with tuberous sclerosis of the brain. Rhabdomyomas usually arise from the myocardium and may extend inward—protruding into the left ventricle—or outward—onto the epicardium. These tumors account for 35% of nonproliferative tumors in children under age 3, most of whom die within the first year of life. Rarer myocardial tumors may include *fibromas, hamartomas,* and *mesotheliomas. Teratomas* and other rare benign cardiac tumors, including angiomas, derive from abnormal embryonic development. Teratomas usually arise from the pericardium, as do rarer benign cardiac tumors, including *leiomyomas* and *neurofibromas.*

Some benign tumors are common to all three cardiac layers.

Signs and symptoms

Overt clinical effects develop only after tumor growth impairs heart function. Benign tumors may produce symptoms that simulate familiar cardiac disorders. For this reason, these tumors have been dubbed the great imitators of cardiovascular disease.

The hallmark of benign intracavitary tumors is disruption of cardiac filling and emptying. Symptoms of left atrial myxoma are due to mitral valve obstruction by the tumor, mimicking mitral stenosis. Clinical effects include syncope (especially with change in position) and shocklike syndrome, resulting from a reduction in cardiac output; pulmonary venous congestion; signs of occlusive vascular disease, resulting from embolization; and possibly, seizures or coma. A murmur of mitral regurgitation may also occur. Right atrial myxoma produces symptoms resulting from rapid and unrelenting right heart failure (fatigue, peripheral edema, hepatomegaly, and neck vein distention) with fever, weight loss, and murmur. Right atrial myxomas mimic constrictive pericarditis, tricuspid stenosis, and other cardiac disorders. Cyanosis and neck vein distention may result from superior vena cava obstruction.

Typical signs of right ventricular myxomas include syncope, fever of unknown origin, and murmurs of pulmonary and tricuspid valve obstruction. Rhabdomyomas may obstruct the right ventricular outflow tract, simulating pulmonary stenosis. Left ventricular tumors, such as fibromas arising from the aortic valve, may produce signs of left heart failure, mimicking aortic stenosis or hypertrophic subaortic stenosis; such tumors cause hemodynamic alterations upon changes in body position. Teratomas and other pericardial tumors mimic acute pericarditis and cause precordial pain, friction rub, and signs of pericardial effusion and tamponade. Myocardial tumors may involve the heart wall, valves, or conduction system. Although these tumors rarely cause obstructive disorders, they may cause dysrhythmias and sudden death.

Diagnosis

A patient history and physical examination showing characteristic clinical findings suggest benign cardiac tumors. However, laboratory tests must rule out other cardiac disorders that produce similar symptoms.

• *Chest X-ray* may reveal an abnormal cardiac silhouette, widening of the mediastinum, and intracavitary tumor calcification, but it cannot distinguish between pericardial effusion and pericardial tumors.

• *EKG* often shows axis deviation or ventricular hypertrophy in ventricular myxomas. In other endocardial myxomas, it may show dysrhythmias and conduction disturbances, such as bundle branch block, abnormal P waves, and ST segment changes.

• *Abnormal laboratory results* in myxomas include increased serum enzymes (lactic dehydrogenase and serum glutamic-oxaloacetic transaminase [SGOT]), erythrocyte sedimentation rate (ESR), and alkaline phosphatase; leukocytosis; hyperglobulinemia; and occasionally, increased hemoglobin in right atrial myxoma (polycythemia).

• *Cardiac catheterization,* the most reliable diagnostic tool, shows filling defects, compression, pressure changes in cardiac chambers, or displacement of the major blood vessels and mediastinal structures. However, it cannot distinguish between benign and malignant tumors or large thrombi. This procedure risks dislodgment of tumor fragments, resulting in embolism.

• *Echocardiography* can identify atrial tumors that occupy the mitral or tricuspid valve leaflets and differentiates left atrial myxomas from mitral stenosis.

Treatment

Depending on tumor size and location, open heart surgery using complete cardiopulmonary bypass can remove many benign cardiac tumors; subsequent valve replacement or septal repair with a Dacron graft may be necessary. Before surgery and for symptomatic relief of pericardial tumors, pericardiocentesis can remove fluid accumulation. Symptomatic treatment for inoperable tumors includes pacemaker for heart block, and digitalis, diuretics, and vasodilators for congestive heart failure.

Nursing management

Benign cardiac tumors necessitate intensive care monitoring before and after surgery.

Provide the following preoperative care:

• Auscultate for friction rubs and murmurs. Note EKG changes; report and treat dysrhythmias. Watch for symptoms of decreased cardiac output (syncope and shock), of left heart failure (dyspnea, cyanosis, and rales in the chest), and of right heart failure (fatigue, peripheral edema, and hepatomegaly). Assess for signs of cardiac tamponade in patients with pericardial tumors. Also watch for signs of pulmonary and systemic embolization.

• Explain all diagnostic procedures carefully. Tell the patient what to expect after surgery (endotracheal and chest tubes, ventilator, cardiac monitor, Foley catheter, and venous and pulmonary arterial lines).

• Instruct the patient to avoid positions that further obstruct cardiac blood flow, causing dizziness and reduced cardiac output.

• Provide the following postoperative care:

• Monitor vital signs, level of consciousness, respiratory status, intake and output, and hemodynamic pressures. Record any chest tube drainage, and suction the endotracheal tube frequently. Watch for, report, and treat dysrhythmias.

• When vital signs stabilize, have the patient turn, cough, and breathe deeply at regular intervals. Give medications (antibiotics, digitalis preparations, and diuretics), as ordered.

• Provide emotional support, especially for parents of infants with rhabdomyomas; many of these infants die soon after birth. Since the word tumor conjures visions of cancer, emphasize the benign nature of these lesions.

Myocardial contusion

In myocardial contusions, the heart is compressed between the sternum and the spinal column, resulting in capillary hemorrhage varying in size from petechial to hemorrhagic involvement of the full thickness of the myocardium. Extravasation of blood and fluid disrupts and separates the myocardial fibers, causing ischemic changes and early necrosis. The patient's clinical picture may resemble myocardial infarction (MI).

Causes
Myocardial contusion results from blunt trauma to the chest—for example, from a direct blow or a fall that results in sternal or anterior thoracic compression. The most frequent cause is steering-wheel impact to the chest when the patient has been in an accident.

Signs and symptoms
The patient has a history of recent blunt anterior chest trauma and may have:
• some degree of angina-like substernal chest pain—refractory to nitroglycerin but responsive to oxygen—unassociated with movement or respiration
• palpitations
• no prior cardiovascular disease or risk factors for MI
• ecchymoses over the sternum
• a rapid heartbeat or an abnormal heart sound, such as an early pericardial friction rub.

Diagnosis
Diagnostic tests must be done to help distinguish myocardial contusion from MI. An EKG may show ST-T wave elevations or depressions. Less common EKG changes include widened QRS complex or acute pathologic Q waves. Atrial flutter or fibrillation, conduction disturbances, and ventricular irritability may have occurred—depending on the area of injury. Creatine phosphokinase (CPK) enzyme levels (especially the MB fraction)—sensitive to myocardial damage—shows the extent of the contusion. Radionuclide scanning (myocardial imaging) may have been positive if myocardial damage was extensive.

(Note: the presence of myocardial contusion is sometimes missed in patients with multiple severe injuries who have no obvious thoracic trauma. Keep this in mind whenever you assess such a patient.)

Treatment

Treatment of myocardial contusion is usually supportive and symptomatic: Analgesics for chest pain and cardiac monitoring are the most important treatment modes used.

Nursing management

Your first nursing priorities are pain relief and close observation of the patient to detect consequences of myocardial contusion and to intervene if they occur. Life-threatening conditions may develop, including cardiac dysrhythmias—such as heart block—and cardiac tamponade, which can follow a myocardial contusion. Watch for their signs and symptoms—jugular vein distention, lowered blood pressure, and muffled heart sounds. Also check for signs and symptoms of reduced cardiac output, because the ischemic areas of the myocardium resulting from myocardial contusion cause a pathophysiologic state similar to that of an MI, ranging from microscopic interstitial hemorrhage to transmural necrosis.

Continue giving supplemental oxygen by nasal cannula at 2 to 6 liters/minute to decrease pain, reduce myocardial irritability, and prevent hypoxemia. To further reduce pain, administer analgesics. Myocardial contusions do not usually respond to nitroglycerin. However, *do not* give these medications intramuscularly. Intramuscular administration elevates CPK levels (mimicking the elevation caused by contusion), and intramuscular absorption is unpredictable when cardiac output is reduced.

Monitor the patient's electrolytes for any imbalance, and watch for signs and symptoms of respiratory insufficiency, which can cause hypoxemia and hypercapnia—and possible subsequent acidosis. These can increase his chances of developing dysrhythmias.

Nursing diagnoses

With the data collected from the patient's history and physical examination, formulate nursing diagnoses and establish related goals and interventions. In cardiomyopathy, your diagnoses typically address physical, emotional, and cognitive problems.

Alteration in cardiac output related to tumor, myocardial contusion, and so forth

After formulating this diagnosis, your goals are to achieve adequate cardiac output, maintain hemodynamic stability, prevent complications, and reduce patient anxiety.

Alteration in comfort (chest pain) resulting from decreased myocardial perfusion

Your goals are to relieve discomfort and prevent complications.

Potential knowledge deficit related to inadequate patient teaching

This diagnosis addresses the patient's lack of knowledge about the cause, effects, and treatment of his disease. Your goals are to increase his understanding of cardiomyopathy and promote compliance with the prescribed treatment.

11

CARDIAC COMPLICATIONS

Once a patient with severe cardiac dysfunction is admitted to a coronary care unit, his chances of survival are reasonably good—unless he develops certain complications. Your first priority is preventing these complications or detecting them in their earliest, most treatable stages. Your next priority is giving appropriate treatments promptly.

Cardiogenic shock

Sometimes called pump failure, cardiogenic shock is a condition of diminished cardiac output that severely impairs tissue perfusion. It reflects severe left ventricular failure and occurs as a serious complication in nearly 15% of all patients hospitalized with acute myocardial infarction (MI). Cardiogenic shock typically affects patients whose area of infarction exceeds 40% of muscle mass; in such patients, the fatality rate may exceed 85%. Most patients with cardiogenic shock die within 24 hours of onset. Prognosis for those who survive is extremely poor.

Causes

Cardiogenic shock can result from any condition that causes significant left ventricular dysfunction with reduced cardiac output, such as MI (most common), myocardial ischemia, papillary muscle dysfunction, or end-stage cardiomyopathy. Regardless of the underlying cause, left ventricular dysfunction sets into motion a series of compensatory mechanisms that attempt to increase cardiac output and, in turn, maintain vital organ function.

As cardiac output falls in left ventricular dysfunction, aortic and carotid baroreceptors initiate sympathetic nervous responses, which increase heart rate, left ventricular filling pressure, and peripheral resistance to flow, to enhance venous return to the heart. These compensatory responses initially stabilize the patient but later cause deterioration with rising oxygen demands of the already compromised myocardium. These events constitute a vicious circle of low cardiac output, sympathetic compensation, myocardial ischemia, and even lower cardiac output.

Signs and symptoms

Cardiogenic shock produces signs of poor tissue perfusion: cold, pale, clammy skin; a drop in systolic blood pressure to 30 mm Hg below baseline, or a sustained reading below 80 mm Hg not attributable to medication; tachycardia; rapid, shallow respirations; oliguria (less than 20 ml urine/hour); restlessness, mental confusion, and obtundation; narrowing pulse pressure; and cyanosis. Although many of these clinical features also occur in congestive heart failure (CHF) and other shock syndromes, they are usually more profound in cardiogenic shock. (See *How to Recognize Cardiogenic Shock,* page 180.)

How to Recognize Cardiogenic Shock

The first sign of cardiogenic shock—or any shock—may be a *fast pulse rate,* 110/minute or over. That signals the heart's effort to compensate for a *declining blood pressure* produced by a falling stroke volume, which is another early sign.

You can count on cardiogenic shock to include the signs of hypoperfusion. First, there is the acute MI, documented by the patient's history, certain EKG changes (usually elevated ST segments, flattened or inverted T waves, or enlarged Q waves), and a characteristic release of enzymes into the blood by the damaged tissue (elevated LDH, SGOT, and CPK, especially CPK-MB, which is a measure of the cardiac muscle fraction released by the damage).

The predominant cause of shock in MI is left ventricle loss of 35% to 70% of the heart's pumping muscle. This means that the muscle remaining has to perform double duty, while its own viability is extremely tenuous. Sometimes the papillary muscle itself has been ruptured, or the septum perforated, or all three layers of the wall caught in the infarct. In any case, the surviving heart probably has a bigger work load than it can handle and needs help badly.

One sign of the inevitable hypoperfusion will be cool, clammy, mottled skin (spelling out the poor tissue bath); another will be decreased or absent peripheral pulses.

At first, you may find pulse, heart sounds, and breath sounds normal. But the ensuing hypotension will affect them rapidly, so you will hear a heart rate of perhaps 110/minute, rales in the lung, and abnormal sounds of heartbeat—usually a third sound or ventricular gallop.

Next, look for a systolic blood pressure less than 80 mm Hg, or—if the patient is hypertensive—30 mm Hg below his normal pressure. Remember, taking the blood pressure by cuff of someone in shock does not usually represent the body's true state of perfusion as well as direct arterial cannulation does. By cuff, only 90 mm Hg spells hypotension.

After that, look for the other effects of poor tissue perfusion: clouded sensorium, altered mentation, hypoxemia, lactic acidosis, and a urinary output less than 20 ml/hour.

Last, eliminate other causes of shock such as trauma, infection, or hypovolemia.

Diagnosis

Auscultation detects gallop rhythm, faint heart sounds, and possibly, if the shock results from rupture of the ventricular septum or papillary muscles, a holosystolic murmur. Other abnormal clinical findings include:

• *pulmonary artery pressure (PAP) monitoring:* increased PAP and increased pulmonary capillary wedge pressure (PCWP), reflecting a rise in left ventricular end-diastolic pressure (preload) and increased resistance to left ventricular emptying (afterload) due to ineffective pumping and increased peripheral vascular resistance. Thermodi-

lution technique measures decreased cardiac index (less than 2.2 liters/minute).

• *invasive arterial pressure monitoring:* hypotension due to impaired ventricular ejection

• *arterial blood gases:* may show metabolic acidosis and hypoxia

• *electrocardiogram (EKG):* possible evidence of acute MI, ischemia, or ventricular aneurysm

• *enzyme levels:* elevated creatine phosphokinase (CPK), lactic dehydrogenase (LDH), serum glutamic-oxaloacetic transaminase (SGOT) and serum glutamic-pyruvic transaminase (SGPT), which point to MI or ischemia and suggest CHF or shock. CPK and LDH isoenzymes determinations may confirm acute MI.

Additional tests determine other conditions that can lead to pump dysfunction and failure, such as cardiac dysrhythmias, cardiac tamponade, papillary muscle infarct or rupture, ventricular septal rupture, pulmonary emboli, venous pooling (associated with venodilators and continuous intermittent positive pressure breathing), and hypovolemia.

Treatment

The aim of treatment is to enhance cardiovascular status by increasing cardiac output, improving myocardial perfusion, and decreasing cardiac work load with combinations of various cardiovascular drugs and mechanical-assist techniques. Drug therapy may include dopamine I.V., a vasopressor that increases cardiac output, blood pressure, and renal blood flow; levarterenol (norepinephrine), when a more potent vasoconstrictor is necessary; and nitroprusside I.V., a vasodilator that may be used with a vasopressor to further improve cardiac output by decreasing peripheral vascular resistance (afterload) and reducing left ventricular end-diastolic pressure (preload). The patient's systemic blood pressure must be adequate if nitroprusside is used. Arterial pressure needs close monitoring. The intraaortic balloon pump (IABP) is a mechanical-assist device that attempts to improve coronary artery perfusion and decrease cardiac work load. The inflatable balloon pump is surgically inserted through the femoral artery into the descending thoracic aorta. The balloon inflates during diastole to increase coronary artery perfusion pressure and deflates before systole (before the aortic valve opens) to reduce resistance to ejection (afterload) and therefore lessen cardiac work load. Improved ventricular ejection, which significantly improves cardiac output, and a subsequent vasodilation in the peripheral vasculature lead to lower preload volume.

Nursing management

• At the first sign of cardiogenic shock, check blood pressure and heart rate. If the patient is hypotensive or has difficulty breathing, make sure he has a patent I.V. line and a patent airway, and provide oxygen to promote adequate oxygenation of tissues. Notify the doctor immediately.

• Monitor arterial blood gases to measure oxygenation and detect acidosis from poor tissue perfusion. Increase oxygen flow as indicated by blood gas measurements. Check complete blood count and electrolytes.

• After diagnosis, monitor cardiac rhythm continuously. Assess skin color, temperature, and other vital signs often. Watch especially for a drop in systolic blood pressure to less than 80 mm Hg (usually results in inadequate coronary artery blood flow, which may produce cardiac ischemia or cardiac dysrhythmias and further compromise cardiac output). Report hypotension immediately.

• A Foley catheter may be inserted to measure urinary output. Notify the doctor if output drops below 30 ml/hour.

• Using a pulmonary artery catheter, closely monitor PAP, PCWP, and if equipment is available, cardiac output. A high PCWP indicates CHF and should be reported immediately.

• When a patient is on the IABP, reposition him often and perform passive range-of-motion exercises to prevent skin breakdown. However, do not flex the "ballooned" leg at the hip, since this may displace or fracture the catheter. Assess pedal pulses and skin temperature and color to make sure circulation to the leg is adequate. Check the dressing on the insertion site frequently for bleeding, and change it according to hospital protocol. Also check the site for hematoma or signs of infection, and culture any drainage.

• After the patient has become hemodynamically stable, the frequency of balloon inflation is gradually reduced to wean him from the IABP. During weaning, carefully watch for monitor changes, chest pain, and other signs of recurring cardiac ischemia and shock.

• Provide psychological support. Since the patient and family may be anxious about the intensive care unit (ICU), the IABP, and other tubes and devices, offer reassurance. To ease emotional stress, plan your care to allow frequent rest periods, and provide for as much privacy as possible.

Cardiac tamponade

In cardiac tamponade, a rapid, unchecked rise in intrapericardial pressure impairs diastolic filling of the heart. The rise in pressure usually results from blood or fluid accumulation in the pericardial sac. If fluid accumulates rapidly, this condition is commonly fatal and necessitates emergency lifesaving measures. Slow accumulation and rise in pressure, as in pericardial effusion associated with malignancies, may not produce immediate symptoms, since the fibrous wall of the pericardial sac can gradually stretch to accommodate as much as 1 to 2 liters of fluid.

Causes
Increased intrapericardial pressure and consequent cardiac tamponade may result from:
• effusion (in malignancy, bacterial infections, tuberculosis, and rarely, acute rheumatic fever)
• hemorrhage from trauma (such as gunshot or stab wounds of the chest or perforation by catheter during cardiac or central venous catheterization or during postcardiac surgery)
• hemorrhage from nontraumatic causes (such as rupture of the heart or great vessels or anticoagulant therapy in a patient with pericarditis)
• acute MI
• uremia
• idiopathic Dressler's syndrome.

Signs and symptoms
Cardiac tamponade classically produces increased venous pressure with neck vein distention, reduced arterial blood pressure, muffled heart sounds on auscultation, and *pulsus paradoxus* (an abnormal inspiratory drop in systemic blood pressure greater than 15 mm Hg). These classic symptoms represent failure of physiologic compensatory mechanisms to override the effects of rapidly rising pericardial pressure, which limits diastolic filling of the ventricles and reduces stroke volume to a critically low level. Generally, ventricular end-systolic volume is not changed significantly, since the contractile force of the ventricles remains intact even in severe tamponade. The increasing pericardial pressure is transmitted equally across the heart cavities, producing a proportionate rise in intracardiac pressure, especially both atrial pressures and end-diastolic ventricular pressures. Cardiac tamponade may also produce dyspnea, tachycardia, narrow pulse pressure, restlessness, and hepatomegaly. Lung fields will be clear.

Diagnosis
Diagnosis usually relies on classic clinical features. Laboratory results may include the following:
• *chest X-ray* shows slightly widened mediastinum and cardiomegaly.
• *EKG* is rarely diagnostic of tamponade but is useful in ruling out other cardiac disorders. It may reveal changes produced by acute pericarditis.
• *pulmonary artery catheterization* detects increased right atrial pressure, right ventricular diastolic pressure, and central venous pressure. As tamponade increases diastolic pressure equilibrates.
• *echocardiography* records pericardial effusion, with signs of right ventricular and right atrial compression.

Treatment
The goal of treatment is to relieve intrapericardial pressure and cardiac compression by removing accumulated blood or fluid. Pericardiocentesis (needle aspiration of the pericardial cavity) or surgical creation of an opening dramatically improves systemic arterial pressure

and cardiac output with aspiration of as little as 25 ml of fluid. (See *Emergency Pericardiocentesis*.) Such treatment necessitates continuous hemodynamic and EKG monitoring in the ICU. Trial volume loading with temporary I.V. normal saline solution with albumin and perhaps an inotropic drug, such as isoproterenol or dopamine, is necessary in the hypotensive patient to maintain cardiac output. Although this drug normally improves myocardial function, it may further compromise an ischemic myocardium after MI.

Depending on the cause of tamponade, additional treatment may include:
• *in traumatic injury:* blood transfusion or a thoracotomy to drain reaccumulating fluid or to repair bleeding sites
• *in heparin-induced tamponade:* the heparin antagonist protamine sulfate
• *in warfarin-induced tamponade:* vitamin K.

Nursing management
If the patient is to undergo pericardiocentesis:
• Explain the procedure to him. Keep a pericardial aspiration needle attached to a 50 ml syringe by a three-way stopcock, an EKG machine, and an emergency cart with a defibrillator at the bedside. Make sure the equipment is turned on and ready for immediate use. Position the patient at a 45° to 60° angle to facilitate correct needle insertion. Connect the precordial EKG lead to the hub of the aspiration needle with an alligator clamp and connecting wire, and assist with fluid aspiration. When the needle touches the myocardium, you will see an ST segment elevation or premature ventricular contractions.
• Monitor blood pressure and central venous pressure (CVP) during and after pericardiocentesis. Infuse I.V. solutions, as ordered, to maintain blood pressure. Watch for a decrease in CVP and a concomitant rise in blood pressure, which indicate relief of cardiac compression.
• Watch for complications of pericardiocentesis, such as ventricular fibrillation, vagovagal arrest, or coronary ar-

Emergency Pericardiocentesis

If the doctor suspects a patient has cardiac tamponade, he may do emergency pericardiocentesis. (This procedure is also used to diagnose pericardial effusion.) Pericardiocentesis involves inserting a 16G to 18G intracardiac needle into the pericardial sac to aspirate fluid and relieve intrapericardial pressure.

Pericardiocentesis may cause life-threatening complications, such as ventricular dysrhythmias, bleeding from the myocardium, and coronary artery laceration. A precordial lead attached to the needle's hub lets the EKG monitor reflect needle position. If the needle contacts the patient's myocardium inadvertently, causing bleeding and ventricular irritability, you will see abnormal waveforms—large and erratic QRS complexes. Elevated ST segments indicate that the needle has contacted the ventricle; prolonged PR intervals indicate that it has touched the atrium.

Monitor the patient's EKG, blood pressure, and central venous pressure (CVP) constantly. Make sure, too, that emergency resuscitation equipment is on hand.

Following the procedure, monitor the patient's vital signs every 5 to 10 minutes. His blood pressure should rise as the tamponade is relieved.

Be alert for signs and symptoms of recurring tamponade (which may require repeated pericardiocentesis):
• decreased blood pressure
• narrowing pulse pressure
• increased CVP
• distended neck veins
• tachycardia
• tachypnea
• muffled heart sounds
• friction rub
• anxiety
• chest pain.

tery or cardiac chamber puncture. Closely monitor EKG changes, blood pressure, pulse rate, level of consciousness, and urinary output.

If the patient is scheduled for thoracotomy:
• Explain the procedure to him, and tell him what to expect postoperatively (chest tubes, drainage bottles, and administration of oxygen). Teach him how to turn, deep breathe, and cough.
• Give antibiotics, protamine sulfate, or vitamin K, as ordered.
• Postoperatively, monitor critical parameters, such as vital signs and arterial blood gases, and assess heart and breath sounds. Give pain medication, as ordered. Maintain the chest drainage system, and be alert for complications, such as hemorrhage, cardiac dysrhythmias, and pulmonary or renal dysfunction.

Cardiac arrest

Cardiac arrest is the sudden cessation of the heart's pumping function. Untreated, it is rapidly fatal; a delay in treatment of only 3 to 5 minutes may produce irreversible brain damage. In the United States, cardiac arrest accounts for more than 350,000 deaths a year—most occurring outside the hospital. However, prompt, aggressive treatment and early entry into the emergency medical services system may prevent many of these deaths.

Causes
Cardiac arrest may result from circulatory collapse caused by a dissociation between mechanical and electrical heart functions (electromechanical dissociation). Although its mechanism is not fully understood, electromechanical dissociation may result from failure in the calcium transport system and is associated with severe myocardial ischemia and necrosis.

Other causes of cardiac arrest include:
• *ventricular fibrillation,* resulting from MI, heart failure, anesthetics, electrical

shock, electrolyte disturbances (hyper- or hypokalemia and acidosis), ventricular irritation (from cardiac pacing wires or cardiac catheterization), or acute hemorrhage
• *ventricular standstill* or *asystole,* from hypoxia, acidosis or hypercapnia, vagal stimulation, and hyperkalemia.

Signs and symptoms
Cardiac arrest does not usually occur without premonitory clues. For example, it is apt to quickly follow loss of peripheral blood pressure, changes in EKG patterns, respiratory failure, or sudden tachycardia or bradycardia. Typically, imminent cardiac arrest produces bradycardia and hypotension, followed by seizure, loss of consciousness, cessation of respiration, and absence of peripheral pulses or heart sounds. Pupillary dilation, a sign of inadequate cerebral perfusion, occurs secondary to cardiac arrest.

Diagnosis
Absence of central pulses (carotid or femoral), respiration, and loss of consciousness confirm cardiac arrest. Treatment must begin immediately to restore vital functions and prevent cerebral damage and death secondary to anoxia. Later, EKG can detect lethal dysrhythmias that may have provoked cardiac arrest, or enzyme studies can confirm MI.

Treatment
Treatment attempts to restore an effective heart rhythm that can sustain cardiac output through basic and advanced life support techniques.

Basic life support (BLS) is emergency first aid treatment for both respiratory and cardiac arrests (see "Cardiopulmonary resuscitation," page 340). It establishes an adequate airway, ventilation through artificial means, and circulatory assistance through external (closed) cardiac massage. BLS, properly administered, continues until the patient recovers, can be transported to receive more advanced life support, or is pronounced dead by a doctor.

Management of cardiac arrest then proceeds to advanced life support (ALS), which provides adjunctive treatment by trained personnel to maintain effective ventilation and circulation. ALS includes cardiac monitoring—especially for dysrhythmias—I.V. therapy, defibrillation, and postresuscitative care.

Nursing management
• Check for early signs of cardiac arrest, such as hypotension and bradycardia in high-risk patients, especially those with ischemic heart disease.
• Achieve certification in cardiopulmonary resuscitation (CPR). Know your hospital's procedure for managing cardiac arrest—its method for alerting a cardiac arrest team, and the location and use of emergency equipment and drugs.
• Assess respiratory status by frequently drawing arterial blood gas samples, and adjust oxygen concentrations accordingly. Mechanical ventilation may be necessary.

During recovery from cardiac arrest:
• Keep I.V. lines patent to ensure rapid administration of drugs. For patients with ventricular dysrhythmias, keep I.V. lidocaine at the bedside for bolus administration.
• Obtain arterial blood gas samples frequently, to monitor metabolic abnormalities. Watch for dysrhythmias, hypoxia, acidosis, hypokalemia, and other conditions that may precipitate a second arrest.
• Evaluate renal status by monitoring hourly urinary output and specific gravity, and daily electrolytes, BUN, or creatinine levels. An osmotic diuretic may be ordered to increase urinary output and reverse acute renal failure.
• Assess cardiac status by monitoring level of consciousness, skin color and temperature, and peripheral pulses. Monitor pulmonary artery catheter readings, cardiac output using thermodilution technique, and direct arterial blood pressure.
• Determine neurologic status by checking for signs of cerebral edema and other central nervous system complications (elevated temperature, wide pulse pressure, diminished responsiveness, or seizure activity).
• Watch for complications of CPR (rib or sternal fractures, cardiac tamponade, or pneumothorax).
• If CPR fails, provide psychologic support for the family.

Ventricular aneurysm

Ventricular aneurysm is an outpouching, almost always of the left ventricle, that produces ventricular wall dysfunction in about 20% of patients after MI. Ventricular aneurysm may develop within weeks after MI or may be delayed for years. Untreated ventricular aneurysm can lead to dysrhythmias, systemic embolization, or CHF and is potentially fatal. Resection (rarely used as sole treatment) improves prognosis in CHF or refractory patients who have developed ventricular dysrhythmias; however, the mortality is very high.

Causes
When MI destroys a large muscular section of the left ventricle, necrosis reduces the ventricular wall to a thin sheath of fibrous tissue. Under intracardiac pressure, this thin layer stretches and forms a separate noncontractile sac (aneurysm). Abnormal muscular wall movement accompanies ventricular aneurysm and includes akinesia (lack of movement), dyskinesia (paradoxical movement), asynergia (decreased and inadequate movement), and asynchrony (uncoordinated movement). During systolic ejection, the abnormal muscular wall movements associated with the aneurysm cause the remaining normally functioning myocardial fibers to increase the force of contraction in order to maintain stroke volume and cardiac output. At the same time, a portion of the stroke volume is lost to passive distention of the noncontractile sac.

Signs and symptoms

Ventricular aneurysm may cause dys-rhythmias—such as premature ventric-ular contractions or ventricular tachy-cardia—palpitations, signs of cardiac dysfunction (weakness on exertion, fa-tigue, or angina), and occasionally, a visible or palpable systolic precordial bulge. This condition may also lead to left ventricular dysfunction, with chronic CHF (dyspnea, fatigue, edema, rales, gallop rhythm, or neck vein dis-tention); pulmonary edema; systemic embolization; and with left ventricular failure, pulsus alternans. Ventricular aneurysms enlarge but rarely rupture.

Diagnosis

Persistent ventricular dysrhythmias, on-set of heart failure, or systemic emboli-zation in a patient with left ventricular failure and a history of MI strongly sug-gests ventricular aneurysm. Indicative tests include the following:
• *Left ventriculography* reveals left ven-tricular enlargement, with an area of akinesia or dyskinesia (during cinean-giography) and diminished cardiac function.
• *EKG* may show persistent ST-T–wave elevations 2 weeks after infarction.
• *Chest X-ray* may demonstrate an ab-normal bulge distorting the heart's con-tour if the aneurysm is large; the X-ray may be normal if the aneurysm is small.
• *Noninvasive nuclear cardiology scan* may indicate the site of infarction and suggest the area of aneurysm.
• *Echocardiogram* will show aberrant left ventricular wall motion.

Treatment

Depending on the size of the aneurysm and the complications, treatment will necessitate either routine medical ex-amination to follow the patient's condi-tion or aggressive measures for intract-able ventricular dysrhythmias, CHF, and emboli.

Emergency treatment of ventricular dysrhythmia includes antiarrhythmics I.V. or electrocardioversion. Preventive treatment continues with oral antiar-rhythmics, such as procainamide, quin-idine, or disopyramide.

Emergency treatment for CHF with pulmonary edema includes oxygen, dig-italis I.V., furosemide I.V., morphine sulfate I.V., and, when necessary, nitro-prusside I.V. and intubation. Mainte-nance therapy may include nitrates, pra-zosin, and hydralazine by mouth. Systemic embolization requires antico-agulation therapy or embolectomy. Re-fractory ventricular tachycardia, heart failure, recurrent arterial embolization, and persistent angina with coronary ar-tery occlusion may necessitate surgery, of which the most effective procedure is aneurysmectomy, with myocardial re-vascularization.

Nursing management

• If ventricular tachycardia occurs, monitor blood pressure and heart rate. If cardiac arrest develops, initiate CPR and call for assistance, resuscitative equip-ment, and medication.
• In a patient with CHF, closely monitor vital signs, heart sounds, intake and out-put, fluid and electrolyte balances, and BUN and creatinine levels. Because of the threat of systemic embolization, fre-quently check peripheral pulses and the color and temperature of extremities. Be alert for sudden changes in sensorium that indicate cerebral embolization and for any signs that suggest renal failure or progressive MI.
• If dysrhythmias necessitate cardiover-sion, use a sufficient amount of conduct-ing jelly to prevent chest burns. If the patient is conscious, give diazepam I.V., as ordered, before cardioversion. Ex-plain that cardioversion is a lifesaving method using brief electroshock to the heart. If the patient is receiving antiar-rhythmics, check appropriate laboratory tests. For instance, if he takes procain-amide, check antinuclear antibodies be-cause this drug may induce lupus ery-thematosus syndrome.

If the patient is scheduled to undergo resection:
• Before surgery, explain expected post-operative care in the ICU (including use

of endotracheal tube, ventilator, hemodynamic monitoring, chest tubes, and drainage bottle).

• After surgery, monitor vital signs, intake and output, heart sounds, and pulmonary artery catheter. Watch for signs of infection, such as fever and excessive drainage from incision.

To prepare the patient for discharge:

• Teach him how to take his pulse (observing for irregularity and rate changes). Urge him to follow his medication regimen strictly (even if he has to set an alarm to take medication during the night) and to watch for side effects.

• Since dysrhythmias can cause sudden death, refer the family to a community-based CPR training program.

• Provide psychological support for the patient and family.

Hypovolemic shock (Hypovolemic shock syndrome)

In hypovolemic shock, reduced intravascular blood volume causes circulatory dysfunction and inadequate tissue perfusion. Without sufficient blood or fluid replacement, hypovolemic shock syndrome may lead to irreversible cerebral and renal damage, cardiac arrest, and ultimately, death. Hypovolemic shock syndrome necessitates early recognition of signs and symptoms and prompt, aggressive treatment to improve prognosis. (See *Pathophysiology of Hypovolemic Shock.*)

Causes

Hypovolemic shock usually results from acute blood loss—about one fifth of total volume. Such massive blood loss may result from gastrointestinal bleeding, internal hemorrhage (hemothorax or hemoperitoneum), external hemorrhage (accidental or surgical trauma), or from any condition that reduces circulating intravascular plasma volume or other body fluids, such as in severe burns. Other underlying causes include intestinal obstruction, peritonitis, acute pancreatitis,

Pathophysiology of Hypovolemic Shock

Normally, the body compensates for a loss of blood or fluid by constricting arteriolar beds, increasing heart rate and contractile force, and redistributing fluids. These compensation mechanisms are effective enough to maintain stable vital signs, even after a 10% blood loss. But by the time blood or fluid loss reaches 15% to 25%, these mechanisms fail to maintain cardiac output, and blood pressure drops.

Baroreceptors (pressure-sensitive stretch receptors) in the aorta and carotid bodies trigger sympathetic nerve fibers. As a result, the adrenal glands release norepinephrine and epinephrine, causing vasoconstriction, which—in turn—sharply reduces the blood flow to peripheral muscle and some of the vital organs (kidneys, liver, and lungs). Some cells, therefore, no longer receive oxygen, and cellular metabolism shifts from aerobic to anaerobic pathways, producing an accumulation of lactic acid, which is not metabolized to yield needed energy. Impaired renal or hepatic function causes this acid to accumulate and results in metabolic acidosis.

To compensate for metabolic acidosis, the patient hyperventilates to exhale more CO_2 and, in doing so, induces respiratory alkalosis. Since he may be unable to maintain the physical exertion required for hyperventilation, the patient may eventually need respiratory support, either oxygen by mask or mechanical ventilation.

Eventually, the compensatory mechanisms that serve to maintain acid-base balance fail, and cellular function is severely impaired, leading to cell death and subsequent organ failure.

ascites and dehydration from excessive perspiration, severe diarrhea or protracted vomiting, diabetes insipidus, diuresis, or inadequate fluid intake.

Signs and symptoms

Hypovolemic shock produces a syndrome of hypotension, with narrowing pulse pressure; decreased sensorium; tachycardia; rapid, shallow respirations; reduced urinary output (less than 25 ml/hour); and cold, pale, clammy skin. Metabolic acidosis with an accumulation of lactic acid develops as a result of tissue anoxia, as cellular metabolism shifts from aerobic to anaerobic pathways. Disseminated intravascular coagulation (DIC) is a possible complication of hypovolemic shock.

Diagnosis

No single symptom or diagnostic test establishes the diagnosis or severity of shock. Laboratory findings include:
• elevated potassium, serum lactate, and blood urea nitrogen levels
• increased urine specific gravity (more than 1.020) and urine osmolality
• decreased blood pH and PO_2 and increased PCO_2

In addition, gastroscopy, aspiration of gastric contents through a nasogastric tube, and X-rays identify internal bleeding sites; coagulation studies may detect coagulopathy from DIC.

Treatment

Emergency treatment measures consist of prompt, adequate blood and fluid replacement to restore intravascular volume and raise blood pressure. Saline solution, then possibly plasma proteins (albumin), other plasma expanders, or lactated Ringer's solution may produce volume expansion until whole blood can be matched. Application of medical antishock trousers may be helpful. Treatment may also include oxygen administration, identification of bleeding site, control of bleeding by direct measures (such as pressure and elevation of an extremity), and possibly, surgery.

Nursing management

Management of hypovolemic shock necessitates prompt, aggressive supportive measures and careful assessment and monitoring of vital signs. Note that measurements of vital signs, urine, blood loss, CVP, and all other parameters will be different in children. Follow these priorities:
• Check for a patent airway and adequate circulation. If blood pressure and heart rate are absent, start CPR.
• Place the patient flat in bed, with his legs elevated about 30° to increase blood flow by promoting venous return to the heart.
• Record blood pressure, pulse rate, peripheral pulses, respirations, and other vital signs every 15 minutes; record EKG continuously. Systolic blood pressure less than 80 mm Hg usually results in inadequate coronary artery blood flow, cardiac ischemia, dysrhythmias, and further complications of low cardiac output. When blood pressure drops below 80 mm Hg, increase the oxygen flow rate, and notify the doctor immediately. A progressive drop in blood pressure, accompanied by a thready pulse, generally signals inadequate cardiac output from reduced intravascular volume. Notify the doctor, and increase the infusion rate.
• Start I.V.s with normal saline or lactated Ringer's solution, using a large-bore catheter (14G), which allows easier administration of later blood transfusions. (*Caution:* Do not start I.V.s in the legs of a patient in shock who has suffered abdominal trauma, since infused fluid may escape through the ruptured vessel into the abdomen.)
• An indwelling (Foley) catheter may be inserted to measure hourly urinary output. If output is less than 30 ml/hour in adults, increase the fluid infusion rate, but watch for signs of fluid overload, such as an increase in PCWP (see Chapter 14, Monitoring Procedures). Notify the doctor if urinary output does not improve. An osmotic diuretic, such as mannitol, may be ordered to increase renal blood flow and urinary output.

Determine how much fluid to give by checking blood pressure, urinary output, CVP, or PCWP. (To increase accuracy, CVP should be measured at the level of the right atrium, using the same reference point on the chest each time.)
• Draw an arterial blood sample to measure blood gas levels. Administer oxygen by face mask or airway to ensure adequate oxygenation of tissues. Adjust the oxygen flow rate to a higher or lower level, as blood gas measurements indicate.
• Draw venous blood for CBC, electrolytes, type and cross match, and coagulation studies.
• During therapy, assess skin color and temperature, and note any changes. Cold, clammy skin may be a sign of continuing peripheral vascular constriction, indicating progressive shock.
• Watch for signs of impending coagulopathy (petechiae, bruising, bleeding or oozing from gums or venipuncture sites).
• Explain all procedures and their purpose. Throughout these emergency measures, provide emotional support to the patient and family.

Nursing diagnoses

After collecting subjective data from the patient interview and objective data from the cardiovascular assessment, formulate nursing diagnoses that clearly explain the patient's problems and allow you to plan appropriate goals and interventions. Typically, your diagnoses reflect the physiologic and psychological consequences that lead up to the complication.

Alteration in cardiac output related to acute MI and altered hemodynamic status of the body

Alteration in gas exchange related to pulmonary edema

Your goals are to provide constant patient monitoring, promptly detect changes in the patient's condition, and prevent sudden death from complications.

Alteration in tissue perfusion related to cardiac arrest, hypovolemic shock, or ventricular aneurysm

Your goal is to prevent ischemic complications by maintaining adequate cardiac output. Watch for and report any signs and symptoms of inadequate tissue perfusion. Monitor vital signs carefully.

12

DIAGNOSTIC PROCEDURES

The continuing proliferation of diagnostic tests has made nursing care of patients with cardiovascular disorders as complex as it is commonplace. More nurses than ever before participate in the diagnosis of these disorders.

Choice of a specific diagnostic test depends on the doctor's clinical suspicions, the kind of information needed, and the risk to the patient. As a rule, noninvasive tests precede invasive ones, since invasive tests are generally more hazardous and costly. However, invasive tests are often necessary to obtain the most diagnostic information.

GRAPHIC RECORDING

Electrocardiography—the most frequently performed graphic recording test—records the conduction, magnitude, and duration of the electrical activity of the heart. It identifies rhythm disturbances, conduction abnormalities and electrolyte imbalances, and contributes information about the size of the heart chambers and the relative position of the heart in the chest. The electrocardiogram (EKG) is useful in documenting the diagnosis and progression of myocardial infarction (MI), ischemia, and pericarditis, and in evaluating the effectiveness of artificial pacemakers and cardiotonic drugs.

Exercise electrocardiography measures the cardiovascular effects of controlled physical stress (bike riding or treadmill walking). During this test, the EKG is checked for evidence of ischemia, dysrhythmias, or conduction ab-

normalities. The exercise EKG can help identify the cause of chest pain and plan therapy for patients with known cardiovascular disease. Both ambulatory and exercise electrocardiography must be preceded by a thorough clinical workup.

Ambulatory (Holter) electrocardiography records the heart's electrical activity for 24 hours or longer as the patient performs his usual activities and experiences normal physical and emotional stress. It can detect intermittent dysrhythmias, gauge the effectiveness of antiarrhythmic drugs, and assess patient progress during recovery from MI. It can also help detect the cause of dizziness, vertigo, palpitations, and chest pain. (See also *Additional Diagnostic Tests,* pages 192 and 193.)

Electrocardiography

The most frequently used procedure for evaluating cardiac status, electrocardiography detects the presence and location of MI, ischemia, conduction delay, chamber enlargement, or dysrhythmias, and helps assess the effects of electrolyte disturbances and cardiac drugs. In the 12-lead EKG, five electrodes attached to the patient's arms, legs, and chest measure the electrical potential generated by the heart. This potential is analyzed from twelve different views, or leads: three standard bipolar limb leads (I, II, III), three unipolar augmented limb leads (aV_R, aV_L, aV_F), and six unipolar chest leads (V_1 to V_6). Lead I measures the electrical potential between the left and right arms; lead II, the electrical potential between the left leg and right arm; and lead III, the electrical potential between the left leg and left arm. Using the same electrode placement, leads aV_R, aV_L, and aV_F measure electrical potential between one augmented limb lead and the electrical midpoint of the remaining two leads (determined electronically by the EKG machine). Both standard and augmented leads view the heart from the front, in the vertical plane. The six unipolar chest leads view it from the horizontal plane, helping to locate pathology in the lateral and posterior walls. The EKG machine averages the electrical potentials of the three limb electrodes (I, II, and III) and compares this with the electrical potential of the chest electrode. Recordings made with the V connection show variations in electrical potential that occur under the chest electrode as its position is changed.

After electrical potentials are transmitted to the EKG machine, these forces are amplified and graphically displayed on a strip chart recorder. The graphic display, or tracing, usually consists of the P wave, the QRS complex, and the T wave. The P wave shows atrial depolarization; the QRS complex, ventricular depolarization; and the T wave, ventricular repolarization.

Purpose

• To help identify primary conduction abnormalities, cardiac dysrhythmias, cardiac hypertrophy, pericarditis, electrolyte imbalance, myocardial ischemia, and the site and extent of MI
• To monitor recovery from MI
• To evaluate the effectiveness of cardiac medication (cardiac glycosides, antiarrhythmics, antihypertensives, and vasodilators)
• To observe pacemaker performance. (See *EKG Strip: What It Shows*, page 195.)

Equipment

Single-channel EKG machine with amplifier and strip chart recorder/recording paper/five lead wires/four limb lead electrodes with rubber straps/one suction cup chest electrode/electrode gel/4″ x 4″ gauze pads/alcohol/disposable ra-

zor/moist cloth towel.

A gauze pad soaked in normal saline solution may be substituted for the electrode gel beneath the limb leads.

Procedure

Explain the procedure to the patient to allay his fears and promote cooperation. Inform him that he need not restrict food or fluids beforehand, and that the procedure takes about 15 minutes. Instruct him to relax, lie still, and breathe normally. Advise him not to talk during the procedure because the sound of his voice may distort the EKG tracing.

Check the patient's history for cardiac drugs, and note any current therapy on the test request form.

Instruct the patient to disrobe to the waist and expose both legs for electrode placement. Drape the female patient's chest until chest leads are applied.

Place the patient in the supine position. However, if he is orthopneic, place him in a semi-Fowler's position. Instruct him to avoid touching the metal handrail of the bed or allowing his feet to touch the footboard, to prevent current leakage that distorts the EKG tracing.

Turn on the EKG machine and set the lead selector to the standby mode to warm up the stylus mechanism. Check the paper supply and center the stylus on the paper.

Cleanse the electrode placement sites with alcohol and shave them, if necessary. Apply electrode gel to the inner aspect of the forearms and the medial aspect of the lower legs. Rub the skin vigorously when applying the electrodes, creating an erythema, to enhance skin contact with the electrode.

Secure the limb electrodes with rubber straps, but avoid overtightening the straps to prevent circulatory impairment and the onset of muscle spasms, which may distort the recording. Position the leg electrodes with their connector ends pointing upward to avoid bending or straining the lead wires.

Connect each lead wire to an electrode by inserting the wire prong into the terminal post and tightening the

Additional Diagnostic Tests

Test	Definition	Diagnostic objectives
Cardiac series	Fluoroscopic visualization of motion and pulsations of heart and great vessels during systole and diastole; largely superseded by echocardiography for most diagnostic purposes	To assess structural abnormalities of heart chambers To detect aortic and mitral valve calcification To evaluate prosthetic valve function To detect abnormalities of aortic arch and esophageal contours
Lower limb venography (ascending contrast phlebography)	Fluoroscopic visualization of veins after injection of contrast medium	To confirm deep vein thrombosis (DVT) To identify cause of dependent edema To assess vascular status before surgery
Phonocardiography	Graphic recording of normal and abnormal sounds of the cardiac cycle—gallops, murmurs, and other heart sounds—and the vibrations of great vessels	To help identify structural valve defects To aid precise timing of cardiac events To evaluate ventricular function by demonstrating systolic time intervals
Apexcardiography	Graphic recording of chest wall movement caused by low-frequency precordial cardiac pulsations	To help evaluate left ventricular function To help identify heart sounds
Vectorcardiography	Graphic recording of variations in electrical potential during cardiac cycle, using two simultaneously recorded lead axes to construct a three-dimensional view of the heart; more commonly used in research than in clinical setting	To detect ventricular hypertrophy, interventricular conduction disturbances, and MI To clarify doubtful EKG results

Test	Definition	Diagnostic objectives
Carotid pulse tracing	Graphic recording of low-frequency carotid artery vibrations, which reflect pressure changes on heart's left side during systole and diastole	To help identify aortic valve disease, idiopathic hypertrophic subaortic stenosis, left ventricular failure, hypertension
Jugular pulse tracing	Graphic recording of low-frequency jugular vein vibrations, which reflect pressure changes on the heart's right side during systole and diastole	To aid diagnosis of right heart failure
Impedance plethysmography (occlusive impedance phlebography)	Graphic recording of changes in electrical resistance (impedance) caused by variations in circulating blood volume—the result of respiration or venous occlusion	To help detect DVT, especially in popliteal and iliofemoral veins
Digital subtraction angiography (DSA)	Arteriography with contrast medium using computerized subtraction technique and fluoroscopy	To detect vascular abnormalities (plaques, tumors, aneurysms, embolisms) To visualize arterial bypass grafts and arterial disease
Magnetic resonance imaging (MRI)	Imaging technique using magnetic waves. Computer analyzes signals from hydrogen atoms in body—safe for children and pregnant women, affects pacemaker function	To visualize blood flow, cardiac chambers, interventricular septum and valves. To detect vascular lesions, plaque, infarctions, and blood clots

screw. Be sure to match each color-coded lead wire to the corresponding electrode.

Turn the lead selector to lead I. Then write the lead number on the paper strip, or push the marking button on the machine to identify the lead with a series of dots and dashes (see *Chest Lead Positions and Marks*, page 196). Record for 3 to 6 seconds, and then return the machine to the standby mode. Repeat the procedure for leads II to aV$_F$.

After completing the aV$_F$ run, turn the lead selector to a neutral position before running chest leads V$_1$ to V$_6$. This prevents the stylus from swinging wildly and possibly damaging the paper.

Connect the chest lead wire to the suction cup electrode, apply electrode gel to the chest lead sites, and press the cup firmly to the V$_1$ position. Apply enough gel to produce efficient suction and low skin resistance.

Return the lead selector to the neutral position, reposition the electrode to V$_2$, and record. Repeat the procedure through V$_6$, always turning the selector to the neutral position before moving the suction cup.

After completing V$_6$, run a rhythm strip on lead II for at least 6 seconds. Assess the quality of the whole series and repeat individual lead tracings as needed. (See *The Standard 12-Lead Electrocardiogram*, page 197.)

Special considerations

• If necessary, replace metal electrodes and straps with suction cups for limb leads to enhance baseline stability. Position the cups on the outer aspect of the upper arms instead of the forearms and on the upper thighs instead of the lower legs.
• Before recording, recheck the lead positions and the lead wire and electrode connections to avoid lead reversal, which produces misleading test results. Become thoroughly familiar with the appearance of normal EKG tracings so you can recognize recording errors. For example, the leads for the right and left

arms, when reversed, may falsely indicate MI. A normal lead I has a positive deflection; similarly, the P waves in lead II normally have a positive deflection. The R waves in the chest leads should appear increasingly positive as they progress from V$_2$ to V$_6$. Avoid positioning V$_3$ at the same level as V$_4$ to V$_6$ to prevent a spurious Q wave tracing.
• If the patient's skin is exceptionally oily, scaly, or diaphoretic, rub the electrode site with alcohol and dry it with a cotton ball before applying the gelled electrode. This may help reduce baseline wander and interference in the tracing.
• If the patient with left ventricular hypertrophy exhibits large R wave tracings that run off the paper, change the sensitivity setting to half-standard, but be sure to mark the run as such. If the patient experiences chest pains during a lead run, note it on the appropriate strip. If he has a pacemaker in place, you can perform electrocardiography with or without a magnet, but be sure to indicate the presence of a pacemaker and the use of the magnet on the strip. (Many pacemakers function only when the heartbeat falls below a preset rate; a magnet makes the pacemaker fire regularly, permitting evaluation of its performance.)

Findings

The lead II waveform, known as the rhythm strip, depicts the heart's rhythm more clearly than any other waveform. In lead II, the normal P wave does not exceed 2.5 mm (0.25 millivolt) in height or last longer than 0.11 second. The P-R interval, which includes the P wave plus the PR segment, persists for 0.12 to 0.2 second for cardiac rates over 60 beats/minute. The Q-T interval varies with the cardiac rate and lasts 0.52 to 0.4 second for rates above 60; the voltage of the R wave in the V$_1$ through V$_6$ leads does not exceed 27 mm. The total QRS interval lasts 0.06 to 0.1 second. (See *Normal EKG Waveforms*, page 198.)

Implications of results

An abnormal EKG may show MI, right

EKG Strip: What It Shows

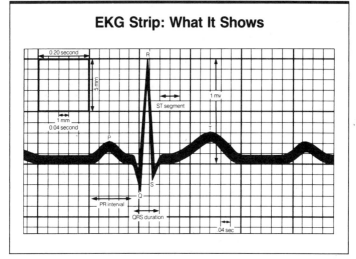

or left ventricular hypertrophy, dysrhythmias, right or left bundle branch block, ischemia, conduction defects or pericarditis, electrolyte abnormalities (such as hypokalemia), or the effects of cardioactive drugs. Sometimes an EKG may reveal abnormal waveforms only during episodes of symptoms such as angina or during exercise.

Documentation

Label each EKG strip with the patient's name and room number (if applicable), the date and time of the procedure, and the doctor's name. Include any special information, such as use of a magnet to test pacemaker function. If you send the strips to the EKG department, fill out the request form completely. Include the patient's age, height, weight, blood pressure, diagnosis, and drug regimen.

Exercise electrocardiography (Stress EKG)

The body responds to exercise by increasing its demand for oxygen—the result of increased respiratory rate, cardiac output, and extraction of oxygen by the tissues. Exercise electrocardiography evaluates these changes by monitoring heart rate, blood pressure, and EKG waveforms as the patient walks on a treadmill or pedals a stationary bicycle. This procedure provides diagnostic information that cannot be obtained from a resting EKG alone. It is used to diagnose the cause of chest pain, to screen for asymptomatic coronary artery disease (CAD), to identify cardiac dysrhythmias during exercise, to determine the functional capacity of the heart after surgery or MI, to help establish limits for exercise, and to evaluate the effectiveness of antiarrhythmic or antianginal drug therapy.

Exercise testing can be performed in single or multiple stages. The single-stage test entails a constant workload throughout the procedure, while the more frequently used multiple-stage test increases the workload at regular intervals until the patient reaches an endpoint, such as a target heart rate or the onset of chest pain or fatigue. Within these protocols, the test may also be submaximal or maximal. The submaximal test does not require the patient to

Chest Lead Positions and Marks

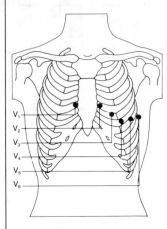

Limb leads		Chest leads	
I:	-	V₁:	— -
II:	–	V₂:	— --
III:	——	V₃:	— ---
aVR:	- —	V₄:	— ——
aVL:	– —	V₅:	— ———
aVF:	—— —	V₆:	— ———

To prevent spurious test results, position chest electrodes as follows:
V₁: fourth intercostal space at right border of sternum
V₂: fourth intercostal space at left border of sternum
V₃: halfway between V₂ and V₄
V₄: fifth intercostal space at midclavicular line
V₅: anterior axillary line (halfway between V₄ and V₆)
V₆: midaxillary line, level with V₄.

Use marking button on EKG machine to identify chest leads (shown above) and limb leads. Depress button to print a code of long and short dashes (shown above) directly on the EKG strip. (*Note:* Since code varies, check manufacturer's instructions.)

reach his highest level of functional aerobic capacity, but stops at an arbitrary endpoint, such as a target heart rate. This test is safer, but yields less diagnostic information than the maximal exercise tests.

Since exercise electrocardiography places considerable stress on the heart, it may be contraindicated in the patient with dissecting aortic aneurysm, uncontrolled dysrhythmias, pericarditis, myocarditis, acute MI, severe anemia, uncontrolled hypertension, unstable angina, congestive heart failure (CHF), second- or third-degree heart block, and severe heart valve disease, or CAD.

Purpose
• To help diagnose the cause of chest pain or other possible cardiac pain
• To determine the functional capacity of the heart after surgery or MI
• To screen for asymptomatic CAD (particularly in men over age 35)
• To help set limitations for an exercise program
• To identify cardiac dysrhythmias that develop during physical exercise
• To evaluate the effectiveness of antiarrhythmic or antianginal therapy.

Equipment
Motor-driven treadmill and controls (or bicycle ergometer with adjustable workload capacity)/EKG recorder and monitor/patient cable/ten electrodes with gel/elastic bandage or nonallergenic tape to secure electrodes/cotton-tipped applicators or 4″ x 4″ gauze sponges/alcohol/disposable razor (or sterilized nondisposable razor)/timing device with elapsed time display/examination table/crash cart containing emergency drugs and equipment/I.V. solutions and tubing / stethoscope / sphygmomanometer / optional: skin-deburring device, acetone, gown with opening in front.

Procedure
Explain the procedure to the patient to allay his fears and promote his cooperation. Instruct him not to eat, smoke, or

The Standard 12-Lead Electrocardiogram

Normally, five electrodes (four limb, one chest) record the heart's electrical potential from twelve different views, or leads. (One of these electrodes may serve as a ground.) Standard bipolar limb leads (I, II, III) detect variations in electrical potential at two points (negative pole and positive pole) and record the difference. When current flows toward the positive pole, the EKG wave deflects upward; when it flows toward the negative pole, the wave inverts. (The arrows, called Einthoven's reference lines, form a triangle indicating the direction electrical current moves to produce a positive [upward] deflection.)

Lead I connects the left and right arms, and the EKG tracing shows an upward deflection since the left arm is positive and the right arm negative. Lead II connects the left leg and right arm, and the tracing deflects upward since the left leg is positive and the right arm negative. Lead III connects the left leg and left arm, and the tracing deflects upward since the left leg is positive and the left arm negative.

The unipolar augmented limb leads (AVR, AVL, and AVF), which use the same electrode placement as standard limb leads, measure electrical potential between one augmented limb lead and the electrical midpoint of the remaining two leads (determined electronically by the EKG machine). Both standard and augmented leads measure electrical potential while viewing the heart from the front, in a vertical plane.

The six unipolar chest leads (V_1 through V_6) view the electrical potential from a horizontal plane that helps locate pathology in the lateral and posterior walls of the heart. The EKG machine averages the electrical potentials of all three limb lead electrodes (I, II, III) and compares this average with the electrical potential of the chest electrode. Recordings made with the V connection show electrical potential variations that occur under the chest electrode as its position is changed.

Normal EKG Waveforms

Lead I

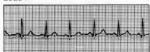

Lead V₁

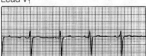

Lead II

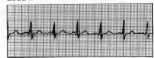

Lead V₂

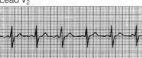

Lead III

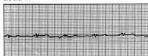

Lead V₃

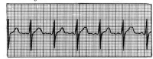

Lead AVR

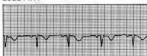

Lead V₄

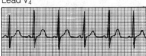

Lead AVL

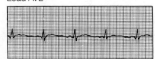

Lead V₅

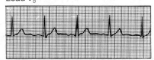

Lead AVF

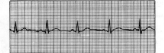

Lead V₆

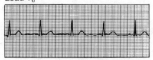

Since each lead takes a different view of heart activity, it generates its own characteristic tracing. The traces shown here are representative of each of the 12 leads. Leads AVR, V_1, V_2, and V_3 normally show strong negative deflections below the baseline. Negative deflections indicate current is flowing away from the positive electrode; positive deflections indicate that the current's flowing toward the positive electrode.

drink alcohol or caffeine-containing beverages for 3 hours before the procedure, but to continue any drug regimen unless the doctor directs otherwise. Tell him this test causes fatigue and slight breathlessness, but assure him that it has few risks. Emphasize that he may stop the test if he feels chest pain or extreme fatigue.

Make sure the patient or a responsible family member understands and signs a consent form. Check the patient's history for a recent physical examination (within 1 week) and for baseline 12-lead EKG results.

Take vital signs. Instruct the male patient to disrobe to the waist; tell the female patient to keep on her bra, and if she is not wearing a lightweight, short-sleeved blouse, give her a gown that opens in the front.

Apply chest electrodes according to the desired lead system.

Turn on the monitor and obtain a baseline rhythm strip with the patient in the supine position, another with him standing, and a third after a short period of hyperventilation, to detect changes in the ST segment that may follow position changes and hyperventilation.

Take blood pressure in supine and standing positions. The doctor then examines the rhythm strips and blood pressure measurements for evidence of resting abnormalities and auscultates the chest to detect S_3 or S_4 gallops, murmurs, or rales.

If you are performing the treadmill test, turn on the machine to a slow speed, and show the patient how to step onto it and use the railing to maintain his balance but *not* to support his weight. Turn off the machine, and then ask the patient to step onto it; turn it on again at slow speed and allow the patient to adjust to walking on it.

If you are performing the ergometer test, ask the patient to sit on the bicycle. If necessary, adjust the seat and handlebars so he can pedal comfortably. Tell him not to grip the handlebars tightly, but to use them only to maintain balance. Instruct him to pedal until he reaches the desired speed indicated on the speedometer.

Depending on the protocol, increase the workload in stages—usually every 2 to 3 minutes. Start the timer when the patient begins the first stage. Observe the monitor continuously for changes in the heart's electrical activity. Check the rhythm strips at 1-minute intervals for premature ventricular contractions (PVCs), dysrhythmias, or ST segment changes, and mark each strip with the test level and the time elapsed. Check the patient's blood pressure after each stage, and note any changes.

Stop the test upon reaching the predetermined endpoint or target heart rate. Tell the patient you will slow the machine, and ask him to continue walking or pedaling at the slower rate for several minutes to prevent nausea and dizziness. Then stop the machine and record another rhythm strip, heart rate, and blood pressure. Note the elapsed time.

Help the patient to the examination table and place him in a supine or semi-Fowler's position, with his legs elevated.

After the doctor listens to the patient's heart and lungs, record rhythm strip every minute and take blood pressure every 1 to 3 minutes for up to 15 minutes, or until blood pressure returns to baseline.

Special considerations

• Stop the test immediately if the patient experiences nausea, exhaustion, dizziness, or faintness, or if you detect any of the following: three consecutive PVCs on the tracing; decrease in systolic pressure to below the resting level; decrease in heart rate to 10 beats per minute below the resting level; or onset of severe hypertension, sustained ventricular tachycardia, severe changes in the ST segment, alternating bundle branch pattern or new onset pattern, or any previously undetected rapid dysrhythmia. Also, depending on the patient's condition and hospital policy, stop the test if the rhythm strip shows bundle branch block or an ST segment depression exceeding 3 mm. Rarely, persistent ST segment elevation may indicate transmural myocardial ischemia and contraindicates further testing. Avoid stopping the test abruptly if the patient has exercised strenuously to prevent a possible vasovagal attack.

• Remember that the predictive accuracy of exercise electrocardiography in detecting CAD varies with patient's history and sex, and that false-positive results occur in 15% to 20% of all cases.

• Assist the patient to a chair, and continue monitoring heart rate and blood pressure for 10 to 15 minutes or until the EKG returns to baseline.

• Auscultate for S_3 or S_4 gallops. Frequently, an S_4 gallop develops after exercise, due to increased blood flow volume and turbulence. However, an S_3 gallop is more significant than an S_4 gallop, indicating transient left ventricular dysfunction.

Findings
In a normal exercise EKG, the P, QRS, and T waves and the ST segment change slightly; slight ST segment depression occurs in some patients, especially women. Heart rate rises in direct proportion to the workload and metabolic oxygen demand; systolic blood pressure also rises as workload increases. The normal patient attains the endurance levels predicted by his age and the appropriate exercise protocol.

Implications of results
Although criteria for judging test results vary, two findings strongly suggest an abnormality: a flat or downsloping ST segment depression of 1 mm or more for at least 0.08 second after the junction of the QRS and ST segments (J point); and a markedly depressed J point, with an upsloping but depressed ST segment of 1.5 mm below the baseline 0.08 second after the J point. Initial ST segment depression on the resting EKG must be further depressed by 1 mm during exercise to be considered abnormal.

Hypotension resulting from exercise, ST depression of 3 mm or more, downsloping ST segments, and ischemic ST segments appearing within the first 3 minutes of exercise and lasting 8 minutes into the post-test recovery period may indicate multivessel or left CAD. ST segment elevation may indicate dyskinetic left ventricular wall motion or severe transmural ischemia.

Documentation
Document the patient's vital signs, tolerance of the procedure, and any abnormal symptoms. Use a flowchart during the test to document the stage of protocol reached by the patient; his heart rate at each minute of exercise; blood pressure at each progressive stage, and every 3 minutes after exercise; adverse symptoms, if any; EKG changes during exercise; and exercise-induced dysrhythmias, if any.

Ambulatory electrocardiography (Holter monitoring)

During Holter monitoring, the patient wears a small reel-to-reel or cassette tape monitor connected to bipolar electrodes applied to his chest, and he keeps a diary of his activities and any associated symptoms, usually for 24 hours. After this period, the tape is analyzed by a microcomputer to permit correlation of cardiac irregularities, such as dysrhythmias and ST segment changes, with the activities noted in the patient's diary. Other monitors can be worn for 5 to 7 days and are activated by the patient to record cardiac cycles only when he experiences symptoms.

Purpose
• To detect the quantity and quality of cardiac dysrhythmias
• To evaluate chest pain
• To evaluate cardiac status after acute MI or pacemaker implantation
• To evaluate effectiveness of antiarrhythmic drug therapy
• To assess and correlate dyspnea, central nervous system symptoms—such as syncope and light-headedness—and

palpitations with actual cardiac events and the patient's activities.

Equipment

Monitor, case, and strap/rechargeable batteries/reel-to-reel or cassette tape/electrodes (three to five, depending on the number of recording channels available)/electrode gel, if necessary/patient cable with lead wires/test cable/EKG machine for recording test strips/alcohol or acetone/4″ x 4″ gauze sponges/disposable razor/nonallergenic adhesive tape/sample and blank patient diaries.

Procedure

Because ambulatory electrocardiography is usually performed on an outpatient, carefully explain the procedure to him to ensure his cooperation, thereby promoting accurate test results. Tell him he may feel transient discomfort during preparation of the electrode sites. Demonstrate the application of the monitor and show him how to position it when he lies down. Advise him to wear loose-fitting clothing and a front-buttoning top.

Tell the patient to follow his daily routine during the monitoring period. If he must bathe, advise a sponge bath to avoid wetting the equipment and dislodging the electrodes.

Show the patient a sample diary, and instruct him to log all his daily activities. For example, tell him to include walking, stair climbing, sleep, elimination, intercourse, emotional upset, physical symptoms (dizziness, palpitation, pain, fatigue), and ingestion of medication. Remind him to wear a watch so he can log his activities accurately.

Special considerations

• If the procedure is performed on an inpatient whose activity is unrestricted, encourage him to walk about and simulate as many of his normal activities as possible. Confining such a patient to bed prevents detection of dysrhythmias that are precipitated by activity.

Findings

When compared with the patient's di-ary, the normal EKG pattern shows no significant dysrhythmias or ST segment changes. Changes in heart rate normally occur during various activities.

Implications of results

Abnormalities of the heart detected by ambulatory electrocardiography include PVC, conduction defects, tachyarrhythmias, bradyarrhythmias, and bradytachyarrhythmia syndrome. Dysrhythmias may be associated with dyspnea and CNS symptoms, such as dizziness and syncope.

Monitoring the MI patient 1 to 3 days before discharge and again 4 to 6 weeks after discharge may detect ST-T wave changes associated with ischemia or dysrhythmias; such information aids patient therapy and rehabilitation and refines prognosis. Monitoring a patient with an artificial pacemaker may detect a dysrhythmia, such as bradycardia, that the pacemaker fails to override.

Although ambulatory electrocardiography correlates patient symptoms and EKG changes, it does not always identify their causes. If initial monitoring proves inconclusive, the test may be repeated.

Documentation

Record the duration of monitoring on outpatient. If monitoring is performed on an inpatient, enter any treatments, activities, and drug administration in the patient's diary. In the nursing cardex, document ongoing monitoring and convey this information to the next shift.

RADIOGRAPHY

Cardiac radiography permits visualization of the position, size, and contour of the heart and great vessels of the circulatory system. Chest X-ray films can show enlargement of the heart, interstitial and alveolar edema, aortic dilatation, left heart failure, and intracardiac calcifications.

Kidney-ureter-bladder (KUB) radiography allows gross visualization of the urinary system. When assessing a patient for the cause of secondary hypertension, this test is often the starting point for the diagnostic workup. Other more definitive tests may be done depending on the results of the KUB.

Renal angiography and excretory urography employ the administration of an I.V. contrast medium. Angiography permits examination of the renal vasculature and parenchyma, while urography allows visualization of the renal parenchyma, calices, and pelvis as well as the ureters, bladder, and in some cases the urethra. (See also *Additional Diagnostic Tests,* pages 192 and 193.)

Cardiac radiography (Chest X-ray)

Among the most frequently used tests for evaluating cardiac disease and its effects on the pulmonary vasculature, cardiac radiography provides images of the thorax, mediastinum, heart, and lungs. In a routine evaluation, posteroanterior and left lateral views are taken. The posteroanterior view is preferable to the anteroposterior view because it places the heart slightly closer to the plane of the film, giving a sharper, less-distorted image. Using portable equipment, chest X-rays may be taken of patients who are bedridden, but such equipment can provide only anteroposterior views.

Purpose
• To help detect cardiac disease and abnormalities that change the size, shape, or appearance of the heart and lungs
• To ensure correct positioning of pulmonary artery and cardiac catheters and pacemaker wires.

Equipment
None at the bedside.

Procedure
Explain to the patient that this test reveals the size and shape of the heart. Tell him who performs the test and where it will be done. Reassure him that it employs little radiation and is harmless.

Instruct the patient to remove jewelry, other metal objects, and clothing above his waist, and to put on a hospital gown with ties instead of metal snaps.

Posteroanterior view: The patient stands erect about 6' (1.82 m) from the X-ray machine, with his back to the machine and his chin resting on top of the film cassette holder. The holder is adjusted to slightly hyperextend the patient's neck. The patient places his hands on his hips, with his shoulders touching the holder, and centers his chest against it. He takes a deep breath and holds it during the X-ray film exposure.

Left lateral view: The patient stands with his arms over his head and his left torso flush against the cassette and centered. He takes a deep breath and holds it during the X-ray film exposure.

Anteroposterior view of a bedridden patient: The head of the bed is elevated as much as possible, and the patient is assisted to an upright position, to reduce visceral pressure on the diaphragm and other thoracic structures. The film cassette is centered under his back. Although the distance between the patient and the X-ray machine may vary, the path between the two should be clear. The patient takes a deep breath and holds it during the X-ray film exposure.

Special considerations
• Cardiac radiography is usually contraindicated during the first trimester of pregnancy. If it is performed during pregnancy, a lead shield or apron should cover the abdomen and pelvic area during the X-ray exposure.
• When X-raying an ambulatory patient, make sure the radiographic order stipulates a posteroanterior view and not an anteroposterior view. Include on the order any pertinent findings from previous cardiac radiographs, as well as the indication for this test.
• When X-raying a bedridden patient, make sure anyone else in the room is protected from the X-rays by a lead

shield, room divider, or sufficient distance.

Findings

Normally, in the posteroanterior view, the thoracic cage appears at least twice as wide as the heart. However, in the anteroposterior view, relative heart size and position may look different, and the cardiac silhouette and vascular markings may increase.

If cardiac radiography is performed to evaluate the position of cardiac catheters and pacemakers, the films should confirm accurate placement and the integrity of their parts.

Implications of results

Cardiac X-ray films must be evaluated in light of the patient's history, physical examination, electrocardiography results, and results of previous radiographic tests for cardiac abnormalities.

An abnormal cardiac silhouette usually reflects left or right ventricular or left atrial enlargement.

Documentation

• Record testing on cardex.

Kidney-ureter-bladder radiography

Usually the first step in diagnostic testing of the urinary system, KUB radiography surveys the abdomen to determine the position of the kidneys, ureters, and bladder, and to detect gross abnormalities. This test does not require intact renal function and may aid differential diagnosis of urologic and gastrointestinal diseases, which often produce similar signs and symptoms. However, a KUB has many limitations and nearly always must be followed by more elaborate tests, such as excretory urography or renal computed tomography. KUB should not follow recent instillation of barium, which obscures the urinary system.

Purpose

• To evaluate the size, structure, and position of the kidneys
• To screen for abnormalities, such as calcifications in the region of the kidneys, ureters, and bladder
• To screen for possible causes of secondary hypertension.

Equipment

None at the bedside.

Procedure

Explain to the patient that this test shows the position of the urinary system organs and helps detect abnormalities in them. Inform him that he need not restrict food or fluids. Tell him who will perform the test, where it will be done, and that it takes only a few minutes.

The patient is placed in a supine position in correct body alignment, on a radiographic table. His arms are extended overhead, and the iliac crests are checked for symmetrical positioning. A single radiograph is taken.

Special considerations

• The male patient should have gonadal shielding to prevent irradiation of the testes. The female patient's ovaries cannot be shielded because they are located too close to the kidneys, ureters, and bladder.
• Gas, feces, contrast medium, or foreign bodies in the intestine may obscure the urinary system.
• Calcified uterine fibromas or ovarian lesions may prevent clear visualization of the kidneys, ureters, and bladder.
• Obesity or ascites may result in a radiograph of poor quality.

Findings

The shadows of the kidneys appear bilaterally, the right slightly lower than the left. Both kidneys should be approximately the same size, with the superior poles tilted slightly toward the vertebral column, paralleling the shadows (or stripes) produced by the psoas muscles. The ureters are not usually visible unless an abnormality, such as calcification, is present. Visualization of the bladder depends on the density of its muscular wall and the amount of urine in the bladder. Generally, a shadow of the bladder can be seen but not as clearly as those of the kidneys.

Implications of results

Bilateral renal enlargement may result from polycystic disease, multiple myeloma, lymphoma, amyloidosis, hydronephrosis, or compensatory hypertrophy. Tumor, cyst, or hydronephrosis may cause unilateral enlargement. Abnormally small kidneys may suggest end-stage glomerulonephritis or bilateral atrophic pyelonephritis. An apparent decrease in the size of one kidney suggests possible congenital hypoplasia, atrophic pyelonephritis, or ischemia. Renal displacement may be due to a retroperitoneal tumor, such as an adrenal tumor. Obliteration or bulging of a portion of the psoas muscle stripe may result from tumor, abscess, or hematoma.

Congenital anomalies, such as abnormal location or absence of a kidney, may be detected. Horseshoe kidney may be suggested by renal axes that parallel the vertebral column, especially if the inferior poles of the kidneys cannot be clearly distinguished. A lobulated edge or border may suggest polycystic kidney disease or patchy atrophic pyelonephritis.

Opaque bodies may reflect calculi or vascular calcification due to aneurysm or atheroma; opacification may also suggest cystic tumors, fecaliths, foreign bodies, or abnormal fluid collection. Calcifications may appear anywhere in the urinary system, but positive identification requires further testing. The only exception is staghorn calculus, which forms a perfect cast of the renal pelvis and calyces.

Documentation

Record on nursing cardex when test was done.

Renal angiography

Renal angiography permits radiographic examination of the renal vasculature and parenchyma following arterial injection of a contrast medium. As the contrast pervades the renal vasculature, rapid-sequence radiographs show the vessels during three phases of filling: arterial, nephrographic, and venous. This procedure virtually always follows standard bolus aortography, which shows individual variations in number, size, and condition of the main renal arteries, aberrant vessels, and the relationship of the renal arteries to the aorta.

Clinical indications for renal angiography include renal masses, pseudotumors, unilateral or bilateral kidney enlargement, nonfunctioning kidneys in patients with acute renal failure, positive urograms in patients with renovascular hypertension, vascular malformations, and intrarenal calcifications of unexplained etiology.

Purpose

• To demonstrate the configuration of total renal vasculature before surgical procedures
• To determine the cause of renovascular hypertension, such as from stenosis, thrombotic occlusions, emboli, and aneurysms
• To evaluate chronic renal disease or renal failure
• To investigate renal masses and renal trauma.

Equipment

Image-intensified fluoroscope with television monitor/high-powered X-ray equipment/pressure-injection device/rapid cassette changer/polyethylene radiopaque vascular catheters/flexible guide wire/contrast material (such as Hypaque, Renografin, Conray, or Isopaque)/preparation tray with 70% alcohol or povidone-iodine solution/emergency resuscitative equipment.

Procedure

Explain to the patient that this test permits visualization of the kidneys, blood vessels, and functional units, and aids in diagnosing renal disease or masses. Instruct him to fast for 8 hours before the test. Tell him who will perform the test, where it will be done, and that it takes approximately 1 hour.

Describe the procedure to the patient, and tell him that he may experience transient discomfort (flushing, burning sensation, and nausea) during injection of the contrast medium.

Make sure the patient or responsible family member has signed a consent form. Check the patient's history for hypersensitivity to iodine-based contrast media or iodine-containing foods, such as shellfish. If the patient has a history of sensitivity, inform the doctor so he can prescribe prophylactic antiallergenics (diphenhydramine or steroids) or have them available during the procedure.

As ordered, administer medication (usually a sedative and a narcotic analgesic) before the test. Instruct the patient to put on a hospital gown and remove all metallic objects that may interfere with test results. He should void before leaving the unit.

The patient is placed in a supine position, and a peripheral I.V. infusion is started. The skin over the arterial puncture site is cleansed with antiseptic solution, and a local anesthetic is injected. Using the Seldinger technique, the femoral artery is punctured and, under fluoroscopic visualization, cannulated. (If a femoral pulse is absent or the artery is convoluted or plaque-ridden, percutaneous transaxillary, transbrachial, or translumbar catheterization may be performed instead.) After passing the flexible guide wire through the artery, the cannula is withdrawn, leaving several inches of wire in the lumen. Next, a polyethylene catheter is passed over the wire and advanced, under fluoroscopic guidance, up the femoroiliac vessels to the aorta. At this juncture, the contrast medium is injected, and screening aortograms are taken before proceeding. On completion of the aortographic study, a renal catheter is exchanged for the former one. The guide wire is removed, and the catheter is flushed with heparinized saline solution to prevent clotting in the tip.

To determine the position of the renal arteries and ensure that the catheter tip is in the lumen, a test bolus of contrast (about 1 ml) is injected immediately. This prevents subintimal injection or arterial spasm that may mimic a renal artery lesion. If the patient has no adverse reaction to the contrast, 20 to 25 ml of contrast is injected just below the origin of the renal arteries so it does not reach the mesenteric vessels first, obscuring the renal arteries. After this, a series of rapid-sequence X-ray films of the filling of the renal vascular tree is exposed.

If additional selective studies are required, the catheter remains in place while the films are examined. If the films are satisfactory, the catheter is removed, and a sterile sponge is firmly applied to the puncture site for 15 minutes. Before the patient is returned to his room, the puncture site is observed for hematoma.

Special considerations

- Renal angiography is contraindicated during pregnancy and in patients with bleeding tendencies, allergy to contrast media, and renal failure due to end-stage renal disease.
- Recent contrast studies (such as a barium enema or an upper gastrointestinal series) may produce a cloudy radiographic image and interfere with accurate interpretation of test results.
- Patient movement during the test may impair radiograph quality.
- Feces and gas in the gastrointestinal tract may impair radiograph clarity and hinder accurate interpretation of results.

Findings

Renal arteriographs show normal arborization of the vascular tree and normal architecture of the renal parenchyma.

Implications of results

Renal tumors usually show hypervascularity; renal cysts typically appear as clearly delineated, radiolucent masses. Renal artery stenosis caused by arteriosclerosis produces a noticeable constriction in the blood vessels, usually within the proximal portion of its length; this is a crucial finding in confirming renovascular hypertension. Renal artery dysplasia, unlike renal artery stenosis, usually affects the middle and distal portions of the vessel. Alternating aneurysms and stenotic regions give this rare disorder a characteristic beads-on-a-string appearance.

In renal infarction, blood vessels may appear to be absent or cut off, with normal tissue replaced by scar tissue. Another typical finding is triangular areas of infarcted tissue near the periphery of the affected kidney. The kidney itself may appear shrunken due to tissue scarring. Other disorders that may be discovered through renal angiography include renal artery aneurysms (saccular or fusiform), and renal arteriovenous fistula with abnormal widening of and direct passage between the renal artery and renal vein. Destruction, distortion, and fibrosis of renal tissue with areas of reduced and tortuous vascularity may be noted in severe or chronic pyelonephritis, and an increase in capsular vessels with abnormal intrarenal circulation may indicate renal abscesses or inflammatory masses.

When angiography is used to evaluate renal trauma, it may detect intrarenal hematoma, parenchymal laceration, shattered kidney, and areas of infarction.

Documentation

Record vital signs every 15 minutes for 1 hour, every ½ hour for 2 hours, then every hour until stable.

Document the appearance or absence of the popliteal and dorsalis pedis pulses.

Record any unusual bleeding or hematoma formation at injection site.

Excretory urography (Intravenous pyelography)

The cornerstone of a urologic workup, this test allows visualization of the renal parenchyma, calices, and pelvis, as well as the ureters, bladder, and in some cases, the urethra, following I.V. administration of a contrast medium. Known traditionally as intravenous pyelography, this common and extremely useful procedure is more accurately called excretory urography, because it shows the entire urinary tract—not just the renal pelvis—as the prefix *pyelo* implies. Clinical indications for this test include suspected renal or urinary tract disease, space-occupying lesions, congenital anomalies, or trauma to the urinary system.

Purpose
• To evaluate the structure and excretory function of the kidneys, ureters, and bladder
• To support a differential diagnosis of renovascular hypertension.

Equipment
Contrast medium (sodium diatrizoate or iothalamate, or meglumine diatrizoate or iothalamate)/50-ml syringe (or I.V. container and tubing)/19G to 21G needle, catheter, or butterfly needle/venipuncture equipment (tourniquet, antiseptic, adhesive bandage)/X-ray table/X-ray and tomographic equipment/emergency resuscitative equipment.

Procedure
Explain to the patient that this test helps evaluate the structure and function of the urinary tract. Be sure the patient is well hydrated, then instruct him to fast for 8 hours before the test. Tell him who will perform the test and where it will be done.

Inform the patient that he may experience a transient burning sensation and metallic taste when the contrast medium is injected. Tell him to report any other sensations. Warn him that the X-ray machine will make loud, clacking sounds during the test.

Make sure the patient or responsible family member has signed a consent form. Check the patient's history for hypersensitivity to iodine, iodine-containing foods, or contrast media containing iodine. If he has such a history, notify the doctor. Administer a laxative, as ordered, the night before the test, to minimize poor resolution of X-ray films due to feces and gas in the gastrointestinal tract.

The patient is placed in supine position on the radiographic table. A KUB radiograph is exposed, developed, and studied for gross abnormalities of the urinary system. In the absence of any such abnormality, contrast medium is injected (dosage varies according to age), and the patient is observed for signs of hypersensitivity (flushing, nausea, vomiting, hives, or dyspnea). The first radiograph, visualizing the renal parenchyma, is obtained about 1 minute after the injection, possibly supplemented by tomography if small space-occupying masses like cysts or tumors are suspected. Films are then exposed at regular intervals—usually 5, 10, and 15 or 20 minutes after the injection. Ureteral compression is performed after the 5-minute film is exposed. This can be accomplished through inflation of two small rubber bladders placed on the abdomen on both sides of the midline and secured by a flannel fastener wrapped around the patient's torso. The inflated bladders occlude the ureters, without causing the patient discomfort, and facilitate retention of the contrast medium by the upper urinary tract. (Ureteral compression is contraindicated by ureteral calculi, aortic aneurysm, or recent abdominal trauma or surgical procedure.) After the 10-minute film is exposed, ureteral compression is released. As the contrast flows into the lower urinary tract, another film is taken of the lower halves of both ureters and then, finally, one is taken of the bladder.

At the end of the procedure, the patient voids, and another film is made immediately to visualize residual bladder content or mucosal abnormalities of the bladder or urethra.

Special considerations
• Premedication with corticosteroids may be indicated for patients with severe asthma or history of sensitivity to the contrast medium.
• End-stage renal disease, fecal matter or gas in the colon, insufficient injection of contrast medium, or recent barium enema or gastrointestinal or gallbladder series may produce films of poor quality that cannot be interpreted accurately.

Findings
The kidneys, ureters, and bladder show no gross evidence of soft- or hard-tissue lesions. Prompt visualization of the contrast medium in the kidneys demonstrates bilateral renal parenchyma and pelvocalyceal systems of normal conformity. The ureters and bladder should be outlined, and the postvoiding radiograph should show no mucosal abnormalities and minimal residual urine.

Implications of results
Excretory urography can demonstrate many abnormalities of the urinary system, including renal or ureteral calculi; abnormal size, shape, or structure of kidneys, ureters, or bladder; supernumerary or absent kidney; polycystic kidney disease associated with renal hypertrophy; redundant pelvis or ureter; space-occupying lesion; pyelonephritis; renal tuberculosis; hydronephrosis; and renovascular hypertension.

Documentation
Record patient's vital signs on return to his room.

Document the formation of a hematoma at the injection site if one develops.

ULTRASONOGRAPHY

Echocardiography, a painless noninvasive test, directs ultra–high-frequency sound waves through the chest wall into the heart, which then reflects these waves to a transducer and a recording device at various frequencies, depending on the density of the cardiac tissue. It shows the movement of cardiac structures and the dimensions of heart chambers. This test evaluates cardiac structure and function, and can reveal valve deformities (mitral prolapse), tumors (left atrial myxoma), septal defects, pericardial effusion, and idiopathic hypertrophic subaortic stenosis.

Ultrasonography of the abdominal aorta also uses high-frequency sound waves. By directing these waves into the abdomen over a wide area, a diagnosis of suspected aortic aneurysm can be confirmed. The test is also used every six months to monitor any changes in the aneurysm's status.

Doppler ultrasonography is a noninvasive test that evaluates blood flow in the major veins and arteries of the arms and legs and in the extracranial cerebrovascular system. Developed as an alternative to arteriography and venography, Doppler ultrasonography is safer and less costly and requires a shorter test period than invasive tests (see also *Additional Diagnostic Tests,* pages 192 and 193).

Echocardiography

This widely used, noninvasive test examines the size, shape, and motion of cardiac structures and is useful for evaluating patients with chest pains, enlarged cardiac silhouettes on X-ray films, electrocardiographic changes unrelated to CAD, and abnormal heart sounds on auscultation.

The techniques most commonly used in echocardiography are motion-mode (M-mode) and two-dimensional (cross-sectional). In M-mode echocardiography, a single, pencil-like ultrasound beam strikes the heart, producing an ice pick or vertical view of cardiac structures. This method is especially useful for precisely recording the motion and dimensions of intracardiac structures.

In two-dimensional echocardiography, the ultrasound beam rapidly sweeps through an arc, producing a cross-sectional or fan-shaped view of cardiac structures. This technique is useful for recording lateral motion and providing the correct spatial relationship between cardiac structures. Often, these techniques complement each other.

Purpose
- To diagnose and evaluate valvular abnormalities
- To measure the size of the heart's chambers
- To evaluate chambers and valves in congenital heart disorders
- To aid diagnosis of hypertrophic and related cardiomyopathies
- To detect atrial tumors
- To evaluate cardiac function or wall motion after MI
- To detect pericardial effusion.

Equipment
None at the bedside.

Procedure
Explain to the patient that this test evaluates the size, shape, and motion of various cardiac structures. Inform him that he need not restrict food or fluids before the test. Tell him who will perform the test, where it will be done, and that it usually takes 15 to 30 minutes. Reassure him that it is safe and painless. Explain that the room may be darkened slightly to aid visualization on the oscilloscope screen, and that other procedures (electrocardiography and phonocardiography) may be performed simultaneously.

The patient is placed in a supine position. Conductive jelly is applied to the third or fourth intercostal space to the left of the sternum, and the transducer is placed directly over it, systematically angled to direct ultrasonic waves at specific parts of the patient's heart. During the test, the oscilloscope screen, which displays the returning echoes, is observed; significant oscilloscopic findings are recorded on a strip chart recorder (M-mode echocardiography) or

Thallium Imaging: What It Shows

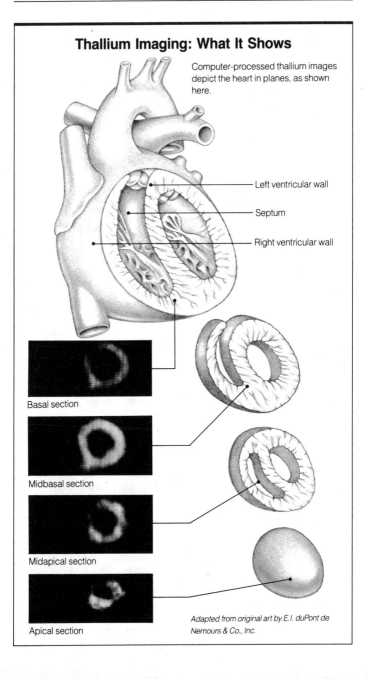

Computer-processed thallium images depict the heart in planes, as shown here.

Left ventricular wall

Septum

Right ventricular wall

Basal section

Midbasal section

Midapical section

Apical section

Adapted from original art by E.I. duPont de Nemours & Co., Inc.

on a videotape recorder (two-dimensional echocardiography).

Special considerations
None.

Findings
An echocardiogram can reveal both the motion pattern and structure of the four cardiac valves. Anterior and posterior mitral valve leaflets normally separate in early diastole, with the anterior leaflet moving toward the chest wall and the posterior leaflet moving away from it. The leaflets attain maximum excursion rapidly, then move toward each other during ventricular diastole; after atrial contraction, they come together and remain so during ventricular systole. On an M-mode echocardiogram, the leaflets appear as two fine lines within the echo-free, blood-filled left ventricular cavity.

An echocardiogram can also show the tricuspid and pulmonary valves. The motion of the tricuspid valve resembles that of the mitral valve; the motion of the pulmonary valve—particularly the posterior cusp—is quite different. During diastole, this cusp gradually moves posteriorly; during atrial systole, it is displaced posteriorly; and during ventricular systole, it quickly moves posteriorly. During right ventricular ejection, the cusp moves anteriorly, attaining its most anterior position during diastole.

An echocardiogram can also help evaluate both the left and the right ventricles. The left ventricular cavity normally appears as an echo-free space between the interventricular septum and the posterior left ventricular wall. Echoes produced by the chordae tendineae and the mitral leaflet appear within this cavity. The right ventricular cavity normally appears as an echo-free space between the anterior chest wall and the interventricular septum.

Implications of results
Valvular abnormalities, especially those affecting the mitral and aortic valves, readily appear on the echocardiogram.

Aortic valve abnormalities—especially aortic insufficiency—can also affect the mitral valve, since the anterior mitral leaflet is just below the aortic cusps. When blood regurgitates through the aortic valve during diastole, it strikes this leaflet, causing the flutter seen in M-mode. Although the aortic valve may appear normal, this characteristic fluttering confirms aortic insufficiency. In stenosis due to conditions such as rheumatic fever or bacterial endocarditis, the aortic valve thickens and thus generates more echoes. However, in rheumatic fever, the valve may thicken slightly and allow normal motion during systole, or it may thicken severely and curtail motion. In bacterial endocarditis, valve motion is disrupted, and shaggy or fuzzy echoes usually appear on or near the valve, due to vegetations.

Other chamber or valve abnormalities may indicate a congenital heart disorder, such as aortic stenosis, which may require further tests. A large chamber size may indicate cardiomyopathy, valvular disorders, or CHF; a small chamber, restrictive pericarditis.

Idiopathic hypertrophic subaortic stenosis can also be identified by the echocardiogram, with systolic anterior motion of the mitral valve and asymmetric septal hypertrophy.

Left atrial tumor, which is most commonly a myxoma, is usually on a pedicle, and can thus shift in and out of the mitral opening. During diastole, the tumor appears as a mass of echoes against the anterior mitral valve leaflet; during ventricular systole, these echoes shift back into the body of the atrium.

In CAD, ischemia or infarction may cause absent or paradoxical motion in ventricular walls that normally move together and thicken during systole. These affected areas may also fail to thicken or may even become thinner, particularly when scar tissue is present.

The echocardiogram is especially sensitive in detecting pericardial effusion. Normally, the epicardium and pericardium are continuous membranes, and thus produce a single or near-single echo. When fluid accumulates between these membranes, it causes an abnormal echo-free space to appear. In large effusions, pressure exerted by excess fluid can restrict pericardial motion. An echocardiogram should be correlated with clinical history and physical examination. Additional procedures may be necessary to clarify results.

Documentation

Record testing on cardex.

Ultrasonography of the abdominal aorta

In this noninvasive test, a transducer directs high-frequency sound waves into the abdomen over a wide area from the xiphoid process to the umbilical region. The sound waves, echoing to the transducer from interfaces between tissue of different densities (acoustic interfaces), are transmitted as electrical impulses and displayed on an oscilloscope or television screen, to reveal internal organs, the vertebral column, and most importantly the size and course of the abdominal aorta and other major vessels.

Ultrasonography helps confirm a suspected aortic aneurysm and is the method of choice for determining its diameter. Several scans may be performed to detect expansion of a known aneurysm, because the risk of rupture is highest when aneurysmal diameter is 7 cm or greater. However, angiography is indicated preoperatively to visualize the extent of atherosclerotic changes; to discover anatomic anomalies, such as three renal arteries; when the extent of the aneurysm cannot be determined precisely with ultrasound; and when diagnosis is unclear. When an aneurysm is detected, ultrasonography is used every 6 months to monitor changes in patient status.

Purpose

• To detect and measure suspected abdominal aortic aneurysm

• To determine the diameter and detect expansion of known abdominal aortic aneurysm

• To confirm/dispell the threat of ruptured, expanding, or leaking aneurysm.

Equipment

None at the bedside.

Procedure

Explain to the patient that this procedure allows examination of the abdominal aorta. Instruct him to fast for 12 hours before the test; this minimizes bowel gas and motility, which interfere with scan results. Tell him who will perform the test and where, that the room light may be reduced to improve visualization of images on the oscilloscope, and that the test takes 30 to 45 minutes.

Tell the patient that mineral oil or a gel will be applied to his abdomen and will feel cool. Explain that a transducer will pass smoothly over his skin, from the costal margins to the umbilicus or slightly below, directing inaudible sound waves into the abdominal vessels and organs. Assure him that this is not harmful or painful but that he will feel slight pressure. If the patient has a known aneurysm, reassure him that sound waves will not cause it to rupture. Instruct him to remain as still as possible during scanning and to hold his breath when requested.

If ordered, give simethicone to reduce bowel gas. Just before the procedure, instruct the patient to put on a hospital gown.

Tell the patient to ask his doctor if he should take prescribed routine oral medications the day of the test (if he is an outpatient).

The patient is placed in a supine position, and acoustic coupling gel or mineral oil is applied to his abdomen. Longitudinal scans are made at 0.5- to 1-cm intervals left and right of the midline until the entire abdominal aorta is outlined. Transverse scans are made at 1- to 2-cm intervals from the xiphoid to the bifurcation at the common iliac arteries. The patient may be placed in right and left lateral positions for some scans. Appropriate views are photographed or recorded on videotape.

Special considerations

• If the patient has an abdominal dressing or draining abdominal wounds, discuss this with radiology before sending the patient for the test.

• If possible, allow the patient to visit the radiology department before the test. Since the thought of having an aneurysm can cause considerable anxiety, emotional support is very important.

• Bowel gas and motility, excessive body movement, surgical wounds, and severe dyspnea may prevent adequate imaging.

• Residual barium from gastrointestinal contrast studies within the past 24 hours and air introduced during endoscopy within the past 12 to 24 hours hinder ultrasound transmission.

• In obese patients, mesenteric fat may impair ultrasound transmission.

Findings

In adults, the normal abdominal aorta tapers from about 2.5 cm to 1.5 cm in diameter along its length from the diaphragm to the bifurcation of the iliac arteries. It descends through the retroperitoneal space, anterior to the vertebral column and slightly left of the midline. Its major branches are usually well visualized: the celiac trunk, the renal arteries, the superior mesenteric artery, and the common iliac arteries.

Implications of results

A luminal diameter of the abdominal aorta greater than 4 cm is aneurysmal; over 7 cm, it is aneurysmal with a high risk of rupture.

Visualization of an abdominal aortic aneurysm implies the disease of atherosclerosis. Atherosclerosis is the leading cause of aortic aneurysm because it damages the aorta by weakening and dilating the vessel walls.

Sizing of the abdominal aortic aneurysm by ultrasound helps the surgeon decide when the aneurysm should be resected. However, although most abdominal aortic aneurysms continue to slowly expand, some never require surgical intervention.

Documentation

Record the patient's vital signs and psychological state.

After establishing what the patient has been told, document any patient teaching, explanations, or emotional support given in relation to his diagnosis.

Doppler ultrasonography

In Doppler ultrasonography, a hand-held transducer directs high-frequency sound waves to the artery or vein being tested. The sound waves strike moving red blood cells (RBCs) and are reflected back to the transducer at frequencies that correspond to the velocity of blood flow through the vessel. The transducer then amplifies the sound waves to permit direct listening and graphic recording of blood flow.

Measurement of systolic pressure during this test helps detect the presence, location, and extent of peripheral arterial occlusive disease. Observation of changes in sound wave frequency during respiration helps detect venous occlusive disease, since venous blood flow normally fluctuates with respiration. Use of compression maneuvers also helps detect occlusion of the veins as well as occlusion or stenosis of carotid arteries.

Pulse volume recorder (PVR) testing may be performed along with Doppler ultrasonography to yield a quantitative recording of changes in blood volume or flow in an extremity or organ.

Purpose

• To aid diagnosis of chronic venous insufficiency and superficial and deep vein thromboses (popliteal, femoral, iliac)

• To aid diagnosis of peripheral artery disease and arterial occlusion

• To monitor patients who have had arterial reconstruction and bypass grafts

• To detect abnormalities of carotid ar-

tery blood flow associated with such conditions as aortic stenosis
• To evaluate possible arterial trauma.

Equipment
Check with the vascular laboratory to determine if special equipment will be used and if special instructions are necessary.

Procedure
Explain that this test helps evaluate blood flow in the arms and legs or neck. Tell the patient who will perform the test and that it takes about 20 minutes.

Reassure the patient that the test does not involve risk or discomfort. Tell him he will be asked to move his arms to different positions and to perform breathing exercises as measurements are taken, to vary blood flow during the exam. Explain that a small ultrasonic probe resembling a microphone is placed at various sites along specific veins or arteries, and that blood pressure is checked at several sites.

Water-soluble conductive jelly is applied to the tip of the transducer to provide coupling between the skin and the transducer.

For *peripheral arterial evaluation*, always performed bilaterally, the usual test sites in the leg include the common femoral, superficial femoral, popliteal, posterior tibial, and dorsalis pedis arteries; in the arm, the subclavian, brachial, radial, ulnar, and, occasionally, the palmar arch and digital arteries.

The patient is instructed to remove all clothing above or below the waist, depending on the test site. After he is placed in supine position on the examining table or bed, with his arms at his sides, brachial blood pressure is measured, and the transducer is placed at various points along the test arteries. The signals are monitored and the waveforms recorded for later analysis.

Segmental limb blood pressure is obtained to localize arterial occlusive disease. For lower extremity tests, blood pressure cuffs are placed snugly around each thigh, calf and ankle area (6 cuffs in all). The cuffs are inflated separately to approximately 65 mm Hg, and waveform tracings are obtained. To obtain systolic pressure at the thigh, calf and ankle of the lower extremity, the PVR or doppler may be used.

For upper extremity testing, a blood pressure cuff is wrapped around the upper arm and the forearm. The cuffs are again inflated to a pressure of 65 mm Hg. For thoracic outlet compression syndrome testing, the patient is placed in a sitting position with the cuffs applied and the arm is moved through various hyperextended and hyperabducted positions. Then the procedure is repeated on the other side.

For *peripheral venous evaluation*, usual test sites in the leg include the popliteal, superficial femoral, and common femoral veins, and the posterior tibial vein at the ankle; in the arm, the brachial, axillary, subclavian, and jugular veins, and occasionally, the inferior and superior venae cavae.

The patient is instructed to remove all clothing above or below the waist, depending on the test site. He is placed in a supine position and instructed to breathe normally. The transducer is placed over the appropriate vein, waveforms are recorded, and respiratory modulations noted.

Proximal limb compression maneuvers are performed and augmentation noted after release of compression, to evaluate venous valve competency. Changes in respiration are monitored. For lower extremity tests, the patient is asked to perform Valsalva's maneuver, and venous blood flow is recorded. The procedure is repeated for the other arm or leg.

For *extracranial cerebrovascular evaluation,* usual test sites include the supraorbital, common carotid, external carotid, internal carotid, and vertebral arteries.

The patient is placed in supine position on the examining table or bed, with a pillow beneath his head for support. Brachial blood pressure is then recorded, using the Doppler probe. Next the transducer is positioned over the test artery, and blood flow velocity is monitored and recorded. The influence of compression maneuvers on blood flow velocity is measured, and the procedure is repeated on the opposite side.

Special considerations

• Do not place the Doppler probe over an open or draining lesion.
• If the patient is uncooperative, test results may be invalid.

Findings

Arterial waveforms of the arms and legs are multiphasic, with a prominent systolic component and one or more diastolic sounds. The ankle-arm pressure index (API)—the ratio between ankle systolic pressure and brachial systolic pressure—is normally equal to or greater than 1. (The API is also known as arterial ischemia index, ankle/brachial index, or pedal/brachial index.) Proximal thigh pressure is normally 20 to 30 mm Hg higher than arm pressure, but pressure measurements at adjacent sites are similar. In the arms, pressure readings should remain unchanged despite postural changes.

Venous blood flow velocity is normally phasic with respiration, and is of a lower pitch than arterial flow. Distal compression or release of proximal limb compression increases blood flow velocity. In the legs, abdominal compression eliminates respiratory variations, but release increases blood flow; Valsalva's maneuver also interrupts venous flow velocity.

In cerebrovascular testing, a strong velocity signal is present. In the common carotid artery, blood flow velocity increases during diastole because of low peripheral vascular resistance of the brain. The direction of periorbital arterial flow is normally anterograde out of the orbit.

Implications of results

Arterial stenosis or occlusion diminishes the blood flow velocity signal, with no diastolic sound and a less prominent systolic component distal to the lesion. At the lesion, the signal is high-pitched and, occasionally, turbulent. If complete occlusion is present and collateral circulation has not taken over, the velocity signal may be absent.

A pressure gradient exceeding 20 to 30 mm Hg at adjacent sites of measurement in the leg may indicate occlusive disease. Specifically, low proximal thigh pressure signifies common femoral or aorto-iliac occlusive disease. An abnormal gradient between the proximal thigh and the above- or below-knee cuffs indicates superficial femoral or popliteal artery occlusive disease; an abnormal gradient between the below-knee and ankle cuffs, indicates tibiofibular disease. Abnormal gradients of arm and forearm pressure readings may indicate brachial artery occlusion.

An abnormal API is directly proportional to the degree of circulatory impairment: mild ischemia, from 1 to 0.75; claudication, 0.75 to 0.50; pain at rest, 0.50 to 0.25; and pregangrene, 0.25 to 0.

If venous blood flow velocity is unchanged by respirations, does not increase in response to compression or Valsalva's maneuver, or is absent, venous thrombosis is indicated. In chronic venous insufficiency and varicose veins, the flow velocity signal may be reversed. Confirmation of results may require venography.

Inability to identify Doppler signals during cerebrovascular examination implies total arterial occlusion. Reversed periorbital arterial flow indicates significant arterial occlusive disease of the extracranial internal carotid artery; in addition, the audible signal may take on the acoustic characteristics of a normal peripheral artery. Stenosis of the internal carotid artery causes turbulent signals. Collateral circulation can be assessed by compression maneuvers.

Oculoplethysmography, carotid phonoangiography, or carotid imaging can further evaluate cerebrovascular disease. Retrograde blood velocity in the vertebral artery can indicate subclavian steal syndrome. Weak velocity signal on comparison of contralateral vertebral arteries can indicate diffuse vertebral artery disease.

Documentation
Record how patient tolerated the procedure.

NUCLEAR MEDICINE

Thallium imaging evaluates myocardial blood flow and the status of myocardial cells after the I.V. injection of the radioisotope thallium-201; healthy myocardial tissue absorbs the radioisotope but ischemic or necrotic tissue does not (thus, the name *cold spot* scanning). This test can detect abnormalities associated with perfusion defects in the coronary arteries and myocardium. *Stress testing* after thallium injection can reveal areas of ischemia resulting from exercise.

Unlike thallium imaging, *technetium pyrophosphate scanning* reveals damaged myocardial tissue as *hot spots*—areas where the radioisotope technetium pyrophosphate accumulates. The test helps to detect acute MI and define its location and size.

Blood pool imaging, in which a radioisotope is tagged to RBCs or albumin and injected I.V., outlines the heart cavities to detect left ventricular regional wall motion abnormalities (commonly seen after MI). In this test, a scintillation camera records the first pass of the radioisotope through the heart; then in subsequent gated or timed imaging, the camera records two or more points in the cardiac cycle, allowing study of left ventricular function. Blood pool imaging also aids diagnosis of left ventricular aneurysm, cardiomyopathies, and intracardiac shunts.

Technetium pyrophosphate scanning (Hot spot myocardial imaging)

Technetium pyrophosphate scanning is used to detect recent MI and determine its extent. In this test, an I.V. tracer isotope (technetium-99m pyrophosphate) accumulates in damaged myocardial tissue (possibly by combining with calcium in the damaged myocardial cells), where it forms a hot spot on a scan made with a scintillation camera. Such hot spots first appear within 12 hours of infarction, are most apparent after 48 to 72 hours, and usually disappear after 1 week. Hot spots that persist longer than 1 week usually suggest ongoing myocardial damage.

This test is most useful for confirming recent MI in patients suffering from obscure cardiac pain, in postoperative cardiac patients, when EKGs are equivocal (as with left bundle-branch block or old myocardial scars), or when serum enzyme tests are unreliable.

Purpose
• To confirm recent MI
• To define the size and location of a recent MI
• To assess prognosis after acute MI.

Equipment
None at the bedside.

Procedure
Explain to the patient that this test helps determine if any areas of the heart muscle are injured. Inform him that he need not restrict food or fluids. Tell him who will perform the test, where it will be done, and that it takes 30 to 60 minutes.

Inform the patient that he will receive a tracer isotope I.V. 2 or 3 hours before the procedure, and that multiple images of his heart will be made. Reassure him that the injection causes only transient discomfort, that the scan itself is painless, and that the test involves less exposure to radiation than chest radiography. Instruct him to remain quiet and motionless while he is being scanned, but assure him that he can talk and move about between views.

Make sure the patient or responsible family member has signed a consent form.

Usually, 20 mCi of technetium-99m pyrophosphate are injected into the antecubital vein. After 2 or 3 hours, the patient is placed in a supine position, and electrocardiography electrodes are attached for continuous monitoring during the test. Generally, scans are taken with the patient in several positions, including anterior, left anterior oblique, right anterior oblique, and left lateral. Each scan takes 10 minutes.

Special considerations
None.

Findings
If normal, this scan shows no accumulation of the isotope in the myocardium.

Implications of results
The isotope is taken up by the sternum and ribs, and the activity of these is compared with that in the heart; 2^+, 3^+, and 4^+ activity (equal to or greater than bone) indicate a positive myocardial scan. The technetium scan can reveal areas of isotope accumulation, or hot spots, in damaged myocardium, particularly 48 to 72 hours after onset of acute MI; however, hot spots are apparent as early as 12 hours after acute MI. In most patients with MI, hot spots disappear after 1 week; in some, they persist for several months if necrosis continues in the area of infarction. Knowing where the infarct is located makes it possible to anticipate complications and to plan patient care. About one fourth of patients with unstable angina pectoris show hot spots due to subclinical myocardial necrosis and may require coronary arteriography and bypass grafting.

Documentation
Record testing on cardex.

Thallium imaging (Cold spot myocardial imaging)

This test evaluates myocardial blood flow and the status of myocardial cells after I.V. injection of the radioisotope thallium-201 (thallous chloride Tl 201, or ²⁰¹TlCl). Thallium, the physiologic analogue of potassium, concentrates in healthy myocardial tissue but not in necrotic or ischemic tissue. Hence, areas of the heart with normal blood supply and intact cells rapidly take up the isotope; areas with poor blood flow fail to take up the isotope and appear as cold spots on a scan. (See *Thallium Imaging: What It Shows*, page 209.)

This test is performed in a resting state or after stress (treadmill exercise). Resting imaging can detect acute MI within the first few hours of symptoms but does not distinguish an old from a new infarct. Stress imaging, performed after the patient exercises on a treadmill until he experiences angina or rate-limiting fatigue, can assess known or suspected CAD and can evaluate the effectiveness of antianginal therapy or balloon angioplasty and the patency of grafts after coronary artery bypass surgery. Complications of stress testing include dysrhythmias, angina pectoris, and MI.

Purpose
- To assess myocardial scarring and perfusion
- To demonstrate the location and extent of acute or chronic MI, including transmural and postoperative infarction (resting imaging)
- To diagnose CAD (stress imaging)
- To evaluate the patency of grafts after coronary artery bypass surgery
- To evaluate the effectiveness of antianginal therapy or balloon angioplasty (stress imaging).

Equipment
None at the bedside.

Right and Left Heart Catheterization

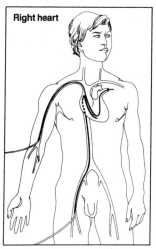

Right heart

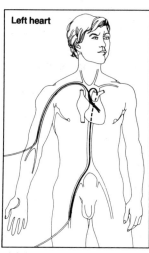

Left heart

The catheter is inserted through veins to the inferior vena cava and the right atrium and ventricle for right-side catheterization, and through arteries to the aorta and into the coronary artery orifices and/or left ventricle for left-side catheterization. Note that both approaches use the antecubital and femoral vessels.

Procedure

Explain to the patient that these tests help determine if any areas of the heart muscle are not receiving an adequate blood supply. For stress imaging, instruct him to restrict alcohol, tobacco, and unprescribed medications for 24 hours before the test and to have nothing by mouth for 3 hours before the test (he may eat a light meal earlier). Tell him who will perform the test, where it will be done, that initial testing takes 45 to 90 minutes and that additional scans may be required.

Tell the patient he will receive a radioactive tracer I.V., and that multiple images of his heart will be scanned. Warn him that he may experience discomfort from skin abrasion during preparation for electrode placement, but reassure him that there is no known radiation danger from the isotope.

Make sure the patient or responsible family member has signed a consent form. For stress imaging, instruct the patient to wear walking shoes during the treadmill exercise and to report fatigue, pain, or shortness of breath immediately.

Stress imaging: The patient, wired with electrodes, walks on a treadmill at a regulated pace that is gradually increased, while EKG, blood pressure, and heart rate are monitored. When the patient reaches peak stress, the examiner injects 1.5 to 3 mCi of thallium into the antecubital vein and flushes it with 10 to 15 ml of normal saline solution. The patient exercises an additional 45 to 60 seconds to permit circulation and uptake of the isotope, then lies on his back under the scintillation camera. If he is asymptomatic, the precordial leads are removed. Scanning begins after 3 to 5 minutes with the patient in anterior, 45° and 60° left anterior oblique, and left lateral positions. Additional scans may be taken after he rests 3 to 6 hours.

Resting imaging: Within the first few hours of symptoms of MI, the patient receives an injection of thallium I.V. Scanning begins after 3 to 5 minutes, with the patient positioned as above.

Special considerations

• Contraindications to stress imaging include impaired neuromuscular function, pregnancy, locomotor disturbances, acute MI and myocarditis, aortic stenosis, acute infection, unstable metabolic conditions (such as diabetes), digitalis toxicity, and recent pulmonary infarction.

• Stress imaging is stopped at once if the patient develops chest pain, dyspnea, fatigue, syncope, hypotension, ischemic EKG changes, significant dysrhythmias, or critical signs (pallor, clammy skin, confusion, or staggering gait).

Findings

Imaging should reveal characteristic distribution of the isotope throughout the left ventricle and no visible defects (cold spots).

Implications of results

Persistent defects generally indicate MI; transient defects (present during peak exercise but not after 3- to 6-hour rest) usually indicate ischemia from CAD. After coronary artery bypass surgery, improved regional perfusion suggests patency of the graft. Increased perfusion after ingestion of antianginal drugs can demonstrate their effectiveness in relieving ischemia. Improved perfusion after balloon angioplasty suggests increased coronary flow.

Documentation

Record patient's vital signs on returning to his room.

Record how patient tolerated the procedure. If he must return for further scanning, record in the nurses' notes when this was done.

Cardiac blood pool imaging

Cardiac blood pool imaging evaluates regional and global ventricular performance after I.V. injection of human serum albumin or RBCs tagged with the isotope technetium-99m (^{99m}Tc) pertechnetate. In first-pass imaging, a scintillation camera records the radioactivity emitted by the isotope in its initial pass through the left ventricle. Higher counts of radioactivity occur during diastole because there is more blood in the ventricle; lower counts occur during systole as the blood is ejected. The portion of isotope ejected during each heartbeat can then be calculated to determine the ejection fraction. The presence and size of intracardiac shunts can also be determined.

Gated cardiac blood pool imaging, performed after first-pass imaging or as a separate test, has several forms; however, most use signals from an EKG to trigger the scintillation camera. In two-frame gated imaging, the camera records left ventricular end-systole and end-diastole for 500 to 1,000 cardiac cycles. Superimposition of these gated images allows assessment of left ventricular contraction to find areas of dyskinesia or akinesia. In multiple-gated acquisition (MUGA) scanning, the camera records 14 to 64 points of a single cardiac cycle, yielding sequential images that can be studied like motion picture films to evaluate regional wall motion and determine the ejection fraction and other indices of cardiac function. In the stress MUGA test, the same test is performed at rest and after exercise to detect changes in ejection fraction and cardiac output. In the nitro MUGA test, the scintillation camera records points in the cardiac cycle after the sublingual administration of nitroglycerin, to assess its effect on ventricular function.

Blood pool imaging is more accurate and involves less risk to the patient than left ventriculography in assessing cardiac function.

Purpose
• To evaluate left ventricular function
• To detect aneurysms of the left ventricle and other myocardial wall-motion abnormalities (areas of akinesia or dyskinesia).

Equipment
None at the bedside.

Procedure
Explain to the patient that this test permits assessment of the heart's left ventricle. Advise him he need not restrict food or fluids. Tell him who will perform the test, where it will be done, that he will receive an I.V. injection of a radioactive tracer, and that a detector positioned above his chest will record the circulation of this tracer through the heart. Reassure him that the tracer poses no radiation hazard and rarely produces side effects.

Make sure the patient or responsible family member has signed a consent form.

The patient is placed in a supine position beneath the detector of a scintillation camera, and 15 to 20 mCi of albumin or RBCs tagged with technetium-99m pertechnetate are injected. For the next minute, the scintillation camera records the first pass of the isotope through the heart, for subsequent localization of the aortic and mitral valves. Then, using an EKG, the camera is gated for selected 60-millisecond intervals, representing end-systole and end-diastole, and 500 to 1,000 cardiac cycles are recorded on X-ray or Polaroid film. To observe septal and posterior wall motion, the patient may be assisted to a modified left anterior oblique position, or he may be assisted to a right anterior oblique position and given 0.4 mg of nitroglycerin sublingually. The scintillation camera then records additional gated images to evaluate abnormal contraction in the left ventricle.

The patient may be asked to exercise as the scintillation camera records gated images.

Special considerations
• Cardiac blood pool imaging is contraindicated during pregnancy.

Findings
Normally, the left ventricle contracts symmetrically, and the isotope appears evenly distributed in the scans. The normal ejection fraction is 55% to 65%.

Implications of results
Patients with CAD usually have asymmetric blood distribution to the myocardium, which produces segmental abnormalities of ventricular wall motion; such abnormalities may also result from preexisting conditions, such as myocarditis. In contrast, patients with cardiomyopathies show globally reduced ejection fractions. In patients with left-to-right shunts, the recirculating radioisotope prolongs the downslope of the curve of scintigraphic data; early arrival of activity in the left ventricle or aorta signifies a right-to-left shunt.

Documentation
Record how patient tolerated the procedure.

Record vital signs when patient returns to his room.

CATHETERIZATION

Cardiac catheterization is the insertion of a catheter into the right or left side of the heart and the injection of contrast medium to permit visualization of cardiac contraction and cardiac structures. Left heart catheterization helps evaluate aortic and mitral valve function, measurement of cardiac output, and coronary artery patency. Right heart catheterization permits evaluation of pulmonary and tricuspid valve function and measurement of cardiac output, right heart pressures, and pulmonary capillary wedge pressure (PCWP). The test can demonstrate valvular efficiency or defects, assess the causes of chest pain, detect congenital heart defects, and help evaluate candidates for coronary artery surgery. It is usually contraindicated in patients with acute MI and acute debilitating conditions.

In *His bundle electrography,* an electrode-tipped catheter is passed into the right atrium and ventricle to record and study the activity of the heart's conduction system. This test allows precise location of bundle branch blocks, detection of dysrhythmias, and evaluation of the effects of antiarrhythmic drugs. This test is contraindicated in patients with severe coagulopathy and acute pulmonary embolism.

Pulmonary artery catheterization permits measurement of PCWP after passage of a balloon-tipped, flow-directed catheter into a small branch of the pulmonary artery; the PCWP reflects both left atrial and left ventricular end-diastolic pressure. This test, performed primarily on patients who have suffered an acute MI, helps assess left ventricular failure and monitors the effects of therapy after complications develop. This test should be performed cautiously in patients with left bundle branch block.

Cardiac catheterization

Cardiac catheterization is the passing of a catheter into the right or left side of the heart. Catheterization can determine blood pressure and blood flow in the chambers of the heart, permit collection of blood samples, or record films of the heart's ventricles (contrast ventriculography) or arteries (coronary arteriography or angiography).

In left heart catheterization, a catheter is inserted into an artery in the antecubital fossa or into the femoral artery through a puncture or cutdown procedure, and, guided by fluoroscopy, the catheter is advanced retrograde through the aorta into the coronary artery orifices or left ventricle. Injection of a contrast medium into the ventricle permits radiographic visualization of the ventri-

cle and coronary arteries and filming (cineangiography) of heart activity. Left heart catheterization assesses the patency of the coronary arteries, mitral and aortic valve function, and left ventricular function. It also aids diagnosis of left ventricular enlargement, aortic stenosis and regurgitation, aortic root enlargement, mitral regurgitation, aneurysm, and intracardiac shunt.

In right heart catheterization, the catheter is inserted into an antecubital vein or the femoral vein and advanced through the inferior vena cava or right atrium into the right side of the heart, and into the pulmonary artery. Right heart catheterization assesses tricuspid and pulmonary valve function and pulmonary artery pressures.

Catheterization permits blood pressure measurement in the heart chambers to determine valve competency and cardiac wall contractility and to detect intracardiac shunts. If thermodilution catheters are used, it allows calculation of cardiac output.

Purpose
• To evaluate valvular insufficiency or stenosis, septal defects, congenital anomalies, myocardial function and blood supply, and cardiac wall motion.

Equipment
None at the bedside.

Procedure
Explain to the patient that this test evaluates the function of the heart and its vessels. Instruct him to restrict food and fluids for at least 6 hours before the test. Tell him who will perform the test, where it will be done, and that it takes 2 to 3 hours. Inform him that he may receive a mild sedative, but he will remain conscious during the procedure.

Tell the patient that the catheter is inserted into an artery or vein in his arm or leg and if the skin above the vessel is hairy, it will be shaved and cleansed with an antiseptic. Tell him he will experience a transient stinging sensation when a local anesthetic is injected to numb the incision site for catheter insertion. He may also feel pressure as the catheter moves along the blood vessel but assure him these sensations are normal. Inform him that injection of a contrast medium through the catheter may produce a hot, flushing sensation or nausea that quickly passes. Instruct him to follow directions to cough or breathe deeply. Tell him that he will be given medication if he has chest pain during the procedure and that he may also receive nitroglycerin periodically to dilate coronary vessels and aid visualization. Assure him that complications such as MI or thromboemboli are rare.

Make sure the patient or responsible family member has signed a consent form. Check patient hypersensitivity to shellfish, iodine, or contrast media used in other diagnostic tests; notify the doctor if such hypersensitivities exist. If the patient is scheduled for right heart catheterization, discontinue any anticoagulant therapy, as ordered, to reduce the risk of complications from venous bleeding. If he is scheduled for left heart catheterization, begin or continue anticoagulant therapy, as ordered, to reduce the risk of arterial catheter-tip clotting. The patient is placed in a supine position on a tilt-top table and secured by restraints. EKG leads are applied for continuous monitoring and an I.V. line, if not already in place, is started with dextrose 5% in water or normal saline solution at keep-vein-open rate. After the local anesthetic is injected at the catheterization site, a small incision or percutaneous puncture is made into the artery or vein, depending on whether left-side or right-side studies are to be performed, and the catheter is passed through the needle into the vessel. The catheter is then guided to the cardiac chambers or coronary arteries using fluoroscopy. When the catheter is in place, the contrast medium is injected through it to visualize the cardiac vessels and structures. (See *Right and Left Heart Catheterization,* page 217.)

The patient may be asked to cough or breathe deeply. Coughing helps counter-

Normal Pressure Curves

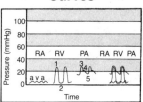

Right-heart chambers

Two pressure complexes are represented for each chamber. Complexes at far right in this diagram represent simultaneous recordings of pressures from the right atrium, right ventricle, and pulmonary artery. The numbered tracings are: 1, RV peak systolic pressure; 2, RV end-diastolic pressure; 3, PA peak systolic pressure; 4, PA dicrotic notch; 5, PA diastolic pressure.

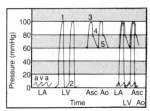

Left-heart chambers

Overall pressure configurations are similar to those of the right heart, but left-heart pressures are significantly higher, because systemic flow resistance is much greater than pulmonary resistance.

KEY

PA = Pulmonary artery
RV = Right ventricle
RA = Right atrium
a wave = Contraction
v wave = Passive filling
LV = Left ventricle
LA = Left atrium
Asc Ao = Ascending aorta

From H. Kasparian et al., "Interpreting Cardiac Catheterization Data," Postgraduate Medicine, 57:4:66 (April 1975).

act nausea or light-headedness caused by the contrast medium and can correct dysrhythmias produced by its depressant effect on the myocardium; deep breathing can ease catheter placement into the pulmonary artery or the wedge position and moves the diaphragm downward, making the heart easier to visualize. During the procedure, the patient may be given nitroglycerin to eliminate catheter-induced spasm or measure its effect on the coronary arteries. Ergonovine maleate, a vasoconstrictor, may be administered to provoke coronary artery spasm (a risky but valuable test in Prinzmetal's angina).

Heart rate and rhythm, respiration, pulse rate, and blood pressure are monitored frequently during the procedure. After completing the procedure, the catheter is removed and a pressure dressing is applied to the incision site.

Special considerations
• Coagulopathy, poor renal function, or debilitation are relative contraindications for both left and right heart catheterization. Unless a temporary pacemaker is inserted to counteract induced ventricular asystole, left bundle branch block contraindicates right heart catheterization. Acute MI once contraindicated left-heart catheterization, but now many doctors perform catheterization and surgically bypass blocked vessels during acute ischemic episodes to prevent myocardial necrosis.
• If the patient has valvular heart disease, prophylactic antibiotic therapy may be indicated to guard against subacute bacterial endocarditis.

Findings
Cardiac catheterization should reveal no abnormalities of heart chamber size and configuration, wall motion and thickness, or direction of blood flow and valve motion. The coronary arteries should have a smooth and regular outline. (See *Normal Pressure Curves*, page 221.)

A normal ejection fraction (60% to 70%) is a good indicator for successful cardiac surgery.

Implications of results
Common abnormalities and defects confirmable by cardiac catheterization include CAD, myocardial incompetency, valvular heart disease, and septal defects.

In *CAD*, catheterization shows constriction of the lumen of the coronary arteries. Constriction greater than 70% is especially significant, particularly in proximal lesions. Narrowing of the left main coronary artery and occlusion or narrowing high in the left anterior descending artery is often an indication for revascularization surgery. (This lesion responds best to coronary bypass grafting.)

Impaired wall motion can indicate *myocardial incompetency* from CAD, aneurysm, cardiomyopathy, or congenital anomalies. Comparing the size of the left ventricle in systole and diastole helps assess the efficiency of cardiac muscular contraction, segmental wall motion, chamber size, and ejection fraction (comparison of the amount of blood pumped out of the left ventricle during systole with the amount of blood remaining at end diastole).

Valvular heart disease is indicated by a gradient, or difference in pressures above and below a heart valve. For example, systolic pressure measurements on both sides of a stenotic aortic valve show a gradient across the valve. The higher the gradient, the greater the degree of stenosis. If left ventricular systolic pressure measures 200 mm Hg and aortic systolic pressure is 120 mm Hg, the gradient across the valve is 80 mm Hg. Since these pressures should normally be equal during systole when the aortic valve is open, a gradient of this magnitude indicates the need for corrective surgery. Incompetent valves can be visualized in ventriculography by watching retrograde flow of the contrast medium across the valve during systole.

Septal defects (both atrial and ventricular) can be confirmed by measuring blood oxygen content in both sides of the heart. Elevated blood oxygen on the right side indicates a left-to-right atrial or ventricular shunt; decreased oxygen on the left side indicates a right-to-left shunt.

Cardiac output can be measured by analyzing blood oxygen levels in the cardiac chambers, by injecting contrast medium into the venous circulation and measuring its concentration as it moves past a thermodilution catheter, or by drawing blood from cardiac chambers.

Documentation

Record patient's vital signs every 15 minutes for the first hour after the procedure, then every hour until stable.

Document any observance of blood loss or hematoma formation at the catheter insertion site.

Record how the patient tolerated the procedure and any analgesics administered.

Record the patient's color, skin temperature, and peripheral pulse below the puncture site.

Document when the post-test EKG was done.

Keep an accurate record of any unusual signs and symptoms that may point to complications. (See *Nurses' Guide to Cardiac Catheterization Complications*, pages 224 to 227.)

His bundle electrography

His bundle electrography permits measurement of discrete conduction intervals by recording electrical conduction during the slow withdrawal of a bipolar or tripolar electrode catheter from the right ventricle through the His bundle to the sinoatrial node. The catheter is introduced into the femoral vein and passed through the right atrium and across the septal leaflet of the tricuspid valve.

The His bundle electrogram can localize disturbances within the atrioventricular conduction system. When an ectopic site takes over as pacemaker of the heart, the electrogram can help pinpoint its origin. The test also aids diagnosis of syncope, evaluates a candidate for permanent artificial pacemaker implantation, and helps select or evaluate antiarrythmic drugs.

Possible complications of His bundle electrography include dysrhythmias, phlebitis, pulmonary emboli, thromboemboli, and catheter-site hemorrhage.

Purpose
• To diagnose dysrhythmias and conduction anomalies
• To determine the need for implanted pacemakers and cardioactive drugs and evaluate their effects on the conduction system and ectopic rhythms
• To locate the site of a bundle branch block, especially in asymptomatic patients with conduction disturbances.

Equipment
None at the bedside.

Procedure
Explain to the patient that this test evaluates the heart's conduction system. Instruct him to restrict food and fluids for at least 6 hours before the test. Tell him who will perform the test, where it will be done, and that it takes 1 to 3 hours.

Inform the patient that after the groin area is shaved, a catheter will be inserted into the femoral vein, and an I.V. line may be started. Tell him that, while he will receive a local anesthetic, he may still feel some pressure upon catheter insertion. Inform him that he will be conscious during the test, and urge him to report any discomfort or pain.

Make sure the patient or responsible family member has signed a consent form. Check the patient's history, and inform the doctor of any ongoing drug therapy. Just before the test, ask the patient to void.

The patient is placed in a supine position on a special X-ray table. Limb electrodes for EKG recording during catheterization are applied, and the insertion site is shaved, scrubbed, and sterilized. The local anesthetic is injected, and a J-tip electrode is introduced I.V. into the femoral vein

Nurses' Guide to Cardiac Catheterization Complications

When your patient returns from the catheterization laboratory, do you know what complications to look for? Use this chart to review your skills.

Cardiac catheterization imposes more risks than most other diagnostic tests. Although the possibility of complications is slight, some complications can be life-threatening. So watch the patient closely during the first 48 hours after the procedure.

Keep in mind that some complications are common to *both* left- and right-sided heart catheterization; others result only from catheterization of one side.

Also note that these are high-risk patients and that MI, cerebrovascular accident (CVA), emboli, and so on, may occur during or around the time of catheterization but may be unrelated to the procedure.

Note: An anaphylactic reaction to the contrast dye used for angiography may occur within 15 minutes of dye injection. Since this complication occurs in the catheterization laboratory, it is not included it in this chart.

RIGHT-SIDED CATHETERIZATION

Possible complication	Possible cause	Signs and symptoms	Nursing considerations
Thrombophlebitis	• Vein damaged during catheter insertion	• Vein is hard, sore, cordlike, and warm to the touch. Vein may look like a red line above catheter insertion site. • Swelling at site	• Elevate limb and apply warm, wet compresses. • Notify doctor. • Administer anticoagulant or fibrinolytic drugs, if ordered. • Document complication and treatment.
Pulmonary embolism	• Catheter tip dislodged blood clot or plaque, which traveled to lungs	• Shortness of breath • Hyperventilation • Increased heart rate • Chest pain	• Notify doctor. • Place patient in high Fowler's position. • Administer oxygen, if ordered. • Monitor vital signs. • Document complication and treatment.
Vagal response	• Vagus nerve endings irritated in sino-atrial node, atrial muscle tissue, or atrioventricular junction	• Hypotension • Decreased heart rate • Nausea	• Notify doctor. • Monitor heart rate closely. • Administer atropine, if ordered. • Keep patient supine and quiet. • Give liquids. • Document complication and treatment.

LEFT-SIDED CATHETERIZATION

Possible complication	Possible cause	Signs and symptoms	Nursing considerations
Arterial embolus or thrombus in limb	• Injury to artery during catheter insertion, causing blood clot • Catheter dislodged plaque from artery wall	• Slow or faint pulse distal to insertion site • Loss of warmth, sensation, and color in limb distal to insertion site	• Notify doctor. He may perform an arteriotomy and Fogarty catheterization to remove embolus or thrombus. • Protect affected limb from pressure. Keep it at room temperature and maintain in a level or slightly dependent position. • Administer vasodilators such as papaverine hydrochloride to relieve painful vasospasm, if ordered. • Document complication and treatment.
Cerebrovascular accident	• Catheter tip dislodged blood clot or plaque, which traveled to brain	• Hemiplegia • Aphasia • Lethargy • Confusion or decreased consciousness level	• Notify doctor. • Monitor vital signs closely. • Keep suctioning equipment nearby. • Give oxygen, as ordered. • Document complication and treatment.

EITHER LEFT- OR RIGHT-SIDED CATHETERIZATION

Possible complication	Possible cause	Signs and symptoms	Nursing considerations
Myocardial infarction	• Emotional stress induced by procedure • Catheter tip dislodged blood clot, which traveled to a coronary artery (left-sided catheterization only) • Air embolism	• Chest pain, possibly radiating to left arm, back, and/or jaw • Cardiac dysrhythmias • Diaphoresis, restlessness, and/or anxiety • Thready pulse • Temperature rise • Peripheral cyanosis, causing cool skin	• Call for code team and begin cardiopulmonary resuscitation (CPR), if necessary. • Notify doctor. • Give oxygen and other drugs, as ordered. • Monitor patient's heart rate closely. • Document complication and treatment.

continued

EITHER LEFT- OR RIGHT-SIDED CATHETERIZATION *(continued)*

Possible complication	Possible cause	Signs and symptoms	Nursing considerations
Dysrhythmias	• Cardiac tissue irritated by catheter	• Irregular heartbeat • Irregular apical pulse • Palpitations	• Notify doctor. • Monitor patient continuously, as ordered. • Administer antiarrhythmic drugs, if ordered. • Document complication and treatment.
Cardiac tamponade	• Perforation of heart wall by catheter	• Dysrhythmias • Increased heart rate • Decreased blood pressure • Chest pain • Diaphoresis • Cyanosis	• Notify doctor. • Give oxygen, if ordered. • Prepare patient for emergency surgery, if ordered. • Monitor patient continuously, as ordered. • Document complication and treatment.
Infection (systemic)	• Poor aseptic technique • Catheter contaminated during manufacturing process, storage, or use	• Fever • Increased pulse rate • Chills and tremors • Unstable blood pressure	• Notify doctor. • Collect samples of patient's urine, sputum, and blood for culture, as ordered. • Document complication and treatment.
Hypovolemia	• Diuresis from angiography dye	• Increased urine output • Hypotension	• Replace fluids by giving patient one or two glasses of water every hour, or maintain I.V. at a rate of 150 to 200 ml/hour, as ordered. • Monitor fluid intake and output closely. • Document complication and treatment.

(occasionally, into a vein in the antecubital fossa). Guided by the fluoroscope, the catheter is advanced until it crosses the tricuspid valve and enters the right ventricle. Then the catheter is slowly withdrawn from the tricuspid area, and recordings of conduction intervals are made from each pole of the catheter, either simultaneously or sequentially. After recordings and measurements are completed, the catheter is removed and a pressure dressing is applied to the site.

Special considerations
• His bundle electrography is contraindicated in patients with severe coagulopathy, recent thrombophlebitis, and acute pulmonary embolism.
• Be sure emergency medication is available, in case the patient develops dysrhythmias during the test.

Values
Normal conduction intervals in adults: H-V interval, 35 to 55 milliseconds; A-

EITHER LEFT- OR RIGHT-SIDED CATHETERIZATION *(continued)*

Possible complication	Possible cause	Signs and symptoms	Nursing considerations
Hematoma, or blood loss at insertion site	• Bleeding at insertion site, from vein or artery damage	• Bloody dressing • Limb swelling • Decreased blood pressure • Increased heart rate	• Elevate limb and apply direct manual pressure. • When bleeding has stopped, apply a pressure bandage. • If bleeding continues, or if vital signs are unstable, notify doctor. • Document complication and treatment.
Dye reaction	• Allergy to iodine base of angiography dye	• Fever • Agitation • Hives • Itching • Decreased urine output, indicating kidney failure	• Notify doctor. • Administer antihistamines to relieve itching, as ordered. • Administer diuretics to treat kidney failure, as ordered. • Monitor fluid intake and output closely. • Document complication and treatment.
Infection at insertion site	• Poor aseptic technique	• Swelling, warmth, redness, and soreness at site • Purulent discharge at site	• Obtain drainage sample for culture. • Clean site and apply antimicrobial ointment, if ordered. Cover site with sterile gauze pad. • Review and improve aseptic technique. • Document complication and treatment.

H interval, 45 to 150 milliseconds; P-A interval, 20 to 40 milliseconds.

Implications of results

A prolonged H-V interval can result from acute or chronic disease. This interval represents the conduction time from the His bundle to the Purkinje fibers. Atrioventricular nodal (A-H interval) delays can stem from atrial pacing, chronic conduction system disease, carotid sinus pressure, recent MI, and drugs. Intra-atrial (P-A interval) delays can result from acquired, surgically induced, or congenital atrial disease and atrial pacing.

Documentation

Record the patient's vital signs every 15 minutes for 1 hour, then every hour for 4 hours.

Document any shortness of breath, chest pain, pallor, or changes in pulse rate or blood pressure.

Record any unusual bleeding from the insertion site.

Document when the post-test EKG was done.

Pulmonary artery catheterization (Swan-Ganz catheterization)

Pulmonary artery catheterization uses a balloon-tipped, flow-directed catheter to provide intermittent monitored occlusion of the pulmonary artery. Once the catheter is in place, this procedure permits measurement of both pulmonary artery pressure (PAP) and pulmonary capillary wedge pressure (PCWP)—also known as pulmonary artery wedge pressure. The PCWP reading accurately reflects left atrial pressure and left ventricular end-diastolic pressure, although the catheter itself never enters the left side of the heart. Such a reading is possible because the heart momentarily relaxes during diastole as it fills with blood from the pulmonary veins; at this instant, the pulmonary vasculature, left atrium, and left ventricle act as a single chamber, and all have identical pressures. Thus, changes in PAP and PCWP reflect changes in left ventricular filling pressure, permitting detection of left ventricular dysfunction.

In this procedure, which is usually performed at bedside in an intensive care unit, the catheter is inserted through the cephalic vein in the antecubital fossa or the subclavian (sometimes, femoral) vein. The catheter is threaded into the right atrium, the balloon is inflated, and the catheter follows the blood flow through the tricuspid valve into the right ventricle and out into the pulmonary artery.

In addition to measuring atrial and pulmonary arterial pressures, this procedure evaluates pulmonary vascular resistance and tissue oxygenation, as indicated by mixed venous oxygen content. It should be performed cautiously in patients with left bundle branch block or implanted pacemakers.

Purpose
• To help assess right and left ventricular failure
• To monitor therapy for complications of acute MI, such as cardiogenic shock, pulmonary edema, fluid-related hypovolemia and hypotension, systolic murmur, unexplained sinus tachycardia, and various cardiac dysrhythmias
• To monitor fluid status in patients with serious burns, renal disease, or shock lung (noncardiogenic pulmonary edema) after open heart surgery
• To monitor the effects of cardiovascular drugs, such as nitroglycerin and nitroprusside.

Equipment
Local anesthetic (1% Xylocaine)/70% alcohol or povidone-iodine solution/antiseptic ointment/heparin/skin preparation set/sterile drape, sterile towels, and tape/sterile stockinette/cutdown tray or percutaneous needle/tuberculin syringe/2.5-ml syringe/two-, three-, or four-lumen catheter/gloves, mask, and gown/I.V. pole and transducer holder/strain gauge transducer with sterile dome/three 3-way stopcocks/two Sorenson Intraflo Valves/ two Cobe pressure tubings/transfer pack/blood recipient set (for transfer pack), or regular I.V. tubing for prepackaged bagged solution/pressure bag including manometer/defibrillator/emergency or code cart/4″ x 4″ gauze pads/500 ml normal saline solution I.V. bottle/3-0 and 4-0 silk sutures/oscilloscope/digital readout recorder.

Procedure
Explain to the patient that this test evaluates heart function and provides information for determining appropriate therapy or managing fluid status. Advise him that he need not restrict food or fluids before the test. Tell him who will perform the test and where it will be done.

Inform the patient that he will be conscious during catheterization and may

Pulmonary Artery Catheters

Four types of pulmonary artery catheters help evaluate cardiovascular and pulmonary functions. The *double-lumen catheter* monitors pulmonary artery pressure (PAP) and pulmonary capillary wedge pressure (PCWP). It is also used for obtaining samples of mixed venous blood and for infusion of solutions. The *triple-lumen catheter* has the same capabilities as the double-lumen catheter, but also allows monitoring of right atrial (central venous) pressure. The *four-lumen, flow-directed thermodilution catheter* has the same capabilities as double- and triple-lumen catheters but also allows evaluation of cardiac output.

The *five-lumen pulmonary catheter* (shown here) has the same capabilities as the other catheters but it also allows atrial, ventricular, and atrioventricular sequential pacing. By performing the same functions that previously required two or more catheters, it helps reduce patient trauma and discomfort. The five-lumen pulmonary catheter is particularly effective in patients who require hemodynamic monitoring and temporary pacing, have suffered acute MI with conduction defects, require cardiac surgery or override of atrial or ventricular dysrhythmias, or require diagnosis of complex dysrhythmias.

**Types of pulmonary
artery catheters**

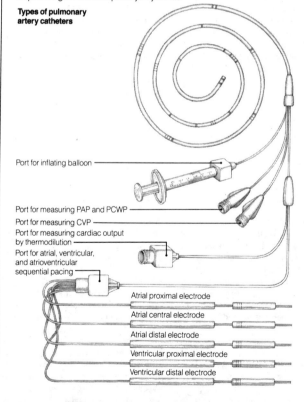

Port for inflating balloon

Port for measuring PAP and PCWP

Port for measuring CVP

Port for measuring cardiac output
by thermodilution

Port for atrial, ventricular,
and atrioventricular
sequential pacing

Atrial proximal electrode

Atrial central electrode

Atrial distal electrode

Ventricular proximal electrode

Ventricular distal electrode

Interpreting Hemodynamic Waveforms

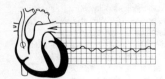

RIGHT ATRIUM
Normal Pressure
Mean: 1 to 6 mm Hg
Physiologic Significance
Right atrial (RA) pressures reflect mean RA diastolic (filling) pressure (equivalent to central venous pressure) and right ventricular (RV) end-diastolic pressure.
Clinical Implications
Increased RA pressure may signal RV failure, volume overload, tricuspid valve stenosis or regurgitation, constrictive pericarditis, or pulmonary hypertension.

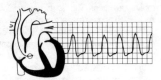

RIGHT VENTRICLE
Normal Pressures
Systolic: 15 to 25 mm Hg
Diastolic: 0 to 8 mm Hg
Physiologic Significance
RV systolic pressure equals pulmonary artery systolic pressure; RV end-diastolic pressure reflects RV function and equals RA pressure.
Clinical Implications
RV pressures rise in mitral stenosis or insufficiency, pulmonary disease, hypoxemia, constrictive pericarditis, chronic congestive heart failure, atrial and ventricular septal defects, and patent ductus arteriosus.

feel transient local discomfort from the administration of the local anesthetic. Tell him catheter insertion takes about 30 minutes, but the catheter will remain in place, causing little or no discomfort, for 48 to 72 hours. Instruct him to report any discomfort immediately.

Make sure the patient or responsible family member has signed a consent form.

The flexible catheter used in this test comes in two-lumen, three-lumen, and four-lumen (thermodilution) modes and in various lengths. (See *Pulmonary Artery Catheters*, page 229.) In the two-lumen catheter, one lumen contains the balloon, 1 mm behind the catheter tip; the other lumen, which opens at the tip, measures pressure in front of the balloon. The two-lumen catheter measures PAP and PCWP and can be used to sample mixed venous blood and infuse I.V. solutions. The three-lumen catheter has an additional proximal lumen that opens 30 cm behind the tip. When the tip is in the main pulmonary artery, the proximal lumen lies in the right atrium, permitting administration of fluids or monitoring of right atrial pressure (central venous pressure). The four-lumen type includes a transistorized thermistor for monitoring blood temperature and

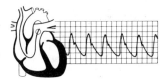

PULMONARY ARTERY PRESSURE
Normal Pressures
Systolic: 15 to 25 mm Hg
Diastolic: 8 to 15 mm Hg
Mean: 10 to 20 mm Hg
Physiologic Significance
Pulmonary artery pressure (PAP) reflects
venous pressure in the lungs and mean
filling pressure in the left atrium and left
ventricle (if the mitral valve is normal), allowing detection of pulmonary congestion. PAP also reflects RV function since,
in the absence of pulmonary stenosis,
systolic PAP usually equals RV systolic
pressure.
Clinical Implications
PAP rises in left ventricular (LV) failure, increased pulmonary blood flow (left or
right shunting as in atrial or ventricular
septal defects), and in any increase in pulmonary arteriolar resistance (as in pulmonary hypertension or mitral stenosis).

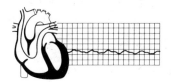

**PULMONARY CAPILLARY WEDGE
PRESSURE**
Normal Pressure
Mean: 5 to 12 mm Hg
Physiologic Significance
Pulmonary capillary wedge pressure
(PCWP) accurately reflects both left
atrial (LA) and LV pressures (if mitral
stenosis is not present), because the
heart momentarily relaxes during
diastole as it fills with blood from pulmonary veins. At this instant, the pulmonary vasculature, left atrium, and
left ventricle act as a single chamber
with identical pressures. Thus,
changes in PAP and PCWP reflect
changes in LV filling pressure.
Clinical Implications
PCWP rises in LV failure, mitral stenosis or insufficiency, and pericardial
tamponade. It decreases in hypovolemia.

allows measurement of cardiac output.

After the patient is positioned, the
catheter balloon is checked for defects
using sterile technique. Then the catheter is introduced into the vein percutaneously or by cutdown. The catheter is
directed to the right atrium, and the
catheter balloon is partially inflated so
that venous flow carries the catheter tip
through the right atrium and tricuspid
valve into the right ventricle and pulmonary artery. While the catheter is
being directed, the oscilloscope screen
is observed for characteristic waveform
changes, and the location of the catheter
tip is found. A printout of each stage of

catheter insertion is obtained for baseline information.

As the catheter is passed into the right
heart chambers, the oscilloscope screen
is observed for frequent PVCs and
tachycardia—the result of catheter irritation of the right ventricle. If irritation
occurs, the catheter may be partially
withdrawn or medication administered
to suppress the dysrhythmia or right
bundle branch block.

To record the PCWP, the catheter balloon is carefully inflated with the specified amount of air or carbon dioxide—
not fluid—using the smallest syringe
possible; the catheter tip will float into

Solving Problems with Pulmonary Artery Lines

PROBLEM	POSSIBLE CAUSES	SOLUTION
Dampened pressures	• Air in system	• Check Intraflow, stopcock, and transducer for bubbles.
	• Blood on transducer	• Flush off or change transducer.
	• Clot in system	• Aspirate blood until it thins; notify doctor.
	• Catheter kinked	• Instruct patient to cough or extend his arm to 90° angle from his body, and gently flush the catheter. If problem, obtain X-ray film.
	• Loose connection	• Check connections for security.
	• Incorrect stopcock position	• Correct stopcock position.
	• Pressure tubing too long	• Shorten distance between patient and transducer.
Transducer imbalance	• Damaged transducer	• Try another transducer.
	• Wrong amplifier	• Check transducer connection to amplifier.
	• Broken amplifier	• Change the amplifier.
	• Set at wrong level (midchest)	• Readjust the transducer.
Waveform drifting	• Short warm-up time	• Allow recommended time for warm-up.
	• Cable air vents kinked or coiled	• Unkink or decompress cable air vents.
False-low reading	• Dampened waveform	• See section on dampened pressures.
	• Transducer imbalance	• Place transducer at heart level.
	• Wrong calibration	• Recalibrate the monitor.

the wedge position, as indicated by an altered waveform on the oscilloscope screen. If a PCWP waveform occurs with less than the recommended inflation volume, do not inflate the balloon further. After the balloon is inflated, the wedge pressure is recorded. Then the air from the balloon is allowed to return to the syringe, which is then deflated. This allows the catheter to float back into the pulmonary artery. The oscilloscope screen is observed for a PA waveform, and the system is flushed and recalibrated.

The balloon should not be overinflated. Overinflation could distend the pulmonary artery, causing vessel rupture. If the balloon cannot be fully deflated after recording the PCWP, it should not be reinflated unless the doctor is present; balloon rupture may cause a life-threatening air embolism. All connections are checked for air leaks that may have prevented balloon inflation, particularly if the patient is confused or uncooperative.

When the catheter's correct positioning and function are established, it is sutured to the skin and antibiotic ointment and an airtight dressing are applied to the insertion site. A chest X-ray film is obtained, as ordered, to verify cathe-

PROBLEM	POSSIBLE CAUSES	SOLUTION
False-high reading	• Transducer imbalance • Flush solution administered too quickly	• Rebalance the transducer. • Pour slow continual flush to 3 to 6 ml/hour.
Configuration	• Improper catheter placement • Transducer needs to be calibrated • Transducer not at right atrial level • Transducer loosely connected to catheter	• Try to wedge catheter. Obtain pulmonary capillary wedge pressure (PCWP). If problem, obtain X-ray film. • Recalibrate transducer. • Reposition and recalibrate transducer. • Secure transducer.
Drifting wedge pressure (with inflated balloon)	• Balloon overinflation • Air in system	• Watch scope while inflating balloon. When waveform changes from a pulmonary artery to a wedge shape, stop inflating. • Remove air from tubing and/or transducer.
PCWP pressure trace unobtainable	• Incorrect amount of balloon air • Ruptured balloon	• Deflate, start again slowly. Check for air to refill syringe during balloon deflation. • With no resistance to inflation, stop inflation. Notify doctor.

ter placement. (The radiology department is notified before the procedure that a catheter is to be inserted.) Alarms are set on the EKG and pressure monitors. Vital signs are monitored, as ordered. PAP waveforms are documented at the beginning of each shift and monitored frequently throughout the shift. PCWP and cardiac output are checked, as ordered (usually every 6 hours). Routine aseptic precautions are taken to prevent infection.

When the catheter is no longer needed, the patient's blood pressure and radial pulse are taken. Then the balloon is deflated, the dressing removed, and

the catheter slowly withdrawn. The EKG is monitored for dysrhythmias. If any difficulty is encountered in removing the catheter, the procedure is stopped at once and the doctor notified.

After the catheter is withdrawn, pressure, an antibiotic ointment, and a sterile dressing are applied to the insertion site. Blood pressure and radial pulse are checked.

Special considerations
• After each PCWP reading, flush and recalibrate the monitoring system and make sure the balloon is completely deflated; if you encounter difficulty in

flushing the system, notify the doctor. Maintain 300 mm Hg pressure in the pressure bag to permit fluid flow of 3 to 6 ml/hour. Instruct the patient to extend the appropriate arm (or leg, if the catheter is inserted into the femoral vein). If the patient develops fever while the catheter is in place, remove the catheter and send the tip to the laboratory for culture.

• Make sure all stopcocks are properly positioned and all connections are secure. Loose connections during the test can allow rapid, massive arterial blood loss, as well as inaccurate pressure measurement.

• Be sure the lumen hubs are properly identified to serve the appropriate catheter ports. Do not add or remove fluids from the distal pulmonary artery port; this may cause pulmonary extravasation or damage the artery.

• If the catheter has not been sutured to the skin, tape it securely to prevent dislodgement.

Values

Normal pressures are as follows:
Right atrial: 1 to 6 mm Hg
Systolic right ventricular: 20 to 30 mm Hg
End-diastolic right ventricular: < 5 mm Hg
Systolic PAP: 20 to 30 mm Hg
Diastolic PAP: about 10 mm Hg
Mean PAP: < 20 mm Hg
PAWP: 6 to 12 mm Hg
Left atrial: about 10 mm Hg.
(See *Interpreting Hemodynamic Waveforms,* pages 230 and 231.)

Implications or results

An abnormally high right atrial pressure can indicate pulmonary disease, right heart failure, fluid overload, cardiac tamponade, tricuspid stenosis and regurgitation, or pulmonary hypertension.

Elevated right ventricular pressure can result from pulmonary hypertension, pulmonary valvular stenosis, right ventricular failure, pericardial effusion, constrictive pericarditis, chronic CHF, or ventricular septal defects.

An abnormally high PAP is characteristic in increased pulmonary blood flow, such as in a left-to-right shunt secondary to atrial or ventricular septal defect; increased pulmonary arteriolar resistance, such as in pulmonary hypertension or mitral stenosis; chronic obstructive pulmonary disease; pulmonary edema or embolus; and left ventricular failure from any cause. Pulmonary artery systolic pressure is the same as right ventricular systolic pressure. Pulmonary artery diastolic pressure is the same as left atrial pressure, except in patients with severe pulmonary disease causing pulmonary hypertension; in such patients, catheterization still provides important diagnostic information.

Elevated PCWP can result from left ventricular failure, mitral stenosis and regurgitation, cardiac tamponade, or cardiac insufficiency; depressed PCWP, from hypovolemia. (See *Solving Problems with Pulmonary Artery Lines,* pages 232 and 233.)

Documenation

Record the patient's vital signs and any changes that might signal complications such as pulmonary emboli, pulmonary artery perforation, heart murmurs, thrombi, and dysrhythmias.

Document any signs of infection at the insertion site, such as redness, swelling, or discharge.

Document how the patient tolerated the procedure.

13

LABORATORY PROCEDURES

aboratory procedures are a critical part of cardiovascular nursing. The numerous blood and urine tests now available give the clinician new insights into diseases and body dysfunctions and help with diagnosis, treatment, and patient teaching. Nurses play an important role in laboratory testing by providing pre- and post-test teaching and psychological support to patients and families, assisting with testing, and sometimes administering tests themselves.

HEMATOLOGIC TESTS

The type of blood sample required— whole blood, plasma, or serum—depends on the nature of the test. *Whole blood*—containing all blood elements— is the sample of choice for blood gas analysis, determination of hemoglobin derivatives, and measurement of red blood cell (RBC) constituents. In addition, most routine hematologic studies, such as complete blood count (CBC), erythrocyte sedimentation rate, and reticulocyte and platelet counts, require whole blood samples. *Plasma* is the liquid part of whole blood, which contains all the blood proteins; *serum,* the liquid that remains after whole blood clots. Plasma and serum samples, which contain most of the physiologically and clinically significant substances found in blood, are used for most biochemical, immunologic, and coagulation studies. They also provide useful electrolyte evaluation, enzyme analysis, and protein determination.

Venous, arterial, and capillary blood

Venous blood returns to the heart through the veins. It carries a high concentration of carbon dioxide from the cells back to the lungs, for exhalation. Since venous blood represents physiologic conditions throughout the body and is relatively easy to obtain, it is used for most laboratory procedures.

Arterial blood, replenished with oxygen from the lungs, leaves the heart through the arteries to distribute nutrients throughout the capillary network. (See *Common Arterial and Venous Puncture Sites,* page 236.) Although arterial puncture increases the risk of hematoma and arterial spasm, pH, PO_2 and PCO_2 determinations, and oxygen saturation studies must be done with arterial blood specimens.

Capillary or peripheral blood does the real work of the circulatory system— exchanging fluids, nutrients, and wastes between the blood and other tissues. The composition of free-flowing capillary blood is similar to that of arteriolar blood. Capillary blood specimens are most useful for studies such as hemoglobin and hematocrit determinations; blood smears; microtechniques for clinical chemistry; and platelet, RBC, and white blood cell (WBC) counts requiring only small amounts of blood.

Quantities and containers

Specimen quantities needed for diagnostic studies depend on the laboratory, available equipment, and the type of test to be conducted. The desired specimen quantity determines the collection procedure and the type and size of the con-

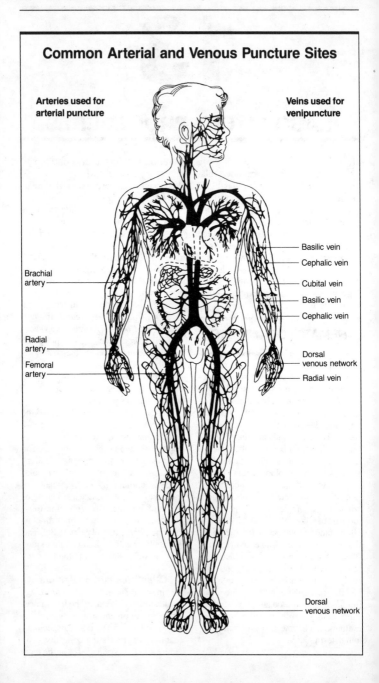

Common Arterial and Venous Puncture Sites

Arteries used for arterial puncture

Veins used for venipuncture

Brachial artery

Radial artery

Femoral artery

Basilic vein

Cephalic vein

Cubital vein

Basilic vein

Cephalic vein

Dorsal venous network

Radial vein

Dorsal venous network

tainer. A single venipuncture with a conventional glass or disposable plastic syringe can provide 15 ml of blood—sufficient for many hematologic, immunologic, chemical, and coagulation tests, but hardly enough for a series of tests.

To avoid multiple venipunctures, an evacuated tube system (Vacutainer, Corvac) with interchangeable glass tubes, optional draw capacities, and a selection of additives should be used. Evacuated tubes are commercially prepared without additives or with a premeasured amount of anticoagulant, and with enough vacuum to draw a predetermined blood volume (2 to 20 ml per tube).

Microanalysis of minute amounts of capillary blood collected with micropipetts or glass capillary tubes allows numerous hematologic and routine laboratory studies to be done on infants, children, and patients with poor veins. Micropipetts are color-coded by specimen capacity, ranging from 30 to 5 µl of whole blood. Glass capillary tubes yield 80 to 130 µl of serum or plasma.

Arterial blood for blood gas analysis is collected in a heparinized syringe, and approximately 10 µl is required.

Collection procedures

The nature of the test and the patient's age and condition determine the appropriate blood specimen, collection site, and technique to be used. Most tests require a venipuncture.

Venous sample

Although venipuncture is a relatively simple procedure, it still must be done carefully to avoid hemolysis or hemoconcentration of the specimen, to prevent hematoma, and to protect the patient's veins for future use. (See *How to Collect a Venous Sample,* page 238.)

Necessary equipment includes:
• tourniquet
• 70% alcohol or povidone-iodine solution.
• sterile syringes or evacuated tubes
• sterile needle—20G or 21G for forearm; 25G for wrist, hand, or ankle, or

for children
• color-coded tubes containing appropriate anticoagulants or additives and identification labels
• 2" x 2" gauze pads
• small adhesive bandage.

Before drawing the specimen:
• Wash your hands thoroughly. Assemble the necessary equipment. Label all test tubes clearly with the patient's name and room number, doctor's name, date, and collection time.
• Explain to the patient what a venipuncture is and why it is being done. Tell him it takes only about 3 minutes. Except for pressure from the tourniquet and the prick of the needle, he should experience no discomfort.
• Patients who have had numerous blood specimens drawn may be able to show you the best venipuncture site. The most common site is the antecubital area. Other sites include the wrist, back of the hand, or dorsum of the foot. To draw the specimen at bedside, instruct the patient to lie on his back with his head slightly elevated, his arms resting at his sides. To draw blood from an ambulatory patient, have him sit in a chair with his arm supported securely on an armrest or table.
• Apply a soft rubber tourniquet above the puncture site to prevent venous blood return and increase venous pressure. This makes veins more prominent and increases the volume of blood at the puncture site. Make sure the tourniquet is snug but not tight enough to constrict arteries.
• Instruct the patient to make a fist several times to enlarge the veins further. Select a vein by palpation and inspection. If you cannot feel a vein distinctly, *do not* try to enter it. Using a tourniquet in patients with large, distended, and highly visible veins may increase the risk of hematoma, so if the patient's veins are visible enough, you may be able to do the venipuncture without a tourniquet.
• Working in a circular motion from the center outward, clean the puncture site with alcohol or antiseptic solution and

How to Collect a Venous Sample

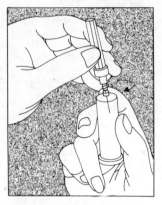
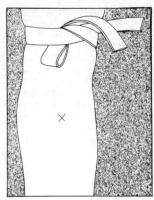
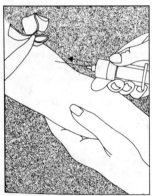
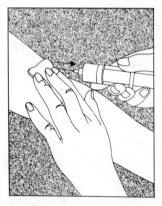

- Select a venipuncture site, usually the antecubital fossa.
- Using a circular motion, cleanse the area first with povidone-iodine solution and then alcohol.
- Screw the Vacutainer needle into the sleeve (top left).
- Apply a soft rubber tourniquet above the venipuncture site (top right).
- Remove the needle cover. With the bevel facing up, insert the needle into the patient's vein at a 15° angle (bottom left). When a drop of blood appears just inside the needle holder, gently push the Vacutainer tube into the needle sleeve, so the blood enters the tube. Try to keep the needle still to prevent it from perforating the patient's vein.
- When the tube is filled, remove the tourniquet, and pull the Vacutainer tube off the needle end. Withdraw the needle, using a dry sponge to apply direct pressure to the puncture site (bottom right). After 2 or 3 minutes, remove the sponge, and cover the site with an adhesive bandage.

dry with a gauze pad. If you must touch the cleansed puncture site again to relocate the vein, palpate with an antiseptically clean finger, and wipe the area again with an alcohol swab.

• Draw the skin taut over the vein by pressing just below the puncture site with your thumb to keep the vein from moving.

• Hold the syringe or tube with the needle bevel up and the shaft parallel to the path of the vein at a 15° angle to the arm. Enter the vein with a single direct puncture of the skin and vein wall. If you use a syringe, venous blood will appear in the hub. Withdraw the blood slowly, gently pulling on the syringe to create steady suction until you obtain the desired amount. If you use an evacuated tube, blood flows into the tube automatically.

• To prevent stasis, release the tourniquet as soon as you establish adequate blood flow. However, if the flow is sluggish, you may want to leave the tourniquet in place.

After drawing the specimen:

• Ask the patient to open his fist as soon as you collect the desired amount of blood. Release the tourniquet. Place a gauze pad over the puncture site, then withdraw the needle slowly and gently. Apply gentle pressure to the puncture site. If the patient is alert and cooperative, tell him to hold the gauze in place for several minutes until the bleeding stops. This will prevent hematoma. If the patient is not alert or cooperative, hold the pad in place or apply a small adhesive bandage.

• If you use a syringe, remove the needle and carefully pour the collected blood into test tubes containing an appropriate anticoagulant, when required, without delay. To avoid foaming and possible hemolysis, *do not* eject blood through the needle or force it out of the syringe.

• Place the appropriate color-coded stoppers on the tubes. Gently invert the tubes containing the anticoagulant several times to mix the specimen thoroughly. *Do not* shake the tubes.

• Before leaving the patient, check his condition. If hematoma develops at the puncture site, apply warm soaks to the area. If he has lingering discomfort or undue bleeding, instruct him to lie down. Watch for signs of anxiety or shock.

• Make sure the specimen is sent to the laboratory immediately.

Arterial sample

Arterial blood is rarely required in routine blood studies. Since arterial puncture can be hazardous, specimens are generally collected by a doctor or a specially trained nurse.

Perform an Allen's test (see *Performing the Allen's Test,* page 55) to assess circulation in the radial artery. Choose either the radial or brachial artery, whichever has the better circulation. *Do not* choose a site where the patient has had a vascular graft or has an atrioventricular fistula in situ.

Before drawing an arterial blood sample, administer a local anesthetic at the puncture site, if necessary.

Note on the laboratory slip the patient's temperature, hemoglobin count, and the type and amount of oxygen he is receiving. Send the sample to the laboratory immediately.

After releasing pressure on the puncture site, tape a bandage firmly over it. (Do not tape the entire wrist, as this may restrict circulation.)

After arterial puncture, observe carefully for signs of circulatory impairment distal to the puncture site, such as swelling, discoloration, pain, numbness, or tingling in the bandaged extremity.

Before drawing an arterial blood sample for blood gas studies, carefully check the patient's oxygen therapy. If arterial blood gas (ABG) levels are being measured to monitor response to withdrawal of oxygen, but the patient continues to receive it, results will be misleading. For the same reason, do not draw an arterial sample immediately after suctioning or after placement on a ventilator. Wait at least 15 minutes to allow circulating blood levels to accurately reflect response to mechanical ventilation.

Capillary sample

Collection of a capillary blood sample requires skin puncture of the fingertip or earlobe of adults, or puncture of the great toe or heel of neonates.

After drawing the sample, wipe away the first drop of blood to reduce the chance of sample dilution with tissue fluid. For the same reason, avoid squeezing the puncture site. After collecting the sample, briefly apply pressure to the puncture site to prevent painful extravasation of blood into the subcutaneous tissues. Ask the adult patient to hold a sterile gauze pad over the puncture site until bleeding has stopped. Then apply a small adhesive bandage.

Interfering factors: The effect of diet and drugs

Food or medications can interfere with test methods, so be sure to check the patient's diet and medication history before tests, and schedule tests after an overnight fast of 12 to 14 hours. Although the concentration of most blood constituents does not change significantly after a meal, fasting is customary because blood collected shortly after eating often appears cloudy (turbid) from a temporary tryglyceride increase that can interfere with many chemical reactions. Dietary-related lipemia usually disappears 4 to 6 hours after a meal, making shorter fasts acceptable.

Numerous drugs and their metabolites affect test results by direct, pharmacologic, or chemical interference. *Direct interference* is the natural or expected effect on the concentration of a particular substance; for example, insulin administered to patients with hyperglycemia or diabetes lowers blood glucose levels. *Pharmacologic interference* results from temporary or permanent drug-induced physiologic change in a blood component; for example, long-term administration of drugs such as erythromycin can damage the liver and alter the results of liver function tests. *Chemical interference* results from a

physical drug characteristic that alters the test reaction; for example, high dosages of ascorbic acid may raise blood glucose levels. Whatever the type of interference, all unexpected changes in blood values require serious attention and careful observation of the patient.

COMPLETE BLOOD COUNT

Hematocrit (Hct)

Hematocrit (Hct), a common, reliable test, may be done by itself or as part of a complete blood count. It measures the percentage, by volume, of packed RBCs in a whole blood sample; for example, an Hct of 40% means that a 100-ml sample contains 40 ml of packed RBCs. This packing is achieved by centrifugation of anticoagulated whole blood in a capillary tube, so that red cells are tightly packed without hemolysis.

Purpose

• To aid diagnosis of abnormal states of hydration, polycythemia, and anemia
• To provide data for calculating red cell indices
• To determine blood viscosity in cardiovascular disorders.

Equipment

Venipuncture: tourniquet/70% alcohol or povidone-iodine solution/sterile syringes or evacuated tubes/sterile needle—20G or 21G for forearm, 25G for wrist, hand, ankle, or for children/color-coded tubes containing appropriate additives/identification labels/2″ x 2″ gauze pads/small adhesive bandage.

Capillary blood: sterile, disposable blood lancet/2″ x 2″ gauze pads/70% alcohol or povidone-iodine solution/ glass slides, heparinized capillary tubes or pipettes/appropriate solutions.

Procedure

Explain to the patient that this test detects anemia and other abnormal conditions of the blood. Inform him he need

Normal Hematocrit Varies According to Age

Newborn	55% to 68%
1 week	47% to 65%
1 month	37% to 49%
3 months	30% to 36%
1 year	29% to 41%
10 years	36% to 40%
Adult men	42% to 54%
Adult women	38% to 46%

not restrict food or fluids, and that the test requires a blood sample. If the patient is an infant or child, explain to the parents (and to the child if he is old enough to understand) that a small amount of blood will be drawn from his finger or earlobe. Reassure him that collecting the sample will take less than 3 minutes.

Macro method: Draw venous blood into a 7-ml *lavender-top* tube.

Micro method: Perform a finger stick using a heparinized capillary tube with a red band on the anticoagulant end.

Macro method: Completely fill the tube, and invert it gently several times to mix the sample and anticoagulant. Do not shake the tube vigorously, since this may cause hemolysis. Send the sample to the laboratory immediately.

Micro method: Avoid excessive squeezing of the finger to obtain blood, as this may alter test results. Fill the capillary tube from the red-banded end to about two-thirds capacity, and seal this end with clay. Send the sample to the laboratory immediately. Or, if you perform the test, place the tube in the centrifuge, with the red end pointing outward.

Special considerations
• Failure to use the proper anticoagulant in the collection tube and to fill it appropriately may interfere with accurate determination of test results.
• Tourniquet constriction for longer than

1 minute causes hemoconcentration and typically raises Hct by 2.5% to 5%.
• Taking the blood sample from the same arm that is being used for I.V. infusion of fluids causes hemodilution.

Values
Hematocrit values vary, depending on the patient's sex and age, type of sample, and the laboratory performing the test. (See *Normal Hematocrit Varies According to Age.*)

Implications of results
Low Hct may indicate anemia or hemodilution; high Hct suggests polycythemia or hemoconcentration due to blood loss.

Documentation
Record testing on cardex.

Total hemoglobin

This test measures the grams of hemoglobin (Hgb) found in a deciliter (100 ml) of whole blood. Hgb concentration correlates closely with the RBC count and is affected by the Hgb-RBC ratio (mean corpuscular hemoglobin [MCH]) and free plasma Hgb. In the laboratory, Hgb is chemically converted to pigmented compounds and is measured by spectrophotometric or colorimetric technique.

The test is usually performed as part of a CBC.

Purpose
• To measure the severity of anemia or polycythemia and monitor response to therapy
• To supply figures for calculating MCH and mean corpuscular hemoglobin concentration
• To aid in diagnosing specific cardiovascular disorders.

Equipment
Venipuncture: tourniquet/70% alcohol or povidone-iodine solution/sterile syringes or evacuated tubes/sterile nee-

dle—20G or 21G for forearm, 25G for wrist, hand, ankle, or for children/color-coded tubes containing appropriate additives/identification labels/2″ x 2″ gauze pads/small adhesive bandage.

Capillary blood: sterile, disposable blood lancet/2″ x 2″ gauze pads/70% alcohol or povidone-iodine solution/ glass slides, heparinized capillary tubes or pipettes/appropriate solutions.

Procedure

Explain to the patient that this test helps determine or assesses his response to treatment. Inform him that he need not restrict food or fluids, and that the test requires a blood sample. If the patient is an infant or a young child, explain to the parents (and to the child if he is old enough to understand) that a small amount of blood will be drawn from his finger or earlobe.

For adults and older children, perform a venipuncture, and collect the sample in a 7-ml *lavender-top* tube. For younger children and infants, collect capillary blood in a pipette.

Special considerations

• Completely fill the collection tube, and invert it gently several times to adequately mix the sample and the anticoagulant.
• Handle the sample gently to prevent hemolysis.
• Failure to use the proper anticoagulant in the collection tube or to adequately mix the sample and anticoagulant may interfere with accurate determination of test results.
• Prolonged tourniquet constriction may cause hemoconcentration.
• Very high white cell counts, lipemia, or red cells that are resistant to lysis will falsely elevate Hgb values.
• Hemodilution in the sample may result from drawing it from the same arm used for intravenous infusion of fluids.

Values

Hgb concentration varies, depending on the patient's age and sex and the type of blood sample drawn. Except for infants,

Normal Hgb Values Vary with Age

		Unit
Newborns	17 to 22	g/dl
1 week	15 to 20	g/dl
1 month	11 to 15	g/dl
Children	11 to 13	g/dl
Men	14 to 18	g/dl
Men after middle age	12.4 to 14.9	g/dl
Women	12 to 16	g/dl
Women after middle age	11.7 to 13.8	g/dl

values for blood groups listed in the accompanying chart are based on venous blood. (See *Normal Hgb Values Vary with Age.*)

Implications of results

Low Hgb concentration may indicate anemia, recent hemorrhage, or fluid retention, causing hemodilution; elevated Hgb suggests hemoconcentration from polycythemia or dehydration.

Documentation

Record testing on cardex.

Erythrocyte sedimentation rate

The erythrocyte sedimentation rate (ESR) measures the time required for erythrocytes in a whole blood sample to settle to the bottom of a vertical tube. As the red cells descend in the tube, they displace an equal volume of plasma upward, which retards the downward progress of other settling blood elements. Factors affecting ESR include red cell volume, surface area, density, aggregation, and surface charge. Plasma proteins (notably fibrinogen and globulin) encourage aggregation, increasing ESR.

The ESR is a sensitive but nonspecific test that is frequently the earliest indicator of disease when other chemical or physical signs are normal. It often rises significantly in widespread inflammatory disorders due to infection or autoimmune mechanisms. Such elevations may be prolonged in localized inflammation and malignancy.

Purpose
• To monitor inflammatory or malignant disease
• To aid detection and diagnosis of myocarditis, endocarditis, pericarditis, rheumatoid heart disease, renal disease from hypertension, aortic arch syndrome, and benign cardiac tumors.

Equipment
Venipuncture: tourniquet/70% alcohol or povidone-iodine solution/sterile syringes or evacuated tubes/sterile needle—20G or 21G for forearm, 25G for wrist, hand, ankle, or for children/color-coded tubes containing appropriate additives/identification labels/2" x 2" gauze pads/small adhesive bandage.

Procedure
Explain to the patient that this test evaluates the condition of RBCs. Inform him that he need not restrict food or fluids and that the test requires a blood sample.

Perform a venipuncture, and collect the sample in a 7-ml *lavender-top*, 4.5-ml *black-top*, or 4.5-ml *blue-top* tube. (Check with the laboratory for its preference.)

Special considerations
• Completely fill the collection tube, and invert it gently several times to adequately mix the sample and anticoagulant.
• Since prolonged standing decreases the ESR, after examining the sample for clots or clumps, send it to the laboratory immediately (it must be tested within 2 hours).
• Handle the sample gently to prevent hemolysis.
• Failure to use the proper anticoagulant in the collection tube, to adequately mix the sample and anticoagulant, and to send the sample to the laboratory immediately may interfere with accurate determination of test results.

Values
Normal sedimentation rates range from 0 to 20 mm/hour for both males and females (Westergren Method).

Implications of results
The ESR rises in pregnancy, acute or chronic inflammation, tuberculosis, paraproteinemias (especially multiple myeloma and Waldenström's macroglobulinemia), rheumatic fever, rheumatoid arthritis, and some malignancies. Anemia also tends to raise the ESR, since less upward displacement of plasma occurs to retard the relatively few sedimenting RBCs. Polycythemia, sickle cell anemia, hyperviscosity, or low plasma protein level tend to depress ESR.

Documentation
Record testing on cardex.

White blood cell differential

Because the WBC differential evaluates the distribution and morphology of white cells, it provides more specific information about a patient's immune system than the WBC count. In this test, the laboratory classifies 100 or more white cells in a stained film of peripheral blood according to two major types of leukocytes—granulocytes (neutrophils, eosinophils, and basophils) and nongranulocytes (lymphocytes and monocytes)—and determines the percentage of each type. The differential count is the relative number of each type

Additional Laboratory Tests

Test
Antistreptolysin-O Test (ASO)
Definition
Serologic testing in patients with acute rheumatic fever to confirm antecedent infection by showing serologic response to streptococcal antigen. Measures the relative serum concentrations of the antibody to streptolysin-O, an enzyme produced by group A beta-hemolytic streptococci.
Diagnostic Objectives
To confirm recent or ongoing infection with beta-hemolytic streptococci.
To help diagnose rheumatic fever.
To distinguish between rheumatic fever and rheumatoid arthritis when joint pains are present.
To aid in the diagnosis of myocarditis.

Test
Blood Culture
Definition
Inoculation of a culture medium with a blood sample and incubating it for isolation and identification of the pathogens of bacteremia and septicemia.
Diagnostic objectives
To identify the causative organisms in bacteremia, septicemia, myocarditis, endocarditis and pericarditis.

Test
Blood Urea Nitrogen (BUN)
Definition
Measures the nitrogen fraction of urea, the chief end product of protein metabolism.
Diagnostic Objectives
To aid in the diagnosis of rheumatic heart disease.
To aid in the diagnosis of hypovolemic shock.

Test
Serum Haptoglobin
Definition
Measures serum levels of haptoglobin, a glycoprotein produced by the liver.
Diagnostic Objectives
To aid in the diagnosis of acute rheumatic fever.

Test
Lymphocyte Transformation Test
Definition
Evaluates lymphocyte competency without injection of antigens into the patient's skin. This is an in vitro test that can accurately assess the ability of lymphocytes to recognize and respond to antigens.
Diagnostic Objectives
To provide histocompatibility typing of both tissue transplant recipients and donors.

of white cell in the blood. By multiplying the percentage value of each type by the total WBC count, the investigator obtains the absolute number of each type of white cell. (See also *Additional Laboratory Tests.*)

Purpose

• To determine and evaluate the body's physiologic capacity to resist and overcome an infection
• To determine the stage and severity of an infection, such as myocarditis, endocarditis, and pericarditis
• To detect and assess the severity of allergic reactions (eosinophil count)
• To detect inflammatory conditions like rheumatic heart disease
• To help detect systemic problems like hypertension.

Equipment

Venipuncture: tourniquet/70% alcohol or povidone-iodine solution/sterile syringes or evacuated tubes/sterile needle—20G or 21G for forearm, 25G for wrist, hand, ankle, or for children/color-coded tubes containing appropriate additives/identification labels/2″ x 2″ gauze pads/small adhesive bandage.

Procedure

Explain to the patient that the test evaluates the immune system. Inform him that he need not restrict food or fluids but should refrain from strenuous exercise for 24 hours. Tell him the test requires a blood sample.

Review the patient's history for use of medications that may alter test results. Perform a venipuncture, and collect the sample in a 7-ml *lavender-top* tube.

Special considerations

• Completely fill the collection tube, and invert it gently several times to mix the sample and the anticoagulant adequately. Handle the tube gently to prevent hemolysis.
• Failure to use the proper anticoagulant, to completely fill the collection tube, or to mix the sample and anticoagulant adequately may influence accu-

rate determination of test results.

Values

Normal values for the five types of WBCs that are classified in the differential—neutrophils, eosinophils, basophils, lymphocytes, and monocytes—are given for adults and children in the accompanying table (see *WBC Reference Values,* page 246). For an accurate diagnosis, differential test results must always be interpreted in relation to the total WBC count.

Implications of results

Evidence for a wide range of disease states and other conditions is revealed by abnormal differential patterns, as shown in the chart.

Documentation

Document any medications the patient is taking that might affect test results.

Hemostasis

Hemostasis is the process whereby the circulatory system protects itself from excessive blood loss. In this process, vascular injury activates a complex chain of events—vasoconstriction, platelet aggregation, and coagulation—leading to clotting that stops the bleeding without hindering blood flow through the injured vessel.

Three crucial steps to blood clotting

Normal clotting proceeds in three stages:
1. Trauma to blood vessels or tissues triggers thromboplastin activity through intrinsic and extrinsic pathways.
2. Thromboplastin activity converts prothrombin to thrombin.
3. Thrombin converts fibrinogen in the surrounding plasma to a fibrin plug.

Bleeding time

This test measures the duration of bleeding after a standardized skin incision.

WBC Reference Values

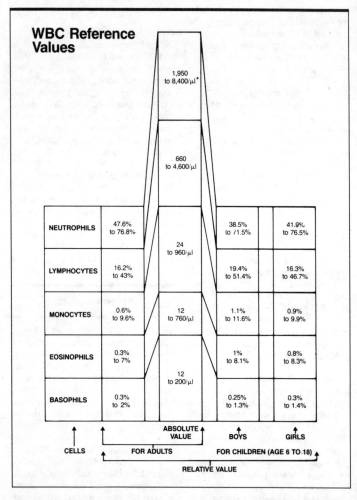

CELLS	FOR ADULTS		ABSOLUTE VALUE	FOR CHILDREN (AGE 6 TO 18)	
	RELATIVE VALUE			BOYS	GIRLS
			1,950 to 8,400/μl*		
			660 to 4,600/μl		
NEUTROPHILS	47.6% to 76.8%		24 to 960/μl	38.5% to 71.5%	41.9% to 76.5%
LYMPHOCYTES	16.2% to 43%			19.4% to 51.4%	16.3% to 46.7%
MONOCYTES	0.6% to 9.6%		12 to 760/μl	1.1% to 11.6%	0.9% to 9.9%
EOSINOPHILS	0.3% to 7%		12 to 200/μl	1% to 8.1%	0.8% to 8.3%
BASOPHILS	0.3% to 2%			0.25% to 1.3%	0.3% to 1.4%

Bleeding time depends on the elasticity of the blood vessel wall and on the number and functional capacity of platelets. Although this test is usually performed on patients with personal or family histories of bleeding disorders, it is also useful for preoperative screening, along with a platelet count.

Purpose

• to assess overall hemostatic function (platelet response to injury and vasoconstriction)
• to detect congenital and acquired platelet function disorders
• to help assess anticoagulant therapy.

Equipment

Blood pressure cuff/disposable lancet/template with 9-mm slits (template method) or 5-mm slits (modified template method)/spring-loaded blade (modified template method)/70% alcohol or povidone-iodine solution/filter paper/small pressure bandage/stopwatch.

Procedure
Explain to the patient that this test measures the time required to form a clot and stop bleeding. Tell him who will perform the test, when it will be done, and that he need not restrict food or fluids.

Check patient history for recent ingestion of drugs that prolong bleeding time. If the patient has taken such drugs, check with the laboratory for special instructions. If the test is being used to identify a suspected bleeding disorder, it should be postponed and the drugs discontinued, as ordered. If it is being used preoperatively to assess hemostatic function, it should proceed as scheduled.

• *Template and modified template methods:* Wrap the pressure cuff around the upper arm and inflate the cuff to 40 mm Hg. Select an area on the forearm that is free of superficial veins, and cleanse it with antiseptic. Allow the skin to dry *completely* before making the incision. Apply the appropriate template lengthwise to the forearm. For the template method, use the lancet to make two incisions 1 mm deep and 9 mm long. For the modified template method, use the spring-loaded blade to make two incisions 1 mm deep and 5 mm long. Start the stopwatch. Taking care not to touch the cuts, gently blot the drops of blood with filter paper every 30 seconds until the bleeding stops in both cuts. Average the bleeding time of the two cuts, and record the result.

• *Ivy method:* After applying the pressure cuff and preparing the test site, make three small punctures with a disposable lancet. Start the stopwatch immediately. Taking care not to touch the punctures, blot each site with filter paper every 30 seconds until the bleeding stops. Average the bleeding time of the three punctures, and record the result.

• *Duke method:* Drape the patient's

shoulder with a towel. Clean the earlobe, and let the skin air-dry. Then, using a disposable lancet, make a puncture wound 2 to 4 mm deep on the earlobe. Start the stopwatch. Being careful not to touch the ear, blot the site with filter paper every 30 seconds until bleeding stops. Record bleeding time.

Special considerations
• If the bleeding does not diminish after 15 minutes, discontinue the test by applying compression to the incision site.
• As ordered, resume administration of medications discontinued before the test. Sulfonamides, thiazides, antineoplastics, anticoagulants, nonsteroidal antiinflammatory drugs, aspirin and aspirin compounds, and some nonnarcotic analgesics may prolong bleeding times.

Values
Normal range of bleeding time is from 2 to 8 minutes in the template method; 2 to 10 minutes in the modified template method; 1 to 7 minutes in the Ivy method; and 1 to 3 minutes in the Duke method.

Implications of results
Prolonged bleeding time may indicate the presence of many disorders associated with thrombocytopenia, such as Hodgkin's disease, acute leukemia, disseminated intravascular coagulation, hemolytic disease of the newborn, Schönlein-Henoch purpura, severe hepatic disease (cirrhosis, for example), or severe deficiency of factors I, II, V, VII, VIII, IX, and XI. Prolonged bleeding time in a person with a normal platelet count suggests a platelet function disorder (thrombasthenia, thrombocytopathia) and requires further investigation with clot retraction, prothrombin consumption, and platelet aggregation tests. (See *Common Coagulation Screening Tests,* page 248.)

Documentation
Record the use of any medications that might alter test results.

Common Coagulation Screening Tests

TEST	WHAT ABNORMAL FINDINGS USUALLY MEAN
Bleeding Time	Prolonged bleeding time: thrombocytopenia, disseminated intravascular coagulation, or von Willebrand's disease. Abnormal bleeding time, with normal platelet count: platelet function disorder.
Capillary Fragility	Excessive number of petechiae in 2″ (5-cm) circle of skin: capillary wall weakness or platelet disorder.
Activated Partial Thromboplastin Time (APTT)	Prolonged APTT: presence of anticoagulant, fibrin split products, fibrinolysins, or antibodies to specific clotting factors; or deficiency of clotting factor other than Factor VII or Factor XIII.
Prothrombin Time (PT)	Prolonged PT: deficiency of fibrinogen (Factor I), prothrombin (Factor II), or factors V, VII, or X; hepatic disease; vitamin K deficiency; or ongoing anticoagulant therapy.
Plasma Thrombin Time	Prolonged thrombin time: hepatic disease, disseminated intravascular coagulation, effective heparin therapy, hypofibrinogenemia or dysfibrinogenemia.
Fibrin Split Products (FSP)	Elevated FSP: pulmonary embolus, myocardial infarction, deep venous thrombosis, disseminated intravascular coagulation, or primary fibrinolysis syndrome.

Platelet count

Platelets, or thrombocytes, are the smallest formed elements in the blood. They are vital to the formation of the hemostatic plug in vascular injury and promote coagulation by supplying phospholipids to the intrinsic thromboplastin pathway. Platelet count is one of the most important screening tests of platelet function.

Purpose
• To evaluate platelet production
• To assess effects of chemotherapy or radiation therapy on platelet production
• To aid diagnosis of thrombocytopenia and thrombocytosis
• To confirm visual estimate of platelet number and morphology from a stained blood film
• To help assess problems in the cardiovascular system.

Equipment
Venipuncture: tourniquet/70%alcohol or povidone-iodine solution/sterile syringes or evacuated tubes/sterile needle—20G or 21G for forearm, 25G for wrist, hand, ankle, or for children/color-coded tubes containing appropriate additives/identification labels/2″x 2″ gauze

pads/small adhesive bandage.

Procedure

Explain to the patient that this test helps determine if his blood clots normally. Inform him that he need not restrict food or fluids before the test and that the test requires a blood sample.

Check patient history for use of medications that may affect test results. Notify the laboratory if such drugs have been used.

Perform a venipuncture, and collect the sample in a 7-ml *lavender-top* tube.

Special considerations

• To prevent hemolysis, handle the sample gently and avoid excessive probing at the venipuncture site.
• Completely fill the collection tube, and invert it gently several times to mix the sample and the anticoagulant adequately.
• Failure to use the proper anticoagulant or mix the sample and anticoagulant promptly and adequately may interfere with the accurate determination of test results.
• Medications that may decrease platelet count include acetazolamide, acetohexamide, antimony, antineoplastics, brompheniramine maleate, carbamazepine, chloramphenicol, ethacrynic acid, furosemide, gold salts, hydroxychloroquine, indomethacin, isoniazid, mephenytoin, mefenamic acid, methazolamide, methimazole, methyldopa, oral diazoxide, oxyphenbutazone, penicillamine, penicillin, phenylbutazone, phenytoin, pyrimethamine, quinidine sulfate, quinine, salicylates, streptomycin, sulfonamides, thiazide and thiazide-like diuretics, and tricyclic antidepressants. Heparin causes transient, reversible thrombocytopenia.
• Platelet counts normally increase at high altitudes, with persistent cold temperature, and during strenuous exercise and excitement; counts decrease just before menstruation.

Values

Normal platelet counts range from 130,000 to 370,000/mm^3.

Implications of results

A decreased platelet count (thrombocytopenia) can result from aplastic or hypoplastic bone marrow; infiltrative bone marrow disease, such as carcinoma, leukemia, or disseminated infection; megakaryocytic hypoplasia; ineffective thrombopoiesis due to folic acid or vitamin B_{12} deficiency; pooling of platelets in an enlarged spleen; increased platelet destruction due to drugs or immune disorders; disseminated intravascular coagulation; Bernard-Soulier syndrome; or mechanical injury to platelets.

An increased platelet count (thrombocytosis) can result from hemorrhage; infectious disorders; malignancies; iron deficiency anemia; recent surgery, pregnancy, or splenectomy; and inflammatory disorders, such as collagen vascular disease. In such cases, the platelet count returns to normal after the patient recovers from the primary disorder. However, the count remains elevated in primary thrombocytosis, myelofibrosis with myeloid metaplasia, polycythemia vera, and chronic myelogenous leukemia. When the platelet count is abnormal, diagnosis usually requires further studies, such as a complete blood count, bone marrow biopsy, direct antiglobulin test (direct Coombs' test), and serum protein electrophoresis.

Documentation

Record the use of any medications that might alter test results.

Whole blood clotting time (Lee-White coagulation time)

Whole blood clotting time measures the interval required for fresh whole blood to clot in vitro at 98.6° F. (37° C.) and grossly evaluates the intrinsic clotting mechanism. Using the same whole blood sample, the clot retraction study measures the time needed for the platelet and fibrinogen network to contract into a firm clot. Successful retraction is based on the number and activity of platelets, fibrinogen and other intrinsic factor levels, and hematocrit.

Purpose
• To assess the intrinsic system of blood coagulation
• To monitor effectiveness of heparin therapy (but less reliable than activated partial thromboplastin time [APTT]).

Equipment
Venipuncture: tourniquet/70% alcohol or povidone-iodine solution/sterile syringes or evacuated tubes/sterile needle—20G or 21G for forearm, 25G for wrist, hand, ankle, or for children/color-coded tubes containing appropriate additives/identification labels/2″ x 2″ gauze pads/small adhesive bandage.

Procedure
Explain to the patient that this test helps determine if his blood clots normally. Inform him he need not restrict food or fluids, and that the test requires a blood sample.

Check the patient's history for medications that may affect test results. Notify the laboratory, when appropriate.

Perform a venipuncture, using a two-syringe technique. Draw 3 ml of blood with a plastic syringe, then disconnect the syringe from the needle and discard it (to minimize contamination of the sample with tissue thromboplastin). Attach a new syringe, and start a stopwatch as soon as blood enters the new syringe. Apply pressure to the puncture site after withdrawing the needle, and ask the patient to continue applying pressure until the bleeding stops.

Remove the needle from the syringe, and immediately transfer 1-ml portions of the sample into three 12 x 75 mm plain glass tubes set in a water bath at 98.6° F. (37° C.). Take the last tube filled and tilt it gently every 30 seconds until a clot forms; do the same with the second tube filled, and finally, with the first. Stop the watch when clotting has occurred in all three tubes, and record the time elapsed as the whole blood clotting time.

Observe the three samples at hourly intervals for signs of clot retraction. Record retraction as complete when the clot has separated from the sides and bottom of the tube.

Special considerations
• If a coagulation defect is suspected, avoid excessive probing during venipuncture; do not leave the tourniquet on too long (it will cause bruising); and apply pressure to the venipuncture site for 5 minutes, or until the bleeding stops.
• Since the inside surface of the collection tube affects clot retraction, use only plain glass tubes.
• Handle the sample gently to prevent hemolysis.
• Failure to record the sample collection time, maintain the sample at 98.6° F. (37° C.), or fill the collection tubes to the proper level may interfere with accurate determination of test results.
• Contamination of the sample with tissue thromboplastin may interfere with accurate determination of test results.
• Use of a plastic or silicone-coated collection tube, instead of glass, prolongs clotting time.
• Depressed fibrinogen levels (less than 100 mg/dl) prolong clotting time.
• Anticoagulants increase clotting time.

Values
Normal whole blood clotting time ranges from 5 to 15 minutes. After 1 hour, the clot becomes firm and retracted from the sides of the tube, occupying about half the original blood volume (most of the serum has been expressed from the clot). Record the retraction as normal, doubtful, or defective; approximately 50% retraction is normal.

Implications of results
Prolonged clotting time indicates a severe deficiency of coagulation factors (except Factor VII and Factor XIII) or the presence of anticoagulants. Abnormal clotting time necessitates further tests, including prothrombin time,

APTT, and specific factor assays.

Slow or incomplete clot retraction may indicate thrombocytopenia; thrombasthenia also produces reduced retraction and a soft clot. Abnormal retraction also occurs in hyperfibrinogenemia and anemia. The clot may appear soft and ill-defined in a patient with secondary fibrinolysis or disseminated intravascular coagulation (DIC).

Documentation
Record the use of any medications that might alter test results.

Activated partial thromboplastin time

The APTT test evaluates all the clotting factors of the intrinsic pathway—except Factor VII and Factor XIII—by measuring the time required for formation of a fibrin clot after the addition of calcium and phospholipid emulsion to a plasma sample. The APTT relies on an activator, such as kaolin, to shorten clotting time. The partial thromboplastin time (PTT) test, which is similar but less sensitive and less frequently performed, does not require an activator; instead, it relies on contact with the glass surface of a test tube to activate the sample. Since most congenital coagulation deficiencies occur in the intrinsic pathway, APTT is particularly valuable in preoperative screening for bleeding tendencies. It is also the test of choice for monitoring heparin therapy.

Purpose
• To screen for deficiencies of the clotting factors in the intrinsic pathways (except Factor VII and Factor XIII)
• To monitor heparin therapy.

Equipment
Venipuncture: tourniquet/70% alcohol or povidone-iodine solution/sterile syringes or evacuated tubes/sterile needle—20G or 21G for forearm, 25G for wrist, hand, ankle, or for children/color-coded tubes containing appropriate additives/identification labels/2″ x 2″ gauze pads/small adhesive bandage.

Procedure
Explain to the patient that this test helps determine if his blood clots normally. Advise him that he need not restrict food or fluids and that the test requires a blood sample.

When appropriate, tell the patient receiving heparin therapy that this test may be repeated at regular intervals to assess response to treatment.

Perform a venipuncture, and collect the sample in a 7-ml *blue-top* tube.

Special consideration
• To prevent hemolysis, avoid excessive probing at the venipuncture site and handle the sample gently.
• Completely fill the collection tube, invert it gently several times, and send it to the laboratory immediately, or place it on ice.
• Failure to use the proper anticoagulant, to fill the collection tube completely, or to mix the sample and anticoagulant adequately may interfere with accurate determination of test results.

Values
Normally, a fibrin clot forms 25 to 36 seconds after addition of reagent.

Implications of results
Prolonged times may indicate a deficiency of plasma clotting factors other than Factor VII and Factor XIII or the presence of heparin, fibrin split products, fibrinolysins, or circulating anticoagulants that are antibodies to specific clotting factors.

Documentation
Record the use of any medications that might alter test results.

Prothrombin time (Pro time)

This test measures the time required for a fibrin clot to form in a citrated plasma sample after addition of calcium ions and tissue thromboplastin (Factor III) and compares this time with the fibrin clotting time in a control sample of plasma. Since the test reaction bypasses the intrinsic coagulation pathway (plasma thromboplastin formation in Stage I) and does not involve platelets, the prothrombin time (PT) indirectly measures prothrombin and is an excellent screening procedure for overall evaluation of extrinsic coagulation factors V, VII, and X, and of prothrombin and fibrinogen. Prothrombin time is the test of choice for monitoring oral anticoagulant therapy.

Although test results are frequently reported as "percent of normal activity," compared with a curve of the clotting rate of normal diluted plasma, this method is inaccurate, because dilution of the sample affects the coagulation mechanism. The most reliably accurate method reports both the patient's and control's clotting times in seconds.

Purpose
• To evaluate the extrinsic coagulation system
• To monitor response to oral anticoagulant therapy.

Equipment
Venipuncture: tourniquet/70% alcohol or povidone-iodine solution/sterile syringes or evacuated tubes/sterile needle—20G or 21G for forearm, 25G for wrist, hand, ankle, or for children/color-coded tubes containing appropriate additives/identification labels/2″ x 2″ gauze pads/small adhesive bandage.

Procedure
Explain to the patient that this test helps determine if his blood clots normally. Advise him that he need not restrict food or fluids, and that the test requires a blood sample.

Check patient history for use of medications that may interfere with accurate determination of test results.

When appropriate, explain to the patient that this test monitors the effects of

medications (oral anticoagulants). Tell him it will be performed daily when therapy begins and will be repeated at longer intervals when medication levels stabilize.

Perform a venipuncture, and collect the sample in a 7-ml *blue-top* tube.

Special considerations
• To prevent hemolysis, avoid excessive probing during venipuncture and handle the sample gently.
• Completely fill the collection tube, and invert it gently several times to mix the sample and the anticoagulant adequately. If the tube is not filled to the correct volume, an excess of citrate appears in the sample.
• Send the sample to the laboratory promptly. If transport is delayed more than 4 hours, and the sample is kept at room temperature, Factor V may deteriorate, prolonging the PT; however, if the sample is refrigerated, Factor VII may be activated, shortening the PT.
• Fibrin or fibrin split products in the sample or plasma fibrinogen levels less than 100 mg/dl can prolong PT.
• Falsely prolonged results may occur if the collection tube is not filled to capacity with blood; then the amount of anticoagulant is excessive for the blood sample.
• Prolonged PT can also result from the use of adrenocorticotropic hormone, alcohol (large quantities), anabolic steroids, cholestyramine resin, heparin I.V. (within 5 hours of sample collection), indomethacin, mefenamic acid, para-aminosalicylic acid, methimazole, oxyphenbutazone, phenylbutazone, phenytoin, propylthiouracil, quinidine, quinine, thyroid hormones, and vitamin A.
• Shortened PT can result from the use of antihistamines, chloral hydrate, corticosteroids, digitalis, diuretics, glutethimide, griseofulvin, progestin-estrogen combinations, pyrazinamide, vitamin K, and xanthines (caffeine, theophylline).
• Prolonged or shortened PT results can follow ingestion of antibiotics, barbiturates, hydroxyzine, sulfonamides, salicylates (more than 1 g/day prolongs PT),

mineral oil, or clofibrate.

Values
Normally, PT values range from 9.6 to 11.8 seconds in males and 9.5 to 11.3 seconds in females. However, values vary, depending on the source of tissue thromboplastin and the type of sensing devices used to measure clot formation. In a patient receiving oral anticoagulants, PT is usually maintained between one and a half and two times the normal control.

Implications of results
Prolonged PT may indicate deficiencies in fibrinogen, prothrombin, or factor V, VII, or X (specific assays can pinpoint such deficiencies); vitamin K deficiency; and hepatic disease. Or it may result from ongoing oral anticoagulant therapy. Prolonged PT that exceeds two and a half times the control value is commonly associated with abnormal bleeding.

Documentation
Record the use of any medications that might alter test results.

Plasma thrombin time (Thrombin clotting time)

The thrombin time test measures how quickly a clot forms when a standard amount of bovine thrombin is added to a platelet-poor plasma sample from the patient and to a normal plasma control sample. After thrombin is added, the clotting time for each sample is compared and recorded. Since thrombin rapidly converts fibrinogen to a fibrin clot, this test allows a quick but imprecise estimation of plasma fibrinogen levels, which are a function of clotting time.

Purpose
• To detect fibrinogen deficiency or defect
• To monitor the effectiveness of treatment with heparin, streptokinase, or urokinase.

Equipment
Venipuncture: tourniquet/70% alcohol or povidone-iodine solution/sterile syringes or evacuated tubes/sterile needle—20G or 21G for forearm, 25G for wrist, hand, ankle, or for children/color-coded tubes containing appropriate additives/identification labels/2″ x 2″ gauze pads/small adhesive bandage.

Procedure
Explain to the patient that this test helps determine if his blood clots normally. Inform him he need not restrict food or fluids, and that the test requires a blood sample.

Perform a venipuncture, and collect the sample in a 7-ml *blue-top* tube.

Special considerations
• To prevent hemolysis, avoid excessive probing during venipuncture and rough handling of the sample.
• Fill the collection tube, invert it gently several times, and send it to the laboratory immediately, or place it on ice.
• Failure to use the proper anticoagulant in the collection tube, to mix the sample and anticoagulant adequately, to send the sample to the laboratory immediately, or to place it on ice may interfere with the accurate determination of test results.
• Administration of heparin may prolong clotting time.

Values
Normal thrombin times range from 10 to 15 seconds. Test results are usually reported with a normal control value.

Implications of results
A thrombin time greater than 1.3 times the control may indicate effective heparin therapy, hepatic disease, DIC, hypofibrinogenemia, or dysfibrinogenemia.

Patients with prolonged thrombin times require quantitation of fibrinogen levels. In suspected DIC, the test for fibrin split products is also necessary.

Documentation

Record the use of any medications that might alter test results.

Fibrin split products (FSP)

After a fibrin clot forms in response to vascular injury, the fibrinolytic system acts to prevent excessive clotting by converting plasminogen into the fibrin-dissolving enzyme plasmin. Plasmin breaks down fibrin and fibrinogen into fragments, or split products, labeled X, Y, D, and E, in order of decreasing molecular weight. These products may combine with fibrin monomers to prevent polymerization; that is, the fragments retain some anticoagulant activity. An excess of such products in circulation leads to abnormally active fibrinolysis and to coagulation disorders, such as DIC.

Fibrin split products (FSP) are detected by an immunoprecipitation reaction, in which the serum left in a blood sample after clotting is mixed on a slide with latex particles that carry D and E split products. These products adhere in clumps if fibrin or fibrinogen degradation products are present in serum.

Purpose

• To detect FSP in the circulation
• To help diagnose DIC and distinguish it from other coagulation disorders
• To determine the degree of fibrinolysis during coagulation
• To help diagnose pulmonary embolus, myocardial infarction (MI), and deep vein thrombosis.

Equipment

3-ml plastic, disposable syringe/laboratory tube containing soybean trypsin inhibitor and bovine thrombin/tourniquet/ 70% alcohol or povidine-iodine solution/sterile needle—20G or 21G for forearm, 25G for wrist, hand, ankle, or children/identification labels/2" x 2" gauze pads/small adhesive bandage.

Procedure

Explain to the patient that this test helps determine if his blood clots normally. Inform him that he need not restrict food or fluids, and that the test requires a blood sample.

Check patient history for use of medications that may interfere with accurate determination of test results.

Perform a venipuncture, and draw 2 ml of blood into a plastic syringe. Transfer the sample to the tube provided by the laboratory, which contains a soybean tryspin inhibitor and bovine thrombin.

Special considerations

• Draw the sample before administering heparin, which may cause false-positive test results.
• Gently invert the collection tube several times to mix the contents adequately; do not shake the tube vigorously or hemolysis may result. The blood clots within 2 seconds and must then be immediately sent to the laboratory to be incubated at 98.6° F. (37° C.) for 30 minutes before testing proceeds.
• Fibrinolytic drugs, such as urokinase, and large doses of barbiturates increase FSP levels.

Values

In a screening assay, serum contains less than 10 mcg/ml of FSP. A quantitative assay shows normal levels of less than 3 mcg/ml.

Implications of results

FSP levels rise in primary fibrinolytic states, due to increased levels of circulating profibrinolysin; in secondary states, due to DIC and subsequent fibrinolysis; and in alcoholic cirrhosis, postcesarean birth, preeclampsia, abruptio placentae, congenital heart disease, sunstroke, burns, intrauterine death, pulmonary embolus, deep-vein thrombosis (transient increase), and MI (after 1 or 2 days). FSP levels usually exceed 100 mcg/ml in active renal disease or renal transplant rejection.

Documentation

Record the use of any medications that might alter test results.

Blood gases and electrolytes

Laboratory analysis of blood gases and electrolytes helps evaluate the respiratory and metabolic states of the body. ABG measurements provide important diagnostic information concerning the adequacy of gas exchange in the lungs, the integrity of the ventilatory control system, and the blood pH and acid-base balance. Measuring serum concentrations of electrolytes also supplies valuable data about the body's acid-base balance and fluid balance. (See *Important Definitions for Understanding Blood Gases and Electrolytes,* page 256.)

Arterial blood gases

Blood gas studies are usually performed on arterial blood, which contains oxygen (O_2) and carbon dioxide (CO_2). ABGs are measurements of the partial pressure (PaO_2 and $PaCO_2$) that each gas exerts in the blood. As the concentration of the gas rises, so does its partial pressure.

Acid-base balance

Enzymes that control vital cellular functions perform most efficiently when the body's pH ranges between 7.35 and 7.45. Therefore, the carbonic acid/bicarbonate buffer system helps maintain body pH at this desirable level. The system may be represented by these equations:

$$CO_2 + H_2O \leftrightarrow H_2CO_3$$

carbon dioxide + water ↔ carbonic acid

In turn, carbonic acid can undergo the following change:

$$H_2CO_3 \leftrightarrow H^+ + HCO_3^-$$

carbonic acid ↔ hydrogen ion + bicarbonate

Bicarbonate and carbonic acid normally exist in a 20:1 ratio. Any change in this ratio causes a blood pH that is abnormally acidic or alkaline.

Clinical significance of ABGs

Abnormal variations in ABGs may result from respiratory or metabolic causes. Compensatory mechanisms, such as those in the lungs and kidneys, automatically attempt to correct an imbalance. But compensation is not correction, and compensatory mechanisms are limited.

Although valuable in assessing overall respiratory and metabolic status, ABG measurements are not diagnostically specific. For example, taken alone, ABG values do not distinguish between pulmonary and cardiac disorders. These values are most useful when considered with other factors, such as cardiac output, regional blood flow, and tissue oxygen consumption.

The significance of ABG studies is also limited by the fact that these studies do not necessarily detect disease. For example, the lungs may continue to function properly, with unchanged ABG values, despite the presence of pulmonary disease. Therefore, other diagnostic screening tests, such as spirometry or chest X-ray, must be performed. When dealing with ABG values, make sure you check the accepted values for your hospital. Normal range may vary, according to the laboratory method. (See *Acid-base Disorders,* page 260.)

Serum electrolytes

Electrolytes are substances that dissociate into ions when dissolved in the blood. Electrolytes that carry a positive charge are called cations; those that carry a negative charge are called anions. Sodium, calcium, chloride, and bicarbonate are the major extracellular electrolytes. Sodium is the most abundant extracellular cation; chloride, the most abundant anion. Potassium, magnesium, and phosphate are the major intracellular electrolytes. Potassium is the most abundant intracellular cation; phosphate, the most abundant anion.

Serum concentrations of electrolytes influence movement of fluid within and

Important Definitions for Understanding Blood Gases and Electrolytes

Partial pressure	A measure of the force that a gas exerts on the fluid in which it is dissolved
Pao$_2$	Partial pressure of oxygen in arterial blood
Paco$_2$	Partial pressure of carbon dioxide in arterial blood
pH	A measure of acid-base balance or the concentration of free hydrogen ions in the blood
O$_2$CT	Oxygen content, or the volume of oxygen combined with hemoglobin in arterial blood
O$_2$ Sat	Oxygen saturation, a measure of the percentage of oxygen combined with hemoglobin to the total amount of oxygen with which hemoglobin could combine
Electrolytes	Substances that dissociate into ions when fused or in solution, and thus conduct electricity
Cations	Positively charged ions
Anions	Negatively charged ions
Acidosis	Metabolic or respiratory changes that result in a loss of base or accumulation of acid
Alkalosis	Metabolic or respiratory changes that result in a loss of acid or accumulation of base

between body compartments. Such movement depends on osmolality—the concentration of electrolytes in the respective fluid compartments. Total electrolyte concentration (usually expressed in milliequivalents [mEq] per liter of serum) plus other dissolved substances, such as glucose, determine the osmolality of a given compartment. During osmosis, water flows from a compartment of lower osmolality to one of higher osmolality, until the osmotic pressure in the two compartments is equal.

Electrolytes help maintain acid-base balance. The kidneys may exchange potassium or sodium for hydrogen and absorb or excrete bicarbonate or chloride ions to maintain a proper pH. Serum electrolyte concentrations affect all metabolic activity in some way. Also, electrolyte concentration differences between intracellular fluid and extracellular fluid regulate neuromuscular function. Consequently, serum electrolyte studies are essential to routine medical evaluation in all hospitalized patients. Abnormal electrolyte values may reflect fluid or acid-base imbalance, or kidney, neuromuscular, endocrine, or skeletal dysfunction. (See *Serum Electrolyte Functions*, page 262.)

Arterial blood gas analysis

Arterial blood gas (ABG) analysis evaluates gas exchange in the lungs by measuring the partial pressures of oxygen (PaO_2) and carbon dioxide ($PaCO_2$) and the pH of an arterial sample. PaO_2 indicates how much oxygen the lungs are delivering to the blood. $PaCO_2$ indicates how efficiently the lungs eliminate carbon dioxide. The pH indicates the acid-base level of the blood, or the hydrogen ion (H^+) concentration. Acidity indicates H^+ excess; alkalinity, H^+ deficit. Oxygen content (O_2CT), oxygen saturation (O_2 Sat), and bicarbonate (HCO_3^-) values also aid diagnosis. A blood sample for ABG analysis may be drawn by percutaneous arterial puncture or from an arterial line.

Purpose
• To evaluate the efficiency of pulmonary gas exchange
• To assess integrity of the ventilatory control system
• To determine the acid-base level of the blood
• To monitor respiratory therapy
• To help monitor cardiac disorders and efficiency of the cardiac pump.

Equipment
10-ml Luer-Lok glass syringe/1-ml ampul heparin/20G, 1½″ short bevel needle/23G, 1″ short bevel needle/rubber stopper or cork/antiseptic swabs/70% alcohol or povidone-iodine solution/2″ x 2″ gauze pads/tape or adhesive bandage/iced specimen container/labels (for syringe and specimen bag) for patient's name and room number (if applicable), doctor's name, date, collection time, and details of oxygen therapy.

Procedure
Explain to the patient that this test evaluates how well the lungs are delivering oxygen to blood and eliminating carbon dioxide. Inform him he need not restrict food or fluids, and that the test requires a blood sample. Also tell him who will perform the arterial puncture, when it will be done, and which site—radial, brachial, or femoral artery—has been selected for the puncture. Instruct the patient to breathe normally during the test. If the radial or brachial artery is used, perform the Allen's Test first. (See *Performing the Allen's Test,* page 55.)

Perform an arterial puncture.

Special considerations
• If the patient has recently had an intermittent positive-pressure breathing treatment, wait at least 20 minutes before drawing arterial blood, because such treatment alters blood gas values.
• If the patient is receiving oxygen therapy, find out whether the order for ABG measurements specifies that these be obtained on room air or oxygen therapy. If the order indicates room air, discontinue oxygen therapy for 15 to 20 minutes before drawing the sample.

Before sending the sample to the laboratory, include the following information on the requisition slip:
• Indicate whether the patient was breathing room air or receiving oxygen therapy when the sample was drawn. If he was receiving oxygen therapy, give the flow rate.
• If the patient is on a ventilator, note the FIO_2 and tidal volume.
• Record the patient's rectal temperature and respiratory rate.
• Exposing the sample to air affects PaO_2 and $PaCO_2$ levels and interferes with accurate determination of results.
• Failure to heparinize the syringe, to place the sample correctly in an iced bag, or to send the sample to the laboratory immediately adversely affects test results.
• Venous blood in the sample may lower PaO_2 and elevate $PaCO_2$.
• Bicarbonate, ethacrynic acid, hydrocortisone, metolazone, prednisone, and thiazides may elevate $PaCO_2$ levels. Acetazolamide, methicillin, nitrofurantoin, and tetracycline may decrease $PaCO_2$ levels.

Values

Normal ABG values fall within the following ranges:

PaO_2	75 to 100 mm Hg
$PaCO_2$	35 to 45 mm Hg
pH	7.35 to 7.42
O_2CT	15% to 23%
O_2 Sat	94% to 100%
HCO_3^-	22 to 26 mEq/liter

Implications of results

Low PaO_2, O_2CT, and O_2 Sat levels, in combination with a high $PaCO_2$ value, may be due to conditions that impair respiratory function, such as respiratory muscle weakness or paralysis (as in Guillain-Barré syndrome or myasthenia gravis); respiratory center inhibition (from head injury, brain tumor, or drug abuse, for example); airway obstruction (possibly from mucous plugs or a tumor); and from cardiac pump failure. Similarly, low readings may result from bronchiole obstruction caused by asthma or emphysema; an abnormal ventilation-perfusion ratio due to partially blocked alveoli or pulmonary capillaries; or from alveoli that are damaged or filled with fluid because of disease, hemorrhage, or near-drowning.

When inspired air contains insufficient oxygen, PaO_2, O_2CT, and O_2 Sat also decrease, but $PaCO_2$ may be normal. Such findings are common in pneumothorax, impaired diffusion between alveoli and blood (due to interstitial fibrosis, for example), or in an arteriovenous shunt that permits blood to bypass the lungs.

Low O_2CT—with normal PaO_2, O_2 Sat, and, possibly, $PaCO_2$ values—may result from severe anemia, decreased blood volume, and reduced hemoglobin oxygen-carrying capacity.

In addition to clarifying blood oxygen disorders, ABGs can give considerable information about acid-base disorders, as shown in the chart on page 260.

Documentation

Record vital signs and any signs of circulatory impairment, such as numbness, tingling, swelling, or discoloration of the limb that was used for the test.

Total carbon dioxide content

This test measures the total concentration of all such forms of CO_2 in serum, plasma, or whole blood samples. Since about 90% of CO_2 in serum is in the form of bicarbonate, this test closely assesses bicarbonate levels. Total CO_2 content reflects the adequacy of gas exchange in the lungs and the efficiency of the carbonic acid-bicarbonate buffer system, which maintains acid-base balance and normal pH. Consequently, this test is commonly ordered for patients with respiratory insufficiency and is usually included in any assessment of electrolyte balance. For maximum clinical significance, test results must be considered with both pH and arterial blood gas values.

Purpose

• To help evaluate acid-base balance.

Equipment

Venipuncture: tourniquet/70% alcohol or povidone-iodine solution/sterile syringes or evacuated tubes/sterile needle—20G or 21G for forearm; 25G for wrist, hand, ankle, or for children/color-coded tubes containing appropriate additives/identification labels/2" x 2" gauze pads/small adhesive bandage.

Procedure

Explain to the patient that this test measures the amount of CO_2 in the blood. Inform him that he need not restrict food or fluids, and that this test requires a blood sample. Check the patient's history for use of medications that may influence CO_2 blood levels.

Perform a venipuncture. Since CO_2 content is usually measured along with electrolytes, a 10- to 15-ml *red-top* tube may be used. When this test is performed alone, a *green-top* (heparinized) tube is appropriate.

Special considerations
Completely fill the tube to prevent diffusion of CO_2 into the vacuum.
• CO_2 levels rise with administration of excessive ACTH, cortisone, thiazide diuretics, or with excessive ingestion of alkalis or licorice.
• CO_2 levels decrease with administration of salicylates, paraldehyde, methicillin, dimercaprol, ammonium chloride, acetazolamide, and accidental ingestion of ethylene glycol or methyl alcohol.

Values
Normally, total CO_2 levels range from 22 to 34 mEq/liter.

Implications of results
High CO_2 levels may occur in metabolic alkalosis (due to excessive ingestion or retention of base bicarbonate), respiratory acidosis (from hypoventilation, for example, as in emphysema or pneumonia), primary aldosteronism, and Cushing's syndrome. CO_2 levels may also rise above normal after excessive loss of acids, as in severe vomiting and continuous gastric drainage.

Decreased CO_2 levels are common in metabolic acidosis (as in diabetic acidosis or renal tubular acidosis resulting from renal failure). Decreased total CO_2 levels in metabolic acidosis also result from loss of bicarbonate (as in severe diarrhea or intestinal drainage). Levels may fall below normal in respiratory alkalosis (from hyperventilation, for example, after trauma).

Documentation
Record the use of any medications that might alter test results.

Serum calcium

This test measures serum levels of calcium, a predominantly extracellular cation that helps regulate and promote neuromuscular and enzyme activity, skeletal development, and blood coagulation.

Purpose
• To aid diagnosis of neuromuscular, skeletal, and endocrine disorders; dysrhythmias; blood-clotting deficiencies; and acid-base imbalance.

Equipment
Venipuncture: tourniquet/70% alcohol or povidone-iodine solution/sterile syringes or evacuated tubes/sterile needle—20G or 21G for forearm, 25G for wrist, hand, ankle, or for children/color-coded tubes containing appropriate additives/identification labels/2″ x 2″ gauze pads/small adhesive bandage.

Procedure
Explain to the patient that this test determines blood calcium levels. Inform him he need not restrict food or fluids, and that the test requires a blood sample.

Perform a venipuncture, and collect the sample in a 10- to 15-ml *red-top* tube.

Special considerations
None.

Values
Normally, serum calcium levels range from 8.9 to 10.1 mg/dl (atomic absorption) or from 4.5 to 5.5 mEq/liter. In children, serum calcium levels are higher than in adults. Calcium levels can rise as high as 12 mg/dl or 6 mEq/liter during phases of rapid bone growth.

Implications of results
Abnormally high serum calcium levels (hypercalcemia) may occur in hyperparathyroidism and parathyroid tumors (due to oversecretion of parathyroid hormone), Paget's disease of the bone, multiple myeloma, metastatic carcinoma, multiple fractures, or prolonged immobilization. Elevated serum calcium levels may also result from inadequate excretion of calcium, as in adrenal insufficiency and renal disease; from excessive calcium ingestion; or from overuse of antacids such as calcium carbonate.

Observe the patient with hypercalcemia for deep bone pain, flank pain due

Acid-base Disorders

DISORDERS AND ABG FINDINGS	POSSIBLE CAUSES	SIGNS AND SYMPTOMS
Respiratory acidosis (excess CO_2 retention) pH < 7.35 HCO_3^- > 26 mEq/liter (if compensating) $Paco_2$ > 45 mm Hg	• Central nervous system depression from drugs, injury, or disease • Asphyxia • Hypoventilation due to pulmonary, cardiac, musculoskeletal, or neuromuscular disease	• Diaphoresis, headache, tachycardia, confusion, restlessness, apprehension
Respiratory alkalosis (excess CO_2 excretion) pH > 7.42 HCO_3^- < 22 mEq/liter (if compensating) $Paco_2$ < 35 mm Hg	• Hyperventilation due to anxiety, pain, or improper ventilator settings • Respiratory stimulation by drugs, disease, hypoxia, fever, or high room temperature • Gram-negative bacteremia	• Rapid, deep respirations; paresthesias; light-headedness; twitching; anxiety; fear
Metabolic acidosis (HCO_3^- loss, acid retention) pH < 7.35 HCO_3^- < 22 mEq/liter $Paco_2$ < 35 mm Hg (if compensating)	• HCO_3^- depletion due to renal disease, diarrhea, or small bowel fistulas • Excessive production of organic acids due to hepatic disease; endocrine disorders, including diabetes mellitus; hypoxia; shock; or drug intoxication • Inadequate excretion of acids due to renal disease	• Rapid, deep breathing; fruity breath; fatigue; headache; lethargy; drowsiness; nausea; vomiting; coma (if severe)
Metabolic alkalosis (HCO_3^- retention, acid loss) pH > 7.42 HCO_3^- > 26 mEq/liter $Paco_2$ > 45 mm Hg (if compensating)	• Loss of hydrochloric acid from prolonged vomiting, gastric suctioning • Loss of potassium due to increased renal excretion (as in diuretic therapy), steroid overdose • Excessive alkali ingestion	• Slow, shallow breathing; hypertonic muscles; restlessness; twitching; confusion; irritability; apathy; tetany; convulsions; coma (if severe)

to renal calculi, and muscle hypotonic-ity. Hypercalcemic crisis begins with nausea, vomiting, and dehydration, leading to stupor and coma, and it can end in cardiac arrest.

Low calcium levels (hypocalcemia) may result from hypoparathyroidism, total parathyroidectomy, or malabsorp-tion. Decreased serum levels of calcium may follow calcium loss in Cushing's syndrome, renal failure, acute pancre-atitis, and peritonitis.

In a patient with hypocalcemia, be alert for circumoral and peripheral numbness and tingling, muscle twitch-ing, Chvostek's sign (facial muscle spasm), tetany, muscle cramping, Trousseau's sign (carpopedal spasm), seizures, and arrhythmias.

Documentation
Record testing on cardex.

Serum chloride

This test, a quantitative analysis, mea-sures serum levels of chloride, the major extracellular fluid anion. Interacting with sodium, chloride helps maintain the osmotic pressure of blood and there-fore helps regulate blood volume and arterial pressure. Chloride levels also affect acid-base balance. Serum concen-trations of this electrolyte are regulated by aldosterone secondarily to regulation of sodium. Chloride is absorbed from the intestines and is excreted primarily by the kidneys.

Purpose
• To detect acid-base imbalance (aci-dosis and alkalosis) and to aid evaluation of fluid status and extracellular cation-anion balance.

Equipment
Venipuncture: tourniquet/70% alcohol or povidone-iodine solution/sterile sy-ringes or evacuated tubes/sterile nee-dle—20G or 21G for forearm, 25G for wrist, hand, ankle, or for children/color-coded tubes containing appropriate ad-ditives/identification labels/2″ x 2″ gauze pads/small adhesive bandage.

Procedure
Explain to the patient that the test eval-uates the chloride content of blood and requires a blood sample. Tell him who will perform the venipuncture, when it will be done, and that he may feel some transient discomfort from the needle puncture and pressure of the tourniquet. Reassure the patient that collecting the sample usually takes only a few minutes.

Check the patient's medication his-tory for recent therapy with drugs that may influence chloride levels.

Perform a venipuncture, and collect the sample in a 10- to 15-ml *red-top* tube.

Special considerations
• Handle the sample gently to prevent hemolysis.
• Elevated serum chloride levels may result from administration of ammo-nium chloride, cholestyramine, boric acid, oxyphenbutazone, phenylbuta-zone, or excessive I.V. infusion of so-dium chloride.
• Serum chloride levels are decreased by thiazides, furosemide, ethacrynic acid, bicarbonates, or prolonged I.V. in-fusion of dextrose 5% in water.

Values
Normally, serum chloride levels range from 100 to 108 mEq/liter.

Implications of results
Chloride levels relate inversely to those of bicarbonate and thus reflect acid-base balance. Excessive loss of gastric juices or of other secretions containing chlo-ride may cause hypochloremic meta-bolic alkalosis; excessive chloride reten-tion or ingestion may lead to hyperchloremic metabolic acidosis.

Elevated serum chloride levels (hy-perchloremia) may result from severe dehydration, complete renal shutdown, head injury (producing neurogenic hy-perventilation), and primary aldoste-ronism.

Low chloride levels (hypochloremia)

are usually associated with low sodium and potassium levels. Possible underlying causes include prolonged vomiting, gastric suctioning, intestinal fistula, chronic renal failure, and Addison's disease. Congestive heart failure (CHF) or edema resulting in excess extracellular fluid can cause dilutional hypochloremia.

Observe a patient with hypochloremia for hypertonicity of muscles, tetany, and depressed respirations. In a patient with hyperchloremia, be alert for signs of developing stupor, rapid deep breathing, and weakness that may lead to coma.

Documentation
Record testing on cardex.

Serum magnesium

This test, a quantitative analysis, measures serum levels of magnesium, the most abundant intracellular cation after potassium. Vital to neuromuscular function, this often overlooked electrolyte helps regulate intracellular metabolism, activates many essential enzymes, and affects the metabolism of nucleic acids and proteins. Magnesium also helps transport sodium and potassium across cell membranes and, through its effect on the secretion of parathyroid hormone, influences intracellular calcium levels. Most magnesium is found in bone and intracellular fluid; a small amount is found in extracellular fluid. Magnesium is absorbed by the small intestine and excreted in the urine and feces.

Purpose
• To evaluate electrolyte status
• To assess neuromuscular or renal function.

Equipment
Venipuncture: tourniquet/70% alcohol or povidone-iodine solution/sterile syringes or evacuated tubes/sterile needle—20G or 21G for forearm, 25G for

Serum Electrolyte Functions

CATIONS

Sodium (Na⁺)
• Maintains osmotic pressure of extracellular fluid
• Helps regulate neuromuscular activity
• Influences acid-base balance and chloride and potassium levels
• Helps regulate water excretion

Potassium (K⁺)
• Maintains cellular osmotic equilibrium
• Helps regulate neuromuscular and enzymatic activity and acid-base balance
• Influences kidney function

Calcium (Ca⁺⁺)
• Helps regulate and promote neuromuscular activity, skeletal development, and blood coagulation

Magnesium (Mg⁺⁺)
• Helps regulate intracellular activity and sodium, potassium, calcium, and phosphorus levels

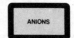

ANIONS

Chloride (Cl⁻)
• Influences acid-base balance
• Helps maintain blood osmotic pressure and arterial pressure

Bicarbonate (HCO₃⁻)
• Acts with carbonic acid in buffer system that regulates blood pH

Phosphate (HPO₄⁻⁻)
• Helps regulate calcium levels, energy metabolism, and acid-base balance

wrist, hand, ankle, or for children/color-coded tubes containing appropriate additives/identification labels/2″ x 2″ gauze pads/small adhesive bandage.

Procedure

Explain to the patient that this test determines the magnesium content of the blood. Instruct him not to use magnesium salts (such as milk of magnesia or Epsom salt) for at least 3 days before the test, but he need not restrict food or fluids. Tell him the test requires a blood sample.

Perform a venipuncture, and collect the sample in a 10- to 15-ml *red-top* tube.

Special considerations

• Handle the sample gently to prevent hemolysis. (*Note:* This is especially important with this test, since 75% of the blood's magnesium is present in RBCs.)

• Excessive use of antacids or cathartics or excessive infusion of magnesium sulfate raises magnesium levels.

• Prolonged I.V. infusions without magnesium suppress magnesium levels. Excessive use of diuretics, including thiazides and ethacrynic acid, decreases levels by increasing magnesium excretion in the urine.

• I.V. administration of calcium gluconate may falsely decrease serum magnesium levels if measured by the Titan yellow method.

Values

Normally, serum magnesium levels range from 1.7 to 2.1 mg/dl (atomic absorption) or from 1.5 to 2.5 mEq/liter.

Implications of results

Elevated serum magnesium levels (hypermagnesemia) most commonly occur in renal failure, when the kidneys excrete inadequate amounts of magnesium. Adrenal insufficiency (Addison's disease) can also elevate serum magnesium.

In suspected or confirmed hypermagnesemia, observe the patient for lethargy, flushing, diaphoresis, decreased blood pressure, slow, weak pulse, diminished deep tendon reflexes, muscle weakness, and slow, shallow respirations.

Suppressed serum magnesium levels (hypomagnesemia) most commonly result from chronic alcoholism. Other causes include malabsorption syndrome, diarrhea, faulty absorption following bowel resection, prolonged bowel or gastric aspiration, acute pancreatitis, primary aldosteronism, severe burns, hypercalcemic conditions (including hyperparathyroidism), and certain diuretic therapy.

In hypomagnesemia, watch for leg and foot cramps, hyperactive deep tendon reflexes, cardiac dysrhythmias, muscle weakness, seizures, twitching, tetany, and tremors.

Documentation

Record testing on cardex.

Serum phosphates

This test measures serum levels of phosphates, the dominant cellular anions. Phosphates help store and use body energy and help regulate calcium levels, carbohydrate and lipid metabolism, and acid-base balance. They are essential to bone formation; about 85% of the body's phosphates are found in bone. The intestine absorbs a considerable amount of phosphates from dietary sources, but adequate levels of vitamin D are necessary for their absorption. The kidneys excrete phosphates and serve as a regulatory mechanism. Since calcium and phosphate interact in a reciprocal relationship, urinary excretion of phosphates increases or decreases in inverse proportion to serum calcium levels. Abnormal concentrations of phosphates result more often from improper excretion than from abnormal ingestion or absorption from dietary sources.

Purpose

• To aid diagnosis of renal disorders and acid-base imbalance in cardiovascular disorders.

Equipment

Venipuncture: tourniquet/70% alcohol or povidone-iodine solution/sterile syringes or evacuated tubes/sterile needle—20G or 21G for forearm, 25G for wrist, hand, ankle, or for children/color-coded tubes containing appropriate additives/identification labels/2" x 2" gauze pads/small adhesive bandage.

Procedure

Explain to the patient that this test determines the blood levels of phosphate. Inform him he need not restrict food or fluids. Tell him this test requires a blood sample, who will perform the venipuncture, when it will be done, and that, although he may feel some discomfort from the needle puncture and the pressure of the tourniquet, collecting the sample takes only a few minutes. Check the patient's medication history for recent therapy with drugs that alter phosphate levels.

Perform a venipuncture, and collect the sample in a 10- to 15-ml *red-top* tube.

Special considerations

Handle the sample gently to prevent hemolysis.

• Excessive vitamin D intake and drug therapy with anabolic steroids and androgens may elevate serum phosphorus levels.

• Suppressed phosphate levels may result from excessive phosphate excretion due to prolonged vomiting and diarrhea, vitamin D deficiency (which interferes with phosphate absorption), extended I.V. infusion of dextrose 5% in water, ingestion of phosphate-binding antacids, and drug therapy with acetazolamide, insulin, and epinephrine.

Values

Normally, serum phosphate levels range from 2.5 to 4.5 mg/dl (atomic absorption) or from 1.8 to 2.6 mEq/liter. Children have higher serum phosphate levels than adults. Phosphate levels can rise as high as 7 mg/dl or 4.1 mEq/liter during periods of increased bone growth.

Implications of results

Since serum phosphate values alone are of limited use diagnostically (only a few rare conditions directly affect phosphate metabolism), they should be interpreted in light of serum calcium results.

Depressed phosphate levels (hypophosphatemia) may result from malnutrition, malabsorption syndromes, hyperparathyroidism, renal tubular acidosis, or treatment of diabetic acidosis. In children, hypophosphatemia can suppress normal growth.

Elevated levels (hyperphosphatemia) may result from skeletal disease, healing fractures, hypoparathyroidism, acromegaly, diabetic acidosis, high intestinal obstruction, and renal failure. Hyperphosphatemia is rarely clinically significant; however, if prolonged, it can alter bone metabolism by causing abnormal calcium phosphate deposits.

Documentation

Record the use of any medications that might alter test results.

Serum potassium

This test, a quantitative analysis, measures serum levels of potassium, the major intracellular cation. Small amounts of potassium may also be found in extracellular fluid. Vital to homeostasis, potassium maintains cellular osmotic equilibrium and helps regulate muscle activity (it is essential in maintaining electrical conduction within the cardiac and skeletal muscles). Potassium also helps regulate enzyme activity and acid-base balance and influences kidney function. Potassium levels are affected by variations in the secretion of adrenal steroid hormones and by fluctuations in pH, serum glucose levels, and serum sodium levels. A reciprocal relationship appears to exist between potassium and sodium; a substantial intake of one element causes a corresponding decrease in the other. Although it readily conserves sodium, the body has no efficient method for conserving potassium.

Since the kidneys daily excrete nearly all ingested potassium, a dietary intake of at least 40 mEq/day is essential. (A normal diet usually includes 60 to 100 mEq potassium.)

Purpose

• To evaluate clinical signs of potassium excess (hyperkalemia) or potassium depletion (hypokalemia)

• To monitor renal function, acid-base balance, and glucose metabolism

• To evaluate neuromuscular and endocrine disorders

• To detect the origin of dysrhythmias

• To evaluate hypertensive therapy with potassium-depleting diuretics.

Equipment

Venipuncture: tourniquet/70% alcohol or povidone-iodine solution/sterile syringes or evacuated tubes/sterile needle—20G or 21G for forearm, 25G for wrist, hand, ankle, or for children/color-coded tubes containing appropriate additives/identification labels/2″ x 2″ gauze pads/small adhesive bandage.

Procedure

Explain to the patient that this test determines the potassium content of blood. Inform him he need not restrict food or fluids, and that the test requires a blood sample.

Check the patient's medication history for use of diuretics or other drugs that may influence test results. If these medications must be continued, note this on the laboratory slip.

Perform a venipuncture, and collect the sample in a 10- to 15-ml *red-top* tube.

Special considerations

• Draw the sample immediately after applying the tourniquet, since a delay may elevate the potassium level by allowing leakage of intracellular potassium into the serum.

• Handle the sample gently to avoid hemolysis.

• Excessive or rapid potassium infusion, spironolactone or penicillin G potassium therapy, or renal toxicity from administration of amphotericin B, methicillin, or tetracycline elevates serum potassium levels.

• Insulin and glucose administration, diuretic therapy (especially with thiazides but not with triamterine, amiloride, or spironolactone), or I.V. infusions without potassium suppress serum potassium levels.

Values

Normally, serum potassium levels range from 3.8 to 5.5 mEq/liter.

Implications of results

Abnormally high serum potassium levels (hyperkalemia) are common in patients with burns, crushing injuries, diabetic ketoacidosis, and MI—conditions in which excessive cellular potassium enters the blood. Hyperkalemia may also indicate reduced sodium excretion, possibly due to renal failure (preventing normal sodium/potassium exchange) or Addison's disease (due to the absence of aldosterone, with consequent potassium buildup and sodium depletion).

Observe a patient with hyperkalemia for weakness, malaise, nausea, diarrhea, colicky pain, muscle irritability progressing to flaccid paralysis, oliguria, and bradycardia. Electrocardiogram (EKG) reveals a prolonged P-R interval, wide QRS, tall, tented T wave, and S-T depression.

Below-normal potassium values often result from aldosteronism or Cushing's syndrome (marked by hypersecretion of adrenal steroid hormones), loss of body fluids (as in long-term diuretic therapy), or excessive licorice ingestion (due to the aldosterone-like effect of glycyrrhizic acid). Although serum values and clinical symptoms can indicate a potassium imbalance, an EKG provides the definitive diagnosis.

Observe a patient with hypokalemia for decreased reflexes; rapid, weak, irregular pulse; mental confusion; hypotension; anorexia; muscle weakness; and paresthesia. EKG shows a flattened T wave, S-T depression, and U wave elevation. In severe cases, ventricular fibrillation, respiratory paralysis, and cardiac arrest can develop.

Documentation
Record the use of any medications that might alter test results.

Serum sodium

This test measures serum levels of sodium, the major extracellular cation. Sodium affects body water distribution, maintains osmotic pressure of extracellular fluid, and helps promote neuromuscular function. It also helps maintain acid-base balance and influences chloride and potassium levels. Sodium is absorbed by the intestines and is excreted primarily by the kidneys; a small amount is lost through the skin.

Since extracellular sodium concentration helps the kidneys regulate body water (decreased sodium levels promote water excretion and increased levels promote retention), serum levels of sodium are evaluated in relation to the amount of water in the body. (See *The Sodium Pump*, page 268.) For example, a sodium deficit (hyponatremia) refers to a decreased level of sodium in relation to the body's water level. The body normally regulates this sodium-water balance through aldosterone, which inhibits sodium excretion and promotes its resorption (with water) by the renal tubules, to maintain balance. Low sodium levels stimulate aldosterone secretion; elevated sodium levels depress aldosterone secretion.

Purpose
• To evaluate fluid-electrolyte and acid-base balance and related neuromuscular, renal, and adrenal functions.
• To monitor hypertensive therapy.

Equipment
Venipuncture: tourniquet/70% alcohol or povidone-iodine solution/sterile syringes or evacuated tubes/sterile needle—20G or 21G for forearm, 25G for wrist, hand, ankle, or for children/color-coded tubes containing appropriate additives/identification labels/2" x 2" gauze pads/small adhesive bandage.

Procedure
Explain to the patient that this test determines the sodium content of blood. Inform him that he need not restrict food or fluids, and that this test requires a blood sample.

Check the patient's medication history for use of diuretics and other drugs that influence sodium levels. If these medications must be continued, note this on the laboratory slip.

Perform a venipuncture, and collect the sample in a 10- to 15-ml *red-top* tube.

Special considerations
• Handle the sample gently to prevent hemolysis.
• Most diuretics suppress serum sodium levels by promoting sodium excretion; lithium, chlorpropamide, and vasopressin suppress levels by inhibiting water excretion.
• Corticosteroids elevate serum sodium levels by promoting sodium retention. Antihypertensives, such as methyldopa, hydralazine, and reserpine, may cause sodium and water retention.

Values
Normally, serum sodium levels range from 135 to 145 mEq/liter.

Implications of results
Sodium imbalance can result from a loss or gain of sodium or from a change in water volume. Remember, *serum sodium results must be interpreted in light of the patient's state of hydration.*

Elevated serum sodium levels (hypernatremia) may be due to inadequate water intake, water loss in excess of sodium (as in diabetes insipidus, impaired renal function, prolonged hyperventilation, and occasionally, severe vomiting and diarrhea), and sodium retention (as in aldosteronism). Hypernatremia can also result from excessive sodium intake.

In a patient with hypernatremia and associated loss of water, observe for signs of thirst, restlessness, dry and sticky mucous membranes, flushed skin, oliguria, and diminished reflexes. However, if increased total body sodium causes water retention, observe for hypertension, dyspnea, and edema.

Abnormally low serum sodium levels (hyponatremia) may result from inadequate sodium intake or excessive sodium loss due to profuse sweating, gastrointestinal suctioning, diuretic therapy, diarrhea, vomiting, adrenal insufficiency, burns, or chronic renal insufficiency with acidosis. Urine sodium determinations are frequently more sensitive to early changes in sodium balance and should always be evaluated simultaneously with serum sodium findings.

In a patient with hyponatremia, watch for apprehension, lassitude, headache, decreased skin turgor, abdominal cramps, and tremors that may progress to convulsions.

Documentation
Record the use of any medications that might alter test results.

Enzymes

Enzymes are reusable proteins that catalyze the thousands of chemical reactions needed to keep a single cell alive and functioning. They accelerate and control reaction rates without being destroyed themselves in the process.

Different kinds of cells produce different enzymes, and most tissues contain many different enzymes. When tissue cells are damaged by disease or some other defect, they release enzymes specific to that area into the blood stream, where they can be readily detected.

Cardiac enzymes and isoenzymes
Creatine phosphokinase, cardiac muscle (CPK-MB) levels rise 4 to 8 hours after onset of infarction, peak after 24

hours, and may remain elevated for as long as 72 hours. *Levels of lactic dehydrogenase (LDH$_1$ and LDH$_2$)* levels usually rise within 24 hours after an episode, tapering off 72 to 96 hours later. Some laboratories also measure *hydroxybutyric dehydrogenase (HBD)* in suspected acute MI when electrophoresis equipment is not available or when the total LDH is not diagnostic. Serum HBD levels rise 8 to 10 hours after infarction, peak in 48 to 96 hours, and return to normal in 16 to 18 days.

Serum glutamic-oxaloacetic transaminase (SGOT) also rises during acute MI, increasing 6 to 10 hours after the infarction and peaking in 24 to 48 hours. The SGOT level may increase to 4 to 10 times normal but returns to normal in 4 to 6 days. In some patients, SGOT rises as a result of severe angina or arrhythmia and does not indicate MI. Thus, correct interpretation of enzyme analyses always requires careful correlation with the patient's clinical status.

Since the diagnostic value of some enzyme tests depends on the sequence of analysis, each sample must be labeled with the time of collection, the date, and the patient's name and room number. For example, in acute MI, the first set of tests is ordered immediately to obtain a baseline. Subsequent sets of tests are ordered serially, perhaps at 6, 12, and 24 hours after the episode and daily thereafter, to monitor enzyme elevations and peaks. Writing "Rule out MI" on the requisition slip helps, but specifying the time the sample was drawn is also essential. Specifying "4 hours post-suspected time of MI" helps place test results in their chronologic order.

Urine enzymes
Because enzymes that circulate in the blood are normally reabsorbed by the renal tubules, with only small amounts excreted in the urine, increased enzyme concentration in the urine may signal renal dysfunction, especially impaired tubular reabsorption.

The Sodium Pump

According to the laws of diffusion, a substance spreads from an area of higher concentration to one of lower concentration. Thus, when stimuli, such as heat, cold, electricity, or mechanical damage, cause the cellular membrane to become very permeable, sodium ions—normally most abundant outside the cells—diffuse inward, and potassium ions—normally most abundant inside the cells—diffuse outward. To combat this ionic diffusion and maintain normal sodium and potassium concentrations, an active sodium transportation mechanism is constantly at work.

Since sodium and potassium cannot easily penetrate the cellular membrane, they are forced to combine with a single lipoprotein carrier. (This carrier is called Y in combination with sodium and X following a chemical transformation allying it with potassium.) In the cellular membrane, sodium from inside the cells combines with carrier Y to form large quantities of NaY, which move toward the cell's outer surface. Because of energy provided by adenosine triphosphate (ATP) and adenosine triphosphatase (ATPase), the sodium is released out-

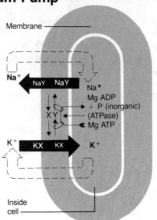

side the cells, and the Y is chemically transformed to X. X joins potassium, forming KX. As the KX within the membrane moves inward, ATP and ATPase provide the energy needed to split K from X. K enters the cells, X is reconverted to Y, and the cycle continues indefinitely. This system, known as the sodium pump, helps prevent cellular swelling, stimulate glandular secretions, and transmit neuromuscular impulses.

Creatine phosphokinase (Creatine kinase)

Creatine phosphokinase (CPK) is an enzyme that catalyzes the creatine-creatinine metabolic pathway in muscle cells and brain tissue. Because of its intimate role in energy production, CPK reflects normal tissue catabolism; an increase above normal serum levels indicates trauma to cells with high CPK content. CPK may be separated into three isoenzymes with distinct molecular structures: CPK-BB (CPK$_1$), CPK-MB (CPK$_2$), and CPK-MM (CPK$_3$). CPK-

BB is found primarily in brain tissue; CPK-MB, in cardiac muscle (a small amount also appears in skeletal muscle); and CPK-MM, in skeletal muscle.

An assay of total serum CPK was once widely used to detect acute MI, but elevated serum CPK levels caused by skeletal muscle damage reduce the test's specificity for this disorder. Fractionation and measurement of CPK isoenzymes is rapidly replacing use of total CPK to accurately localize the site of increased tissue destruction.

Purpose

• To detect and diagnose acute MI and reinfarction (CPK-MB primarily used)

• To evaluate possible causes of chest pain and monitor the severity of myocardial ischemia after cardiac surgery, cardiac catheterization, or cardioversion (CPK-MB primarily used).

Equipment
Venipuncture: tourniquet/70% alcohol or povidone-iodine solution/sterile syringes or evacuated tubes/sterile needle—20G or 21G for forearm, 25G for wrist, hand, ankle, or for children/color-coded tubes containing appropriate additives/identification labels/2″ x 2″ gauze pads/small adhesive bandage.

Procedure
Explain to the patient that this test helps assess myocardial and skeletal muscle function, and that multiple blood samples are required to detect fluctuations in serum levels. Inform him that he need not restrict food or most fluids.

Withhold alcohol, aminocaproic acid, and lithium, as ordered, before the test. If these substances must be continued, note this on the laboratory slip.

Perform a venipuncture, and collect the sample in a 7-ml *red-top* tube.

Special considerations
• Draw the sample before or within 1 hour of giving I.M. injections, as muscle trauma raises total CPK levels.
• Obtain the sample on schedule. Note on the laboratory slip the time the sample was drawn and the hours elapsed since onset of chest pain.
• Handle the collection tube gently to prevent hemolysis, and send the sample to the laboratory immediately (CPK activity diminishes significantly after 2 hours at room temperature).
• Failure to draw the samples at the scheduled time, missing peak levels, may interfere with accurate determination of test results.
• Halothane and succinylcholine, alcohol, lithium, and large doses of aminocaproic acid reportedly cause elevated CPK levels. Injections, cardioversion, invasive diagnostic procedures, surgery, trauma, recent vigorous exercise or

muscle massage, and severe coughing also increase total CPK values.

Values
Total CPK values determined by ultraviolet or kinetic measurement range from 23 to 99 u/liter for men and 15 to 57 u/liter for women. CPK levels may be significantly higher in very muscular people. Infants up to age 1 have levels two to four times higher than adult levels, possibly reflecting birth trauma and striated muscle development. Normal ranges for isoenzyme levels are as follows: CPK-BB, undetectable; CPK-MB, undetectable to 7 IU/liter; CPK-MM, 5 to 70 IU/liter.

Implications of results
CPK-MM constitutes over 99% of total CPK normally present in serum. Detectable CPK-BB isoenzyme may indicate brain tissue injury, certain widespread malignant tumors, severe shock, or renal failure. However, such elevations do not confirm a specific diagnosis.

CPK-MB isoenzyme greater than 5% of total CPK (or more than 10 IU/liter) indicates MI, especially if the LDH_1/LDH_2 isoenzyme ratio is greater than 1 (flipped LDH). In acute MI and following cardiac surgery, CPK-MB begins to rise in 2 to 4 hours, peaks in 12 to 24 hours, and usually returns to normal in 24 to 48 hours. Persistent elevations or increasing levels indicate ongoing myocardial damage. Total CPK follows roughly the same pattern but rises slightly later. CPK-MB levels do not rise in CHF or during angina pectoris not accompanied by myocardial cell necrosis (not all investigators agree on this, however). Serious skeletal muscle injury that occurs in certain muscular dystrophies, polymyositis, and severe myoglobinuria may produce mild CPK-MB elevation, since a small amount of this isoenzyme is present in some skeletal muscles.

Rising CPK-MM values follow skeletal muscle damage from trauma, such as surgery and I.M. injections, or from diseases, such as dermatomyositis and muscular dystrophy (values may be 50 to 100 times normal). A moderate rise in CPK-MM levels develops in patients with hypothyroidism; sharp elevations occur with muscular activity caused by agitation, such as an acute psychotic episode.

Total CPK levels may be elevated in patients with severe hypokalemia, carbon monoxide poisoning, malignant hyperthermia, postconvulsions, alcoholic cardiomyopathy, and occasionally, in those who have suffered pulmonary or cerebral infarctions.

Documentation
Document the time of the patient's chest pain and when the blood was drawn. Record the use of any medications that might alter test results.

Lactic dehydrogenase

LDH is an enzyme that catalyzes the reversible conversion of muscle lactic acid into pyruvic acid. This essential final step in the Embden-Meyerhof glycolytic pathway provides the metabolic bridge to the Krebs cycle (citric acid or tricarboxylic acid cycle), ultimately producing cellular energy. Because LDH is present in almost all body tissues, cellular damage causes an elevation of total serum LDH, thus limiting the diagnostic usefulness of LDH. However, five tissue-specific isoenzymes can be identified and measured, using heat inactivation or electrophoresis. Two of these isoenzymes, LDH_1 and LDH_2, appear primarily in the heart, RBCs, and kidneys; LDH_3, primarily in the lungs; and LDH_4 and LDH_5, in the liver and the skeletal muscles.

The specificity of LDH isoenzymes and their distribution pattern is useful in diagnosing hepatic, pulmonary, and erythrocytic damage. But its widest clinical application (with other cardiac enzyme tests) is in diagnosing acute MI. LDH isoenzyme assay is also useful when CPK has not been measured within 24 hours of an acute MI. The

myocardial LDH level rises later than CPK (12 to 48 hours after infarction begins), peaks in 2 to 5 days, and drops to normal in 7 to 10 days, if tissue necrosis does not persist.

Purpose
• To aid differential diagnosis of MI, pulmonary infarction, anemias, and hepatic disease
• To support CPK isoenzyme test results in diagnosing MI or to provide diagnosis when CPK-MB samples are drawn too late to display elevation.

Equipment
Venipuncture: tourniquet/70% alcohol or povidone-iodine solution/sterile syringes or evacuated tubes/sterile needle—20G or 21G for forearm, 25G for wrist, hand, ankle, or for children/color-coded tubes containing appropriate additives/identification labels/2" x 2" gauze pads/small adhesive bandage.

Procedure
Explain to the patient that this test is used primarily to detect tissue alterations. Inform him he need not restrict food or fluids, and that the test requires a blood sample. Tell the patient suspected of having an MI that the test will be repeated on the next two mornings to monitor progressive changes.

Perform a venipuncture, and collect the sample in a 7-ml *red-top* tube.

Special considerations
• Draw the samples on schedule to avoid missing peak levels, and mark the collection time on the laboratory slip.
• Handle the sample gently to prevent artifact blood sample hemolysis, since RBCs contain LDH_1.
• Send the sample to the laboratory immediately, or if transport is delayed, keep the sample at room temperature. Changes in temperature reportedly inactivate LDH_5, thus altering isoenzyme patterns.
• Recent surgery or pregnancy can cause elevated LDH levels. Prosthetic heart valves may also increase LDH levels, as

a result of chronic hemolysis.

Values

Total LDH levels normally range from 48 to 115 IU/liter. Normal distribution is as follows:

LDH_1	18.1% to 29% of total
LDH_2	29.4% to 37.5% of total
LDH_3	18.8% to 26% of total
LDH_4	9.2% to 16.5% of total
LDH_5	5.3% to 13.4% of total

Implications of results

Since many common diseases cause elevations in total LDH levels, isoenzyme electrophoresis is usually necessary for diagnosis. In some disorders, total LDH may be within normal limits, but abnormal proportions of each enzyme indicate specific organ tissue damage. For instance, in acute MI, the concentration of LDH_1 is greater than LDH_2 within 12 to 48 hours after onset of symptoms. This reversal of normal isoenzyme patterns is typical of myocardial damage and is referred to as flipped LDH. (See *Isoenzymes of Lactic Dehydrogenase*, page 272.)

Documentation

Document the time of the patient's chest pain and when the blood was drawn.

Document any medications used that might alter test results.

Hydroxybutyric dehydrogenase

Hydroxybutyric dehydrogenase (HBD) is actually total LDH that is tested using a hydroxybutyric acid substrate instead of lactic or pyruvic acid. With this substrate, the electrophoretically fast-moving LDH_1 and LDH_2 (cardiac) isoenzymes exhibit more activity than the slow-moving LDH_5 (liver) fraction, so that HBD activity roughly parallels LDH_1 and LDH_2 activity. Measurement of serum HBD is sometimes used as a substitute for LDH isoenzyme fractionation.

Although HBD concentration predominately reflects LDH_1 and LDH_2 activity, it may also show LDH_5 activity, if enough isoenzyme is present (as it is in some forms of hepatic disease). Therefore, this test is not consistently reliable in distinguishing between myocardial and hepatic cellular damage and is less popular than it once was.

Purpose

- To aid diagnosis of MI when LDH isoenzyme assay is unavailable
- To monitor cardiac isoenzyme activity after LDH_1 is proven to be elevated
- To detect MI after other enzyme levels drop to normal (HBD remains elevated longer)
- To aid in differentiating between cardiac and hepatic cellular damage when total LDH is elevated (LDH/HBD ratio is commonly used).

Equipment

Venipuncture: tourniquet/70% alcohol or povidone-iodine solution/sterile syringes or evacuated tubes/sterile needle—20G or 21G for forearm, 25G for wrist, hand, ankle, or for children/color-coded tubes containing appropriate additives/identification labels/2″ x 2″ gauze pads/small adhesive bandage.

Procedure

Explain to the patient that this test evaluates heart or liver function. Inform him he need not restrict food or fluids, and that the test requires a blood sample. Tell the patient suspected of having an MI that the test will be repeated on subsequent mornings to monitor his progress.

Perform a venipuncture, and collect the sample in a 7-ml *red-top* tube.

Special considerations

- For patients with MI, draw blood at the same time each morning.
- Handle the collection tube gently to prevent hemolysis, since RBCs contain LDH_1. Because HBD activity is unstable at room temperature, send the sample to the laboratory immediately or refrigerate it at 32° to 39.2° F. (0° to 4° C.).

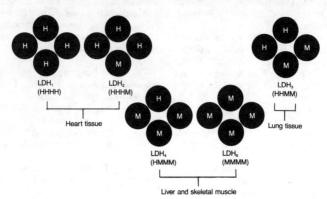

Isoenzymes of Lactic Dehydrogenase

LDH₁ (HHHH)

LDH₂ (HHHM)

LDH₃ (HHMM)

LDH₄ (HMMM)

LDH₅ (MMMM)

Heart tissue

Lung tissue

Liver and skeletal muscle

Individual monomers of the five lactic dehydrogenase (LDH) isoenzymes carry the letter H, for those subunits that appear most consistently in heart tissue, or the letter M, for those predominant in skeletal muscle tissue. Injury to almost any tissue stimulates the release of isoenzymes with a tetrametric pattern peculiar to the injured tissue and roughly parallel to the degree of damage. For instance, in myocardial infarction, blood levels of LDH_1 (HHHH) and LDH_2 (HHHM) are elevated. Damage to pulmonary tissue causes the release of LDH_3 (HHMM); injury to the liver and skeletal muscle, LDH_4 (HMMM) and LDH_5 (MMMM).

• Extensive surgery or cardioversion can elevate HBD levels.

Values

Serum HBD values range from 114 to 290 u/ml. Ratio of serum LDH to HBD normally varies from 1.2:1 to 1.6:1.

Implications of results

In MI, HBD levels peak 72 hours after onset of chest pains and remain elevated for 2 weeks. The LDH/HBD ratio is decreased due to greater activity of LDH_1 and LDH_2, as reflected in HBD levels; total LDH rises less markedly. HBD levels are also raised by artifact blood sample hemolysis, hemolytic or megaloblastic anemia, muscular dystrophy, and moderate-to-severe acute hepatocellular damage. Acute hepatitis increases the LDH/HBD ratio, since HBD levels are less sensitive to hepatocellular damage than LDH levels, which increase moderately.

Documentation

Record testing on cardex.

Serum glutamic oxaloacetic transaminase

Although a high correlation exists between MI and elevated serum glutamic oxaloacetic transaminase (SGOT), this test is sometimes considered superfluous for diagnosing MI because of its relatively low organ specificity—it does not enable differentiation between acute MI and the effects of hepatic congestion due to heart failure.

Purpose

• To detect recent MI (together with CPK and LDH)
• To monitor patient progress and prognosis in cardiac and hepatic diseases.

Procedure

Explain to the patient that this test helps assess heart and liver function. Inform him that he need not restrict food or fluids, and that the test usually requires three venipunctures: one at admission and one each day for the next 2 days.

Withhold morphine, codeine, meperidine, chlorpropamide, methyldopa, sulfamethoxypyridazine, phenazopyridine, and antitubercular drugs (isoniazid, para-aminosalicylates, and pyrazinamide), as ordered. If such medications must be continued, note this on the laboratory slip.

Perform a venipuncture, and collect the sample in a 7-ml *red-top* tube.

Special considerations

• To avoid missing peak SGOT levels, draw serum samples at the same time each day.
• Handle the collection tube gently to prevent hemolysis, and send the sample to the laboratory immediately.
• Chlorpropamide, opiates, methyldopa, erythromycin, sulfonamides, pyridoxine, dicumarol, antitubercular agents, large doses of acetaminophen, salicylates, vitamin A, and many other drugs known to affect the liver cause elevated SGOT levels. Strenuous exercise and muscle trauma caused by I.M. injections also raise SGOT levels.

Values

SGOT levels range from 8 to 20 u/liter. Normal values for infants are as high as four times those of adults.

Implications of results

SGOT levels fluctuate in response to the extent of cellular necrosis and therefore may be transiently and minimally elevated early in the disease process and extremely elevated during the most acute phase. Depending on when during the course of the disease the initial sample was drawn, SGOT levels can rise—indicating increasing disease severity and tissue damage—or fall—indicating disease resolution and tissue repair. Thus, the relative change in SGOT values

serves as a reliable monitoring mechanism.

High levels (ranging from 10 to 20 times normal) may indicate severe MI, severe infectious mononucleosis, and alcoholic cirrhosis. High levels also occur during the prodromal or resolving stages of conditions that cause maximal elevations.

Moderate-to-high levels (ranging from 5 to 10 times normal) may indicate Duchenne muscular dystrophy, dermatomyositis, and chronic hepatitis. Moderate-to-high levels also occur during prodromal and resolving stages of diseases that cause high elevations.

Low-to-moderate levels (ranging from 2 to 5 times normal) may indicate hemolytic anemia, metastatic hepatic tumors, acute pancreatitis, pulmonary emboli, delirum tremens, and fatty liver. SGOT levels rise slightly after the first few days of biliary duct obstruction. Also, low-to-moderate elevations occur at some time during any of the preceding conditions or diseases.

Documenatation

Record the time of day the blood was drawn.

Record any use of medications that might alter test results.

Plasma renin activity

Renin secretion is the first stage of the renin-angiotensin-aldosterone cycle that controls the body's sodium-potassium balance, fluid volume, and blood pressure. Renin is released by the juxtaglomerular cells of the kidneys into the renal veins in response to sodium depletion and blood loss. It catalyzes the conversion of angiotensinogen, an alpha$_2$-globulin plasma protein, to angiotensin I, which in turn is converted by hydrolysis into angiotensin II, a vasoconstrictor that stimulates aldosterone production in the adrenal cortex. When present in excessive amounts, angiotensin II causes renal hypertension.

The plasma renin activity (PRA) test

is a screening procedure for renovascular hypertension but does not unequivocally confirm it. When supplemented by other special tests, the PRA can help establish the cause of hypertension. For instance, sampling blood obtained from both renal veins by renal vein catheterization and analyzing the renal venous renin ratio can identify renovascular disorders. Indexing renin levels against urinary sodium excretion can help identify primary aldosteronism.

Some experts believe that essential hypertension with low, normal, and high renin levels should be treated differently, and the PRA test can categorize the disease for appropriate therapy.

Purpose

• To screen for renal origin of hypertension
• To help plan the best treatment of essential hypertension, a genetic disease often aggravated by excess sodium intake
• To help identify hypertension linked to unilateral (sometimes bilateral) renovascular disease by renal vein catheterization
• To help identify primary aldosteronism (Conn's syndrome) resulting from aldosterone-secreting adrenal adenoma
• To confirm primary aldosteronism (sodium-depleted plasma renin test).

Equipment

Venipuncture: tourniquet/70% alcohol or povidone-iodine solution/sterile syringes or evacuated tubes/sterile needle—20G or 21G for forearm, 25G for wrist, hand, ankle, or for children/color-coded tubes containing appropriate additives/identification labels/2″ x 2″ gauze pads/small adhesive bandage.

Procedure

Explain to the patient that this test helps determine the cause of hypertension. As ordered, tell the patient to discontinue use of diuretics, antihypertensives, vasodilators, oral contraceptives, and licorice for 2 to 4 weeks before the test and to maintain a normal-sodium diet (3 g/ day) during this period. (See *Patient-Teaching Aid: Low-Sodium Diet for Renin Testing,* page 280.) For the sodium-depleted renin test, tell the patient he will receive furosemide or, if he has angina or cerebrovascular insufficiency, that he will receive chlorthiazide and follow a low-sodium diet for 3 days. Tell him the test requires a blood sample.

If a recumbent sample is ordered, instruct the patient to remain in bed until it is obtained. (Posture influences renin secretion.) If an upright sample is ordered, instruct him to stand or sit upright for 2 hours before the test.

If renal catheterization is ordered, make sure the patient has signed a consent form. Tell him the procedure will be done in the X-ray department and that a local anesthetic will be given.

Peripheral vein sample: Perform a venipuncture, and collect the sample in a 7-ml *lavender-top* tube.

Renal vein catheterization: A catheter is advanced to the kidneys through the femoral vein, under fluoroscopic control, and samples are obtained from both renal veins and the vena cava.

Special considerations

• Since renin is very unstable, the sample must be drawn into a chilled syringe and collection tube, placed on ice, and sent to the laboratory immediately.
• Completely fill the collection tube, and invert it gently several times to mix the sample and anticoagulant.

Values

Levels of plasma renin activity and aldosterone decrease with advancing age.

Sodium-depleted, upright, peripheral vein: For ages 20 to 39, the range is from 2.9 to 24 ng/ml/hour; mean, 10.8 ng/ml/hour. For age 40 and over, the range is from 2.9 to 10.8 ng/ml/hour; mean, 5.9 ng/ml/hour.

Sodium-replete, upright, peripheral vein: For ages 20 to 39, the range is from 0.1 to 4.3 ng/ml/hour; mean, 1.9 ng/ml/hour. For age 40 and over, the range is from 0.1 to 3 ng/ml/hour; mean, 1 ng/ml/hour.

In renal vein catheterization, the renal venous renin ratio (the renin level in the renal vein compared to the level in the inferior vena cava) is less than 1.5 to 1.

Implications of results

Elevated renin levels may occur in essential hypertension (uncommon), malignant and renovascular hypertension, cirrhosis, hypokalemia, hypovolemia due to hemorrhage, renin-producing renal tumors (Bartter's syndrome), and adrenal hypofunction (Addison's disease). High renin levels may also be found in chronic renal failure with parenchymal disease, end-stage renal disease, and transplantation rejection. Decreased renin levels may indicate hypervolemia due to a high-sodium diet, salt-retaining steroids, primary aldosteronism, Cushing's syndrome, licorice ingestion syndrome, or essential hypertension with low renin levels.

High serum and urine aldosterone levels, with low plasma renin activity, help identify primary aldosteronism. In the sodium-depleted renin test, low plasma renin confirms this and differentiates it from secondary aldosteronism (characterized by increased renin).

Documentation

Renal vein catheterization: record vital signs every half hour for 2 hours, then every 2 hours for the next 4 hours.

Document any pain, bleeding, or hematoma at the catheter insertion site.

Lipids and lipoproteins

Lipids, also called fats, are organic substances with a hydrophobic side chain or steroid nucleus—or with both these molecular features—that causes them to be insoluble in water. The major lipids are triglycerides, free cholesterol, cholesterol esters, and phospholipids. For transportation through the body, lipids must combine with plasma proteins into a lipid-protein molecular complex called lipoproteins. Nonesterified fatty acids

(free fatty acids) bind to albumin; other blood lipids (free and esterified cholesterol), triglycerides, and phospholipids) bind to globulin.

Clinical implications

Lipoprotein determinations are also useful in evaluating the risk of coronary artery disease (CAD). At one time, total blood cholesterol—the amount of cholesterol in all lipoproteins—was considered the major indicator of CAD for patients under age 50. However, the Framingham Heart Study found that high levels of high-density lipoproteins (HDL)-cholesterol actually help prevent CAD, whereas high levels of low-density lipoproteins (LDL)-cholesterol increase the risk. Apparently, HDLs help the enzyme lecithin cholesterol acyltransferase remove cholesterol from arterial walls. Further study has shown that patients with angina pectoris or MI generally have lower HDL-cholesterol than healthy persons, and that low HDL-cholesterol levels—which can be hereditary—are not just associated with CAD but precede it. Low HDL-cholesterol levels are also connected with diabetes mellitus, hypertension, cigarette smoking, obesity, and lack of exercise.

Although HDL-cholesterol and LDL-cholesterol are good indicators of CAD risk, a full lipoprotein profile is a more useful measure. This battery of tests includes total cholesterol, total triglycerides, and lipoprotein phenotyping.

Triglycerides

This test provides quantitative analysis of triglycerides—the main storage form of lipids—which constitute about 95% of fatty tissue. Although not in itself diagnostic, serum triglyceride analysis permits early identification of hyperlipemia (characteristic in nephrotic syndrome and other conditions) and risk of CAD.

Purpose

• To screen for hyperlipemia

- To help identify nephrotic syndrome
- To determine the risk of CAD.

Equipment

Venipuncture: tourniquet/70% alcohol or povidone-iodine solution/sterile syringes or evacuated tubes/sterile needle—20G or 21G for forearm, 25G for wrist, hand, ankle, or for children/color-coded tubes containing appropriate additives/identification labels/2″ x 2″ gauze pads/small adhesive bandage.

Procedure

Define triglycerides for the patient, and explain that this test helps detect disorders of fat metabolism. Advise the patient to abstain from food for 12 to 14 hours before the test and from alcohol for 24 hours; he does not need to abstain from water. Tell him the test requires a blood sample.

As ordered, withhold medications that may alter test results (antilipemics, steroids, estrogen, and some diuretics).

Perform a venipuncture, and collect a serum sample in a 7-ml *red-top* tube. A plasma sample is acceptable if a serum sample cannot be collected but gives values that are usually slightly higher and that do not correlate reliably with the normal range in serum.

Special considerations

- Send the sample to the laboratory immediately.
- A plasma sample may produce slightly higher values than a serum sample.
- Failure to comply with dietary restrictions may interfere with accurate determination of test results.
- Ingestion of alcohol within 24 hours of the test may cause elevated triglyceride levels. In fact, excessive consumption of alcohol is a common cause of excess concentration of triglycerides. Alcohol is heavily hydrogenated. As a result, this hydrogen has to be disposed of during alcohol metabolism, and most of it ultimately ends up in triglyceride. Fatty liver is an early manifestation of this phenomenon.
- Certain drugs lower cholesterol levels

but raise or may have no effect on triglyceride levels. All antilipemics lower serum lipid concentration in the bloodstream, although their mechanism of action may differ. Cholestyramine lowers cholesterol; it raises or may have no effect on triglycerides. Colestipol lowers cholesterol; it raises or may have no effect on triglycerides.

- Long-term use of corticosteroids raises triglyceride levels, as do oral contraceptives, estrogen, ethyl alcohol, furosemide, and miconazole.
- Clofibrate, dextrothyroxine, gemfibrozil, and niacin lower cholesterol and triglyceride levels.
- Certain drugs have a variable effect. Probucol inhibits transport of cholesterol from the intestine and may also affect cholesterol synthesis. It lowers cholesterol but has a variable effect on triglycerides.

Values

Triglyceride values are age-related. Some controversy exists over the most appropriate normal ranges, but the following are fairly widely accepted:

Age	Triglycerides, mg/dl
0 to 29	10 to 140
30 to 39	10 to 150
40 to 49	10 to 160
50 to 59	10 to 190

Implications of results

Increased or decreased serum triglyceride levels merely suggest a clinical abnormality, and additional tests are required for definitive diagnosis. For example, measurement of cholesterol may also be necessary, since cholesterol and triglycerides vary independently. High levels of triglyceride and cholesterol reflect an exaggerated risk of CAD.

A mild-to-moderate increase in serum triglyceride levels indicates biliary obstruction, diabetes, nephrotic syndrome, endocrinopathies, or overconsumption of alcohol. Markedly increased levels without an identifiable cause reflect congenital hyperlipoproteinemia and necessitate lipoprotein phenotyping to confirm diagnosis.

Documentation
Record the use of any food, alcohol, or medications that may alter test results.

Total cholesterol

This test, the quantitative analysis of serum cholesterol, measures the circulating levels of free cholesterol and cholesterol esters; it reflects the level of the two forms in which this biochemical compound appears in the body. Total cholesterol is the only cholesterol routinely measured.

Cholesterol, a structural component in cell membranes and plasma lipoproteins, is a precursor of glucocorticoids, sex hormones, and bile acids. On the average, two thirds of blood cholesterol is absorbed from the diet and one third is synthesized in the liver.

A diet high in saturated fat raises cholesterol levels by stimulating absorption of lipids, including cholesterol, from the intestine; a low–saturated-fat diet lowers them. High serum cholesterol levels may be associated with an increased risk of CAD.

Purpose
• To assess the risk of CAD.

Equipment
Venipuncture: tourniquet/70% alcohol or povidone-iodine solution/sterile syringes or evacuated tubes/sterile needle—20G or 21G for forearm, 25G for wrist, hand, ankle, or for children/color-coded tubes containing appropriate additives/identification labels/2″ x 2″ gauze pads/small adhesive bandage.

Procedure
Explain to the patient that this test determines the body's fat metabolism. If the patient is hospitalized, enforce overnight fast and abstention from alcohol for 24 hours. Tell the patient the test will require a blood sample.

As ordered, withhold drugs that influence cholesterol levels.

Perform a venipuncture, and collect the sample in a 7-ml *red-top* tube.

Special considerations
• Send the sample to the laboratory immediately, since cholesterol is not stable at room temperature.
• Cholesterol levels are lowered by cholestyramine, clofibrate, colestipol, dextrothyroxine, haloperidol, neomycin, niacin, and chlortetracycline. Levels are raised by epinephrine, chlorpromazine, trifluoperazine, oral contraceptives, and trimethadione. Androgens may have a variable effect on cholesterol levels.
• Failure to follow dietary restrictions may interfere with test results.

Values
Total cholesterol concentrations vary with age and sex and may range from 120 mg/dl to 330 mg/dl.

Implications of results
Elevated serum cholesterol (hypercholesterolemia) may indicate risk of CAD, as well as incipient hepatitis, lipid disorders, bile duct blockage, nephrotic syndrome, obstructive jaundice, pancreatitis, and hypothyroidism. Hypercholesterolemia due to high dietary intake requires modification of eating habits and, possibly, medication to retard absorption of cholesterol.

Low serum cholesterol (hypocholesterolemia) is commonly associated with malnutrition, cellular necrosis of the liver, and hyperthyroidism. Abnormal cholesterol levels frequently necessitate further testing to pinpoint the disorder, depending on the type of abnormality and the presence of overt signs. Abnormal levels associated with cardiovascular diseases, for example, may necessitate lipoprotein phenotyping.

Documentation
Record the use of any food, alcohol, or medications that may alter test results.

Lipoprotein-cholesterol fractionation

Cholesterol fractionation tests isolate and measure the major lipids in serum—

chylomicrons, very low-density lipoproteins, LDLs, and HDLs—by ultracentrifugation or electrophoresis. The cholesterol in LDL and HDL fractions is the most significant, since the Framingham Heart Study has shown that cholesterol in HDL is inversely related to the incidence of CAD—the higher the HDL level, the lower the incidence of CAD; the higher the LDL level, the higher the incidence of CAD.

Purpose
• To assess the risk of CAD.

Equipment
Venipuncture: tourniquet/70% alcohol or povidone-iodine solution/sterile syringes or evacuated tubes/sterile needle—20G or 21G for forearm, 25G for wrist, hand, ankle, or for children/color-coded tubes containing appropriate additives/identification labels/2" x 2" gauze pads/small adhesive bandage.

Procedure
Tell the patient that this test helps determine the risk of CAD. Instruct him to maintain his normal diet for 2 weeks before the test, to abstain from alcohol for 24 hours, and to fast and avoid exercise for 12 to 14 hours. Tell him the test requires a blood sample.

As ordered, withhold thyroid hormones, oral contraceptives, and antilipemics, which alter test results.

Perform a venipuncture, and collect the sample in a 7-ml *red-top* tube.

Special considerations
Send the sample to the laboratory immediately, since spontaneous redistribution of cholesterol occurs among the lipoproteins and can alter test results. If the sample cannot be transported immediately, it should be refrigerated but not frozen.

• Values are lowered by antilipemic medications, such as clofibrate, cholestyramine, colestipol, dextrothyroxine, niacin, probucol, and sitosterols.

• Oral contraceptives, disulfiram, alcohol, miconazole, and high doses of phe-

nothiazines may increase values.
• Estrogens usually increase values.
• Collecting the sample in a heparinized tube may produce false elevation of values through activation of the enzyme lipase, which, in turn, causes the release of fatty acids from triglycerides.
• Presence of bilirubin, hemoglobin, salicylates, iodine, vitamins A and D, and some other substances may affect accurate determination of values. Some procedures (for example, Abell-Kendall) are less susceptible to interference than others.
• Concurrent illness, especially if accompanied by fever, recent surgery, or MI, may interfere with accurate determination of test results.

Values
Since normal cholesterol values vary according to age, sex, geographic region, and ethnic group, check the laboratory for the normal values in your hospital. An alternate method (measuring cholesterol and triglyceride levels, and separating out HDL by selective precipitation and using these values to calculate LDL) provides normal HDL-cholesterol levels that range from 29 to 77 mg/100 ml and normal LDL-cholesterol levels that range from 62 to 185 mg/100 ml.

Implications of results
High LDL levels increase the risk of CAD. Elevated HDL levels generally reflect a healthy state but can also indicate chronic hepatitis, early-stage primary biliary cirrhosis, or alcohol consumption. Rarely, a sharp rise (to as high as 100 mg/dl) in a second type of HDL (alpha$_2$-HDL) may signal CAD. Although cholesterol fractionation provides valuable information about the risk of heart disease, remember that other sources of such risk—diabetes mellitus, hypertension, cigarette smoking—are at least as important.

Documentation
Record the use of any medications that would alter test results.

Lipoprotein phenotyping

For transportation through the blood, most lipids must combine with water-soluble proteins (apoproteins) to form lipoproteins. Several types of lipoproteins normally exist in the body, but in certain familial disorders, the blood levels of these types change. Classification of patients by the pattern of their lipoprotein levels identifies hyperlipoproteinemias and hypolipoproteinemias.

Purpose
• To determine classification of hyperlipoproteinemia or hypolipoproteinemia
• To help assess risk of CAD.

Equipment
Venipuncture: tourniquet/70% alcohol or povidone-iodine solution/sterile syringes or evacuated tubes/sterile needle—20G or 21G for forearm, 25G for wrist, hand, ankle, or for children/color-coded tubes containing appropriate additives/identification labels/2" x 2" gauze pads/small adhesive bandage.

Procedure
Explain to the patient that this test helps determine how the body metabolizes fats. Instruct him to abstain from alcohol for 24 hours and to fast after midnight before the test. Tell him this test requires a blood sample. Provide a low-fat meal the night before the test.

Check the patient's drug history for use of heparin. As ordered, withhold antilipemics, such as cholestyramine, about 2 weeks before the test.

Notify the laboratory if the patient is hospitalized for any other condition that might significantly alter lipoprotein metabolism, such as diabetes mellitus, nephrosis, or hypothyroidism.

Perform a venipuncture, and collect the sample in a 7-ml *lavender-top* tube.

Special considerations
• When drawing multiple samples, collect the sample for lipoprotein phenotyping first, since venous obstruction for 2 minutes can affect test results.
• Fill the collection tube completely, and invert it gently several times to mix the sample and the anticoagulant.
• Handle the sample gently to prevent hemolysis.
• Failure to observe diet and alcohol restrictions, or recent use of antilipemics, which lower lipid levels, may interfere with accurate determination of values.
• Administration of heparin (which activates the enzyme lipase, producing fatty acids from triglycerides) or collection of the sample in a heparinized tube may falsely elevate values.

Values
Types of hyperlipoproteinemias or hypolipoproteinemias are identified by characteristic electrophoretic patterns. The laboratory reports the type of lipoproteinemia present.

Implications of results
Familial lipoprotein disorders are classified as either hyperlipoproteinemias or hypolipoproteinemias.

The hyperlipoproteinemias break down into six types—I, IIa, IIb, III, IV, and V. Types IIa, IIb, and IV are relatively common. In contrast, all hypolipoproteinemias are rare and include hypobetalipoproteinemia, abetalipoproteinemia (Bassen-Kornzweig syndrome), and alpha-lipoprotein deficiency (Tangier disease).

Documentation
Record the use of any medications that might alter test results.

Adrenal hormones

Hormones are powerful, complex chemicals normally produced by the endocrine system and transported through the bloodstream to stimulate or inhibit the metabolic activity of target glands or organs.

The *adrenal glands* secrete mineralo-

Patient-Teaching Aid

Low-Sodium Diet for Renin Testing

Dear Patient:
Before undergoing renin testing, you must severely restrict your intake of sodium for 3 days. This restriction is important to the accuracy of the test. If you are following this diet at home, observe these precautions:

• Eat only the foods included in the meal plan provided by the doctor.
• Measure all portions, using standard measuring cups and spoons.
• Use 4 oz (112 g) *unsalted* beefsteak or ground beef for lunch and 4 oz (112 g) *unsalted* chicken for dinner. (Amount refers to weight before cooking.)
• You may eat the following *unsalted* (fresh or frozen) vegetables: asparagus, green or wax beans, cabbage, cauliflower, lettuce, and tomatoes.
• Use only the specified amount of coffee.
• If you are thirsty between meals, drink distilled water (no other food or beverage is allowed).
• Prepare all foods without salt; do not use salt at the table.

Breakfast:
1 egg, poached, boiled, or fried in *unsalted* fat
2 slices *unsalted* toast
1 shredded wheat biscuit or ⅔ cup *unsalted* cooked cereal
4 oz (120 ml) half-and-half or milk
8 oz (240 ml) coffee
Sugar, jam or jelly, and *unsalted* butter, as desired.

Lunch:
4 oz (120 ml) *unsalted* tomato juice
4 oz (112 g) *unsalted* beefsteak or ground beef; may be broiled, or fried in *unsalted* fat
½ cup *unsalted* potato
½ cup *unsalted* green beans or other allowed vegetable
1 serving fruit
8 oz (240 ml) coffee
1 slice *unsalted* bread
Sugar, jam or jelly, and *unsalted* butter, as desired

Dinner:
4 oz (112 g) *unsalted* chicken; baked, broiled or fried in *unsalted* fat
½ cup *unsalted* potato
1 slice *unsalted* bread
Lettuce salad (vinegar and oil dressing)
1 serving fruit
8 oz (240 ml) coffee
Sugar, jam or jelly, and *unsalted* butter, as desired

Reprinted with permission of Mayo Foundation.
This patient-teaching aid may be reproduced by office copier for distribution to patients.

corticoids (aldosterone) to maintain salt and water balance; glucocorticoids (primarily cortisol) to regulate carbohydrate, fat, and protein metabolism; and catecholamines to regulate reaction to stress. The adrenal cortex secretes the mineralocorticoids and the glucocorticoids that are essential to life. The adrenal medulla secretes catecholamines (mainly epinephrine, norepinephrine, and dopamine) in moments of danger, as part of the body's fight-or-flight response.

Serum aldosterone

This test measures serum aldosterone levels by quantitative analysis and radioimmunoassay. Aldosterone, the principal mineralocorticoid secreted by the zona glomerulosa of the adrenal cortex, regulates ion transport across cell membranes in the renal tubules to promote reabsorption of sodium and chloride in exchange for potassium and hydrogen ions. Consequently, it helps to maintain blood pressure and blood volume and regulate fluid and electrolyte balance.

Aldosterone secretion is controlled primarily by the renin-angiotensin system and the circulating concentration of potassium. Thus, high serum potassium levels elicit secretion of aldosterone through a potent feedback system; similarly, hyponatremia, hypovolemia, and other disorders that provoke the release of renin stimulate aldosterone secretion.

This test identifies aldosteronism and, when supported by plasma renin levels, distinguishes between the primary and secondary forms of this disorder. Thus, it is helpful in identifying adrenal adenoma and adrenal hyperplasia, causes of primary aldosteronism. Secondary aldosteronism is commonly associated with salt depletion, potassium excess, CHF with ascites, or other conditions that characteristically increase activity of the renin-angiotensin system.

Purpose
• To aid diagnosis of primary and sec-

ondary aldosteronism, adrenal hyperplasia, hypoaldosteronism, and salt-losing syndrome.

Equipment
Venipuncture: tourniquet/70% alcohol or providone-iodine solution/sterile syringes or evacuated tubes/sterile needle—20G or 21G for forearm, 25G for wrist, hand, ankle, or for children/color-coded tubes containing appropriate additives/identification labels/$2'' \times 2''$ gauze pads/small adhesive bandage.

Procedure
Explain to the patient that this test helps determine if symptoms are due to improper hormonal secretion. Instruct him to maintain a low-carbohydrate, normal-sodium diet (135 mEq or 3 g/day) for at least 2 weeks or, preferably, for 30 days before the test. Tell him that the test requires a blood sample. Collecting the sample takes only a few minutes, but the laboratory requires at least 10 days to complete the multistage analysis.

As ordered, withhold all drugs that alter fluid, sodium, and potassium balance—especially diuretics, antihypertensives, steroids, cyclic progestational agents, and estrogens—for at least 2 weeks or, preferably, 30 days before the test. Also, withhold all renin inhibitors (such as propranolol) for 1 week before the test. If these medications must be continued, note this on the laboratory slip. Licorice produces an aldosterone-like effect and should be avoided for at least 2 weeks before the test.

While the patient is still supine after a night's rest, perform a venipuncture. Collect the sample in a 7-ml *red-top* collection tube, and send it to the laboratory. To evaluate the effect of postural change, draw another sample 4 hours later, after the patient has been up and about, while he is standing. Collect the second sample in a 7-ml *red-top* collection tube, and send it to the laboratory.

Special considerations
• Handle the sample gently to prevent hemolysis.

• Record on the laboratory slip whether the patient was supine or standing during the venipuncture. If the patient is a premenopausal female, specify the phase of her menstrual cycle, since aldosterone levels may fluctuate during the cycle.

• Hemolysis due to rough handling of the sample may interfere with accurate determination of test results.

• Failure to observe restrictions of diet, medications, or posture may interfere with accurate determination of test results. Some antihypertensives—methyldopa, for example—promote sodium and water retention and may reduce aldosterone levels. Diuretics promote sodium excretion and may raise aldosterone levels. Some corticosteroids—fludrocortisone, for example—mimic mineralocorticoid activity and may lower aldosterone levels.

• A radioactive scan performed within 1 week before the test may influence test results.

Values

Normally, serum aldosterone levels (in a standing, nonpregnant patient) range from 1 to 21 ng/dl. Specifically, a normal serum aldosterone level for an adult male or female who has been supine for at least 2 hours is 7.4 ± 4.2 ng/dl; for an adult male or female who has been standing for at least 2 hours, 13.2 ± 8.9 ng/dl.

Implications of results

Excessive aldosterone secretion may indicate a primary or secondary disease. Primary aldosteronism (Conn's syndrome) may result from adrenocortical adenoma or carcinoma or bilateral adrenal hyperplasia. Secondary aldosteronism can result from renovascular hypertension, CHF, cirrhosis of the liver, nephrotic syndrome, idiopathic cyclic edema, or the third trimester of pregnancy.

Depressed serum aldosterone levels may indicate primary hypoaldosteronism, salt-losing syndrome, toxemia of pregnancy, or Addison's disease.

Documentation

Record any food, medication or previous tests that might alter test results.

Document the time of day the specimen was taken and the posture the patient was in at that time.

Plasma cortisol

Cortisol—the principal glucocorticoid secreted by the zona fasciculata of the adrenal cortex, primarily in response to adrenocorticotropic hormone (ACTH) stimulation—helps metabolize nutrients, mediate physiologic stress, and regulate the immune system. Cortisol secretion normally follows a diurnal pattern: levels rise during the early morning hours, peak around 8 a.m., then decline to very low levels in the evening and during the early phase of sleep. Production of this hormone is influenced by physical or emotional stress, which activates ACTH. Thus, intense heat or cold, infection, trauma, exercise, obesity, and debilitating disease influence cortisol secretion.

This radioimmunoassay, a quantitative analysis of plasma cortisol levels, is usually ordered for patients with signs of adrenal dysfunction, but dynamic tests, suppression tests for hyperfunction, and stimulation tests for hypofunction are generally required for confirmation of diagnoses.

Purpose

• To aid in the diagnosis of Cushing's disease, Cushing's syndrome, Addison's disease, and secondary adrenal insufficiency.

Equipment

Venipuncture: tourniquet/70% alcohol or povidone-iodine solution/sterile syringes or evacuated tubes/sterile needle—20G or 21G for forearm, 25G for wrist, hand, ankle, or for children/color-coded tubes containing appropriate additives/identification labels/2″ × 2″ gauze pads/small adhesive bandage.

Procedure
Explain to the patient that this test helps determine if his symptoms are due to improper hormonal secretion. Instruct him to maintain a normal salt diet (2 to 3 g/day) for 3 days before the test and to fast and limit physical activity for 10 to 12 hours before the test. Tell him a blood sample is required, who will perform the venipuncture, and when it will be done. Give reassurance that collecting the sample takes only a few minutes, although the laboratory requires at least 2 days to complete the analysis.

As ordered, withhold all medications that may interfere with plasma cortisol levels, such as estrogens, androgens, and phenytoin, for 48 hours before the test. If the patient is receiving replacement therapy and is dependent on exogenous steroids for survival, note this on the laboratory slip, as well as any other medications that must be continued.

Make sure the patient is relaxed and recumbent for at least 30 minutes before the test.

Between 6 and 8 a.m., perform a venipuncture. Collect the sample in a *green-top* tube, label appropriately, and send to the laboratory immediately. For diurnal variation testing, draw another sample between 4 and 6 p.m. Collect it in a *green-top* tube, label appropriately, and send to the laboratory immediately.

Special considerations
• Handle the sample gently to prevent hemolysis.
• Record the collection time on the laboratory slip.
• Failure to observe restrictions of diet, medications, or physical activity may interfere with accurate determination of test results. Plasma cortisol levels are falsely elevated by estrogens (during pregnancy or in oral contraceptives), which increase plasma proteins that bind with cortisol. Obesity, stress, or severe hepatic or renal disease may also increase these levels. Plasma cortisol levels may be decreased by androgens and phenytoin, which decrease cortisol-binding proteins.

• Radioactive scan performed within 1 week before the test may influence the results.

Values
Normally, plasma cortisol levels range from 7 to 28 mcg/dl in the morning and from 2 to 18 mcg/dl in the afternoon. (The afternoon level is usually half the morning level.)

Implications of results
Increased plasma cortisol levels may indicate adrenocortical hyperfunction in Cushing's disease (a rare disease due to basophilic adenoma of the pituitary gland) or in Cushing's syndrome (glucocorticoid excess from any cause). In most patients with Cushing's syndrome, the adrenal cortex tends to secrete independently of any natural rhythm. Thus, absence of diurnal variation in cortisol secretion is a significant finding in almost all patients with Cushing's syndrome; in these patients, little difference in values, if any, is found between morning samples and those taken in the afternoon. Diurnal variations may also be absent in otherwise healthy persons who are under considerable emotional or physical stress.

Decreased cortisol levels may indicate primary adrenal hypofunction (Addison's disease), most often due to idiopathic glandular atrophy (a presumed autoimmune process). Tuberculosis, fungal invasion, and hemorrhage can cause adrenocortical destruction. Low cortisol levels resulting from secondary adrenal insufficiency may occur in conditions of impaired ACTH secretion, such as hypophysectomy, postpartum pituitary necrosis, craniopharyngioma, or chromophobe adenoma.

Documentation
Record the use of any food or medications that might alter test result.

Record history of any previous tests or surgical procedures that might alter test results.

Document the time and posture of the patient when the specimen was drawn.

Plasma catecholamines

This test, a quantitative (total or fractionated) analysis of plasma catecholamines, has significant clinical importance in patients with hypertension and signs of adrenal medullary tumor and in those with neural tumors that affect endocrine function. Elevated plasma catecholamine levels necessitate supportive confirmation by urinalysis that shows catecholamine degradation products such as vanillylmandelic acid and metanephrine.

Major catecholamines include the hormones epinephrine, norepinephrine, and dopamine, which are produced almost exclusively in the brain, sympathetic nerve endings, and adrenal medulla. When secreted into the bloodstream, adrenal medullary catecholamines prepare the body for the fight-or-flight reaction to stress by increasing heart rate and contractility, constricting peripheral and visceral blood vessels, redistributing circulating blood toward the skeletal and coronary muscles, mobilizing carbohydrate and lipid reserves, and sharpening mental alertness. These effects are similar to those produced by direct stimulation of the sympathetic nervous system, although greatly intensified and prolonged.

Since many factors influence catecholamine secretion, diurnal variations are common; for example, plasma levels may fluctuate in response to temperature, stress, postural change, diet, smoking, and many drugs.

Purpose
• To rule out pheochromocytoma (adrenal medullary or extra-adrenal) in patients with hypertension
• To help identify neuroblastoma, ganglioneuroblastoma, and ganglioneuroma
• To distinguish between adrenal medullary tumors and other catecholamine-producing tumors, through fractional analysis. Urinalysis for catecholamine degradation products is recommended to support diagnosis
• To aid diagnosis of autonomic nervous system dysfunction, such as idiopathic orthostatic hypotension.

Equipment
Venipuncture: tourniquet/70% alcohol or povidone-iodine solution/sterile syringes or evacuated tubes/sterile needle—20G or 21G for forearm, 25G for wrist, hand, ankle, or for children/color-coded tubes containing appropriate additives/identification labels/2″ × 2″ gauze pads/small adhesive bandage.

Procedure
Explain to the patient that this test helps determine if hypertension or other symptoms are related to improper hormonal secretion. Because the action of catecholamines is so transitory, advise him to strictly follow pretest instructions for a reliable test result: to refrain from using self-prescribed medications (especially cold or hay fever remedies that may contain sympathomimetics) for 2 weeks; to exclude amine-rich foods and beverages (such as bananas, avocados, cheese, coffee, tea, cocoa, beer, and Chianti) for 48 hours; to abstain from smoking for 24 hours; and to fast for 10 to 12 hours.

Inform the patient that this test requires two blood samples, and tell him who will perform it and when it will be done. Collecting the samples takes less than 20 minutes, but the laboratory requires at least 1 week to complete the analysis.

If the patient is hospitalized, withhold medications that affect catecholamine levels, such as amphetamines, phenothiazines (chlorpromazine), sympathomimetics, and tricyclic antidepressants, as ordered.

Also, as ordered, insert an indwelling venous catheter (heparin lock) 24 hours before the test. This may be necessary, since the stress of the venipuncture itself may significantly raise catecholamine levels. Make sure the patient is relaxed and recumbent for 45 to 60 minutes before the test. If necessary, provide blankets to keep him warm; low temperatures stimulate catecholamine secretion.

Perform a venipuncture between 6 a.m. and 8 a.m. Collect the sample in a 10-ml chilled tube containing sodium metabisulfite solution (EDTA), which can be obtained from Mayo laboratory on request. Then have the patient stand for 10 minutes, and draw a second sample into another tube. If a heparin lock is used, you may have to discard the first 1 or 2 ml of blood. Check with the laboratory for the preferred procedure.

Special considerations

• After collecting each sample, roll the tube slowly between your palms to distribute the EDTA without agitating the blood. Then pack the tube in crushed ice to minimize deactivation of catecholamines, and send it to the laboratory immediately. Indicate on the laboratory slip whether the patient was supine or standing and the time the sample was drawn.

• Failure to observe pretest restrictions may interfere with accurate determination of test results.

• Epinephrine, levodopa, amphetamines, phenothiazines (chlorpromazine), sympathomimetics, decongestants, and tricyclic antidepressants raise plasma catecholamine levels. Reserpine lowers plasma catecholamine levels.

• A radioactive scan performed within 1 week before the test may influence results, since plasma catecholamine levels are determined by radioimmunoassay.

Values

In fractional analysis, catecholamine levels range as follows:

• supine: epinephrine, undetectable to 110 pg/ml; norepinephrine, 70 to 750 pg/ml; dopamine, undetectable to 30 pg/ml

• standing: epinephrine, undetectable to 140 pg/ml; norepinephrine, 200 to 1,700 pg/ml; dopamine, undetectable to 30 pg/ml.

Implications of results

High catecholamine levels may indicate pheochromocytoma, neuroblastoma, ganglioneuroblastoma, or ganglioneuroma. Similar elevations are possible in thyroid disorders, hypoglycemia, or cardiac disease but do not directly confirm these disorders. Electroshock therapy, or shock resulting from hemorrhage, endotoxins, or anaphylaxis also causes catecholamine levels to rise.

In the patient with normal or low baseline catecholamine levels, failure to show increased catecholamine levels in the sample taken after standing suggests autonomic nervous system dysfunction. No known dysfunction is associated with insufficiency of the adrenal medulla.

Fractional analysis helps identify the specific abnormality that is producing elevated catecholamine levels. For example, adrenal medullary tumors secrete epinephrine; ganglioneuromas, ganglioblastomas, and neuroblastomas secrete norepinephrine.

Documentation

Record the use of any food or medications that might alter test results.

Record any history of previous tests or surgery that might alter test results.

Document the time and position of the patient when the specimen was drawn.

Urine tests

Routine urinalysis and special studies of renal function provide valuable information about the integrity of renal and urinary functions and also serve as sensitive indicators of overall health. To understand the significance of such tests and their clinical applications, you need to know how urine is normally formed, what elements it contains, and the mechanisms that regulate urine volume.

Urine formation

The kidneys, through the activity of the nephrons, continuously remove metabolic wastes, drugs and other foreign substances, excess fluids, inorganic salts, and acid and base substances from the blood for eventual excretion in the urine. Each kidney has approximately 1 million nephrons; in turn, each nephron consists of a vascular ultrafilter called a *glomerulus* and a *renal tubule,* an epithelial-lined conduit for reabsorption of recyclable matter and secretion of foreign and waste substances. The nephrons form urine through three mechanisms—*glomerular filtration, tubular reabsorption,* and *tubular secretion.*

Blood enters each kidney through the renal artery, passing through progressively smaller vascular channels and eventually entering the glomeruli through the afferent glomerular arterioles. These arterioles subdivide into clusters of capillary loops, each of which is partly enclosed in a membranous covering called Bowman's capsule. The walls of the capillaries are semipermeable, so dissolved substances can pass by simple filtration from the plasma through the glomerular capillaries and into the capsule space.

Blood leaves the glomeruli through the efferent glomerular arterioles and travels to a network of peritubular capillaries, which encircle the renal tubules. Glomerular filtrate leaves the Bowman's capsules and enters the proximal convoluted tubules, where approximately 65% is selectively reabsorbed by the peritubular capillaries. (Reabsorbed substances include water, glucose, some proteins, amino acids, acetoacetate ions, vitamins, and hormones.) The remaining 35% of the filtrate proceeds through the loops of Henle and the distal convoluted tubules, where sodium and water are reabsorbed as needed.

During secretion, fluid and solutes such as potassium, uric acid, exogenous substances (such as drugs), and other waste material move from the peritubular capillaries back into the glomerular filtrate. As the liquid filtrate evolves, it is continuously modified by filtration, reabsorption, and secretion. The end product is urine.

Urine composition

Although the actual composition of normal urine changes—depending on diet, physical activity, and emotional stress—it always includes water, urea, uric acid, and sodium chloride. Urine also usually contains other nonprotein nitrogen compounds, citric acid, other organic acids, catecholamines, sulfur-containing compounds, phosphate, potassium, calcium, magnesium, reducing substances, mucoproteins, vitamins, and hormones.

In the presence of disease, urine may contain protein, glucose, ketone bodies, hemoglobin, lipids, bacteria, pus, urobilinogen, or calculi. Microscopic examination of centrifuged urine sediment can detect cells, casts, crystals, bacteria, yeasts and parasites, spermatozoa, or contaminants and artifacts.

Urine volume

Urine volume, closely regulated by the kidneys, reflects overall fluid homeostasis. Actual volume depends on fluid intake, the concentration of solutes in the filtrate, cardiac output, hormonal influences, and fluid loss through the lungs, the large bowel, and the skin. In adults, urine volume normally ranges from 800 to 2,000 ml/day and averages 1,200 to 1,500 ml/day. In children, volume ranges from 300 to 1,500 ml/day; however, a child's urine output is three to four times greater per kilogram of body weight than that of an adult.

Polyuria, urine volume that exceeds 2,000 ml/day, is typical of many abnormal conditions. *Oliguria* is the excretion of less than 500 ml of urine volume/day; *anuria,* the absence of urine excretion. *Nocturia,* urine volume greater than 500 ml at night, with a specific gravity of less than 1.018, is characteristic of chronic glomerulonephritis or heart or liver failure.

Clearance principle

Abnormal findings from routine urinalysis suggest renal disease or dysfunction, but tests for filtration, reabsorption, and secretion permit more precise evaluation. Clearance, the volume of plasma that can be cleared of a substance per unit of time, is the principle used to assess urine-forming mechanisms; it is also a measure of renal plasma flow, which, if diminished, impairs renal function.

Clearance depends on how efficiently the renal tubular cells handle the substance that has been filtered by the glomerulus. If the tubules do not reabsorb or secrete the substance, clearance equals the glomerular filtration rate (GFR). If the tubules reabsorb it, clearance is less than the GFR. If the tubules secrete it, clearance is greater than the GFR. If the tubules reabsorb and secrete the substance, clearance is less than, equal to, or greater than the GFR.

Routine urinalysis

Routine urinalysis is an important, commonly used screening test for urinary and systemic pathologies. Normal urine findings suggest the absence of major disease, while abnormal findings suggest its presence and mandate further urine or blood tests to identify a specific disorder. The elements of routine urinalysis include the evaluation of physical characteristics (color, odor, and opacity); the determination of specific gravity and pH; the detection and rough measurement of protein, glucose, and ketone bodies; and the examination of sediment for red and white blood cells, casts, and crystals.

Laboratory methods for detecting or measuring these elements include visual examination for appearance; reagent strip screening for pH, protein, glucose, and ketone bodies; refractometry for specific gravity; and microscopic inspection of centrifuged sediment for cells, casts, and crystals.

Purpose
• To screen for renal or urinary tract disease
• To help detect metabolic or systemic disease unrelated to renal disorders.

Equipment
For random specimen: bedpan or urinal with cover, if necessary/graduated container/specimen container with lid/label/laboratory request slip.

For clean-catch midstream specimen: basin/soap and water/towel/sterile gloves/three sterile 2″ × 2″ gauze pads/povidone-iodine solution/sterile specimen container with lid/label/bedpan or urinal, if necessary/laboratory request slip. (Commercial clean-catch kits containing antiseptic towelettes, sterile specimen container with lid and label, and instructions for use in several languages are widely used.)

For indwelling catheter specimen: 10-ml syringe/21G or 22G 1½″ needle/tube clamp/sterile specimen cup with lid/alcohol sponge/label/laboratory request slip.

Procedure
Explain to the patient that this test aids diagnosis of renal or urinary tract disease and helps evaluate overall body function. Advise him he need not restrict food or fluids before the test, and that the test requires a urine specimen. Check the history for recent ingestion of medications that may affect test results.

Collect a random urine specimen of at least 15 ml. If possible, obtain a first-voided morning specimen, since this contains the greatest concentration of solutes.

Special considerations
• Send the specimen to the laboratory immediately, or refrigerate it if analysis will be delayed longer than 1 hour.
• Failure to follow proper collection procedure, send the specimen to the laboratory immediately, or refrigerate the specimen may interfere with accurate determination of test results.
• Strenuous exercise before routine urinalysis may cause transient myoglobinuria, producing misleading results and inaccurate diagnosis.
• Many drugs can influence the results of this test.

Values

Macroscopically, normal urine is straw colored, slightly aromatic, and clear in appearance. There is no presence of protein, ketones, glucose, or other sugars. Specific gravity is 1.025 to 1.030, and pH ranges 4.5 to 8.

Microscopically, there are few RBC's, WBC's, and epithelial cells. Casts and crystals are seen occasionally.

Implications of results

Nonpathologic variations in these values may result from diet, nonpathologic conditions, specimen collection time, and other factors. For example, specific gravity influences urine color and odor. As specific gravity increases, urine becomes darker and its odor becomes stronger; as it decreases, urine lightens. Specific gravity is highest in the first-voided morning specimen.

Urine pH, which is greatly affected by diet and medications, influences the appearance of urine and the composition of crystals. An alkaline pH (above 7.0)—characteristic of a diet high in vegetables, citrus fruits, and dairy products but low in meat—causes turbidity and formation of phosphate, carbonate, and amorphous crystals. An acid pH (below 7.0)—typical of a high-protein diet—produces turbidity and formation of oxalate, cystine, amorphous urate, and uric acid crystals.

Although protein is normally absent from the urine, it can appear in orthostatic (postural) proteinuria. This benign condition is most common during the second decade of life, is intermittent, appears after prolonged standing, and disappears after recumbency.

Transient benign proteinuria can also occur with fever, exposure to cold, emotional stress, or strenuous exercise. Sugars, also usually absent from the urine, may appear under normal conditions. The most common sugar in urine is glucose. Transient, nonpathologic glycosuria may result from emotional stress or pregnancy and may follow ingestion of a high-carbohydrate meal. Other sugars—fructose, lactose, and pentose—rarely appear in urine under nonpathologic conditions. (Lactosuria, however, can occur during pregnancy and lactation.)

The three important elements present in centrifuged urine sediment are cells, casts, and crystals. Red cells do not commonly appear in urine without pathologic significance, but hematuria may occasionally follow strenuous exercise.

The following abnormal findings generally suggest pathologic conditions:
- *Color:* Changes in color can result from diet, drugs, and many metabolic, inflammatory, or infectious diseases.
- *Odor:* In diabetes mellitus, starvation, and dehydration, a fruity odor accompanies formation of ketone bodies. In urinary tract infection, a fetid odor is common, especially if *Escherichia coli* is present.
- *Turbidity:* Turbid urine may contain red or white cells, bacteria, fat, or chyle and may reflect renal infection.
- *Specific gravity:* Low specific gravity (< 1.005) is characteristic of diabetes insipidus, nephrogenic diabetes insipidus, acute tubular necrosis, and pyelonephritis. Fixed specific gravity, in which values remain 1.010 regardless of fluid intake, occurs in chronic glomerulonephritis with severe renal damage. High specific gravity (> 1.020) occurs in nephrotic syndrome, dehydration, acute glomerulonephritis, CHF, liver failure, and shock.
- *pH:* Alkaline urine pH may result from Fanconi's syndrome, urinary tract infection, and metabolic or respiratory alkalosis. Acid urine pH is associated with renal tuberculosis, pyrexia, phenylketonuria and alkaptonuria, and all forms of acidosis.
- *Protein:* Proteinuria suggests renal diseases.
- *Sugars:* Glycosuria usually indicates diabetes mellitus but may also result from pheochromocytoma, Cushing's syndrome, and increased intracranial pressure. Fructosuria, galactosuria, and pentosuria generally suggest rare hereditary metabolic disorders. However, an

alimentary form of pentosuria and fructosuria may follow excessive ingestion of pentose or fructose, resulting in hepatic failure to metabolize the sugar. Since the renal tubules fail to reabsorb pentose or fructose, these sugars spill over into the urine.

• *Ketones:* Ketonuria occurs in diabetes mellitus when cellular energy needs exceed available cellular glucose. In the absence of glucose, cells metabolize fat, an alternate energy supply. Ketone bodies—the end products of incomplete fat metabolism—accumulate in plasma and are excreted in the urine. Ketonuria may also occur in starvation states and in conditions of acutely increased metabolic demand associated with decreased food intake, such as diarrhea or vomiting.

• *Cells:* Hematuria indicates bleeding within the genitourinary tract and may result from infection, obstruction, inflammation, trauma, tumors, glomerulonephritis, renal hypertension, lupus nephritis, renal tuberculosis, renal vein thrombosis, hydronephrosis, pyelonephritis, scurvy, malaria, parasitic infection of the bladder, subacute bacterial endocarditis, polyarteritis nodosa, and hemorrhagic disorders. Numerous white cells in urine usually imply urinary tract inflammation, especially cystitis or pyelonephritis. White cells and white cell casts in urine suggest renal infection. An excessive number of epithelial cells suggests renal tubular degeneration.

• *Casts* (plugs of gelled proteinaceous material [high–molecular-weight mucoprotein]): Casts form in the renal tubules and collecting ducts by agglutination of protein cells or cellular debris and are flushed loose by urine flow. Excessive numbers of casts indicate renal disease. Hyaline casts are associated with renal parenchymal disease, inflammation, and trauma to the glomerular capillary membrane; epithelial casts, with renal tubular damage, nephrosis, eclampsia, amyloidosis, and heavy metal poisoning; coarse and fine granular casts, with acute or chronic renal failure, pyelonephritis, and chronic lead intoxication; fatty and waxy casts, with nephrotic syndrome, chronic renal disease, and diabetes mellitus; RBC casts, with renal parenchymal disease (especially glomerulonephritis), renal infarction, subacute bacterial endocarditis, vascular disorders, sickle cell anemia, scurvy, blood dyscrasias, malignant hypertension, collagen disease, and acute inflammation; and WBC casts, with acute pyelonephritis and glomerulonephritis, nephrotic syndrome, pyogenic infection, and lupus nephritis.

• *Crystals:* Some crystals normally appear in urine, but numerous calcium oxalate crystals suggest hypercalcemia. Cystine crystals (cystinuria) reflect an inborn error of metabolism.

• *Other components:* Yeast cells and parasites in urinary sediment reflect genitourinary tract infection, as well as contamination of external genitalia. Yeast cells, which may be mistaken for red cells, can be identified by their ovoid shape, lack of color, variable size, and frequently, signs of budding. The most common parasite in sediment is *Trichomonas vaginalis,* a flagellated protozoan that commonly causes vaginitis, urethritis, and prostatovesiculitis.

Documentation

Record specimen collection and laboratory transport. Note the appearance, odor, color, and any unusual characteristics of the specimen. If necessary, record the volume on the patient's intake and output chart.

Urine hormones and metabolites

Hormones are complex chemicals produced and secreted primarily by the endocrine glands to promote and regulate the activity of target organs and tissues. To directly determine circulating levels of hormones, laboratory methods commonly measure hormone concentrations in blood. But many hormones and their metabolites are also conveniently studied in urine.

Measuring urine hormone and metabolite levels provides a reliable estimate of the amount of circulating hormone. Moreoever, timed, long-term urine measurements offer an advantage. Unlike a blood sample, which determines hormone levels only at the time of venipuncture, a 24-hour urine specimen reflects total daily secretion, offsets diurnal variations, and masks temporary fluctuations.

Chemical classes

Chemically, hormones can be classified into three groups: *steroids* (such as estrogens and androgens), *amines* (such as dopamine and epinephrine), and *proteins* (such as human chorionic gonadotropin). Each group has a marked structural specificity.

Hormone metabolites

Although hormones have specific and characteristic functions, they rarely act independently. Quite the contrary, hormones are linked in an intricate series of complex interactions, including positive and negative feedback mechanisms that enable them to function efficiently and maintain homeostasis. Perhaps the most important of these interactions is the formation of hormone metabolites. These metabolites can be degradation products or essential precursors with individual hormonal effects.

Urine levels of hormone metabolites reflect the secretory rates of the hormones from which these metabolites are derived and serve as valuable diagnostic indicators when the hormones themselves are not excreted in measurable quantities. Metabolite levels also provide important information about the integrity of degradation pathways.

The hormones produced by the endocrine glands and their metabolites that are commonly measured in the urine include the following:

• *Adrenocortical hormones:* These hormones and metabolites are steroids, synthesized and secreted primarily by the adrenal cortex. Formed from acetyl-coenzyme A, cholesterol, and a variety of other precursors, adrenocortical hormones and metabolites fall into three major groups: 1. *Glucocorticoids, 17-hydroxycorticosteroids,* particularly cortisol, maintain carbohydrate, protein, and fat metabolism. 2. *Mineralocorticoids,* principally aldosterone, help regulate blood pressure and fluid and electrolyte balance. 3. *Adrenal androgens* (sex hormones), the most potent of which is dehydroepiandrosterone, aid development of male secondary sex characteristics.

• *Adrenal medullary hormones:* The adrenal medullae synthesize and secrete the catecholamines *norepinephrine* and *epinephrine,* which help mediate stress. Although these hormones are less vital to life than the adrenocortical hormones, determinations of urine levels of the catecholamines and their principal metabolite, *VMA,* can be extremely useful in the detection of catecholamine-producing tumors.

• *Dopamine and other amines:* A catecholamine secreted primarily by the basal ganglia of the brain, dopamine is the precursor of norepinephrine and epinephrine. When a pheochromocytoma, a catecholamine-secreting tumor, is suspected, measurement of urine levels of dopamine and its major metabolite, homovanillic acid, can aid diagnosis.

• *Gonadal and placental hormones:* Urine levels of gonadal and placental hormones, which are principally steroids, are clinically useful for detecting hormone-secreting tumors and pregnancy.

Urine aldosterone

This test measures urine levels of aldosterone, the principal mineralocorticoid secreted by the zona glomerulosa of the adrenal cortex. Aldosterone promotes retention of sodium and excretion of potassium by the renal tubules, thereby helping to regulate blood pressure and fluid and electrolyte balance. In turn, aldosterone secretion is controlled by the renin-angiotensin system. Renin, an enzyme released in the kidneys in response to low plasma volume, stimulates production of angiotensin I, which is converted to angiotensin II, a powerful vasopressor that directly stimulates the adrenal cortex to secrete aldosterone. Potassium levels also influence aldosterone secretion: increased potassium concentration stimulates the adrenal cortex, triggering a substantial increase in aldosterone secretion to promote potassium excretion. This feedback mechanism is vital to maintaining fluid and electrolyte balance.

Urine aldosterone levels, measured through radioimmunoassay, are usually evaluated after measurement of serum electrolyte and renin levels.

Purpose
• To aid diagnosis of primary and secondary aldosteronism.

Equipment
Large collection bottle with cap or stopper or commercial plastic container/preservative, if necessary/bedpan or urinal, if patient does not have an indwelling catheter/graduated container, if patient is on intake and output measurement/ice-filled container, if a refrigerator is not available/label/laboratory request slip/four patient-care reminders. Check with the laboratory to see what preservatives may be needed in the urine specimen.

Procedure
Explain to the patient that this test evaluates hormonal balance. Instruct him to maintain a normal sodium diet (3 g/day) before the test; to avoid sodium-rich foods, such as bacon, barbeque sauce, corned beef, bouillon cubes or powder, and olives; and to avoid strenuous physical exercise and stressful situations during the collection period. Tell him the test requires collection of a 24-hour urine specimen.

Explain the procedure to the patient's family members to enlist their cooperation and prevent accidental disposal of urine during the collection period. Emphasize that loss of even *one* urine specimen during the collection time invalidates the collection and requires that it begin again.

Place patient-care reminders over the patient's bed, in his bathroom, on the bedpan hopper in the utility room, and on the urinal or indwelling catheter collection bag. Include his name and room number, the date(s), and the collection interval.

Instruct the patient to save all urine during the collection period, to notify you after each voiding, and to avoid contaminating the urine with stool or toilet tissue. (If he is to continue the urine collection at home, provide written instructions for the appropriate method.) Explain any dietary or drug restrictions.

Check the patient's medication history for drugs that may affect aldosterone levels. Review your findings with the laboratory, then notify the doctor; he may want to restrict these medications before the test.

Ask the patient to void. Then discard this urine so he starts the collection time with an empty bladder. Record the time.

After pouring the first urine specimen into the collection bottle, add the required preservative. Then refrigerate the bottle or keep it on ice until the next voiding.

Collect all urine voided during the prescribed period. Just before the collection period ends, ask the patient to void again, if possible. Add this last specimen to the collection bottle, pack it in ice to inhibit deterioration of the specimen, and immediately send it to the laboratory. Include a properly completed laboratory request slip.

Special considerations
• Refrigerate the specimen or place it on ice during the collection period. When the collection is completed, send the specimen to the laboratory immediately.
• Antihypertensive drugs promote sodium and water retention and may suppress urine aldosterone levels. Diuretics and most steroids promote sodium ex-

cretion and may raise aldosterone levels. Some corticosteroids, such as fludrocortisone, mimic mineralocorticoid activity and consequently may lower aldosterone levels.

• Patient failure to maintain a normal dietary intake of sodium can influence test results. Failure to collect *all* urine during the 24-hour specimen collection period or to store the specimen properly can interfere with accurate determination of test results.

• Patient failure to avoid strenuous physical exercise and emotional stress before the test stimulates adrenocortical secretions and thus increases aldosterone levels.

• A radioactive scan performed within 1 week before the test may interfere with the accurate determination of aldosterone levels using this radioimmunoassay method.

Values
Normally, urine aldosterone levels range from 2 to 16 mcg/24 hours.

Implications of results
Elevated urine aldosterone levels suggest primary or secondary aldosteronism. The primary form usually arises from an aldosterone-secreting adenoma of the adrenal cortex but may also result from adrenocortical hyperplasia. Secondary aldosteronism, the more common form, results from external stimulation of the adrenal cortex, such as that produced when the renin-angiotensin system is activated by hypertensive and edematous disorders. The major systemic pathologies that result in secondary aldosteronism are malignant hypertension, CHF, cirrhosis of the liver, nephrotic syndrome, and idiopathic cyclic edema.

Low urine aldosterone levels may result from Addison's disease, salt-losing syndrome, and toxemia of pregnancy. These levels normally rise during pregnancy but rapidly decline following parturition.

Documentation
In the cardex and in your notes, record the date(s), interval of collection, and disposition of the specimen.

Urine catecholamines

This test uses spectrophotofluorometry to measure urine levels of the major catecholamines—epinephrine, norepinephrine, and dopamine. Epinephrine is secreted by the adrenal medulla; dopamine, by the central nervous system; and norepinephrine, by both. Catecholamines help regulate metabolism and prepare the body for the fight-or-flight response to stress. Certain tumors can also secrete catecholamines. One of the most common of these tumors is a pheochromocytoma, which usually causes intermittent or persistent hypertension.

The specimen of choice for this test is a 24-hour urine specimen, since catecholamine secretion fluctuates diurnally and in response to pain, heat, cold, emotional stress, physical exercise, hypoglycemia, injury, hemorrhage, asphyxia, and drugs. However, a random specimen may be useful for evaluating catecholamine levels after a hypertensive episode.

For a complete diagnostic workup of catecholamine secretion, urine levels of catecholamine metabolites are measured concurrently. These metabolites—metanephrine, normetanephrine, homovanillic acid (HVA), and VMA—normally appear in the urine in greater quantities than the catecholamines.

Purpose
• To aid diagnosis of pheochromocytoma in a patient with unexplained hypertension.

Equipment
For 24-hour specimen: Large collection bottle with cap or stopper, or commercial plastic container/preservative, if necessary/bedpan or urinal, if patient does not have an indwelling catheter/graduated container, if patient is on in-

take and output measurement/ice-filled container, if a refrigerator is not available/label/laboratory request slip/four patient-care reminders. Check with the laboratory to see what preservatives may be needed in the urine specimen.

For random specimen: bedpan or urinal with cover, if necessary/graduated container/specimen container with lid/label/laboratory request slip.

Procedure

Explain to the patient that this test evaluates adrenal function. Inform him that he need not restrict food or fluids before the test but should avoid stressful situations and excessive physical activity during the collection period. Tell him that either a 24-hour or random specimen is required, and explain the collection procedure.

Check the patient's drug history for medications (such as those listed below) that may affect catecholamine levels. Review your findings with a laboratory technician, then notify the doctor. He may want to restrict such medications before the test.

Collect a 24-hour urine specimen in a bottle containing a preservative to keep the specimen acidified to a pH of 3.0 or less. (If a random specimen is ordered, collect it immediately after a hypertensive episode.)

Special considerations

• Refrigerate a 24-hour specimen or place it on ice during the collection period. At the end of the period, send the specimen to the laboratory immediately.

• Caffeine, insulin, nitroglycerin, aminophylline, ethanol, sympathomimetics, methyldopa, tricyclic antidepressants, chloral hydrate, quinidine, quinine, tetracycline, B-complex vitamins, isoproterenol, levodopa, and monoamine oxidase inhibitors may raise urine catecholamine levels.

• Clonidine, guanethidine, reserpine, and iodine-containing contrast media may suppress urine catecholamine levels.

• Phenothiazines, erythromycin, and methenamine compounds may raise or suppress levels.

• Failure to comply with drug restrictions, collect all urine during the test period, or store the specimen properly may interfere with test results.

• Excessive physical exercise or emotional stress raises catecholamine levels.

Values

Normally, urine catecholamine values range from undetectable to 135 mcg/24 hours, or from undetectable to 18 mcg/dl in a random specimen.

Implications of results

In a patient with undiagnosed hypertension, elevated urine catecholamine levels following a hypertensive episode usually indicate a pheochromocytoma. With the exception of HVA—a metabolite of dopamine—catecholamine metabolites may also be elevated. Abnormally high HVA levels rule out a pheochromocytoma because this tumor mainly secretes epinephrine, whose primary metabolite is VMA, not HVA. If tests indicate a pheochromocytoma, the patient may also be tested for multiple endocrine neoplasia.

Elevated catecholamine levels without marked hypertension may be due to a neuroblastoma or a ganglioneuroma, although HVA levels reflect these conditions more accurately. Neuroblastomas and ganglioneuromas primarily composed of immature cells secrete large quantities of dopamine and HVA. Myasthenia gravis and progessive muscular dystrophy commonly cause urine catecholamine levels to rise above normal, but this test is rarely performed to diagnose these disorders.

Consistently low-normal catecholamine levels may indicate dysautonomia, marked by orthostatic hypotension.

Documentation

In the cardex and in your notes, record the date(s), interval of collection, and the disposition of the specimen.

Urine vanillylmandelic acid

Using spectrophotofluorometry, this test determines urine levels of VMA, a phenolic acid. VMA is the catecholamine metabolite that is normally most prevalent in the urine and is the product of hepatic conversion of epinephrine and norepinephrine. Urine VMA levels reflect endogenous production of these major catecholamines. Like the test for urine total catecholamines, this test helps detect catecholamine secreting tumors—most prominently pheochromocytoma—and helps evaluate the function of the adrenal medulla, the primary site of catecholamine production. This test is performed preferably on a 24-hour urine specimen (not a random specimen) to overcome the effects of diurnal variations in catecholamine secretion. Other catecholamine metabolites—metanephrine, normetanephrine, and HVA—may be measured at the same time.

Purpose
• To help detect pheochromocytoma, neuroblastoma, and ganglioneuroma
• To evaluate the function of the adrenal medulla.

Equipment
Large collection bottle with cap or stopper or commercial plastic container/preservative, if necessary/bedpan or urinal, if patient does not have an indwelling catheter/graduated container, if patient is on intake and output measurement/ice-filled container, if a refrigerator is not available/label/laboratory request slip/four patient-care reminders. Check with the laboratory to see what preservatives may be needed in the urine specimen.

Procedure
Tell the patient that this test evaluates hormonal secretion. Instruct him to restrict foods and beverages containing phenolic acid, such as coffee, tea, bananas, citrus fruits, chocolate, and vanilla, for 3 days before the test, and to avoid stressful situations and excessive physical activity during the urine collection period. Inform him the test requires collection of a 24-hour urine specimen.

Explain the procedure to the patient and his family to enlist their cooperation and prevent accidental disposal of urine during the collection period. Emphasize that loss of even one urine specimen during the collection time invalidates the collection and requires that it begin again.

Place patient-care reminders over the patient's bed, in his bathroom, on the bedpan hopper in the utility room, and on the urinal or indwelling catheter collection bag. Include his name, room number, the date(s), and the collection interval.

Instruct the patient to save all urine during the collection period, to notify you after each voiding, and to avoid contaminating the urine with stool or toilet tissue. (If he is to continue the urine collection at home, provide written instructions for the appropriate method.) Explain any dietary or drug restrictions.

Check the patient's medication history for drugs that may affect test results. Review your findings with the laboratory, then notify the doctor; he may want to withhold these drugs before the test.

Ask the patient to void. Then discard this urine so he starts the collection time with an empty bladder. Record the time.

After pouring the first urine specimen into the collection bottle, add the required preservative. Then refrigerate the bottle or keep it on ice until the next voiding.

Collect all urine voided during the prescribed period. Just before the collection period ends, ask the patient to void again, if possible. Add this last specimen to the collection bottle, pack it in ice to inhibit deterioration of the specimen, and immediately send it to the laboratory. Include a properly completed laboratory request slip.

Special considerations
• Refrigerate the specimen or keep it on ice during the collection period. When the collection is completed, send the specimen to the laboratory immediately.
• Epinephrine, norepinephrine, lithium carbonate, and methocarbamol may raise urine VMA levels. Chlorpromazine, guanethidine, reserpine, monoamine oxidase inhibitors, and clonidine may lower VMA levels. Levodopa and salicylates may raise or lower VMA levels.
• Failure to observe drug and dietary restrictions, collect all urine during the test period, or store the specimen properly may interfere with test results.
• Excessive physical exercise or emotional stress may raise VMA levels.

Values
Normally, urine VMA values range from 0.7 to 6.8 mg/24 hours.

Implications of results
Elevated urine VMA levels may result from a catecholamine-secreting tumor. Further testing, such as measurement of urine HVA levels to rule out pheochromocytoma, is necessary for precise diagnosis. If pheochromocytoma is confirmed, the patient may be tested for multiple endocrine neoplasia, an inherited condition commonly associated with pheochromocytoma. (Family members of a patient with confirmed pheochromocytoma should also be carefully evaluated for multiple endocrine neoplasia.)

Documentation
In the cardex and in your notes, record the date(s), interval of collection, and disposition of the specimen.

14
MONITORING PROCEDURES

Cardiac and hemodynamic monitoring techniques have greatly enhanced effective assessment of the patient's cardiovascular status and his response to therapy. Cardiac monitoring includes hardwire monitoring for continuous monitoring of the patient confined to bed and telemetry monitoring for continuous monitoring of the convalescent patient who has some freedom of movement in the hospital. It also guides cardiac drug therapy with pressors and inotropic agents.

Hemodynamic monitoring demands strict attention to detailed equipment preparation and a good understanding of cardiovascular anatomy and physiology. Monitoring of central venous pressure (CVP), arterial pressure, pulmonary artery and capillary wedge pressure, or cardiac output is frequently performed on the patient with myocardial infarction (MI) or congestive heart failure (CHF).

Monitoring techniques are constantly being studied and improved to obtain the best results with the least risk to the patient.

Cardiac monitoring

Cardiac monitoring is used to continuously observe the heart's electrical activity in patients who may have a symptomatic dysrhythmia or any cardiac pathology that may lead to life-threatening dysrhythmias. It is also used to evaluate the effects of therapy. Like other forms of electrocardiography, this procedure uses electrodes applied to the patient's chest to pick up patterns of cardiac impulses for display and analysis on a monitor screen. The monitoring is done in several ways. Hardwire monitoring permits continuous observation of a patient directly connected to the monitor console. Telemetry monitoring permits continuous monitoring of an ambulatory patient not connected to a monitor; his cardiac impulses travel from a small transmitter he wears to antenna wires in the ceiling that relay the patterns to the monitor screen.

Cardiac monitors usually perform three functions: they display the patient's cardiac rhythm and heart rate, they sound an alarm if heart rate rises above or falls below the allowable per-minute setting; and they provide printouts of cardiac rhythms for documentation. (See *Continuous Cardiac Monitoring*.)

Equipment
Alcohol sponges/4″x4″ gauze sponges/cardiac monitor/nonallergenic tape/patient cable/three lead wires/three disposable pregelled electrodes. (The number of electrodes varies from three to five, depending on the manufacturer.) Optional: shaving equipment (razor, basin, warm water, soap, towel, washcloth).

Procedure
Explain the procedure to the patient and provide privacy. Wash your hands.

Determine electrode positions on the patient's chest. Select the lead that displays the appropriate QRS complex, P waves, and pacing stimulus. If you select *lead II* (provides a tall, positive QRS

Continuous Cardiac Monitoring

If patient's EKG tracings deviate from normal, he will probably need to be monitored continuously for rhythm disturbances. In most cases, a single-lead cardiac monitor (three electrodes and three wires) is used.

Pros and cons.

The two leads most commonly used for continuous monitoring are Lead II and MCL_1. Here's how they compare.

• *Lead II.* This is a bipolar lead specific to heart rhythm monitoring. To set it up, place the positive electrode over the heart's apex (in the left midclavicular line at the fourth intercostal space). Then place the negative electrode beneath the patient's right clavicle. Place the ground beneath the left clavicle or elsewhere on the chest. You can usually see P waves clearly with this lead. However, when an EKG shows an abnormal QRS complex, Lead II tracings of bundle branch blocks and ventricular ectopic beats may be indistinguishable.

• *MCL_1.* This lead simulates V_1 of the standard 12-lead EKG. Unlike V_1, however, MCL_1 is a *bipolar* lead. To set it up, place the positive electrode at the right sternal border at the fourth intercostal space; the negative electrode just below the middle of the left clavicle; and the ground below the right clavicle.

MCL_1 offers more diagnostic advantages than does Lead II. For example, it may help

• distinguish between left ventricular ectopy and right ventricular ectopy
• identify right and left bundle branch blocks (RBBB and LBBB)
• clearly reveal P waves, usually best seen in a right chest lead
• differentiate left ventricular ectopy from RBBB aberration.

When one is not enough.

MCL_1 unfortunately cannot identify the development of hemiblock or reveal the full polarity of the P wave. Although fairly minor, these drawbacks can interfere with assessing heart function. The doctor may decide to supplement MCL_1 tracings with an MCL_6 lead.

MCL_6 simulates the V_6 lead of the 12-lead EKG. To set it up, place a positive electrode at the fifth intercostal space in the midaxillary line.

Note: A single-lead EKG is not always sufficient. A 12-lead EKG may be necessary to clarify diagnosis, especially if the patient's status changes during monitoring.

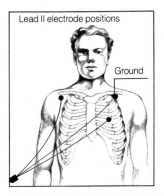

Lead II electrode positions

Ground

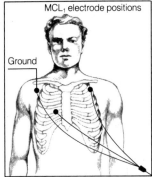

MCL_1 electrode positions

Ground

complex and a positive P wave), place the negative electrode on the right sternal border at the first intercostal space. Then place the positive electrode at the fourth intercostal space, left of the midclavicular line, and place the ground electrode at the fourth intercostal space, right sternal border.

If necessary, shave an area about 4″ (10.16 cm) in diameter around each electrode site. Clean the area with an alcohol sponge and dry it completely to remove skin secretions that may interfere with proper electrode function. Gently abrade the dried area by rubbing it briskly until it reddens to remove dead skin cells and promote better electrical contact with living cells. (Some electrodes have a small rough patch for abrading the skin; otherwise, use a dry washcloth or a dry gauze sponge.)

Apply the electrode to the site, being careful to firmly press the adhesive part to ensure a tight seal.

Using the gain control on the monitor, adjust the size of the QRS complexes that appear on the screen. Calibrate the monitor by pushing the calibration button, which causes a waveform 1 mv high to appear. If necessary, adjust the gain control to make the R wave of the QRS complex higher than the 1-mv waveform. Then center the waveform on the monitor screen.

Set the upper and lower limits of the heart rate alarm, based on assessment of each patient's cardiac status. Most monitoring systems allow the rate to be set on the bedside monitor or the central console. Since these are integrated circuits, the monitor will automatically calibrate the whole system. Put the alarm on automatic so that it sounds whenever the patient's heart rate exceeds or falls below the preset limits.

Make sure the monitor counts each QRS complex. If an audible alarm or flashing light does not occur when each complex appears on the screen, increase the gain setting until each complex is sufficiently high to trigger the audible alarm and the rate light every time.

Demonstrate the alarm system to the patient and tell him that it may be triggered by movement or a loose electrode, as well as by rhythm disturbances. Emphasize that the machine is not a part of therapy, and that he can move about in bed despite the alarm. (See *Troubleshooting Cardiac Monitors*, pages 300 and 301.)

Special considerations
• Avoid removing the paper backing of the electrodes until just before application to prevent them from drying out. Position electrodes on the patient's chest so they will not interfere with application of defibrillator paddles if emergency defibrillation is required.
• Make sure all electrical equipment and outlets are grounded properly.
• If the patient has an allergic reaction to the monitoring electrodes, secure them with hypoallergenic tape. If the electrode itself is irritating, change its location daily and keep its site as clean and dry as possible. If you use only 3 leads of a 4- or 5-lead cable, unused lead receptacles must be plugged to prevent interference.

Documentation
Record the date and time that monitoring begins and the lead used. Document cardiac rhythm and rate at least every hour and whenever arrhythmias occur. Mark the rhythm strip with the patient's name, date, time, and the lead used. Document lead changes by running a printout of the new pattern, and include reasons for the changes.

Arterial pressure monitoring

Arterial pressure monitoring provides continuous and accurate arterial pressure readings from an existing arterial line through a transducer that converts blood pressure into electrical impulses. These electrical impulses are displayed on a monitor screen and recorded on paper tape. In addition, a visible and audible alarm sounds when pressure exceeds preset limits. Arterial monitoring also shows blood pressure wave configuration, providing information about circulatory system physiology and function.

This procedure is commonly indicated in patients receiving vasoactive drugs and those with an altered hemodynamic status related to variations in cardiac output, hypertensive crisis, dysrhythmias, or shock. The transducer for arterial pressure monitoring may simply be added to an existing arterial line, or all necessary equipment may have to be assembled. Arterial pressure monitoring itself has no contraindications; however, insertion of an arterial line is contraindicated in a patient with severe coagulopathy unless the benefits outweigh the risks of bleeding and thrombosis.

Equipment

To add a standard transducer: transducer dome/transducer/transducer mount/3′ to 4′ pressure tubing/2 three-way stopcocks/monitoring equipment.

To add a miniature transducer: transducer/three-way stopcock/monitoring equipment/isolation dome (optional).

To assemble a complete setup: transducer, dome, and mount (or miniature transducer with isolation dome, if desired)/pressure cuff/500-ml bag of normal saline solution/heparin injectable 1:1,000/I.V. pole/3-ml syringe with 22G 1″ needle/alcohol sponges/medication-added label/nonvented administration set with microdrip chamber/3′ to 4′ pressure tubing (for standard transducer)/continuous flush device/6″ extension pressure tubing/5 three-way stopcocks (3 for standard transducer, 2 for miniature transducer)/male adapter plugs/dead-end caps/monitoring equipment.

Prepackaged I.V. equipment is available in various combinations, including complete sets. Some sets include two stopcocks, one for each side of the continuous flush device. Isolation units,

which act as a dome for the miniature transducer, eliminate the need for sterilization.

Procedure

To add a standard transducer to an existing arterial line:

Explain the procedure to the patient.

Attach a stopcock to the long length of pressure tubing and activate the fast flush release to clear the existing line.

Turn off the stopcock in the fluid line to the patient and disconnect the continuous flush device. Then connect the stopcock on the pressure tubing to the continuous flush device, open it to the fluid, and activate the fast flush release until the tubing and stopcock fill.

Turn the stopcock off to the pressure tubing, hold the stopcock port venting to air upright until filled, and put on a dead-end cap. Turn it off to this port.

Connect the free end of the pressure tubing to the patient and open the distal stopcock to the patient and fluid.

Attach the transducer dome to the transducer, following the manufacturer's instructions, and mount it on the I.V. pole.

Place a stopcock on one dome port (the upright one, if present), and open it to air and the dome.

Plug the transducer into the monitor; then zero and calibrate the monitor according to the manufacturer's instructions.

Turn the stopcock on the continuous flush device so it is shut off to the patient. Remove the dead-end cap from the device and attach it to the free port on the transducer dome. Then activate the fast flush release and fill the dome with fluid until it flows from the stopcock. Shut off this stopcock so that fluid flows from both ports, and place dead-end caps on these ports.

Turn the stopcock on the continuous flush device so it is shut off to the free port; then activate the fast flush release to clear the line.

Adjust the stopcock port on the transducer dome to the height of the right atrium. To do this, first locate the level

Troubleshooting Cardiac Monitors

PROBLEM	POSSIBLE CAUSES	SOLUTIONS
Artifact (waveform interference)	• Patient experiencing seizures, chills, or anxiety	• Notify doctor and treat patient as ordered. Keep patient warm and reassure him.
	• Patient movement	• Help patient relax.
	• Electrodes applied improperly	• Check electrodes and reapply, if necessary.
	• Static electricity	• Make sure cables do not have exposed connectors. Change static-causing bedclothes.
	• Electrical short circuit in lead wires or cable	• Replace broken equipment. Use stress loops when applying lead wires.
	• Interference from decreased room humidity	• Regulate humidity to 40%.
Broken lead wires or cable	• Stress loops not used on lead wires	• Replace lead wires and retape them, using stress loops.
	• Cables and lead wires cleaned with alcohol or acetone, causing brittleness	• Clean cable and lead wires with soapy water. *Do not allow cable ends to become wet.* Replace cable as necessary.
60-cycle interference (fuzzy baseline)	• Electrical interference from other equipment in room	• Attach all electrical equipment to common ground. Check plugs to make sure prongs are not loose.
	• Patient's bed improperly grounded	• Attach bed ground to the room's common ground.

PROBLEM	POSSIBLE CAUSES	SOLUTIONS
False high-rate alarm	• Monitor interpreting large T waves as QRS complexes, doubling the rate. • Skeletal muscle activity	• Reposition electrodes to lead where QRS complexes are taller than T waves. • Place electrodes away from major muscle masses.
False low-rate alarm	• Shift in electrical axis from patient movement, making QRS complexes too small to register • Low amplitude of QRS • Poor contact between electrode and skin	• Reapply electrodes. Set *gain* so height of complex is greater than 1 millivolt. • Increase gain. • Reapply electrodes.
Low amplitude	• Gain dial set too low • Poor contact between skin and electrodes; dried gel; broken or loose lead wires; poor connection between patient and monitor; malfunctioning monitor; physiologic loss of QRS amplitude	• Increase gain. • Check connections on all lead wires and monitoring cable. Replace as necessary. Reapply electrodes, if required.
Wandering baseline	• Poor position or contact between electrodes and skin • Thoracic movement with respirations	• Reposition or replace electrodes. • Reposition electrodes.

of the fourth intercostal space at the sternum. Next, measure the depth of the chest at this level and place a mark at one half the anterior-posterior distance (midaxillary line). Finally, adjust the stopcock port on the transducer on the pole to the proper height.

To add a miniature transducer:
Explain the procedure to the patient.

Plug the transducer into the monitor, then zero and calibrate the monitor according to the manufacturer's instructions.

Activate the fast flush release to clear the line; then shut off the stopcock to the patient. Remove the dead-end cap from the continuous flush device and attach one side port of another stopcock. Open this stopcock's middle port to air and activate the fast flush release until fluid flows from it. Place a dead-end cap on this port, prime the opposite port, and attach the miniature transducer.

Open both stopcocks to the line and close them to the free port; then activate the fast flush release to clear the line.

Make sure the transducer is level with the patient's right atrium.

For any assembly:
Record systolic, diastolic, and mean pressure readings and obtain strip chart recordings, if desired.

Observe the pressure waveform on the monitor screen. Notify the doctor of any changes.

Set the monitor alarms about 20 mm Hg above and below the patient's normal pressures, depending on his condition. Keep the alarms on at all times.

Activate the fast flush release at intervals specified by institution policy to prevent thrombus formation. Take pressure readings, as ordered.

Frequently check the patient's pulse and color and the temperature of the involved extremity. Notify the doctor of any changes.

Special considerations
• Always use aseptic technique and observe electrical hazard precautions. Remember that pressure readings can be altered by a clot in the catheter, occlusion of the catheter tip against the artery wall, or air or a leak in the system. Prevent these by checking all connections, removing all air from the system, flushing the line at specified intervals, and making sure the pressure cuff reaches 300 mm Hg.

• Generally, you should recalibrate the monitoring equipment at the beginning of your shift. If there is any doubt as to the accuracy of the monitored arterial pressure, take a cuff pressure reading.

• Inspect and redress the insertion site with povidone-iodine ointment every 24 hours, using aseptic technique and gloves. Mark the dressing with the date, time, and your initials. The monitoring apparatus that contacts the I.V. fluid should be replaced every 24 to 48 hours to aid infection control.

• Dextrose 5% in water is sometimes used as the I.V. solution, because it is not a plasma expander and does not conduct electricity. (See *Troubleshooting Hemodynamic Pressure Monitoring*, pages 304 and 305.)

Documentation
Begin a flowchart of pressure readings. Record the date and time of monitoring, the type of arterial line, and the arterial wave shape and changes.

Pulmonary artery and capillary wedge pressure monitoring

This procedure uses a balloon-tipped, flow-directed catheter, connected to a transducer and a monitor, to measure pulmonary artery pressure (PAP) and pulmonary capillary wedge pressure (PCWP). Monitoring these pressures helps assess ventricular capacity to receive and eject blood. It is also helpful in detecting complications of acute MI, as well as providing information about vascular volume status and evaluating the effectiveness of drug therapy.

The pulmonary artery catheter can have two to five lumens for multiple measurements and wires for atrial or ventricular pacing. It is inserted by the doctor either percutaneously into the subclavian, jugular, or femoral vein, or through a venous cutdown in the antecubital fossa, and threaded to the junction of the vena cava and right atrium. After the balloon is inflated, venous circulation carries the catheter tip through the right atrium and ventricle to a branch of the pulmonary artery, where the balloon will wedge in a vessel lumen smaller than itself. When the balloon is deflated, the catheter drifts out of this wedged position and into its normal resting place. Catheter progress is usually followed by changes in waveforms on a cardiac monitor; it can also be tracked fluoroscopically. Once the catheter is in place, PAP can be monitored continuously and PCWP taken as required. Pulmonary artery catheterization must be performed carefully in a patient with an implanted pacemaker or left bundle branch block.

Equipment
Balloon-tipped, flow-directed pulmonary artery catheter/pressure cuff/500-ml bag of normal saline solution/heparin injectable 1:1,000/3-ml syringe with 22G 1″ needle/alcohol sponges/medication-added label/nonvented I.V. administration set with microdrip chamber/3′ to 4′ pressure tubing/continuous flush device/transducer/transducer dome/6″ extension pressure tubing/3 three-way stopcocks/male adapter plug/two dead-end caps/I.V. pole with transducer mount/monitor/razor, washcloth, basin, and towel (if femoral insertion site is used)/250 ml of normal saline solution heparinized with 1 unit heparin, 1:1,000/ml/introducer, one size larger than catheter/sterile gowns/masks/sterile gloves/sterile tray containing instruments for procedure/two 10-ml syringes/one 5-ml syringe/povidone-iodine solution/1% to 2% lidocaine/25G ½″ needle/1″ and 3″ tape/emergency resuscitation equipment/electrocardiogram (EKG) monitor/EKG electrodes/syringe for taking PCWP/armboard for antecubital insertion/lead aprons (if insertion is done under fluoroscopic guidance)/carbon dioxide for balloon inflation (optional).

Prepackaged equipment for the fluid line is available in various combinations, including complete sets. Some sets incorporate an additional stopcock—one for each side of the continuous flush device. If a miniature transducer is being used, the long length of pressure tubing, one stopcock, and the transducer dome and mount are not necessary, since the transducer is strapped to the patient's arm, and usually does not require a dome. However, transducer domes are now available and are used so the miniature transducer will not require sterilization.

Procedure
Explain the procedure to the patient to allay his fears and promote his cooperation. Make sure he has signed a consent form and that he understands what it means.

Place the EKG electrodes on the patient, if they are not already in place, and connect them to the monitor. For a subclavian approach, keep the electrodes on the opposite side of the patient's chest from the insertion site.

Bring the equipment to the same side of the patient as the insertion site.

To zero and calibrate the system:

Place the transducer dome at the height of the right atrium, and locate the level of the fourth intercostal space at the sternum. Then measure the depth of the chest at this level, and place a mark at one-half the anterior-posterior distance (midaxillary line). Next, adjust the transducer on the pole to the proper height. This usually is not necessary with a miniature transducer as long as it is taped to the patient's arm.

Plug the transducer cable into the monitor.

Remove the dead-end cap and open the stopcock on the transducer dome (if you are using a miniature transducer, open the stopcock closest to the dome) to open the transducer to air.

Troubleshooting Hemodynamic Pressure Monitoring

PROBLEM	POSSIBLE CAUSES	SOLUTIONS
No wave-form	• Power supply turned off. • Monitor screen pressure range set too low. • Loose connection in line • Transducer not connected to amplifier. • Stopcock off to patient. • Catheter occluded or out of blood vessel.	• Check power supply. • Raise monitor screen pressure range, if necessary. Rebalance and recalibrate equipment. • Tighten loose connections. • Check and tighten connection. • Position stopcock correctly. • Use fast-flush valve to flush line. • Try to aspirate blood from catheter. If the line still will not flush, notify the doctor and prepare to replace the line.
Drifing waveforms	• Improper warm-up • Electrical cable kinked or compressed. • Temperature change in room air or I.V. flush solution.	• Allow monitor and transducer to warm up for 10 to 15 minutes. • Place monitor's cable where it cannot be stepped on or compressed. • Routinely zero and calibrate equipment 30 minutes after setting it up. This allows I.V. fluid to warm to room temperature.
Line fails to flush	• Stopcocks positioned incorrectly. • Inadequate pressure from pressure bag • Kink in pressure tubing or blood clot in catheter	• Make sure stopcocks are positioned correctly. • Make sure pressure bag gauge reads 300 mm Hg. • Check pressure tubing for kinks. • Try to aspirate the clot with a syringe. • If the line still will not flush, notify the doctor and prepare to replace the line, if necessary. *Important:* Never use a syringe to *flush* a hemodynamic line.
Artifact (waveform interference)	• Patient movement • Electrical interference • Catheter fling (tip of pulmonary artery catheter moving rapidly in large blood vessel or heart chamber)	• Wait until the patient is quiet before taking a reading. • Make sure electrical equipment is connected and grounded correctly. • Notify the doctor. He may try to reposition the catheter.

PROBLEM	POSSIBLE CAUSES	SOLUTIONS
Falsely high readings	• Transducer balancing port positioned below patient's right atrium.	• Position balancing port level with the patient's right atrium.
	• Flush solution flow rate is too fast.	• Check flush solution flow rate. Maintain it at 3 to 4 ml/hour.
	• Air in system	• Remove air from the lines and the transducer.
	• Catheter fling (tip of pulmonary artery catheter moving rapidly in large blood vessel or heart chamber)	• Notify the doctor. He may try to reposition the catheter.
Falsely low readings	• Transducer balancing port positioned above right atrium.	• Position balancing port level with the patient's right atrium.
	• Transducer imbalance	• Make sure the transducer's flow system is not kinked or occluded, and rebalance and recalibrate the equipment.
	• Loose connection	• Tighten loose connections.
Damped waveform	• Air bubbles	• Secure all connections. • Remove air from lines and transducer. • Check for and replace cracked equipment. • Refer to "Line fails to flush" above.
	• Blood clot in catheter	• Make sure stopcock positions are correct.
	• Blood flashback in line	• Tighten loose connections and replace cracked equipment. • Flush line with fast-flush valve. • Replace the transducer dome if blood backs up into it. • Reposition if the catheter is against vessel wall.
	• Transducer position	• Try to aspirate blood to confirm proper placement in the vessel. If you cannot aspirate blood, notify the doctor and prepare to replace the line. *Note:* Bloody drainage at the insertion site may indicate catheter displacement. Notify the doctor immediately.

Zero and calibrate the monitor according to the manufacturer's directions. Then replace the dead-end cap and close the stopcock to this port.

Make sure all stopcocks are set properly.

Observe the monitor for pulmonary artery systolic (PAS) and diastolic (PAD) waveforms, and obtain waveform strips for documentation and baseline reference.

Record PAS, PAD, and mean values (some monitors record this continuously; others require manual setting).

To take a PCWP reading:

Make sure the machine is set to monitor mean pressure.

To the balloon port, attach a syringe of the size specified on the catheter shaft, filled with the maximum amount of air or carbon dioxide.

Slowly inject the gas from the syringe into the balloon while observing the monitor screen, and inject only until the PAP waveform changes to the PCWP waveform. The PCWP waveform often occurs before the maximum amount of gas is injected but depends on the size of the pulmonary artery. Close the port lock to hold pressure in the balloon until a mean pressure is obtained.

Record the mean pressure.

Remove the syringe and leave the port lock in the open position to allow gas to escape and to prevent the balloon from remaining inflated accidentally.

Check on the monitor waveform screen to verify that the catheter has returned to a pulmonary artery position.

According to hospital policy, activate the fast flush release to flush the catheter, which helps reposition the catheter tip.

Set the high and low rate alarms about 20 mm Hg above and below the patient's normal pressures, depending on his condition. Keep the alarms on at *all* times.

Activate the fast flush release at intervals specified by the institution's policy to prevent thrombus formation.

Take pressure readings, as ordered, and ensure that the pressure cuff maintains 300 mm Hg of pressure. Zero and

calibrate the monitor as specified by the manufacturer.

Frequently check the involved extremity for pulse, color, temperature, and sensation, and notify the doctor of any changes.

Change the catheter dressing when it becomes wet or soiled or at intervals specified by the institution's policy.

Special considerations

• Use aseptic technique throughout the procedure to prevent infection. Prevent exsanguination from a disconnection in the system by using Luer-Loks or other positive locks at all connections, keeping the catheter and all parts of the system unobscured and making sure the monitor is on at all times. Always observe electrical hazard precautions.

• Tubing, stopcocks, continuous flush devices, and fluid for infusion should be changed every 24 to 48 hours, depending on the institution's policy, to aid infection control.

• Positive pressure ventilation may alter the patient's reading in any direction. Pressures should be recorded with the patient on the ventilator.

• Dextrose 5% in water is sometimes used as the I.V. solution because it is not a plasma expander and doesn't conduct an electrical current.

• Note the volume of gas needed to achieve a wedge. Because carbon dioxide diffuses through the balloon at approximately ½ ml/minute, it may be difficult to estimate this, and it may be hard to achieve a wedge. If the volume of gas required for a wedge is significantly below that indicated on the catheter, notify the doctor, since the catheter may have migrated distally. You should feel resistance when inflating the balloon. If you do not, notify the doctor immediately—the balloon may have ruptured.

• Never introduce air into a balloon if you suspect it is ruptured; this can cause an air embolus. Prevent balloon rupture by knowing the maximum volume of the balloon, and avoid overinflating the balloon or aspirating from it. Do not leave the balloon wedged for more than 1 to 2 minutes—even less in the elderly patient or one with pulmonary hypertension. Air in the flush system can also cause an embolus.

• If the waveform will not return to pulmonary arterial from a wedge, or if it is dampening with low numbers and decreased PAS-PAD differential, check for equipment problems. Then check the patient's blood pressure and pulse. If these are not changed, the catheter is probably wedged. Because a permanent wedge can cause pulmonary infarct and necrosis, immediately activate the fast flush release, which can push the catheter tip away from a vessel wall. Then check for a slowed drip rate and increased pressure readings—signs that the catheter is still wedged. If it is, turn the patient on his right side and instruct him to cough as you flush the line. If the waveform does not return to pulmonary arterial, turn the patient onto his left side and repeat the procedure. If there is still no change, notify the doctor immediately.

• Large volumes of fluid and drugs should not be given through the distal port, since vessel spasm or rupture may result.

• Thrombosis can result from local irritation from the catheter; the heparinized flush helps prevent thrombus formation. Thromboembolus can occur if a thrombus breaks off and lodges in the circulatory system.

Documentation

Record the time, size and type of catheter inserted, insertion site, vital signs, administration of drugs (if any), initial PAP and PCWP readings and tracings, and the patient's tolerance of the procedure. Start a flowsheet of PAP readings and tracings, noting any changes.

Central venous pressure monitoring

CVP measurements are monitored with a manometer connected to a catheter that is threaded through the subclavian or jugular vein (or, less commonly, the basilic, cephalic, or saphenous veins) and placed in or near the right atrium. This procedure allows accurate determination of right atrial blood pressure, which reflects right ventricular pressure; in effect, this indicates the capacity of the right heart to receive and eject blood. CVP is also used to assess blood volume.

Because CVP rises only after significant changes have occurred in the left heart or pulmonary venous system due to a relatively great amount of damage or for reasons other than left heart changes, CVP monitoring is being replaced in many hospitals by monitoring through the pulmonary artery or (PA) catheterization for assessing rapidly changing cardiovascular status. PA catheterization detects cardiovascular changes immediately, before they cause changes in the CVP. However, CVP measurement is still the procedure of choice for postoperative monitoring during hemorrhage or for assessing hydration status to determine fluid replacement.

CVP usually ranges from 3 to 15 cmH_2O, but it varies with the patient's size, and whether he's on his side. Only relative changes in CVP are significant.

Equipment

Disposable CVP manometer set with stopcock, extension tubing, and leveling device/I.V. pole/container of I.V. solution, as ordered/I.V. tubing/optional: nonallergenic tape, indelible marker.

Procedure

Explain the procedure to the patient to allay his fears and promote cooperation.

Loosen the protective cover on the distal end of the extension tubing (from the stopcock to the patient), and ask the patient to perform Valsalva's maneuver to avoid formation of an air embolus. Quickly disconnect the existing I.V. tubing, remove the protective covering from the new tubing, and connect it to the patient's catheter.

If the patient is unconscious, wait until he inhales fully and begins to exhale, and then quickly connect the tubing. Lowering the head of the bed is also helpful in preventing an air embolus in a patient who is unable to cooperate. Finally, adjust the flow clamp to the desired infusion rate.

Place the patient in the supine position. Research shows that adjusting the bed to the horizontal position is not necessary for accurate monitoring as long as the zero mark on the manometer remains at the zero reference point.

Adjust the position of the manometer so that the stopcock aligns horizontally with the right atrium.

To find the position of the right atrium, first locate the fourth intercostal space at the sternum. Then measure the depth of the patient's chest from front to back at this level. Divide the depth in half and mark the site with an indelible marker or a strip of nonallergenic tape. This site becomes the *zero reference point*—the location for all subsequent readings.

If the manometer has a leveling rod, extend it between the zero reference point and the zero mark at the bottom of the manometer scale. If the rod has a small viewing window, a bubble will appear between two lines in the window when the rod is horizontal. If a leveling rod is not available, use a yardstick with a level attached. With this you can also watch the bubble for the level.

Recheck the level before each pressure reading. If an adjustment is necessary, first raise or lower the bed and then readjust the manometer on the I.V. pole, if necessary, to maintain alignment with the atrium.

Check the patency of the line by briefly increasing the infusion rate. If the line is not patent, notify the doctor. To avoid possible release of a thrombus, never irrigate a clogged CVP line. If the line is patent, proceed.

Turn the stopcock to the container-to-manometer position to slowly fill the manometer with I.V. solution, as before.

Turn the stopcock to the manometer-to-patient position; the fluid level then falls with inspiration, as intrathoracic pressure decreases, and rises slightly with expiration.

When the fluid column stabilizes (usually between 3 and 15 cmH$_2$O), tap the manometer lightly to dislodge air bubbles that may distort pressure readings. Then position yourself so that the top of the fluid column is at eye level. Expect the column to rise and fall slightly during breathing. Note the *lowest* level the fluid reaches, and take your reading from the base of the meniscus. If the manometer has a small ball floating on the fluid surface, take the reading from the ball's midline. If the fluid fails to fluctuate during breathing, the end of the catheter may be pressed against the vein wall. Ask the patient to cough to change the catheter's position slightly.

Maintain catheter patency by returning the stopcock to the container-to-patient position as soon as you take the reading.

Readjust the infusion rate and be sure all connections are secure to minimize the risk of hemorrhage or an air embolus. (Some hospital policies recommend taping all connections for these reasons.)

Return the patient to a comfortable position.

Special considerations

• If the patient is connected to a ventilator and is receiving positive end-expiratory pressure, expect high CVP readings. To detect significant changes, record all pressure readings while the patient is connected to the ventilator. However, if the patient's condition permits, some hospitals allow you to disconnect the ventilator for all CVP readings and reconnect it immediately after the procedure.

• Report any deviations from the prescribed CVP range to the doctor. Remember that the patient with chronic obstructive pulmonary disease (COPD) usually has a high CVP.

Alternate Methods of Measuring Cardiac Output

In the **dye dilution test,** a known volume and concentration of dye is injected into the pulmonary artery and measured by simultaneously sampling the amount of dye in the brachial artery. To calculate cardiac output, these values are entered into a formula or plotted into a time–and–dilution-concentration curve. A minicomputer like the one used for the thermodilution test does the computation. Dye dilution measurements are particularly helpful in detecting intracardiac shunts and valvular regurgitation.

In the **Fick method,** the blood's oxygen content is measured before and after it passes through the lungs. First, blood is removed from the pulmonary and the brachial arteries and is analyzed for oxygen content. Then, a spirometer measures oxygen consumption—the amount of air entering the lungs each minute. After this, cardiac output is calculated by the following formula:

$$CO \text{ (liter/min)} = \frac{\text{oxygen consumption (ml/min)}}{\text{arterial oxygen content} - \text{venous oxygen content (ml/min)}}$$

A doctor usually performs this procedure at the patient's bedside, using a pulmonary artery catheter. The Fick method is especially useful in detecting low cardiac output levels.

Documentation

Record the time, date, and pressure reading on either a flow sheet or nursing cardex.

Cardiac output measurement

Measuring cardiac output—the amount of blood ejected from the heart—helps evaluate cardiac function. Normal output is 4 to 8 liters/minute. Low cardiac output can result from decreased myocardial contractility due to MI, drugs, acidosis, or hypoxia. Other possible causes are decreased left ventricular filling pressure due to fluid depletion or increased systemic vascular resistance due to arteriosclerosis or hypertension. Cardiac output can also fall below normal as a result of decreased blood flow from the ventricles due to valvular heart disease. High cardiac output can occur with some arteriovenous shunts or from hyperthyroidism or anxiety; it may be normal in athletes.

Cardiac output is usually measured indirectly by the thermodilution technique. Two other methods—the Fick technique and the dye dilution test—are used mostly in research and in some cardiac catheterization laboratories. In the thermodilution technique, a balloon-tipped, flow-directed catheter with four or five lumens is inserted into a vein. Normal venous circulation carries the catheter tip through the right side of the heart and into the pulmonary artery. A chilled or room temperature solution is injected into the right atrium through the proximal lumen of the catheter. A minicomputer then calculates cardiac output from temperature changes detected by a thermistor in the catheter tip, and the cardiac output is displayed on a digital readout. Two nurses are usually needed to perform this procedure—one to inject the solution, the other to operate the minicomputer. However, this procedure can be done by one nurse, depending on the type of equipment available.

Equipment

Cardiac output minicomputer/centigrade thermometer (if the minicomputer does not have a temperature probe)/basin/two bags of dextrose 5% in water or normal saline solution/heparin inject-able/3-ml syringe with 1″ needle/straight I.V. administration set/three-way stop-cock/10-ml syringe/large-gauge needle/alcohol sponges/gun injector (optional). If desired, an additional piece of I.V. tubing can be used to lengthen the setup. Some new minicomputers measure tem-perature directly from the pulmonary artery, making it unnecessary to inject a solution unless the patient is connected to a respirator, has an erratic breathing pattern, or has an estimated cardiac out-put of more than 10 liters/minute.

Procedure

Wash your hands.

Explain the procedure to the patient and provide privacy. Inform him that you are going to inject a solution through the catheter to help evaluate cardiac function. Assure him that he will not experience any discomfort.

After the doctor inserts the thermo-dilution catheter, connect the minicom-puter cable to the catheter thermistor port. Then take the patient's tempera-ture and record it.

Immerse both bags of solution (ex-cept for the ports) in the ice water.

Open the main port of the bag with-out the heparin, and pierce it with the large-gauge needle.

Place the thermometer probe or the centigrade thermometer into the pierced port. The probe or thermometer deter-mines the baseline temperature of the solution.

Using an alcohol sponge, clean the main port of the bag containing the hep-arin. Insert the administration set spike.

Attach the sterile stopcock to the op-posite end of the tubing and, if desired, add additional tubing to the parallel stopcock port.

Hold the bag with the port upright, open the flow clamp, and squeeze air from the bag to avoid introducing an air embolus.

Invert the bag and prime the tubing. Then move the stopcock to all positions.

Next, connect the additional tubing or the stopcock itself to the catheter's prox-imal hub.

Attach the 10-ml syringe to the stop-cock's free port and rest it on the mini-computer cart or a table to avoid strain-ing the line.

Turn on the minicomputer and cali-brate it according to the manufacturer's instructions.

When the temperature of the solution reaches 32° F. (0° C.), turn the stopcock toward the patient and fill the syringe with exactly 10 ml of solution. Then turn the stopcock toward the bag of solution.

Start to inject the solution as your assistant depresses the start button on the minicomputer. Inject the solution within 2 to 3 seconds so it reaches the circulation as a bolus. Otherwise, the thermistor will not accurately detect the peak temperature change, causing inac-curate results.

Record the cardiac output and, after 1 minute, inject more solution. Then record output again, wait 1 minute, and inject more solution.

After measuring the patient's cardiac output, turn the stopcock off to all posi-tions.

Special considerations

• Place the patient in the supine position or with his head slightly elevated for this procedure. Before injecting the solution, make sure the catheter is not wedged in the pulmonary artery, because this can cause false high readings and can also damage the artery. If ordered, calculate the cardiac index—cardiac output/square meter of body surface area—since it is a more specific and useful measurement than cardiac output. (See *Alternate Methods of Measuring Car-diac Output*, page 309.)

Documentation

Record the average or highest cardiac output, as dictated by institution policy. Document the amount and type of solu-tion on the input and output sheet.

15

TREATMENT PROCEDURES

Today, more nurses than ever before participate in the diagnosis, treatment, and prevention of cardiovascular disorders. Their responsibilities may include procedures unknown a decade ago. To accommodate these expanding responsibilities, many states have revised their Nurse Practice Acts. Qualified nurses may now routinely perform such complex procedures as carotid massage, cardiopulmonary resuscitation (CPR), and defibrillation; they may also assist with pericardiocentesis and pacemaker implantation. These role changes have expanded nursing accountability. Today, you're legally required to fully understand the doctor's orders, correctly perform ordered procedures, monitor the patient's response to therapy, and know how to use sophisticated equipment.

NONINVASIVE THERAPY

Carotid massage

Carotid massage is the application of manual pressure to the left or right carotid sinus to slow the heart rate. The carotid sinuses are located slightly above the bifurcations of the carotid arteries in the neck; their nerve endings respond to changes such as pressure as to an increase in blood pressure and relay this message to the vasomotor centers in the brain stem. This, in turn, stimulates the autonomic nervous system to increase vagal tone and slows the heart rate. Peripheral blood vessels then dilate, reducing cardiac output and lowering arterial pressure as much as 20 mm Hg in a normal patient.

Carotid massage is used to diagnose and treat sinus, atrial, and junctional tachydysrhythmias. Although usually performed by a doctor, it is occasionally done by a specially trained nurse under a doctor's supervision. This procedure requires continuous electrocardiogram (EKG) monitoring as pressure is applied, first to one sinus and then to the other, each time for no longer than 5 seconds. Pressure should never be applied simultaneously to both sinuses, because this may cause complete asystole or significant impairment, or both, of cerebral blood flow. Massage is stopped when any sign of rhythm change appears on the EKG monitor.

Carotid massage is contraindicated in patients with systolic blood pressure below 100 mm Hg, cerebrovascular disease or carotid artery disease (CAD), or hypersensitive carotid sinuses.

Equipment
EKG monitor/crash cart/I.V. setup with dextrose 5% in water/cardiotonic drugs, as ordered.

Procedure
Explain the procedure to the patient to allay his fears and ensure his cooperation. Place him in the supine position.

Prepare the patient's skin appropriately and attach EKG electrodes.

Start an I.V. line with dextrose 5% in water at a keep-vein-open rate, as ordered, to provide a route for emergency drug administration.

Auscultate both carotid arteries to detect bruits; if present, do not perform carotid massage.

Locate the bifurcation of the carotid

artery on the right side of the patient's neck by turning his head slightly to the left and hyperextending his neck. This brings the carotid artery closer to the skin and moves the sternocleidomastoid muscle away from the carotid artery.

Using a circular motion, gently massage the right carotid sinus between your fingertips and the transverse processes of the spine for 3 to 5 seconds. Monitor the EKG throughout the procedure and release the artery as soon as any evidence of a rhythm change appears.

If this procedure has no effect within 5 seconds, stop massaging the right carotid sinus and massage the left. If this also fails, administer cardiotonic drugs, as ordered.

Always stop after 5 seconds (or sooner if conversion to sinus rhythm or unacceptable bradycardia occurs) or if the ventricular rate slows sufficiently to permit diagnosis of the rhythm. If severe bradycardia persists or asystole occurs, be prepared to give emergency treatment.

Special considerations

• Avoid vigorous massage, especially if carotid atherosclerosis is present, because this procedure may cause embolization of plaque material and cerebrovascular accident. Although arterial pressure may fall profoundly during massage, especially in the elderly patient with heart disease, it usually rises quickly afterward.
• If the procedure is successful, continue to monitor the patient for several hours. Be aware that conversion to normal sinus rhythm may be preceded by brief asystole or several premature ventricular contractions, or both.

Documentation

Record the date and time of the procedure; your name; frequency and duration of massage; EKG rhythm changes and drug administration, if applicable; and changes in the patient's condition.

Elective cardioversion

Like defibrillation, elective cardioversion attempts to restore the sinoatrial (SA) node to its function as the heart's natural pacemaker. This procedure is performed in much the same way as defibrillation, except that the synchronizer switch is activated and much less energy is needed (25 to 50 joules, or watt-seconds). The discharge buttons on the paddles or defibrillator must be held down because the shock is not triggered until the next QRS complex occurs. This helps prevent ventricular fibrillation, which may result from an improperly timed shock. Usually performed by a doctor, the procedure is elective, requiring the patient's consent; he is then sedated before cardioversion begins.

Cardioversion is used to convert refractory atrial, junctional, and ventricular tachydysrhythmias to normal sinus rhythm. It is contraindicated in patients with digitalis toxicity.

Equipment

EKG monitor/I.V. infusion equipment/cardioverter with synchronizer/emergency drug cart/suction equipment.

Procedure

Explain the procedure to the patient and provide privacy. To avoid alarming him, do not use the word "shock" in your explanation. Instead, tell him that cardioversion uses an electric current to slow down the heart rate and relieve symptoms.

Make sure he or a responsible family member understands and signs a consent form.

Instruct the patient to abstain from food and fluids for at least 7 or 8 hours, and withhold digitalis for 24 to 36 hours. If you suspect digitalis toxicity, the doctor will probably order the patient's digitalis level taken. Cardioversion usually is delayed until the digitalis level is normal. In many institutions, a potassium blood level is obtained and documented

Glossary of Terms

If you are unfamiliar with pacemaker terminology, the subject will seem more complex than necessary. To make things easier, get acquainted with these common terms.

Capture. A pacemaker's ability to cause atrial or ventricular depolarization.

Competition. Paced beats occurring simultaneously with spontaneous beats—a risk with fixed-rate pacemakers. If competition occurs during the vulnerable period of the cardiac cycle (indicated on EKG by a spike on the T wave), it could trigger ventricular tachycardia or ventricular fibrillation.

MA. An abbreviation for *milliampere*, the voltage measurement used for setting threshold.

Noncapture. Failure of a pacemaker to cause atrial or ventricular depolarization.

Oversensing. Inappropriate pacemaker inhibition from the pacemaker's sensing (and being inhibited by) something other than intrinsic atrial or ventricular depolarization; for example, electrical activity from skeletal muscle contraction or T waves.

Pacemaker syndrome. Fatigue, dizziness, and dyspnea associated with a fall in sinus rate at the onset of ventricular pacing. Caused by loss of AV synchrony, it may follow exercise.

Sensing. A pacemaker's ability to detect atrial or ventricular depolarization.

Threshold (stimulation threshold). The electrical energy needed to obtain capture. Threshold is affected by such factors as fibrosis at the catheter tip, myocardial ischemia, and electrolyte imbalance. As a result, the doctor sets threshold at two to three times the minimum energy needed for capture.

---

prior to this procedure.

Start a peripheral I.V. to administer a sedative or emergency drugs, as ordered.

Attach the patient to the EKG monitor and run a 12-lead tracing to detect dysrhythmias. Leave the limb electrodes in place for later recordings. Place chest electrodes in position to obtain the tallest R wave; in most patients this chest lead would be modified lead II or midclavicular. Make sure the electrodes do not interfere with cardioverter paddle placement.

Attach the cardioverter to the monitor and turn on the synchronizer switch or button. Make sure the synchronizer artifact falls on the R wave; if the cardioverter does not recognize the R wave, it will not discharge. To increase the R wave, increase sensitivity, but make sure not to increase the T wave to the height where the cardioverter recognizes it; or select another lead that shows a larger R wave.

Place the patient in the supine position, and avoid raising his head more than 30°. Have an emergency crash cart ready in case symptomatic bradycardia or ventricular dysrhythmias occur. If the patient has loosely fitting dentures, remove them to prevent airway obstruction after sedation. However, if they fit properly, leave them in place to make airway management easier.

Bare the male patient's chest, but cover the female patient's breasts with a towel until paddle electrodes are in position.

Administer a sedative, as ordered.

Set the energy level on the cardioverter as ordered (usually 25 or 50 joules). Lubricate the anterior/posterior (A/P) paddle electrodes as for defibrillation. The doctor should now be present to check the patient's sedation level and to perform cardioversion. Make sure the patient is adequately ventilated, and record baseline vital signs prior to car-

Setting the Stimulation Threshold

After a pacemaker is inserted, the stimulation threshold must be determined to maintain myocardial contractions. Turn on the EKG monitor and set the pacemaker's sensitivity control to *fixed* or *demand*, as ordered. During this procedure, run EKG monitor strips as needed and note the MAs on each strip as you adjust the MA level. To determine the stimulation threshold:

• Increase the pacemaker rate above the patient's heart rate, as ordered.

• Increase the MA, as ordered, and watch the EKG carefully for "capture" (as indicated by a pacemaker spike followed by a QRS complex). Stop increasing the MA when 100% capture is achieved. Slowly decrease the MA until you lose capture (electrical stimulus fails to generate a QRS complex).

• Record the threshold as *the lowest MA that achieves capture.*

• Set the MA and pacemaker rate as ordered.

Note the settings on the nursing cardex. As the patient's condition changes, these settings may need to be altered.

cordium, directly over the heart. Apply 20 to 25 pounds of pressure to the electrodes to ensure good skin contact and to prevent burns. Announce "ready stand back," making sure everyone present is away from the bed to prevent inadvertent grounding and shocks.

Depress the discharge button on the anterior paddle electrode, and hold that position until the energy is delivered. (You may have to hold the button a second or more.) Remove the paddle electrodes immediately after the shock. Make sure a normal sinus rhythm is present; if it is not, repeat the procedure at a higher energy level, as ordered.

Special Considerations

• Take a 12-lead EKG and compare it to the preconversion (baseline) EKG. Take the patient's vital signs, immediately after cardioversion and every 15 minutes for at least 1 hour or until stable, and observe his level of consciousness. Make sure his respiratory rate and excursive movements are adequate.

• Observe cardiac rhythm until it stabilizes.

• Watch for complications of cardioversion: ventricular fibrillation, asystole, rhythm disturbances, skin burns, pulmonary edema or embolus, respiratory depression or arrest, hypotension, and ST segment changes.

• When the patient's condition permits, tell him he may begin to eat and move about.

Documentation

Record how patient tolerated the procedure with respect to vital signs, anxiety level, and postconversion assessment.

dioversion, because the sedative may cause apnea or hypotension.

Make sure the cardioverter is still synchronized with the R wave. Push the charge button to raise the machine to the prescribed energy level. (Most machines have a needle indicator that shows energy level.) Turn on the strip chart recorder to document the cardioversion. Also document a strip that validates synchronization of electric impulse with the R wave prior to cardioversion.

If you are performing the procedure, apply A/P paddles. Put the flat paddle under the patient's body, behind the heart and slightly below the left scapula. Place the other paddle over the left pre-

---

INVASIVE THERAPY

Temporary pacemaker insertion and care

When the heart's natural pacemakers fail to maintain a normal heart rate, and cardioactive drugs prove ineffective, an artificial pacemaker may be needed to restore an effective rate. A temporary pacemaker consists of a battery-powered pulse generator which the patient wears on his chest, waist, or upper arm. An electrode catheter transmits electrical impulses from the pacemaker to the patient's heart, and from the heart back to the pacemaker. Pacemakers come in two types: fixed rate, which fires continuously without regard to the patient's heart rate; and demand, the more common type, which senses the patient's rate and fires accordingly. (See *Glossary of Terms*, page 313.)

Usually aided by a fluoroscope, a doctor inserts the electrode catheter percutaneously into a peripheral vein, through the vena cava and right atrium, and into the apex of the right ventricle. In an emergency, a transthoracic approach may be used. The nurse assists by monitoring catheter insertion with the electrocardiograph (EKG) and by maintaining sterile technique. Femoral insertion is contraindicated in patients with thrombophlebitis, recent pulmonary embolism, or severe coagulopathy.

Equipment

Pacemaker pulse generator with battery/ pacemaker catheter/electrode wires/ EKG monitor with oscilloscope and strip chart recorder/emergency resuscitation equipment/alligator clamp/Velcro strap, elastic bandage, or gauze (for securing the pulse generator to the patient)/armboard (if necessary)/tape/shave preparation kit/povidone-iodine and benzoin solutions/1% lidocaine for anesthesia/3- and 5-ml syringes/21G and 25G needles/sterile gloves, gowns, and drapes/ sphygmomanometer/peripheral I.V. setup/4" × 4" sterile gauze sponges/ linen-saver pad.

For insertion of pacemaker by a doctor: vein dilators/large-bore plastic venous catheter/introducer sheaths/Cournand needle/scalpel/suture/venesection tray (these supplies may come prepackaged).

Assessing Capture

When the pacemaker sends an electrical impulse to the heart, it appears on the EKG strip as a vertical line, commonly called the pacemaker spike. When the spike is followed by a QRS complex or P wave, *capture* has occurred.

If the pacemaker electrode rests in the ventricle, a spike appears in front of every QRS complex that is stimulated by the pacemaker. These complexes appear wide and bizarre—similar to those caused by premature ventricular contractions, except that they will not be early. If the electrode's in the atrium, a spike before a P wave indicates that capture has occurred; the P wave may be inverted or may differ in shape from a spontaneous P wave. If electrodes are pacing both the atria and ventricles, spikes will appear before both QRS complexes and P waves.

Because spikes may not appear in every EKG lead, verify capture by checking more than one lead. A lead that reveals pacing spikes well is aVR, because the QRS complexes are small and less likely to obscure the spike.

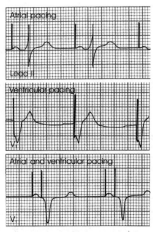

Procedure

Explain the procedure to the patient. Tell him that he will feel some local discomfort at the catheter insertion site. Assure him that the catheter will be in place only temporarily. Inform him that when the catheter is withdrawn, it seldom causes discomfort. Ask if he is allergic to local anesthetics.

Make sure the patient or a responsible family member understands what this procedure involves and signs the consent form.

Provide sedation, as ordered.

Establish an I.V. line at a keep-vein-open rate in the patient's left arm for possible administration of emergency drugs in case of ventricular dysrhythmia.

Connect the patient to the EKG monitor and turn it on.

Establish baseline vital signs and a baseline EKG reading.

Clean the insertion site with povidone-iodine solution, wiping in a circular motion away from the insertion site to minimize the risk of infection. (Some doctors do this themselves.)

The doctor anesthetizes the insertion site and inserts the pacemaker catheter into the vein. Follow the movement of the catheter through the vein on the fluoroscope and watch for dysrhythmias. When the catheter reaches the right atrium, large P waves and small QRS complexes will appear; when it reaches the right ventricle, the QRS complexes become very large and the P waves become smaller. When it contacts the right ventricular endocardium, the monitor will show elevated ST segments (injury current).

Once the catheter is in place, insert the pacemaker leads tightly into their respective slots in the pacemaker generator.

Check the patient's stimulation threshold (see *Setting the Stimulation Threshold*, page 314). When a 1-to-1 capture is achieved, set the milliamperage and pacemaker rate as ordered. (See *Assessing Capture*, page 315.)

The doctor sutures the catheter to the insertion site. He then makes a stress loop of the remaining lead wire and tapes it to the patient's chest.

Secure the pulse generator to the patient's chest, waist, or upper arm, using the Velcro strap, elastic bandage, or elastic gauze.

Place the cap supplied by the manufacturer over the pacer controls to avoid an accidental change in the setting.

After catheter insertion:

Make the patient comfortable and administer pain medication as ordered.

If a femoral or brachial approach was used, immobilize the extremity to avoid stressing the pacing wires. The patient should wiggle fingers or toes to increase circulation and prevent stiffness.

The doctor may order postinsertion studies such as an EKG and chest X-ray. Continuously monitor the patient's heart rhythm and take rhythm strips every hour for 24 hours.

Be sure to note pacemaker settings and include the rate, mode (demand or fixed-rate), and output in milliamperes. (See *Pacemaker Codes: What They Mean,* page 317, and *DDD Versus VVI: Comparing Two Types,* page 319.) Record this information at every shift change; also note if the pacemaker malfunctions or if dysrhythmias occur. The doctor should check the pacemaker's output daily because drugs, electrolyte changes, or ischemia can alter the patient's threshold.

Continue to observe the patient for signs and symptoms of pacemaker malfunction, such as *any* change in pulse rate, dyspnea, fatigue, chest pain, vertigo, distended neck veins, and crepitant rales at the base of the lungs.

Clean the insertion site daily and inspect it for signs of infection, as ordered. Apply povidone-iodine ointment to the site and cover it with a new dressing, as ordered.

Assess circulation in the extremity below the site of insertion by evaluating the distal pulse, color, temperature, and sensation.

Special considerations
• Watch for signs of pacemaker malfunction. (See *Troubleshooting Pacemaker Problems,* pages 320 to 322.)
• Make sure all electrical equipment is grounded with three-pronged plugs inserted in the right receptacles. This protects the patient from accidental shocks to the heart that may cause ventricular fibrillation. Also, cover all exposed metal parts of the pacemaker setup, such as electrode connections or pacemaker terminals, with nonconductive tape to insulate them, or place the pacing unit in a dry rubber surgical glove. Instruct the patient not to use an electric razor or any other nonessential electrical equipment.
• If emergency defibrillation should be necessary, make sure the pacemaker can withstand this procedure before starting it; if not, disconnect it to avoid damaging the generator.
• Protect the pacemaker and its connections from moisture.
• If the patient is disoriented or uncooperative, restrain his arms to prevent accidental removal of pacemaker wires.
• If any evidence of infection is present during catheter implantation, culture disposable pacemaker catheter tips after they are removed.
• Potential complications include: dysrhythmias (asystole following abrupt cessation of pacing; ventricular irritability, resulting in ventricular dysrhythmias, such as ventricular tachycardia); thrombus/embolus (lead-related thrombus or embolism, or inactivity-related thrombus or embolus, both of which may lead to pulmonary embolism); and ventricular rupture (cardiac tamponade resulting from myocardial lead-related hemorrhage, which may lead to cardiac arrest). Complications at the insertion site may include infection, phlebitis, blood vessel occlusion, hemorrhage, or an allergic reaction to the local anesthetic. Pericarditis may also occur.

Documentation
Document the type of pacemaker used; date of insertion; doctor's name; control

Pacemaker Codes: What They Mean
As pacemakers have become more sophisticated, a coding system has been developed to identify their capabilities. The code has five letters, which have the following significance:
• The first letter indicates which heart chamber the pacemaker paces: *A* (atrium), *V* (ventricle), or *D* (dual, or both chambers).
• Using the same abbreviations, the second letter identifies the chamber sensed. (If the second letter of a fixed rate pacemaker is *O*, it has no sensing ability.)
• The third letter indicates pacemaker response to the sensed event. An *I* (inhibited response) means that the pacemaker cannot deliver a stimulus during a preset time interval when it senses spontaneous cardiac activity. A *T* (triggered response) means the pacemaker delivers a stimulus whenever it senses electrical activity. A *D* means that the pacemaker is inhibited and triggered by both atrial and ventricular events. An *O* means no sensing response capability. An *R* (meaning reverse) indicates the ability to respond to a rapid (rather than slow) rate; pacemakers with this capability treat some tachydysrhythmias.
• The fourth letter indicates the pacemaker's ability to be reprogrammed noninvasively.
• The fifth letter indicates how the pacemaker responds to tachycardias; this letter is most significant for antitachycardia pacemakers.
  Most pacemakers are identified by only the first three letters; for example, VVI. Using the preceding information, you can easily interpret such a code: the pacemaker paces the ventricle (V), senses ventricular activity (V), and is inhibited (I) by R waves produced by spontaneous ventricular activity.

settings used; whether or not the pacemaker successfully treated the patient's dysrhythmias, and other pertinent observations. Attach significant portions of the EKG rhythm strip to the record.

Permanent pacemaker insertion and care

Unlike a temporary pacemaker, a permanent pacemaker is self-contained and designed to operate for 3 to 20 years. A surgeon implants a permanent pacemaker in a pocket beneath the patient's skin. This is usually done in the operating room with local or general anesthesia. The nurse assists catheter placement by monitoring the EKG and by maintaining sterile technique.

Permanent pacemakers may be of the fixed rate or demand type; some with an external hand-held unit can be programmed by the doctor to function in either mode after they have been implanted. Candidates for permanent pacemakers include heart attack victims with persistent bradyarrhythmia and patients with complete heart block or slow ventricular rates from congenital or degenerative heart disease or after cardiac surgery. Patients who suffer Stokes-Adams attacks, as well as those with Wolff-Parkinson-White syndrome or sick sinus syndrome, may also benefit from permanent pacemaker implantation.

Equipment
Sphygmomanometer / stethoscope / thermometer/EKG monitor (with oscilloscope and strip-chart recorder)/sterile dressing tray/povidone-iodine ointment/skin preparation kit with razor/sterile gauze dressing/alcohol sponges/nonallergenic tape/emergency resuscitation equipment/scrub gown/mask

Procedure
Explain the procedure to the patient. Provide and review with him literature from the manaufacturer or the American Heart Association so he can learn about the pacemaker and how it works. (See *Patient-Teaching Aid: How to Care for Your Pacemaker*, page 324.) Emphasize that the pacemaker merely augments his natural heart rate and that he will not be in any grave danger if the pacemaker stops working.

Make sure the patient or a responsible family member signs a consent form.

Ask the patient if he is allergic to anesthetics or iodine.

For transvenous pacemaker insertion, shave the patient's chest from the axilla to the midline and from the clavicle to the nipple line on the side selected by the doctor. If the pacemaker is to be inserted in the axilla, shave that area; for epicardial placement, shave from the nipple line to the umbilicus.

Establish an I.V. line at a keep-vein-open rate in the patient's left arm to administer emergency drugs in case of ventricular dysrhythmia.

Establish baseline vital signs and a baseline EKG recording.

Provide sedation, as ordered.

For postoperative care:

Monitor the patient's EKG to check for dysrhythmias. Record a rhythm strip every hour for 24 hours to check for effective pacemaker function.

Also monitor the I.V. flow rate; the I.V. line is usually kept in place for 24 to 48 hours postoperatively to allow for possible emergency treatment of dysrhythmias.

Check the dressing for signs of bleeding, infection, swelling, redness, or exudate. The doctor may order prophylactic antibiotics for up to 7 days after the implantation.

Change the dressing and apply povidone-iodine ointment at least once every 24 hours, or according to doctor's orders and institution policy. If the dressing becomes soiled or the site is exposed to air, change the dressing immediately, regardless of when you last changed it.

Check the patient's vital signs and level of consciousness every 15 minutes for the first hour, every hour for the next 4 hours, every 4 hours for the next 48

DDD Versus VVI: Comparing Two Types

The newest pacemaker type—known by its code, DDD—paces the atria and ventricles, mimicking normal cardiac function. Also called a *universal* pacemaker, a DDD pacemaker stimulates an atrial contraction if the sinoatrial node fails to do so. Then, if the ventricles do not respond spontaneously, it stimulates a ventricular contraction. This system ensures atrial contribution to ventricular filling; it also provides a backup in case the ventricles fail to respond properly.

Because it mimics normal cardiac electrical function, the DDD has these benefits:
• increases ventricular filling time, which in turn increases stroke volume
• increases force of myocardial contractions
• minimizes regurgitation by allowing complete AV valve closure.

Although the DDD has compelling advantages, it is not indicated for everyone. You are more apt to encounter the VVI (ventricular demand) pacemaker, which senses and paces the ventricle at a set rate, unless inhibited by a spontaneous QRS complex. By doing so, it prevents heart rate from slowing dangerously but permits the heart to pace itself when the spontaneous rate is higher than the preset pacemaker rate.

The VVI, although helpful for patients with third-degree AV block, has several disadvantages:
• Because pacemaker activity does not mimic natural function, it does not vary with exercise or rest. Also, paced beats are ectopic, so they do not travel along the normal conduction pathway. This can reduce cardiac output significantly.
• Lack of AV synchrony may contribute to reduced cardiac output and pacemaker syndrome. In addition, spontaneous atrial contractions that occur simultaneously with paced ventricular contractions may cause mitral and tricuspid regurgitation, producing dyspnea.

The diagram below shows how to decipher the codes DDD and VVI. (See also *Pacemaker Codes: What They Mean,* page 317.)

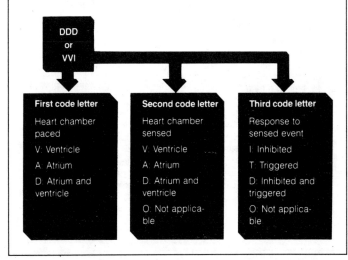

DDD or VVI

First code letter	Second code letter	Third code letter
Heart chamber paced	Heart chamber sensed	Response to sensed event
V: Ventricle	V: Ventricle	I: Inhibited
A: Atrium	A: Atrium	T: Triggered
D: Atrium and ventricle	D: Atrium and ventricle	D: Inhibited and triggered
	O: Not applicable	O: Not applicable

Troubleshooting Pacemaker Problems

Use the following chart as a guide to identifying and dealing with some common problems that affect both permanent and temporary pacemakers. Keep in mind that the return of the patient's original signs and symptoms probably indicates complete failure of the pacemaker.

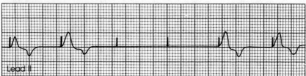

NONCAPTURE
Signs and symptoms
• Bradycardia
• Hypotension, dyspnea, chest pain, dizziness, fatigue, and other signs of low cardiac output
• On an EKG, pacemaker spikes are not followed by QRS complexes (if the electrode is ventricular) or by P waves (if the electrode is atrial).
Possible causes
• Electrode tip out of position
• Pacemaker voltage too low
• Lead wire fracture
• Battery depletion
• Edema or scar tissue formation at electrode tip
• Myocardial perforation by lead wire.
Intervention
• Reposition the patient on his side; if the electrode tip is malpositioned, this

may correct the problem.
• Reprogram the pacemaker to increase voltage (MAs), if necessary.
• Obtain a chest X-ray to check for electrode wire fracture, malpositioned electrode tip, or myocardial perforation.
• If the patient's heart rate is extremely slow, administer a positive chronotropic drug (such as isoproterenol hydrochloride [Isuprel] or atropine sulfate), as ordered.
• Prepare the patient for surgery to replace a reposition equipment, if necessary.
• Monitor the patient for signs and symptoms of cardiac tamponade (such as hypotension, tachycardia, and pulsus paradoxus), a possible result of myocardial perforation.

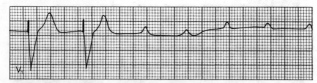

PACEMAKER RATE TOO SLOW OR PACEMAKER STOPS PACING
Signs and symptoms
• Bradycardia or a heart rate that is slower than the preset pacemaker rate
• Hypotension and other signs of low cardiac output.
Possible causes
• Battery failure

• Circuitry failure.
Intervention
• Replace the battery or temporary pacemaker generator (for a temporary pacemaker).
• Prepare the patient for surgery to replace equipment (for a permanent pacemaker).

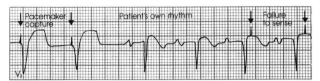

NONSENSING
Signs and symptoms
• Palpitations, skipped beats, ventricular tachycardia, or ventricular fibrillation (rare)
• On an EKG, spikes may fall on T waves; or they may fall regularly but at points where they should not appear.
Possible causes
• Battery depletion
• Electrode tip out of position
• Lead wire fracture
• Increased sensing threshold from edema or fibrosis at electrode tip.
Intervention
• Reposition the patient on his side; this may reposition the electrode tip.
• Obtain a chest X-ray to check for lead wire fracture or electrode malposition.
• Replace the battery, if necessary.
• Prepare the patient for surgery to replace or reposition the lead wire, if necessary.
• Adjust the pacemaker's sensitivity setting, if necessary.

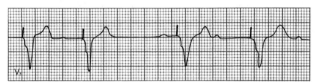

OVERSENSING
Signs and symptoms
• Pacemaker pacing at a rate slower than the set rate
• No paced beats at all (even though spontaneous rate is slower than the pacemaker's set rate).
Possible causes
• Myopotentials (with unipolar leads only). The pacemaker may sense (and be inhibited by) skeletal muscle contractions.
• Electromagnetic interference.
Intervention
• Perform the external magnet test, as ordered.
• Prepare the patient for surgical insertion of a bipolar lead, if ordered.
• Adjust the pacemaker's sensitivity setting, if necessary.

(continued)

Troubleshooting Pacemaker Problems *continued*

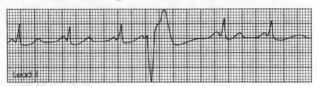

Lead II

PREMATURE VENTRICULAR CONTRACTIONS (PVCs)
Signs and symptoms
• Patient complaining of skipped beats
• PVCs visible on an EKG.
Possible cause
• Electrode causing irritable ventricular focus.
Note: PVCs occur normally within the first 24 hours after pacemaker insertion; they are not treated during this time unless they cause symptoms.
Intervention
• Initiate continuous cardiac monitoring.
• Administer antiarrhythmic drugs, as ordered.
• Prepare the patient for surgery to reposition the lead wire, if necessary.

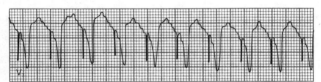

PACEMAKER TACHYCARDIA
Signs and symptoms
• On an EKG, tachycardia with pacemaker spikes preceeding each QRS complex.
Possible cause
• Retrograde conduction through the AV node, repolarizing the atria and triggering rapid pacemaker firing; most common with DDD pacemakers.
Intervention
• Slow the heart rate by holding a magnet over the pulse generator; this converts a demand pacemaker into a fixed-rate pacemaker.
Note: You may have to continue holding the magnet in place until the pacemaker is reprogrammed.
• Monitor the patient for ventricular tachycardia and fibrillation.
• The doctor or a specially trained nurse or technician will reprogram the pacemaker's PR interval to increase the refractory period.

DIAPHRAGMATIC STIMULATION
Signs and symptoms
• Hiccups
• Artifact on an EKG.
Possible causes
• Stimulation of phrenic nerve by electrode tip
• Myocardial perforation by lead wire
• Excessive pacemaker voltage (MAs).
Intervention
• Reposition patient; his hiccups may disappear when he lies on his side.
• Closely monitor the patient for signs of cardiac tamponade.
• Decrease the MAs, if necessary.
• Prepare the patient for surgery to reposition the lead wire, if necessary.

hours, and then once every shift. (Confused, elderly patients with second-degree heart block will not show immediate improvement in level of consciousness.)

Watch for signs and symptoms of a perforated ventricle, with resultant cardiac tamponade: persistent hiccups, distant heart sounds, pulsus paradoxus, hypotension with narrow pulse pressure, increased venous pressure, cyanosis, distended neck veins, decreased urine output, restlessness, or complaints of fullness in the chest. If any of these develop, notify the doctor immediately because a perforated ventricle requires immediate surgery.

Relieve patient discomfort with analgesics, as ordered.

Teach the patient how to take his own pulse daily before he is discharged from the hospital. Make sure he understands that he must take a resting pulse rate. Tell him what constitutes an acceptable and unacceptable discrepancy between pulse readings and whom to call if the discrepancy is unacceptable. The lower rate limit is usually 5 beats per minute below the pulse generator setting; the upper limit is usually 90 to 100 beats per minute.

Special considerations

• If the patient is a hunter, the doctor usually places the pacemaker battery on the side opposite the one where the gun is held to avoid damaging it during recoil. If the patient wears a hearing aid, the pacemaker battery is placed on the opposite side accordingly.
• Watch for signs of pacemaker malfunction. (See "Temporary pacemaker insertion and care," pages 314 to 318.)
• Provide the patient with an identification card that lists the pacemaker type and manufacturer, serial number, pacemaker rate setting, date implanted, and the doctor's name.
• After epicardial placement, the patient risks the complications associated with thoracotomy and general anesthesia. Complications of endocardial placement include thrombus and embolus for-

mation and cardiac tamponade due to perforation of the ventricular wall. Both methods of implantation may cause infection or dysrhythmia. Other complications involving the pacemaker itself, such as battery failure or a displaced electrode wire, are the same as for a temporary pacemaker.

Documentation

Document the type of pacemaker used, the serial number and manufacturer's name, the pacing rate, the date of implantation, and the doctor's name. Note whether or not the pacemaker successfully treated the patient's dysrhythmias, and include other pertinent observations, such as condition of the incision site.

Intraaortic balloon pump insertion and care

The intraaortic balloon pump (IABP) consists of a single-chamber or multi-chamber polyurethane balloon attached to an external pump console by means of a large-lumen catheter. A surgeon advances the balloon catheter up the patient's descending thoracic aorta to a point just distal to the left subclavian artery. The pumping console inflates the balloon with helium or carbon dioxide during diastole and deflates it during systole. This inflation-deflation cycle, called *counterpulsation,* is triggered by the patient's EKG projected on the console's oscilloscope. The IABP increases systemic circulation, improves coronary perfusion, and decreases afterload.

The balloon inflates early in diastole, just after the aortic valve closes. Normally, about 70% to 80% of coronary perfusion occurs during diastole. Balloon inflation forces blood toward the aortic valve, which increases pressure in the aortic root and augments diastolic pressure to enhance coronary perfusion. It also forces blood through the brachiocephalic, common carotid, and subclavian arteries arising from the aortic trunk, which increases peripheral circulation.

How to Care for Your Pacemaker

Dear Patient:

Your doctor has inserted a pacemaker in your chest to produce the electrical impulses necessary to keep your heart working properly. Now that you have a pacemaker, you must learn how to take care of it. Here are some things you should know:

• Keep the incision clean and dry until it heals (usually 7 to 10 days). After that, you may wash as usual.

• Wear loose clothing to avoid putting pressure on the pacemaker. For example, a woman with a pacemaker should not wear a tight bra.

• Normally, the implantation bulges slightly. If it reddens, swells, drains, or becomes warm or painful, *notify the doctor immediately.*

• Depending on which type of pacemaker you have, it should give 3 to 4 years' service. See the doctor regularly, usually every week during the first month or sooner if you have problems. Call the doctor if you experience chest pain, dizziness, shortness of breath, prolonged hiccups, muscle

twitching, nausea, vomiting, diarrhea, or a *very fast* or *very slow* heart rate. He may have you check your pacemaker periodically by transtelephonic monitoring, which enables you to transmit your EKG over the phone.

• To check your pacemaker, count your pulse at least once a day for a full minute *after you have been at rest for at least 15 minutes.* A good time to take a resting pulse rate is first thing in the morning. Your pulse rate reflects the number of times your heart pumps. The nurse will teach you how to count your pulse and tell you what pulse rate to expect. Report any discrepancy to the doctor immediately. Also, record all your pulse rates; include the number of beats, the date, and the time.

• Take your heart medication, as prescribed. This, along with your pacemaker, ensures a regular heart rate. As a reminder, note on a calendar the times when you should take your medication.

• Follow the doctor's orders concern-

During systole, blood pressure in the left ventricle must exceed that in the aorta to allow the aortic valve to open and eject blood into the system. The aortic resistance that must be overcome is called *afterload*. The balloon rapidly deflates just before systole, which reduces aortic volume and decreases aortic pressure and afterload. Since aortic pressure is decreased, the left ventricle need not work as hard to open the aortic valve. This decreased workload reduces the heart's oxygen requirement and, combined with the more efficient myocardial perfusion provided by the IABP, prevents or reduces myocardial ischemia.

The IABP console can assist the heart at preset rates—for example, it can inflate/deflate every one to four beats, depending on the patient's need and the

type of machine used. It also shuts off automatically in the presence of ventricular dysrhythmias.

The balloon catheter can be inserted surgically at the patient's bedside, in the operating room, or in a cardiac catheterization laboratory. Or, it can be inserted percutaneously at the patient's bedside with or without fluoroscopic guidance. If insertion is performed in the unit, strict aseptic technique must be followed. In some hospitals, technicians assist the doctor with balloon catheter insertion and removal and troubleshooting problems, and the nurse is usually responsible for patient assessment and management; otherwise, the nurse may care for the patient and operate the IABP machine as well.

Before insertion of the balloon catheter, a Swan-Ganz pulmonary artery

ing diet and physical activity. You should exercise every day, but the doctor will tell you how much exercise is right for you. You can participate in any physical activity in accordance with the doctor except a contact sport, such as football. *Do not overdo it.* Be especially careful not to stress the muscles near the pacemaker.

• Do not get too close to gasoline engines, electric motors, or poorly shielded microwave ovens. Do not use an electric shaver directly over the pacemaker. Also, stay away from high-voltage fields created by overhead electric lines. Most other electric equipment will not interfere with your pacemaker.

• If you go to the dentist or any other health care professional, tell him you are wearing a pacemaker. If you need dental work or surgery, you might require a prophylactic antibiotic to prevent infections. Consult the doctor before undergoing any procedure that involves electricity, such as cautery or diathermy.

• Always carry your pacemaker emergency card. The card lists your doctor, hospital, type of pacemaker (model, serial number, lead type), and date of implantation.

• You can drive a car a month after your pacemaker is implanted, but avoid long trips for at least 3 months and when the time for your battery replacement nears. Tell the doctor of your travel plans in advance, and carry a list of doctors and hospitals in the area where you will be traveling.

• If you are traveling by plane, you must pass through an airport metal detector. Before doing so, be sure to alert the authorities that you have a pacemaker.

• If you have a *nuclear* pacemaker and plan to travel abroad, the Nuclear Regulatory Commission requires that you inform the pacemaker manufacturer of your travel itinerary, means of travel, and the name of your doctor.

• Periodic short-term hospitalization is usually necessary for battery changes or pacemaker replacement.

catheter, a Foley catheter, and an arterial line should be inserted. A peripheral I.V. or subclavian line should also be in place for administering fluids and medications as needed. A transducer connected to the IABP console projects a visible arterial pressure waveform on the oscilloscope. A separate monitor and transducer may be required to display pulmonary artery pressures.

Common indications for the IABP include left ventricular failure and cardiogenic shock caused by acute myocardial infarction (AMI), unstable or preinfarction angina, and high-risk cardiac surgery. The IABP may also be used to provide preoperative support to the patient undergoing cardiac catheterization.

Use of the IABP is contraindicated by the inability to place the catheter

through arteriosclerotic vessels, and in patients with irreversible brain damage, cardiomyopathy, incompetent aortic valve, dissecting aortic aneurysm, or ventricular fibrillation.

Equipment
For insertion at the bedside:
IABP console and balloon catheters/ Dacron patch (for surgically inserted balloon)/EKG electrodes/gas source for pump (helium or CO_2)/I.V. solution and infusion set/arterial line catheter/heparin flush solution, transducer and intraflo setup/Swan-Ganz pulmonary artery catheter setup/temporary pacemaker setup/sterile drape /sterile gloves/ suture material/povidone-iodine solution and saline or sterile water for irrigation/suction setup /oxygen setup and respirator, if necessary/defibrillator and

Intraarterial Balloon Catheter Placement

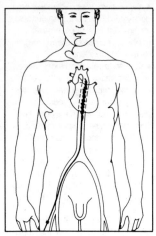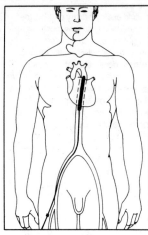

To insert a balloon catheter percutaneously, the doctor punctures the patient's femoral artery with an angiographic needle. He then makes an incision where the needle exits the skin and inserts a dilator to expand the vessel. Next, he removes that dilator and replaces it with the percutaneous introducer dilator and sheath. Just before inserting the balloon catheter, the doctor removes the introducer dilator. He then feeds the balloon catheter into the sheath and through the femoral artery, as shown at left.

The balloon is tightly wound for insertion. Balloon size varies from patient to patient because the inflated balloon must never completely occlude the artery. Once in place, the balloon is unwound to facilitate inflation, shown at right. Before removal, the balloon must be deflated and rewound.

emergency drugs/EKG monitor/Foley catheter/urimeter/arterial blood gas kits and tubes for laboratory studies/dressing materials/iodophor solution or swabs and ointment/4″ x 4″ gauze sponges/disposable razor or commercially available skin preparation kit/forms necessary for charting frequent measurements.

Three IABP devices are currently in use: the Datascope, Kontron, and SMEC. Each requires its own specific preparation for operation. The information provided here generally applies to all units.

Procedure

To prepare for IABP insertion:

Explain the procedure to the patient. Inform him that the balloon catheter temporarily reduces the heart's workload to promote rapid healing of the ventricular muscle, and that it will be removed after his heart can resume an adequate workload. (See *Intraarterial Balloon Catheter Placement*.)

Make sure the patient or responsible family member understands and signs a consent form.

Obtain baseline vital signs, including pulmonary artery pressures if the line is already inserted. Obtain a baseline EKG.

Apply chest electrodes in a standard lead II position or in whatever position produces the largest R wave on the oscilloscope needed to trigger the inflation/deflation cycle.

Assess respiratory status and administer oxygen as necessary.

Prepare and insert a peripheral I.V. line to deliver medications as ordered.

Insert a Foley catheter to allow accurate measurement of urinary output and assessment of fluid balance and renal function.

Shave the patient from the lower abdomen to the lower thigh bilaterally, including the pubic area, to reduce the risk of infection. Although the catheter is usually inserted on the left side, it may be inserted on the right side if the left artery is diseased.

If bradycardia occurs, give atropine or prepare the patient for pacemaker insertion, as ordered. The balloon pump is ineffective if the patient has bradycardia.

Prepare for and assist with insertion of an arterial line, as indicated, to allow arterial pressure monitoring. The augmented pressure waveform demonstrates elevated diastolic and lowered systolic pressure and allows you to check proper timing of the inflation/deflation cycle. (Remember, the balloon should inflate during diastole and deflate during systole.)

Prepare for and assist with insertion of a pulmonary artery line, as indicated, to allow measurement of pulmonary artery pressure, to permit aspiration of blood samples, and to perform cardiac output studies. Increased pressures indicate increased myocardial workload and ineffective balloon pumping. Comparison cardiac output studies may be done on and off the IABP to determine patient progress and potential for weaning.

Administer a sedative, as ordered.

To insert the intraaortic balloon:

The surgeon may insert a special intraaortic balloon catheter percutaneously through the femoral artery into the descending thoracic aorta. This simplified procedure may be performed in the unit or in a cardiac catherization laboratory.

If the surgeon chooses not to insert the catheter percutaneously, he inserts the balloon through a femoral arteriotomy using strict aseptic technique. This procedure is best performed in an operating room.

PTCA: Weighing Both Sides

PTCA is designed to reduce anginal pain and improve exercise tolerance. But before recommending the procedure, the doctor weighs its disadvantages against its intended benefits. Other factors he evaluates include the following:

Advantages
• Dilates artery immediately
• Requires only about 2 hours to perform (in a catheterization laboratory)
• Requires a shorter hospital stay than coronary artery bypass surgery
• Allows patient to resume activities of daily living almost immediately
• Provides symptomatic relief of angina in patients for whom coronary artery bypass grafting is contraindicated because of advanced age or such preexisting conditions as diabetes, cancer, or previous MI.

Disadvantages
• May lead to complications, including acute myocardial infarction, dysrhythmias, coronary vasospasm, or coronary artery dissection with perforation
• Does not eliminate the possibility of restenosis
• Necessitates patient preparation for coronary artery bypass surgery in the event of complications or procedure failure
• Demands patient selectivity on the basis of coronary condition (only one in ten candidates for coronary artery bypass grafting is also a PTCA candidate).

Percutaneous Transluminal Coronary Angioplasty (PTCA)

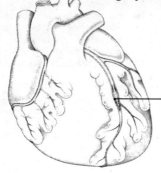

A balloon-tipped catheter (with balloon inflated) rests in a stenosed coronary artery. The close-ups below show, first, catheter placement in the stenotic artery and then, how balloon inflation widens the vessel lumen.

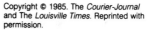

Inflated balloon

Copyright © 1985. The *Courier-Journal* and The *Louisville Times*. Reprinted with permission.

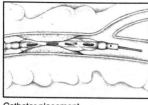

Catheter placement

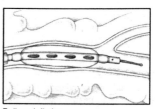

Balloon inflation

After making the incision and isolating the artery, he attaches a Dacron graft to a small opening in the arterial wall, passes the catheter through this graft, and with optional fluoroscopic guidance, advances it up the descending thoracic aorta and positions the catheter tip between the left subclavian artery and the renal arteries.

He then sews the Dacron graft around the catheter at the insertion point and connects the other end of the catheter to the pumping console.

To monitor the patient after IABP insertion:

Obtain a chest X-ray to determine correct balloon placement.

Observe the arterial pressure pattern every 30 minutes for diastolic augmentation, to verify correctly timed counterpulsation.

Measure blood pressure every 15 minutes to 1 hour to determine the effectiveness of therapy and anticipate the need for vasopressors or vasodilators, such as dopamine or nitroprusside (Nipride).

Take apical pulse at least every hour, noting rate and rhythm. Increased or decreased pulse rate alters the effectiveness of the pump and may require drugs, such as atropine, or pacemaker therapy.

Check temperature every hour. If it is elevated, obtain blood specimens for culture, send them to the laboratory immediately, and notify the doctor.

Measure intake and output hourly.

Observe for ischemia in the limbs—especially the affected limb—every hour. Be alert for changes in pulse, color, temperature, and sensation.

Watch for pump interruptions, which may result from loose EKG electrodes or broken wires, static or 60-cycle interference, kinked catheters, and improper body alignment. Elevate the head of the bed no more than 45°, keeping the patient's leg unflexed at the groin to prevent catheter kinking or displacement.

If the IABP is inadvertently shut off for more than 5 minutes, notify the doctor immediately to determine the need for heparinization before restarting the balloon. Resumed pumping without adequate anticoagulant precipitates emboli.

Observe for optimal timing. Balloon inflation should begin when the aortic valve closes or at the dicrotic notch on the arterial wave form. Deflation should occur just before systole. Improper timing includes late inflation, which reduces coronary artery perfusion, and prolonged deflation, which dangerously increases the resistance against which the left ventricle must pump. In both situations, readjust timing according to the manufacturer's guidelines or notify the person responsible for the balloon pump adjustments.

Check for gas leaks from the catheter or the balloon. This may be indicated by an alarm on the pump console. If the balloon ruptures, blood will appear in the catheter. If this happens, shut off the pump console and notify the doctor.

If you suspect balloon rupture, promptly place the patient in Trendelenburg's position to prevent gas embolus from reaching the brain.

Measure left arterial pressure and pulmonary capillary wedge pressure (PCWP) every 1 to 2 hours, or as ordered. A rising PCWP indicates increased ventricular pressure and workload; notify the doctor if this occurs. Some patients require the administration of I.V. nitroprusside in addition to the IABP to reduce preload and afterload.

Redress the balloon site, as ordered, and observe for signs of inflammation or excessive bleeding. Apply pressure to control bleeding.

Prevent constipation to avoid strain on the patient's heart.

If angina occurs, notify the doctor

Laser Phototherapy Vaporizes Plaques

Laser beams, already used for cauterization and excision of tissues, are now being tested experimentally to clear occluded arteries in animals and cadavers. So far, lipoid, fibrous, and calcified plaques have been safely vaporized without damaging adjacent vessel walls; the pulse of laser energy can be adjusted to the size of the occlusion.

In a typical procedure, an angina patient would report to an outpatient clinic or a cardiac catheterization laboratory, where a doctor would insert a fiberoptic catheter through the femoral artery and thread it through the aortic arch to the occlusion site in a coronary artery. Once the catheter is in position, the doctor would trigger a burst of laser light through the fiberoptic scope to vaporize the plaque, a few millimeters at a time. The restored coronary artery perfusion would free the patient of pain and greatly reduce the risk of MI.

immediately, as the IABP is not effective.

Watch for signs and symptoms of a dissecting aortic aneurysm, such as a difference in blood pressure between arms; elevated blood pressure; pain in the chest, abdomen, or back; syncope; pallor; diaphoresis; dyspnea; throbbing abdominal mass; and decreased red blood cell count and increased white blood cell count. If you suspect an aortic aneurysm, notify the doctor.

To wean the patient from the IABP:

Assess cardiac index, systemic blood pressure, and PCWP to evaluate readiness for weaning.

To begin weaning, gradually decrease the frequency of balloon augmentation to 1:2, 1:4, and 1:8 as ordered, and measure the cardiac index at each ratio. (Output is frequently measured both on

Intracoronary Streptokinase Therapy

Intracoronary streptokinase turns AMI treatment from a defensive to an offensive effort aimed at attacking the blockage directly. To ensure administering the best care possible with this drug, you must know how the therapy is accomplished, what its risks are, and which AMI victims it is most likely to help.

Procedure. Intracoronary streptokinase infusion requires cardiac catheterization, including coronary angiography to pinpoint the obstructed artery. Before administering streptokinase, the doctor may insert a temporary pacemaker and give:
• heparin, to prevent clotting
• hydrocortisone, to reduce the chances of allergic reaction
• nitroglycerin, to relieve coronary spasm

Streptokinase administration protocols vary but usually begin with a loading dose of 25,000 units, followed by an infusion of 2,000 to 4,000 units/minute in a dextrose 5% solution. The doctor directs the infusion into the occluded artery, as close to the blockage as possible. An infusion pump maintains an infusion rate of 2 to 4 ml/minute. Every 15 minutes, he checks progress by coronary angiography and EKG. After evidence of reperfusion appears, he continues the infusion for 30 to 60 minutes more. Next, he obtains another EKG, a coronary angiogram, and a complete hemodynamic profile.

The doctor then withdraws the infusion catheter but may leave pacing or balloon catheters in place for another 24 hours. He will continue heparin for 3 to 5 days.

Potential problems. As the chart at right indicates, thrombolytic therapy can cause complications. Streptokinase disrupts the normal clotting process, so hemorrhage is a common hazard. Precautions to lessen the chances of bleeding include immobilizing the catheterization site for 24 hours, checking the site every 15 minutes for color and temperature changes, and administering drugs orally or I.V. rather than by intramuscular injection.

Since streptokinase is a foreign protein, it triggers allergic reactions in a few patients (especially if a previous streptococcal infection has set up a reaction potential). Symptoms of an allergic reaction may include nausea, itching, flushing, fever, musculoskeletal pain, shortness of breath, bronchospasms, and edema. If ordered, administer sympathomimetic drugs, vasopressors, or corticosteroids.

Because ventricular dysrhythmias commonly accompany reperfusion, they are considered reliable indicators of returned circulation. Although certain dysrhythmias can be dangerous, prompt recognition and treatment usually corrects the problem.

and off the machine.) Some doctors prefer to wean the patient by decreasing balloon volume; however, this must be done cautiously to avoid reducing volume so much that the balloon cannot inflate and deflate forcibly enough to repel platelets. The possibility of increased potential for emboli with this method is controversial, and some doctors choose to administer I.V. heparin or low-molecular-weight dextran when using this method.

To remove the IABP:

The surgeon removes the balloon catheter when augmentation is no longer necessary (such as if cardiac output improves during weaning; or, if angina is absent, PCWP returns to normal, and systolic pressure increases when the machine is turned off). He also removes it if circulation to the limb is seriously compromised; if the patient's condition is diagnosed as inoperable during cardiac catheterization; or if the patient's condition deteriorates beyond recovery. Then he closes the Dacron graft and sutures the insertion site. If a percutaneous catheter is in place, the surgeon usually removes it. Pressure must be applied to the site for 15 to 30 minutes or until bleeding stops; in some hospitals, this is the doctor's responsibility.

After removal of the IABP, give necessary wound care.

Special considerations
• Turn and position the patient every 2 hours. Provide oral hygiene at least every 4 hours, or as needed. Give pain medication for insertion site discomfort, as ordered.
• Aortic or femoral artery dissection or perforation may occur during balloon insertion.
• Ischemia or loss of pulses may occur in extremities (especially the legs) due to compromised circulation. Thrombi may form on the balloon, predisposing the patient to emboli. Platelets are destroyed during balloon pumping, causing a decrease in circulating platelets (thrombocytopenia).
• A gas embolus can occur from balloon rupture. Infection may occur at the balloon insertion site.

Documentation
Document all aspects of patient assessment and management. If you are responsible for the IABP device, document all routine checks, problems, and troubleshooting measures. If a technician is responsible for the IABP device, record only when and why the technician was notified, as well as the result of his actions on the patient, if any.

Percutaneous transluminal coronary angioplasty

Percutaneous transluminal coronary angioplasty (PTCA) is a radiologic technique used to dilate an obstructed coronary artery without opening the chest. Performed under fluoroscopic

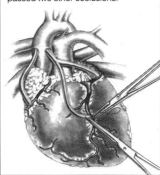

Coronary Artery Bypass Graft (CABG)
Bypassing a coronary artery occlusion, the doctor sutures a graft into place. Note that he has already bypassed two other occlusions.

guidance, it involves passing a tiny catheter through a guiding catheter into the narrowed section of artery and there inflating the catheter's balloon tip. The inflated balloon compresses the obstruction against the arterial walls to allow increased blood flow.

PTCA requires three catheters: an introducer catheter, to lead the guiding catheter into the peripheral artery; a guiding catheter, which is positioned in the ascending aorta at the *coronary ostium*, or opening of the obstructed coronary artery; and a balloon catheter, which is advanced to the obstruction. Once the balloon is positioned, the doctor inflates it with saline solution and contrast medium for several seconds, one or more times, while observing the fluoroscope. He measures pressures at the distal and proximal ends of the lesions to determine the pressure gradient. As the obstruction is compressed, the pressure gradient decreases.

After successful dilation, the doctor removes the balloon. He leaves the introducer sheath in place for several hours after the procedure to maintain access for intravenous drug administra-

Bypassing Coronary Artery Disease

The heart-lung machine provides cardiopulmonary bypass to an extracorporeal circuit during open-heart surgery, with a minimum of hemolysis and trauma. As shown in this simplified diagram, cannulas inserted in the inferior and superior venae cavae divert blood into the machine from its normal path to the right

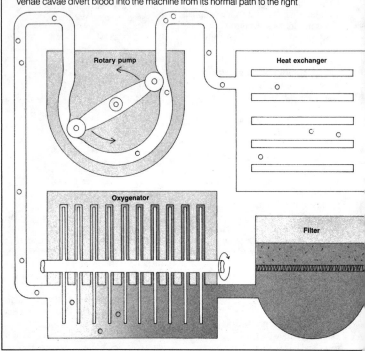

tion or reintroduction of the dilating catheter if the artery reoccludes.

Not every patient with CAD is a candidate for PTCA. The obstruction must be in the distal or proximal part of one or more major arteries, discrete, less than 2 cm long, uncalcified, not totally occluded, and not located at a bifurcation. Also, the affected artery should not be tortuous or sharply angled. Ideally, the patient should have a history of angina for less than 2 years. (See *PTCA: Weighing Both Sides*, page 327.) Since PTCA may cause acute arterial occlusion, the patient must also be a candidate for immediate emergency coronary

artery bypass grafting (CABG).

PTCA has an overall mortality of 1%—lower in patients with single vessel disease; higher in those with multivessel disease because of decreased myocardial reserve; and still higher in those who have had previous bypass surgery. Only 3% to 6% of patients require emergency bypass surgery after the procedure. About 10% of dilted arterial lesions become stenotic (roughly the same percentage as after bypass surgery), but they can be reopened. Current records suggest that a vessel that remains open for 6 months after dilation is likely to remain open indefinitely.

atrium. Also, when the heart is opened, blood is continuously aspirated and returned to the heart-lung machine along with venous blood.

The circuit returns filtered, oxygenated blood to the arterial system through an arterial cannula, which usually is placed in the ascending aorta.

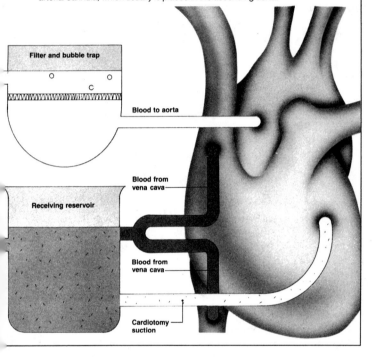

Filter and bubble trap

Blood to aorta

Blood from vena cava

Receiving reservoir

Blood from vena cava

Cardiotomy suction

After PTCA, the patient requires careful follow-up, including monitoring of anticoagulant therapy. An exercise EKG is performed during hospitalization, and again after 4 months, with or without a thallium scan, to confirm successful arterial clearance.

Equipment
Sphygmomanometer / stethoscope / thermometer

Procedure
Explain the procedure to the patient to allay his fears.

Make sure the patient or a responsible family member signs a consent form.

Take and record baseline vital signs.

Establish an I.V. line at a keep-vein-open rate to administer emergency drugs.

As in cardiac catheterization, the doctor inserts a guide wire and then inserts a double-lumen balloon-tipped catheter into the femoral or brachial artery, watching the catheter's progress by fluoroscope. One lumen monitors blood pressure at the catheter tip, helping him to assess blood flow at the stenosed area.

When the doctor believes the catheter is in the stenotic artery, he injects contrast dye through the second lumen to

The Jarvik-7 Artificial Heart

THE JARVIK-7 ARTIFICIAL HEART AT WORK

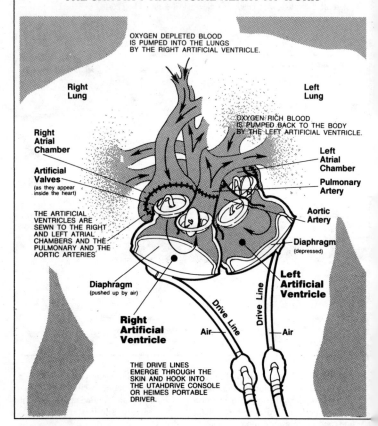

OXYGEN DEPLETED BLOOD IS PUMPED INTO THE LUNGS BY THE RIGHT ARTIFICIAL VENTRICLE.

Right Lung

Left Lung

OXYGEN RICH BLOOD IS PUMPED BACK TO THE BODY BY THE LEFT ARTIFICIAL VENTRICLE.

Right Atrial Chamber

Left Atrial Chamber

Artificial Valves
(as they appear inside the heart)

Pulmonary Artery

THE ARTIFICIAL VENTRICLES ARE SEWN TO THE RIGHT AND LEFT ATRIAL CHAMBERS AND THE PULMONARY AND THE AORTIC ARTERIES

Aortic Artery

Diaphragm
(depressed)

Left Artificial Ventricle

Diaphragm
(pushed up by air)

Right Artificial Ventricle

Drive Line

Drive Line

Air

Air

THE DRIVE LINES EMERGE THROUGH THE SKIN AND HOOK INTO THE UTAHDRIVE CONSOLE OR HEIMES PORTABLE DRIVER.

---

visualize the obstruction. As soon as the balloon is properly placed across a narrowed segment of the artery, he inflates the balloon to 4 to 6 atmospheres. (During balloon inflation, the patient may complain of anginal pain.) Inflated, the balloon exerts a force that compresses atheromas and widens the lumen. (See *Percutaneous Transluminal Coronary Angioplasty [PTCA]*, page 328.)

After 5 to 15 seconds, the doctor deflates the balloon and takes pressure readings on either side of the obstruction. If the procedure is successful, blood flow improves distal to the obstruction. However, if the readings remain high (indicating an unsuccessful or partially successful attempt), the doctor may inflate and deflate the balloon several more times.

During the procedure, the patient receives an anticoagulant, to prevent em-

HOW BLOOD IS PUMPED

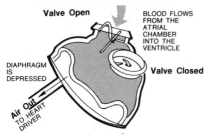

Valve Open

BLOOD FLOWS FROM THE ATRIAL CHAMBER INTO THE VENTRICLE

DIAPHRAGM IS DEPRESSED

Valve Closed

Air Out TO HEART DRIVER

THE DIAPHRAGM IS ACTIVATED BY AIR WHICH IS INTERMITTENTLY PULSED IN AND OUT OF EACH VENTRICLE BY THE EXTERNAL HEART DRIVE SYSTEM.

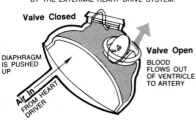

Valve Closed

DIAPHRAGM IS PUSHED UP

Valve Open

BLOOD FLOWS OUT OF VENTRICLE TO ARTERY

Air In FROM HEART DRIVER

THE DRIVE LINE

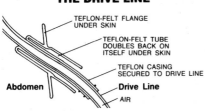

TEFLON-FELT FLANGE UNDER SKIN

TEFLON-FELT TUBE DOUBLES BACK ON ITSELF UNDER SKIN

TEFLON CASING SECURED TO DRIVE LINE

Abdomen

Drive Line

AIR

THE DRIVE SYSTEMS

The HEIMES Portable Heart Driver

AFFORDS GREATER FREEDOM OF MOVEMENT TO THE ARTIFICIAL HEART RECIPIENT. THE PORTABLE DRIVER IS CONTAINED IN A SHOULDER CARRIED CASE AND WEIGHS APPROXIMATELY 11.4 POUNDS. THE MAIN POWER SUPPLY IS A RECHARGEABLE BATTERY WHICH WILL OPERATE THE SYSTEM FOR UP TO FIVE HOURS. THE BATTERY CAN BE CHANGED WITHIN SECONDS WITHOUT INTERRUPTING THE DRIVER'S OPERATION. THE UNIT CONTAINS TWO COMPLETE AIR COMPRESSORS. A MICROPROCESSOR IN THE SYSTEM AUTOMATICALLY ADJUSTS THE RATE AT WHICH THE HEART BEATS TO MEET THE BODY'S NEEDS.

The UTAHDRIVE Heart Controller

IS THE PRIMARY DRIVE SYSTEM FOR THE JARVIK-7 ARTIFICIAL HEART. THE DRIVER PUMPS AND REGULATES AIR SUPPLIED BY A NEARBY AIR COMPRESSOR. THE CONSOLE CONTAINS PRIMARY AND BACKUP SYSTEMS WITH MANUAL CONTROLS FOR REGULATING THE PATIENT'S HEART AS WELL AS MEASURING AND RECORDING DEVICES. IT IS CUMBERSOME BUT CAN BE ROLLED FROM ROOM TO ROOM AND ALONG HOSPITAL CORRIDORS.

Reprinted with permission from *The Courier-Journal* and *The Louisville Times.*

bolism, and nitroglycerin, to prevent coronary artery spasm. Following the procedure, he may continue on anticoagulant therapy or begin antiplatelet therapy. He may also require a vasodilator.

Special Considerations

Before and after PTCA, the patient needs the same nursing care as someone undergoing cardiac catheterization.

Check vital signs frequently, as ordered, and monitor carefully for these possible problems:

• *Bleeding.* Because the patient is taking anticoagulant medication, be especially alert for signs of internal or external bleeding. Externally, check at and around the catheter site; also check the bed sheets for blood stains. If you see signs of bleeding, apply direct pressure over the site for 10 to 15 minutes. Also

Nursing Care after Open-Heart Surgery

Your immediate priority after open-heart surgery is to transfer the patient to the recovery room and stabilize his condition. First, connect the endotracheal or nasotracheal tube to assisted or controlled mechanical ventilation. Then, connect all venous and arterial lines and drainage receptacles. Next, draw blood samples and check vital signs and hemodynamic pressures. Examine dressings and measure urine output.

Systematic assessment

After stabilizing the patient's condition, begin a continuous, systematic assessment.

Respiratory status. Observe for signs of hypoxia, such as cyanosis of the extremities, restlessness, and hyperventilation. Check arterial blood gases as needed, to maintain pH, PCO_2, and PO_2 within the patient's physiological limits. Suction the endotracheal or nasotracheal tube as often as every 2 hours, and note the color of secretions. If they are red, rule out trauma; if pink, rule out pulmonary edema. Listen to breath sounds as needed; be especially alert for decreased breath sounds in the left lung, which could indicate that the endotracheal tube has slipped into the right mainstem bronchus. (If breath sounds decrease, order an immediate chest X-ray.) Take a chest X-ray daily to check for hemothorax, pleural effusion, atelectasis, pulmonary congestion, or widening of the mediastinum. Assess the patient's discomfort and administer analgesics, as ordered.

To keep the patient's chest tubes patent, milk and strip them as needed. Measure chest drainage at least every 2 hours and check hemoglobin and hematocrit every 2 to 4 hours. Observe for excessive drainage, which may indicate cardiac tamponade. Replace drainage with blood, as ordered.

Cardiovascular status. Check vital signs every 15 minutes initially, every 30 minutes when the patient is stable, then every hour. Maintain systolic blood pressure at 90 to 120 mm Hg, diastolic at 70 to 80 mm Hg. Lower

look closely for hematomas. If present, mark the area around the hematoma with a felt-tipped pen and watch for a change in size. If you can not control bleeding or you notice that the hematoma is increasing in size, call the doctor. After the patient stabilizes, continue to check vital signs as before.

• *Decrease or absence of peripheral pulses.* To accurately assess pulses, you must know the patient's baseline pulse characteristics prior to PTCA. Be sure to record the site used in PTCA (for example, femoral, popliteal, brachial, or radial). If you observe a sudden decrease in pulse amplitude or quality, or the absence of a peripheral pulse that was present previously, contact the doctor. Also, be alert for color and temperature changes in the arm or leg used during the procedure. If changes occur, notify the doctor.

• *Hypotension.* If this occurs, place the patient in a supine position and elevate his legs. Then, increase the I.V. flow rate, if ordered, and call the doctor.

• *Hives or respiratory distress.* Either may occur if the patient experiences a reaction to the contrast dye used during arteriography. If hives appear, call the doctor. If the patient is having difficulty breathing, elevate the head of the bed and be prepared to administer epinephrine and Benadryl, as ordered. *Note:* Respiratory distress may also result from pulmonary edema. So be sure to evaluate the patient carefully for the cause of his problem.

readings may impair cerebral and renal perfusion. Watch for dysrhythmias, which are usually associated with excessive bleeding, hypertension, ischemia, MI, acid-base imbalances, or abnormal serum potassium levels. Set the appropriate alarms on the cardiac monitor; if dysrhythmias develop, notify the doctor, and administer antiarrhythmics as ordered. Record an EKG daily, compare results with previous EKGs, and report any changes. Check cardiac enzyme levels daily for 3 days, since abnormally high levels may indicate MI. Watch for increased central venous pressure, which suggests fluid overload, cardiac failure, or cardiac tamponade. After CABG, check pedal and femoral pulses frequently. Diminished pulse may indicate embolized or separated graft. Ensure that the elastic bandage on the donor leg allows adequate circulation.

Fluid status. If the patient excretes less than 30 ml of urine per hour for 2 consecutive hours, notify the doctor. (This may indicate inadequate car-

diac output due to hypovolemia.) If brisk diuresis develops, test urine glucose frequently to rule out osmotic diuresis, which may cause hypokalemia. Keep intake below 2,000 ml for the first 24 hours to prevent cardiac overload. Check his weight daily to detect excessive fluid loss or retention.

Neurologic status. Regularly check pupil reactivity, general movement, strength of extremities, and level of consciousness. Evaluate for symptoms of postperfusion psychosis, which may result from disturbances in cerebral circulation following cardiopulmonary bypass. Reassure the patient's family that this condition is usually transient.

Preparation for convalescence and discharge

During convalescence, encourage progressive ambulation, within the limits of the patient's cardiac capability. To prepare for discharge, discuss diet, exercise, medications, and reportable symptoms of angina with the patient and his family.

• *Nausea or syncope.* These complications usually occur as a result of bradycardia. Recheck the patient's blood pressure and pulse. Contact the doctor. Be ready to administer atropine, fluids, vasopressors, or antiemetics, as ordered.
• *Decreased urine output.* Record the patient's fluid intake and output for at least 24 hours.

Documentation

Document all aspects of patient assessment. Record vital signs and intake and output carefully. (See also *Intracoronary Streptokinase Therapy,* page 330, and *Laser Phototherapy Vaporizes Plaques,* page 329.)

Coronary artery bypass grafting

In this surgical procedure, the doctor grafts a segment of one of the patient's veins (usually a saphenous vein) above and below the coronary artery blockage, providing a bypass that restores blood flow to the myocardium. If successful, CABG surgery relieves pain and improves myocardial performance.

Although CABG surgery can dramatically improve the patient's quality of life in the short run, the long-term outlook is uncertain. According to some reports, 10% to 15% of grafts close within a year after surgery.

Equipment

None.

Procedure

Explain to the patient that he may be shaved from his chin to his toes to eliminate potential infection sources.

Advise him that he will not be permitted to eat or drink after midnight the evening before surgery, but that he can have a sleeping pill if he wants one.

Explain that on the morning of surgery he will receive medication by injection to help him relax. Then, he will be transported to the operating room by stretcher.

Explain the equipment he will see and the noises he will hear in the recovery room and the intensive care unit (ICU). Inform him that a nurse will check him frequently, and assure him that this is not a sign of problems. If time permits, arrange for the patient and his family to tour the ICU before surgery.

Explain that he will be attached to a ventilator and a cardiac monitor following surgery. Familiarize him with the special equipment he will have in place after surgery; for example, an indwelling (Foley) catheter, chest tubes, and a pulmonary artery catheter.

Instruct the patient in deep breathing and coughing, and explain their importance during recovery. Show him how to use an incentive spirometer. Then, arrange a meeting with the physical therapist who will implement the postoperative exercise program.

Begin discharge planning.

Surgical techniques vary according to the doctor's preferences, the patient's condition, and the number of arteries being bypassed. But in general, surgery progresses as follows:

First, the doctor makes a series of longitudinal incisions in the inner aspect of the patient's calf, from the knee to the ankle. The doctor then removes a saphenous vein segment. (Its length depends on the number of arteries he plans to bypass.) If he does not find a suitable vein in one leg, he will repeat the procedure in the other. *Note:* As an alter-

native, the doctor may use an internal mammary artery segment.

As soon as he harvests the vein, the doctor makes a midline sternotomy and exposes the heart. Next, he positions cannulas in the inferior and superior vena cava to divert venous blood to a heart-lung machine. (See *Bypassing Coronary Artery Disease,* pages 332 and 333.) Oxygenated blood returns to the arterial system through an arterial cannula, usually positioned in the ascending aorta. (See *Coronary Artery Bypass Graft [CABG],* page 331.)

During surgery, the doctor induces hypothermia to reduce myocardial oxygen demands: a body temperature to 82.4° F. (28° C.) reduces oxygen consumption by 50%. He also induces *cardioplegia* (heart immobilization) with a cold potassium solution.

When the patient is fully prepared, the doctor joins one end of a saphenous vein segment to the ascending aorta and the other a coronary artery distal to the occlusion. (See *Coronary Artery Bypass Graft [CABG],* page 331.) He repeats this procedure for each artery he bypasses.

Special Considerations

• If CABG is successful, it improves blood supply to the heart and relieves anginal pain, improving the patient's exercise tolerance and quality of life. But like any major surgical procedure, CABG has risks and disadvantages.

It requires a 10- to 14-day hospital stay with scrupulous postoperative care. Complications can develop. The benefits of surgery may be only temporary. And postpericardiotomy syndrome (increased chest pain, fatigue, sinus tachycardia, or palpitations) develops in up to 30% of patients.

The doctor will consider these indications and contraindications before arriving at one of the following decisions.

He will probably perform CABG surgery for a patient with:

• atherosclerosis affecting one or more

To Help the Failing Heart—or to Replace It?

When a patient's heart fails or undergoes cardiogenic shock after open-heart surgery, it may not respond to drug therapy or insertion of an intraaortic balloon pump. In such instances, two experimental devices may be available to surgeons; the ventricular assist pump and the artificial heart.

The Pierce ventricular assist pump, one of several current designs, is being used in some centers to support the circulation in patients who cannot be weaned from cardiopulmonary bypass after open-heart surgery. The sac-type pump is fitted with tilting disk valves and powered pneumatically by periodic compression of the flexible sac. One or both ventricles may be assisted at one time. A cannula inserted into each atrial appendage drains blood from the atria into the pumps. One pump propels blood into the pulmonary artery; the other propels it into the aorta.

An alternative to ventricular assist pumping is heart transplantation, in which an irreparably diseased heart is replaced by a donor heart from a brain-dead patient. However, although about 75,000 patients a year need new hearts, only 1,000 to 2,000 potential donors are available each year.

An obvious solution is to implant an artificial heart, and one of the latest designs is shown on pages 334 and 335. Designed by Dr. Robert Jarvik of the University of Utah, the device consists of a pair of mechanical ventricles that are attached to sleeves stitched to the patient's aorta, pulmonary artery, and atria. The heart is powered by compressed air, which activates internal diaphragms and valves to pump blood. Once it is successfully implanted, the artificial heart must function for the rest of the patient's life without malfunctioning or causing blood clots.

coronary arteries (if the patient's experiencing severe angina despite medical therapy)
• an AMI that develops during cardiac catheterization, arteriography, or PTCA
• an AMI with a papillary muscle rupture, septal rupture, or persistent pain
• some uncontrollable ventricular dysrhythmias, particularly when a left ventricular aneurysm is present
• left main coronary artery stenosis greater than 50%, narrowing of several coronary arteries, or triple-vessel CAD.

The doctor will not perform CABG surgery for a patient with:
• an uncomplicated transmural infarct
• severe left ventricular dysfunction
• distal coronary arteries that are diseased and too small for successful graft placement.

Documentation

Record all pertinent data in order of importance.

Documentation will change with the passage of postoperative days. (See *Nursing Care after Open-Heart Surgery,* pages 336 and 337.)

16
EMERGENCY PROCEDURES

Cardiac emergencies can arise from chest trauma or from preexisting disorders, such as CAD. They require immediate assessment and intervention because they can disrupt basic life processes.

Advanced life-support techniques are often needed to treat the patient with an impending or overt cardiopulmonary emergency. Selection of specific techniques, such as cardiopulmonary resuscitation (CPR) and defibrillation, depends on the patient's condition, but all emergency techniques require thorough knowledge of cardiovascular anatomy and physiology, familiarity with technical equipment, and well-developed assessment and intervention skills.

Cardiopulmonary resuscitation

CPR is an emergency procedure that may restore and maintain a patient's respiration and circulation after his breathing and heartbeat have stopped. CPR must begin as soon as possible after cardiac and respiratory arrest since brain damage or death occurs if circulation is not restored in 3 to 6 minutes. The patient may not be restored to his previous central nervous system status if he has been in arrest for more than 10 minutes. However, if there is any doubt about how long pulse and respirations have been absent, CPR is still performed in an attempt to revive him.

The easiest way to remember the basic CPR procedure is to follow the ABC scheme (see *The ABCs of CPR,* pages 342 to 344.): open the Airway, restore Breathing, then restore Circulation. After airway, breathing, and circulation have been restored, diagnosis by EKG and definitive treatment, including drugs or defibrillation, or both, may follow. (See *Advanced Life Support,* pages 346 and 347.) CPR is contraindicated in "no code" patients.

Equipment
Cardiac arrest board, if available. If not available, use any hard, flat surface under the patient.

Procedure
To verify the patient's unresponsiveness, gently shake him, call out to him in a loud voice (use his name if you know it), and ask if he is all right. Speak directly into each ear in case he has unilateral deafness.

If you are alone, call for help; if you are outside the hospital and other people are around, ask someone to stand by in case you need help.

If the patient is not lying on a hard surface, place the cardiac arrest board (or the headboard of the bed, if detachable; or some other flat, rigid support) under his back so that subsequent compression steps will be effective. If you are outside the hospital, place him in a supine position on the floor or pavement. If the patient needs to be turned from a prone or side-lying position, he should be "logrolled" to avoid causing any further injury.

(A) To open the airway:
Position yourself on one side of the patient's head. Place one hand on the patient's forehead and place your other

hand under his neck, close to the back of his head. Tilt his head back while lifting under the neck. This causes the lower jaw to drop, which makes the tongue fall forward from the back of the throat and opens the airway.

Look toward the patient's feet and put your ear over his mouth and nose. To confirm that he has stopped breathing, watch for chest and stomach movement while listening for sounds of breathing and feeling for breath on your cheek.

(B) To restore breathing:

If the patient is not breathing, use the hand on his forehead to pinch his nostrils closed with your thumb and index finger. Continue to maintain backward pressure on his forehead with the heel and remaining fingers of this hand.

Take a deep breath, cover the patient's mouth with yours (be sure to seal your mouth tightly over his), and give four breaths in rapid succession to maintain positive pressure in the patient's lungs and to reopen collapsed alveoli. After each breath, quickly turn your head slightly toward the patient's chest and take a breath of fresh air. Do not let his lungs deflate completely between breaths.

Move your other hand from under the patient's neck, and use it to palpate for the carotid artery on the side of his neck nearest to you. Check carefully for a pulse since it may be very slow or weak. Allow 5 to 10 seconds for this step. Use the carotid artery because it is closest to you and usually accessible, and it is palpable longer than peripheral pulses.

At this time, if you are in a hospital, activate the emergency medical system. If you are outside the hospital and someone is available, instruct him to call an appropriate emergency number, report a medical emergency, give the exact location, describe the medical emergency, and return immediately so you know he made the call. If you are alone and assistance is not expected, perform CPR for 1 minute, then quickly telephone for help if a phone is available. If none is, continue with CPR.

(C) To restore circulation:

Remove your hands from the patient's head and neck and position yourself beside his chest. If you are on the floor, place your knees beside his chest, your hands in the correct position for chest compression.

Lock your elbows, bring your shoulders directly over your hands, and apply firm, downward pressure, compressing the chest about 1½" to 2" (3.8 to 5 cm). Count aloud *"one* and *two* and *three,"* and so on. Compress the chest on each number and release the pressure completely on each *and,* without removing your hands from the patient's chest to prevent position changes between compressions. Compress at the rate of slightly more than one per second.

After 15 compressions, perform the head-tilt/neck-lift maneuver again. Apply your mouth to the patient's, and give two full breaths in rapid succession (within a period of 4 to 5 seconds) without allowing full exhalation between breaths. Observe the chest rise.

Repeat this 15 compressions/2 breath cycle three more times.

Palpate the carotid artery for 5 seconds to see if the patient's pulse has returned. Also, put your ear over his mouth and nose again to check for breathing.

If there is no pulse, give 2 breaths and resume the pattern of 15 compressions to 2 breaths. Check for the the return of the carotid pulse every 4 to 5 minutes. Do not stop for more than 5 seconds unless the patient revives or is being transferred to a stretcher, another person trained in CPR relieves you, a doctor assumes responsibility, or you are unable to continue due to physical exhaustion.

If another person trained in CPR arrives while you are still able to continue, you should perform the 15 compressions while the other rescuer checks the patient's carotid pulse to monitor the effectiveness of the compressions. The second rescuer then gives two ventilations. The person doing the ventilations also instructs other rescuers to stop compressions, checks the patient's sta-

The ABCs of CPR

Once you have determined that the victim actually has suffered respiratory and cardiac arrest, recall the ABCs of CPR: open the Airway, restore Breathing, and restore Circulation. Administer cardiopulmonary resuscitation (CPR) until one of the following occurs:

• the victim responds with spontaneous breathing and circulation
• another qualified person takes over life-support efforts
• the victim has been transferred to an emergency medical facility, where qualified personnel take over
• you are too exhausted to continue giving CPR.

To give CPR effectively you should complete a course taught by a certified CPR instructor. The drawings below review the CPR techniques currently recommended by the American Heart Association.

Establish unresponsiveness
• When you first discover the victim, look at him closely. Shake him gently by the shoulders and loudly call out "Are you okay?" This shaking and shouting will establish whether or not he is unconscious. If he is unconscious and you are alone, call for help. Begin the CPR procedure until help arrives.
• If the victim is not lying on a hard surface, place a cardiac arrest board or some other flat, rigid support under his back to ensure that subsequent compression steps will be effective.

Open the airway
• Open the victim's airway. The most common cause of airway obstruction in an unconscious person is his tongue, which has relaxed and fallen into the airway. Because the tongue is attached to the lower jaw, moving the lower jaw forward will lift the tongue away from the back of the throat, thereby opening the airway.

You can use three methods to open the victim's airway: the head-tilt/chin-lift (the method recommended by the National Conference on Cardiopulmonary Emergency Cardiac Care), the head-tilt/neck-lift (the most commonly used method), or the jaw-thrust without head-tilt.
• To use the head-tilt/chin-lift method,

place your hand that is closer to the victim's head on his forehead, and tilt his head slightly. Then, place the fingertips of your opposite hand under his lower jaw on the bony part near the chin. Next, gently lift the victim's chin up, taking care not to close his mouth.

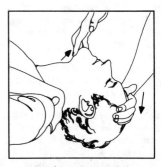

• To use the head-tilt/neck-lift method, place the palm of your hand that is closer to the victim's shoulders under his neck. Place the hand lifting his neck close to the back of his head to minimize cervical-spine extension. Then gently press back on the victim's forehead while lifting up and supporting his neck. (See illustration above.)
• Use the jaw-thrust without head-tilt method if you suspect the victim has a neck or spinal injury. Kneel at the victim's head, facing his feet. Place your

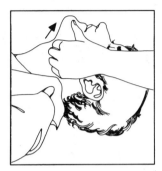

thumbs on his mandible near the corners of his mouth, pointing your thumbs toward his feet. Then, position the tops of your index fingers at the angles of his jaw. (See illustration above.)

Now, push your thumbs down as you lift up with the tips of your index fingers. This action should open the victim's airway.

• After opening the airway, see if this action has restored breathing. Put your ear over the victim's mouth and nose while you look toward his chest and abdomen. Then, listen for air movement and observe if his chest or abdomen is moving up and down. Next, feel with your cheek for any flow of air. If the victim has started to breathe, maintain his airway until help arrives.

Restore breathing
• If the victim has not started to breathe, close his nostrils with the thumb and index finger of your hand on his forehead. (See illustration at right.)
• Open your mouth wide and place it over the victim's mouth, sealing it tightly so no air can escape.
• When using the head-tilt/neck-lift method, support his neck with one hand while you pinch his nares.

• Deliver four quick full breaths, but do not allow the victim to exhale between these breaths. These four breaths maintain positive pressure in the airway. Even if the victim has stopped breathing for only a short time, some of the lungs' alveoli may have already collapsed. Positive pressure helps reinflate them. When you see the victim's chest rise and then fall after your fourth breath, you have verified that air is entering and escaping from his lungs.

If the victim wears dentures, keeping them in place will usually make ventilation easier. However, if his dentures start to slip, be sure to remove them.

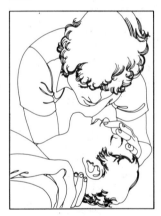

Restore circulation
• Keep your hand on the victim's forehead to maintain the head-tilt position. Use your other hand to find the carotid artery on the side closest to you, in the groove beside the larynx. Use your index and middle fingers to palpate the artery gently for 5 to 10 seconds.

If you find a pulse, do not give cardiac compressions, but do ventilate the patient at the rate of 1 breath ev-

The ABCs of CPR *(continued)*

ery 5 seconds (12 breaths per minute). Continue to check his pulse after every 12 breaths.

If you find no pulse, prepare to begin cardiac compression. Position yourself close to the victim's side, with your knees apart. This position gives you a broad base of support.

• Use the fingers of your hand that is closer to the victim's feet to find the correct hand position. Locate the lower margin of his rib cage and trace it to the notch where his ribs meet his sternum. Place your middle finger on the notch.

• Place your index finger of the same hand next to your middle finger. Then place the heel of your other hand next to your index finger on the long axis of the victim's sternum, as shown. This is the correct position for cardiac compression. If your hands are placed incorrectly, you may deliver an ineffective compression that could lacerate the victim's liver, fracture a rib, or break off the xiphoid process.

• Place the hand you used to locate the notch over the heel of your other hand. Interlock or extend your fingers to keep them off the victim's ribs and to maintain vertical pressure through the heel of the hand touching his sternum. Align your shoulders over your hands, keeping your elbows straight. Keeping your fingers off the victim's ribs and your shoulders aligned ensures that you will compress downward, not laterally. Lateral compressions will not deliver sufficient pressure.

Using the weight of your upper body, compress downward about 1½" to 2" (3.8 to 5 cm), concentrating the pressure through the heels of your hands. (See illustrations above and at right.) Do not deliver bouncing compressions, because they are less effective and could injure the victim. Then, relax the pressure completely to

let the heart fill with blood, but do not remove your hands from his chest or you will lose your hand position.

• If you are the only rescuer, time your compressions at a rate of 80 per minute. Count "one and two and three" and so on, up to the count of fifteen. Then deliver two quick breaths without allowing the victim to exhale between them. (Actually, you will be delivering 60 compressions per minute, because of the delay needed to ventilate the victim.) Perform CPR for 1 minute, and check pulse for 5 seconds. If it is absent, resume CPR with two ventilations to ensure that oxygen is in the lungs before beginning compressions.

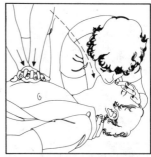

If another person trained in CPR arrives while you can still continue, one of you can perform compressions while the other ventilates the victim and checks his carotid pulse to monitor effectiveness of compressions. The person doing ventilations also instructs the person doing compressions to stop them, checks for spontaneous pulse and respirations, describes the patient's status, and gives one breath. The compressor then resumes compressions. Apply five compressions to one ventilation. Perform at least two cycles before rescuer and compressor switch positions.

tus for the other rescuer, and gives one breath. Compressions are then resumed.

When performing two-person CPR, use a cycle of five compressions (counting "one-one-thousand, two-one-thousand," and so on), followed by one breath, which is given on the release of the fifth compression.

If the person doing the compression becomes tired, change positions as smoothly as possible. To call for a switch in positions after a 5:1 cycle, say *"Switch*-one-thousand, two-one-thousand..." At this signal, the second person (who has been ventilating the patient) gives a breath at the end of the five compressions and then moves immediately to the chest position. The first person takes his place at the patient's head and takes no more than 5 seconds to check for spontaneous pulse and breathing. Meanwhile, the second person positions himself properly to resume compressions at once. If the patient is pulseless and not breathing, the first person gives one breath and signals the second person to resume compressions. Check the patient's pulse every few minutes and change positions whenever necessary.

Special considerations

• If respirations are absent but an adequate pulse is present, give ventilations alone, without compressions. Do not, however, give compressions without ventilations, since ventilation is needed to deliver oxygenated blood to tissues.

• If doing CPR alone, perform compressions at the rate of 80 per minute to compensate for the time you must take to give breaths. Two-person CPR requires a rate of 60 compressions per minute.

• Another way to open the airway is to tilt the head back, place the fingers of the other hand under the lower jaw on the bony part near the chin, and bring the chin forward (the head-tilt/chin-lift maneuver). If you suspect a neck or spinal injury, perform the jaw-thrust maneuver instead of the head-tilt/neck-lift, since the jaw-thrust maneuver does not hyperextend the neck.

• If the patient has false teeth, leave them in because they give a better seal around the mouth. If you cannot open the patient's mouth, if the mouth is injured, or if you cannot get a tight mouth-to-mouth seal, give mouth-to-nose ventilations. Tilt the head back and lift the lower jaw to close the mouth. Give a breath through the nose, then remove your mouth to allow the air to escape and to avoid a buildup of carbon dioxide.

• If the patient has a stoma or temporary tracheostomy, pinch the nostrils with one hand, close the mouth with the other hand, and give mouth-to-stoma or mouth-to-tube ventilations. If the tracheostomy tube has a cuff, inflate it so you will not have to seal the nose and mouth.

• When performing chest compressions, try to make each compression equal in duration. Quick jabs increase the possibility of injury and result in inadequate blood flow.

• If possible, check pupillary reaction, too, to determine the effectiveness of CPR. If the pupils constrict, oxygenated blood is reaching the brain.

The most common complication of CPR, even when performed correctly, is fractured ribs. If a fractured rib punctures a lung, tension pneumothorax or hemothorax may result. Fractures of the sternum can also occur during CPR. Both types of fractures can precipitate fat or bone marrow emboli.

Overzealous compressions can cause cardiac contusions. Compressions of the xiphoid process through improper hand placement can lacerate the liver or spleen.

Gastric distention, another common complication, results when excessive pressure is used to inflate the lungs. This can decrease lung volume and cause regurgitation. If distention occurs, recheck the patient's airway and reposition the airway open. If distention interferes with ventilation and a changed position does not correct it, turn the patient on his side and press gently on the epigastrium to remove air and prevent aspira-

Advanced Life Support

Advanced life support (ALS) measures support CPR by treating the physical changes and complications that can occur after cardiac arrest. These measures include the use of special techniques and equipment to help establish and maintain ventilation and circulation, the use of cardiac monitors to detect abnormal heart rate and rhythm, the insertion of a peripheral I.V. line, drug therapy, cardiac defibrillation, and the insertion of an artifical pacemaker. When the patient's condition stabilizes, the cause of cardiac arrest can be treated. Many ALS techniques, including defibrillation and drug administration, can be initiated by a specially trained nurse under standing orders; some techniques may be performed only by a doctor.

The techniques and equipment used in ALS depend on the patient's needs and on the setting. Usually, the following sequence of ALS procedures is required:

• First, alert co-workers and obtain a crash cart, which usually contains all equipment necessary for ALS.

• Because CPR requires a firm surface to be effective, place a cardiac arrest board or other flat, rigid support under the patient's back. Start CPR immediately *to ensure oxygenation and perfusion of vital organs.* Continue CPR while other ALS equipment is being set up. During later ALS procedures, avoid interrupting CPR for longer than 15 seconds.

• Set up the EKG machine *to monitor cardiovascular status continuously and to help determine proper therapy.* Because the EKG does not indicate the effectiveness of cardiac compression, take central (carotid or femoral) pulses frequently.

• Attempt to obtain a medical history from the patient's family or companion *to learn the probable cause of the arrest and to determine contraindications for resuscitation.*

• Insert a peripheral I.V. line for fluid and emergency drug administration. Use a large blood vessel, such as the brachial vein, *because smaller peripheral vessels tend to collapse quickly during arrest.* Use a large-gauge needle *to prevent dislodgment or injury to the vein, with extravasation and vessel collapse.* Use dextrose 5% in water to start the infusion; other fluids, such as normal saline solution, counteract circulatory collapse caused by hypovolemia and may be ordered as appropriate later.

• Perform defibrillation and adminis-

tion of stomach contents.

If the patient vomits, turn him on his side, wipe his mouth, and then return him to the supine position to continue CPR.

Documentation

Record the time and the reason for starting CPR.

Record the time CPR was stopped and the patient's status past CPR.

Document the times and types of advanced life support measures, if used.

Cardiac defibrillation (Direct-current countershock)

During defibrillation, a strong electric current is passed through a patient's heart by application of two electrode paddles applied to the chest. The resulting shock, which completely depolarizes the myocardium, usually allows the sinoatrial node to resume control of a heart that is in coarse ventricular fibrillation. This emergency procedure may also successfully convert ventricular

ter appropriate drugs, such as epinephrine, isoproterenol, and calcium chloride, which stimulate cardiac pacemaker discharge. These drugs treat asystole without defibrillation but can cause dysrhythmias, such as ventricular fibrillation, which require defibrillation. (Although cardiac monitoring should be started before defibrillation, a single countershock delivered to the heart without monitoring is not harmful, and immediate "blind" defibrillation may prove lifesaving; however, blind defibrillation of children is not recommended.

• If the patient fails to respond quickly to CPR, a single countershock, and basic drug therapy, insert a ventilatory device, such as an endotracheal tube or oxygen cannula. After the device is in place, discontinue mouth-to-mouth breathing but maintain respiratory assistance with an Ambu bag. Oxygen is used jointly with most of these devices.

• Remove oral secretions with portable or wall suction, and insert a nasogastric tube *to relieve or prevent gastric distention.*

• If the patient responds to the preceding treatments and has severe bradycardia with reduced cardiac output (as in acute heart block), vasopressors may be given. If these do not sufficiently raise heart rate and cardiac output, the doctor may insert a temporary cardiac pacemaker to boost the heart's faltering electrical activity to a near-normal rate.

• In most cases, when the patient's condition begins to stabilize or when preliminary ALS steps have been taken, he may be transported to a special-care area. If necessary, use a circulatory assist device, such as a manual or automatic chest compressor, *to provide external cardiac compression during transport.* Because the device compresses the sternum about 1½″ to 2″ (3.8 to 5 cm), position the patient carefully *to avoid accidental compression of the ribs or epigastric area, resulting in rib fracture and possible liver laceration.*

• Begin direct therapy as ordered *to treat the underlying cause of the patient's arrest.* For example, if arrest resulted from an acute hypovolemic crisis, replace blood volume and apply Medical antishock trousers *to redirect circulating blood from the extremities into the central circulation.* Or use acute dialysis to clear endogenous or exogenous toxins that may have caused the arrest.

---

tachycardias that fail to respond to drugs or other therapy; it can also be used to convert other abnormal cardiac rhythms, as in elective cardioversion (See "Elective cardioversion," page 312.)

Cardiac defibrillation is most successful when begun as soon as possible after onset of dysrhythmia to minimize acidosis or hypoxia and to restore normal sinus rhythm. Thus, although hospital policy determines who may defibrillate a patient, a specially trained nurse can perform it when necessary since she is often the first person to recognize the need for defibrillation. (See *Knowing Your Role in a Code,* page 348.)

Equipment

Defibrillator with electrode paddles/conductive jelly or paste, or saline-soaked 4″ x 4″ gauze sponges/emergency resuscitation equipment (including resuscitation bag, oxygen, and mask; resuscitation board; resuscitation drugs; needles and syringes; suction equipment)

Electrode paddles come in adult and infant sizes and anterior and anterior/

Knowing Your Role in a Code

Recorder nurse
• Observes and documents resuscitation efforts, using special code forms if required
• Helps document postarrest progress notes with basic rescuer number one

Medication nurse
• Prepares all I.V. medications as ordered
• May administer I.V. medications as ordered

Equipment nurse
• Sets up emergency equipment
• Assists with emergency procedures

Director (usually a doctor)
• Directs all major lifesaving interventions
• Oversees resuscitation efforts
• Only one with authority to make decision to stop

Basic rescuer number one
(usually the person who finds patient)
• Calls for help
• Starts one-man CPR

Basic rescuer number two
• Calls for advanced life-support (ALS) personnel
• Performs two-man CPR with basic rescuer number one
• The go-between after ALS team arrives

Anesthetist/anesthesiologist
• Intubates patient
• Ventilates patient

posterior (A/P) types. Anterior infant paddles have 1½″ (3.8 cm) steel disks; anterior adult paddles, 3″ (7.6 cm) steel disks. A/P paddles are usually used for elective cardioversion.

Many hospitals store all this equipment in a "crash cart." In that case, bring the cart to the bedside.

Procedure

The nurse who recognizes the emergency alerts other staff members and performs CPR until the defibrillator is ready to assure coronary and cerebral arterial blood flow. (See "Cardiopulmonary resuscitation," pages 340 to 346.)

Turn the defibrillator on and be sure the current indicator lights up. (See *How to Defibrillate*, pages 350 and 351.) If it does not, check the battery or other power source. (In some units, the on/off/charge switches are located on the paddle handles; in others, on the front instrument panel.) If the defibrillator can also be used for cardioversion, make sure it is set to defibrillate or is on the asynchronous mode. If it is set to synchronize, the paddles will not discharge, since there is no R wave in ventricular fibrillation for the synchronous mode to respond to.

Set the unit to the prescribed energy level (in joules, or watt-seconds) and charge the paddles to 200 to 400 joules for the adult patient; to 2 to 3.5 joules per kilogram of body weight for the neonatal or pediatric patient. (In severe chest trauma or open heart surgery, when the heart is exposed, the doctor uses special sterile paddles to deliver 5 to 20 joules directly to the myocardium.)

Make sure the electrode paddles are fully charged. This may be indicated by a light that blinks until full charge is reached, by an audible alarm, by a needle on a panel meter, or by a digital readout.

Lubricate the paddles to enhance conduction and prevent burns. Squeeze a ring of lubricant around one paddle disk, then rub the disks together to spread the lubricant over the entire disk surface. Or, use a gelpad or four saline-soaked 4″ x 4″ gauze sponges to lubricate each disk. Be sure to wipe any lubricant from your hands before discharging the paddles because the electric current can arc from the bottom of the paddles to your hands, causing a shock or burn. Excessive amounts of lubricant can also cause the paddles to slip from the patient's chest.

If the patient is wearing a nitroglycerin patch on his chest, remove it before defibrillation. An electrical arc can develop between the defibrillator paddle and the aluminum covering of the transdermal patch, causing an "explosion" and a burn to the patient.

To position anterior paddles on the patient, put one paddle (sometimes marked "sternum") slightly to the right of the upper sternum and below the clavicle at the level of the second to third intercostal space. For the adult male or pediatric patient, place the other paddle (sometimes marked "apex") slightly to the left of the left nipple at the level of the fifth to sixth intercostal space in the anterior axillary line (corresponding to the V_5 chest lead). For the adult female patient, place the left paddle at the mid- or anterior-axillary level, not over the breasts.

When positioning or lubricating the paddles, avoid placing your fingers on the discharge buttons, to prevent an accidental discharge.

To position A/P paddles, place the flat posterior paddle under the patient's body beneath the heart and immediately below the scapulae (but not under the vertebral column). Place the anterior paddle directly over the heart at the left precordium.

Position infant paddles as you would an adult's.

Rotate the paddles slightly to spread the lubricant outside the disk diameter, to help prevent skin burns if electrical current arcs off the sides of the paddles onto the patient's skin. Make sure that the paddles are correctly positioned before discharge and that lubricated areas do not touch each other, to prevent a short circuit.

Apply paddles to the chest wall using 20 to 25 pounds of forearm pressure. (Shoulder pressure could cause the paddles to slip, especially when the patient's body jolts during the discharge; insufficient pressure could cause sparks.)

If oxygen is being administered, disconnect it and shut it off before discharging the paddles to avoid possible fire hazard.

Although some EKG monitors are protected against defibrillator shocks, others may be damaged by the surge of current. If the patient is connected to a monitor, disconnect the patient cable as a precaution, and reconnect it immediately after defibrillation to record the new heart rhythm.

When you are ready to deliver electric shock, instruct staff members to stand clear of the patient and the bed to avoid the risk of grounding the current and causing a shock.

Discharge the paddles by pushing both handle buttons simultaneously or by pressing the appropriate button on the paddle or instrument panel of the defibrillator.

If the first defibrillation fails to convert the rhythm, make sure the paddles are adequately lubricated and fully recharged and repeat the procedure at the same energy level. If the patient still fails to respond, his heart may be hypoxic, acidotic, or ischemic. Restart CPR and give supplementary oxygen to ensure maximum oxygenation of myocardial tissue in case of hypoxia or ischemia, or administer sodium bicarbonate I.V. to correct acidosis and epinephrine I.V. to stimulate the sinoatrial node. If oxygen is in use, shut it off, then defibrillate again at 360 to 400 joules when the drugs achieve peak action. Continue CPR and oxygen administration until you detect a carotid pulse. Do not leave oxygen on during actual defibrillation.

After defibrillation:

Check carotid pulse, reconnect the EKG cable, and check cardiac rhythm. Reconnect oxygen and continue CPR, if necessary, or prepare to defibrillate again.

If the paddles have been recharged but not used again, clear the charge by turning off the machine and turning the discharge control to zero or by pressing the "bleed" button if there is one. Avoid discharging the paddles against each

How to Defibrillate

Before defibrillation, check the manufacturer's specifications for the difference between the stored energy and the charge delivered through the paddles. Then, set the dial to the level needed for defibrillation. (Note: Some EKG machines and temporary pacemakers are not defibrillator-shielded. Disconnect such units before defibrillation.)

• *Lubricate the paddles to facilitate conduction and prevent burns.* You can use cream, paste, a gel pad, or saline-soaked gauze sponges. If you are using cream or paste, squeeze a ring of lubricant around the disk, then rub the disks together to spread the lubricant over the entire disk surface. Or use one gel pad or four sponges per paddle to lubricate each disk.

• *Wipe any lubricant off your hands before discharging the paddles,* to prevent arcing, which can cause a shock or burn.

• *To start the charging cycle, activate the charge control button.* The meter needle will move gradually to the selected energy level; when it stops, the machine is charged. (Some machines have a digital readout; others sound an alarm when fully charged.)

• *Position the paddles.* To position standard paddles on a man, put one paddle beneath the clavicle, to the right of the upper end of the sternum; put the other paddle on the left lateral chest wall, to the left of the cardiac apex. To position paddles on a woman, place them at the mid- or anterior-axillary level, not over the breasts. (Note: When positioning paddles, keep your fingers off the discharge buttons, so that you do not discharge them accidentally.)

To position A/P paddles, put the flat paddle under the patient's body, behind the heart and just below the left scapula. Put the other paddle over the left precordium, directly over the heart. The discharge button is located on the anterior paddle only. *Never use standard paddles for A/P placement.*

• *Before discharging standard paddles,* look around to be sure no one is touching the patient or the bed (be sure you are standing clear, too) and say loudly, "Stand clear." Give other members of the code team time to step away.

• *Discharge the paddles by pressing*

other or into the air.

Using soap and water, wipe the lubricant from the patient's chest. Treat any burns, as ordered. Clean lubricant from the paddles with soap and water, to avoid corrosion damage to the disks that can cause arcing.

Prepare the defibrillator for immediate reuse. If necessary, restock the machine with more lubricant and other supplies. Be sure to return a battery-powered machine to its recharger.

Special considerations

• Since defibrillators vary in their setup and operation, familiarize yourself with your institution's equipment. The defibrillator should be checked by the charge nurse at every shift change and inspected regularly by the hospital's engineering department or the manufacturer's service representative.

• Remember that the amount of energy required for defibrillation depends on electrode size and placement, lubricant, type of waveform (Lown or Edmark), technique (single or multiple shocks), nature of underlying cardiac disease, and size and metabolic status of the patient at defibrillation. The larger the patient, the more energy required.

• If you carry your stethoscope around your neck, remove it during defibrillation to prevent shock. Avoid using distilled water or alcohol to wet gauze sponges for lubricating the paddles; wa-

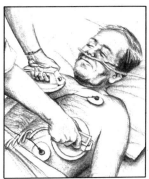

both buttons simultaneously with at least 20 to 25 pounds of forearm pressure per paddle. (A discharging control is usually on both handles but may be on only one.) Be sure to use arm pressure rather than shoulder pressure so that the paddles will not slip out of position.

Defibrillate adults at 200 watt-seconds (or joules), as ordered. If unsuccessful, defibrillate again at the same setting.

• *After defibrillation, check the patient's pulse, and check for any changes on the monitor.* He may need sodium bicarbonate or epinephrine. If the patient requires a third shock, increase the energy level to 360 watt-seconds.

• *If the paddles have been recharged but not used, clear the charge by turning off the machine or pressing the "bleed" button, if applicable.* Do not discharge paddles into each other or into the air.

• *Clean the lubricant off the patient's skin and the paddle disks with soap and water.* Residual lubricant can corrode the metal paddles and cause arcing of the electrical current.

• *Document the procedure and any changes in the patient's heart rhythm.* Record the date, time, lead, and watt-seconds (or joules) on the recording strip or code form. Treat any burns as ordered; document their size and appearance and your care.

• *Prepare the defibrillator unit for reuse, and restock necessary supplies.* Someone should check the defibrillator unit at the beginning of every shift to be sure it is working. The hospital's engineering department should regularly check it and the EKG machine and make needed repairs.

ter is a poor conductor, and alcohol may ignite, causing severe burns.

• Remember that defibrillation is successful only when a patient's heart shows *coarse* ventricular fibrillation (as opposed to *fine* ventricular fibrillation) on the EKG monitor. If his heart is in fine ventricular fibrillation, administer 0.5 mg epinephrine or calcium chloride first, to produce coarse ventricular fibrillation before attempting defibrillation.

• If you have any information about the patient's potassium level, whether hypokalemic or hyperkalemic, inform the doctor responding to the cardiac arrest. Similarly, inform the doctor if you have any knowledge of the patient's digoxin level. Patients who have digitalis toxicity will frequently respond well when defibrillated at a lower energy level.

• Continue to monitor the patient for dysrhythmias and emergency care instituted if defibrillation is successful. Usually, the successfully defibrillated patient is admitted to the intensive care unit if he is not already there.

Documentation

Document the time of cardiac arrest, the personnel performing defibrillation, the amount of energy used (watt-seconds, or joules), the number of shocks, and the patient's response. Record the time and response to CPR and the administration of drugs. Include all monitored rhythm strips taken during the procedure. Note the size and appearance of any burns that may have occurred.

Emergency control of hemorrhage

Hemorrhage results from vascular tissue injury—externally from a laceration, amputation, fracture, crush trauma, or nosebleed; internally from a bleeding ulcer, ruptured spleen, or abdominal and chest trauma. Uncontrolled arterial bleeding can rapidly cause shock, and death can occur. In contrast, venous bleeding, even though heavy at first, is usually controlled quickly by clotting unless the patient is receiving anticoagulant therapy or has a bleeding tendency. However, it still requires prompt treatment to prevent heavy blood loss.

Direct pressure over a bleeding vessel is the action of choice for external bleeding; it may help stop blood flow long enough to allow clot formation. If this fails to stop bleeding, applying pressure to the major artery proximal to the injury may slow or stop blood flow and perfusion into the tissues. A tourniquet should be used to control bleeding only if all other measures fail, since its use may cause gangrene and possibly necessitate amputation of the affected limb.

Equipment

In an emergency, equipment consists of whatever is readily available and adaptable for immediate use. External hemorrhage requires thick pads of sterile gauze, sanitary pads, or clean soft cloths. If dressings are not available, use your hands to stop excessive bleeding until dressings can be obtained. Tourniquets require a wide fold of cloth or other broad material, such as a belt, blood pressure cuff, scarf, or large handkerchief; a stick or pencil to tighten the tourniquet; and a marking pen or lipstick to identify the patient. Avoid using narrow material (wire or rope) to minimize tissue damage.

Procedure

Explain the procedure to the patient—even if he is comatose or in shock—to help allay his fears and promote cooperation.

To control external bleeding:

If necessary, cut the patient's clothing to expose the wound.

Elevate an affected extremity above heart level to stop venous and capillary bleeding.

Apply steady, direct pressure on the wound with a clean dressing of heavy gauze, a sanitary pad, or clean, soft cloths. If nothing else is available, use your hand. Apply ice to the wound, if possible.

If direct pressure fails to stop bleeding or cannot be applied because of a fracture, apply digital pressure to the arterial pressure point nearest the wound (see *Locating Arterial Pressure Points,* page 353). If you are not skilled at locating a pressure point precisely, apply pressure with the heel of your hand to cover the area where the pressure point is located. If you have applied pressure correctly, you will be unable to detect a pulse below the pressure point, and the patient will feel local tingling or numbness.

If you have controlled the bleeding, apply a compression dressing. Using sterile gauze or clean cloths, prepare a compress six to eight layers thick. Tie it in place with any available cloth, such as a scarf, stocking, or strip of clothing. If blood soaks through the dressing, do not remove it; apply additional dressings over the soaked ones and rebandage.

If bleeding persists, prepare to apply a tourniquet. Position the tourniquet on the limb between the site of injury and the heart. Wrap the tourniquet around the extremity, about 2″ (5 cm) above the wound (the tourniquet should not touch the wound edges), tie it with a half knot, then place the stick over the half knot and tie a square knot over it. Tighten the tourniquet by twisting the stick until bleeding stops. Secure the stick in this position with the loose tourniquet ends or an additional piece of cloth. Leave the tourniquet uncovered, and call attention to it by writing a large "T" with a pen or lipstick on the patient's forehead. Indicate tourniquet location and the time of application. Avoid loosening the tourniquet until the patient reaches the hospital. Doing so may cause a massive hemorrhage that could be lethal to an already hypovolemic patient, and it may release dangerous toxins from injured tissues.

To control internal bleeding:

If you suspect internal bleeding, keep the patient calm. Do not give liquids unless medical attention will be delayed and there is no gastrointestinal bleeding. If possible, apply ice packs to the affected area to reduce swelling. Place the patient in Trendelenburg's position to increase cerebral blood flow.

After any type of hemorrhage, when bleeding is controlled, take vital signs and observe for other major injuries.

Special considerations

Make sure you apply the tourniquet properly; a loose tourniquet may actually increase blood loss since arterial bleeding continues, but the tourniquet prevents venous return.

Transport the patient to the hospital without delay. If you suspect spinal injury, make sure that the patient is tied to a backboard before movement. Handle a partially severed limb with extreme care to avoid increasing the extent of injury. A completely severed limb should be transported with the patient. Indicate on the tourniquet or the patient's forehead that the severed limb accompanies the victim.

Cardiac arrest can result from hypovolemia with secondary anoxia. Even correct application of a tourniquet may cause gangrene and loss of a limb.

Documentation

Record vital signs and all treatments performed including the time and whether the procedure was successful in stopping the bleeding.

Assess and document the patient's level of consciousness.

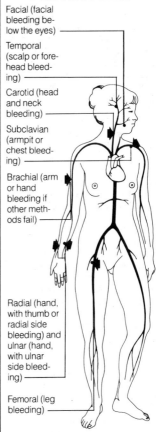

Locating Arterial Pressure Points

Facial (facial bleeding below the eyes)

Temporal (scalp or forehead bleeding)

Carotid (head and neck bleeding)

Subclavian (armpit or chest bleeding)

Brachial (arm or hand bleeding if other methods fail)

Radial (hand, with thumb or radial side bleeding) and ulnar (hand, with ulnar side bleeding)

Femoral (leg bleeding)

To control hemorrhage, compress the appropriate pressure point—the site at which a large blood vessel can be compressed against bone. Compression of a pressure point controls bleeding in a distinct area (indicated in parentheses after the pressure point).

Antishock trousers

Medical antishock trousers (MAST suit, also known as Jobst G Antigravity Suit) is a 3-chambered suit made of inflatable bladders sandwiched between double layers of fabric. When inflated, the suit places external pressure on the lower extremities and abdomen, creating an autotransfusion effect by squeezing blood superiorly and increasing blood volume to the heart, lungs, and brain by up to 30%. The MAST suit is used to treat shock when systolic blood pressure falls below 80 mm Hg or below 100 mm Hg when accompanied by signs of shock. It can control abdominal and lower extremity hemorrhage by creating internal pressure and external tamponade effects; it can also help stabilize and splint pelvic and femoral fractures.

Use of the MAST suit is contraindicated in patients with cardiogenic shock, congestive heart failure, pulmonary edema and tension pneumothorax. It should be used cautiously during pregnancy. The MAST suit must be deflated slowly, with continuous blood pressure monitoring, to prevent potentially irreversible shock from hypovolemia. It should not be removed until the patient's blood volume is restored, his condition is stabilized, or he is being prepared for surgery. If necessary, the MAST suit can be deflated by stages in the operating room.

Equipment

A MAST suit with footpump is the only necessary equipment. MAST suits come in a pediatric size (for patients 3.5′ to 5′ [1.05 to 1.5 m] tall) and an adult size (for patients taller than 5′).

Procedure

To apply a MAST suit:

Explain the procedure to the patient to allay his fears and ensure his cooperation.

Take vital signs to establish baseline measurements.

Assess the patient's injuries to determine whether he can be turned from side to side. If he cannot be, slide the MAST suit under him. If he can be turned, place the MAST suit next to him and logroll him onto it. You can also set up the MAST suit on a gurney or stretcher and place the patient on it in a supine position.

Examine the patient for sharp objects, such as pieces of glass or stones, that could injure him or puncture the suit when it is inflated.

Arrange the MAST suit so the upper edge is just below the patient's rib cage. Pressure above this area could decrease chest expansion, causing respiratory problems.

Fasten the MAST suit around both legs, then around the abdomen. (The suit may not cover a tall patient's lower legs.)

Doublecheck the stopcocks to make sure they are all open so the MAST suit will inflate uniformly. Connect the foot pump to all three (abdomen, right leg, left leg) MAST compartments.

Inflate the legs of the MAST suit first, then the abdominal segment, to about 20 to 30 mm Hg to start. Monitor blood pressure and pulse. Continue to inflate the suit slowly while monitoring vital signs. Stop inflating when systolic blood pressure reaches the desired level, usually 100 mm Hg.

Close all stopcocks to prevent loss of air and accidental deflation. Do not remove the foot pump while the suit is inflated.

Monitor the patient's blood pressure, pulse, and respirations every 5 minutes to determine his response to application of the MAST suit. Check his pedal pulses and temperature periodically. Notify the doctor if the circulation in his feet appears impaired. Also auscultate the patient's lungs frequently for any signs of pulmonary edema.

Make preparations for determining and treating the patient's medical problem, because the MAST suit is only a temporary treatment.

To remove a MAST suit:

Before deflation, make sure that I.V. lines are patent, and that a doctor is in attendance and emergency resuscitation equipment is immediately available. Removing a MAST suit may cause the patient's blood pressure to drop rapidly.

Open the abdominal stopcock and start releasing small amounts of air. Closely monitor the patient's systolic blood pressure as you do this. If it drops 5 mm Hg, close the stopcock.

Deflating the suit too quickly can allow circulating blood to rush to the abdomen or extremities, causing potentially irreversible shock.

If you have to stop deflating the MAST suit because of a drop in blood pressure, increase the flow rate of I.V. solutions to help stabilize blood pressure.

If blood pressure is stable, continue to deflate the MAST suit slowly. After you finish deflating the abdominal section, deflate the legs simultaneously.

When the MAST suit becomes loose enough, gently pull it off.

Clean the MAST suit as required, but do not autoclave it or use solvents.

Special considerations

• Generally, you should see a therapeutic response to treatment when the MAST suit is inflated to 25 mm Hg. A so-called morbidity effect, caused by a change in local circulation, occurs at about 50 mm Hg. Most types of MAST suits have Velcro straps, pop-off valves, or gauges that prevent inflation beyond 104 mm Hg. Normally, the MAST suit should not be left inflated for more than 2 hours, although occasionally it is used for as long as several days. A range of 25 to 50 mm Hg can usually be maintained for up to 48 hours. For prolonged use, the MAST suit may be inflated at a lower pressure than normal.

• A MAST suit is radiolucent and allows X-rays while the patient wears it.

• Vomiting can result from compression of the abdomen. Anaerobic metabolism, which can result from the MAST suit's pressure being higher than the patient's systolic pressure, can lead to metabolic acidosis. Skin breakdown may follow prolonged use. When used with severe leg fractures for long periods, tissue sloughing and necrosis caused by increased compartmental pressures have necessitated amputation.

Documentation

Record the time of application and removal, and the patient's vital signs before application, during treatment, and after removal.

17

CARDIAC DRUG THERAPY

The cardiovascular system can compensate for many defects that arise within itself. However, when it fails to do so, we can intervene with the best cardiovascular drugs. Current drug therapy specifically used for cardiovascular disorders includes cardiac glycosides, antiarrhythmics, antianginals, antihypertensives, vasodilators, and antilipemics. These drug classes and the relevant individual drugs which comprise them are the subjects of this chapter.

CARDIAC GLYCOSIDES

The cardiac (cardiotonic or digitalis) glycosides, which are extracted from plants of the genus Digitalis or chemically synthesized from the plant extract, are used to treat congestive heart failure (CHF) and tachyarrhythmias. All the cardiac glycosides act similarly on the cardiac system; however, they differ in extent of absorption, metabolism, and excretion.

The range between therapeutic and toxic doses is extremely narrow. Toxicity may be due to altered absorption, serum electrolyte concentrations, renal or hepatic dysfunction, drug interactions, or other factors. The choice of cardiac glycoside and route of administration depend on the disorder and the desired onset of activity.

Major uses

Cardiac glycosides increase cardiac output in acute or chronic CHF. They control the rate of ventricular contraction in atrial flutter or fibrillation. The cardiac glycosides are also used to prevent or treat paroxysmal atrial tachycardia and angina that is associated with CHF.

Mechanism of action

• Cardiac glycosides act directly on the myocardium to increase the force of contraction (to produce a positive inotropic effect) by two mechanisms:

They promote movement of calcium from extracellular to intracellular cytoplasm. The force of contraction is directly related to the concentration of calcium in the myocardial cytoplasm.

They also inhibit adenosine triphosphatase (ATPase), the enzyme that regulates potassium and sodium electrolyte concentrations in myocardial cells. Inhibition of ATPase increases intracellular sodium concentration, which in turn increases the force of contraction.

• The glycosides decrease conduction velocity through the atrioventricular (AV) node to slow heart rate.

• They prolong the effective refractory period of the AV node by both direct and sympatholytic effects on the sinoatrial (SA) node.

Absorption, distribution, metabolism, and excretion

• Deslanoside is given I.V. or I.M. only because absorption from the GI tract is erratic or incomplete. It is primarily excreted unchanged in the urine. Use with caution in patients with renal dysfunction.

• Digitoxin is 90% to 100% absorbed after oral administration. Passing through the enterohepatic circulation, the drug is extensively metabolized in the liver into inactive metabolites and is excreted by the kidneys. Neither the drug nor its metabolites accumulate in the

nor its metabolites accumulate in the renal parenchyma when renal function is impaired, since biliary and fecal elimination increase.

• Digoxin is 60% to 85% absorbed after oral administration. (Absorption varies with manufacturer.) Although 80% is absorbed after I.M. administration, this route may cause pain and irritation at the injection site.

Digoxin is excreted primarily unchanged in the urine. Use with caution in patients with renal dysfunction.

• None of the cardiac glycosides are distributed to adipose tissues. In obese patients, dosage should be based on ideal body weight.

Onset and duration
See table on page 359.

Side effects
The following are signs of toxicity that may occur with all cardiac glycosides (those in italics are common or life threatening):

CNS: fatigue, generalized muscle weakness, agitation, hallucinations, headache, malaise, dizziness, vertigo, stupor, paresthesias

CV: increased severity of CHF, arrhythmias (most commonly conduction disturbances with or without AV block, premature ventricular contractions, and supraventricular dysrhythmias), hypotension

Toxic effects on heart may be life-threatening and require immediate attention.

EENT: yellow-green halos around visual images, blurred vision, light flashes, photophobia, diplopia

GI: anorexia, nausea, vomiting, diarrhea

Nursing considerations
Consider the following when administering any cardiac glycoside:

• These drugs are contraindicated in the presence of any digitalis-induced toxicity, ventricular fibrillation, or ventricular tachycardia unless caused by CHF. Administering calcium salts to digitalized patients is also contraindicated. Calcium affects cardiac contractility and excitability in much the same way that glycosides do and may lead to serious dysrhythmias in digitalized patients. Use with extreme caution in the elderly and in patients with acute myocardial infarction, incomplete AV block, chronic constrictive pericarditis, idiopathic hypertrophic subaortic stenosis, renal insufficiency, severe pulmonary disease, or hypothyroidism.

• Hypothyroid patients are very sensitive to glycosides; hyperthyroid patients may need larger doses.

• Obtain baseline data (heart rate and rhythm, blood pressure, electrolytes) before giving the first dose.

• Question the patient about recent use of cardiac glycosides (within the previous 2 to 3 weeks) before administering a loading dose. Always divide loading doses over the first 24 hours unless the clinical situation indicates otherwise.

• The dose is adjusted to the patient's clinical condition and is monitored by serum levels of cardiac glycoside, calcium, potassium, magnesium, and by electrocardiogram (EKG).

• Take an apical-radial pulse for a full minute. Record and report to the doctor any significant changes (sudden increase or decrease in rate, pulse deficit, irregular beats, and particularly regularization of a previously irregular rhythm). Check blood pressure and obtain a 12-lead EKG with these changes.

• Excessive slowing of the pulse rate (60 beats/minute or less) may be a sign of digitalis toxicity. Hold the drug and notify the doctor.

• Observe eating patterns. Ask the patient about nausea, vomiting, anorexia, visual disturbances, and other symptoms of toxicity.

• Monitor serum potassium carefully. Take corrective action *before* hypokalemia occurs.

deslanoside
(Cedilanid-D)

Indications and dosage

CHF, paroxysmal atrial tachycardia, atrial fibrillation and flutter—
Adults: loading dose 1.2 to 1.6 mg I.M. or I.V. in 2 divided doses over 24 hours; for maintenance, use another glycoside. Not recommended for children.

Interactions

Amphotericin B, carbenicillin, ticarcillin, corticosteroids, and diuretics (including chlorthalidone, ethacrynic acid, furosemide, metolazone, and thiazides): hypokalemia, predisposing patient to digitalis toxicity. Monitor serum potassium.
Parenteral calcium, thiazides: hypercalcemia and hypomagnesemia, predisposing patient to digitalis toxicity. Monitor serum calcium and serum magnesium.

Specific considerations

• I.M. injection is painful; give I.V. if possible.

digitoxin
(Crystodigin, Purodigin)

Indications and dosage

CHF, paroxysmal atrial tachycardia, atrial fibrillation and flutter—
Adults: loading dose 1.2 to 1.6 mg I.V. or P.O. in divided doses over 24 hours; maintenance 0.1 mg daily
Children 2 to 12 years: loading dose 0.03 mg/kg or 0.75 mg/m² I.M., I.V., or P.O. in divided doses over 24 hours; maintenance ¹⁄₁₀ loading dose or 0.003 mg/kg or 0.075 mg/m² daily. Monitor closely for toxicity.
Children 1 to 2 years: loading dose 0.04 mg/kg over 24 hours in divided doses; maintenance 0.004 mg/kg daily. Monitor closely for toxicity.
Children 2 weeks to 1 year: loading dose 0.045 mg/kg I.M., I.V., or P.O. in divided doses over 24 hours; mainte-
nance 0.0045 mg/kg daily. Monitor closely for toxicity.
Premature infants, neonates, severely ill older infants: loading dose 0.022 mg/kg I.M., I.V., or P.O. in divided doses over 24 hours; maintenance 0.0022 mg/kg daily. Monitor closely for toxicity.

Interactions

Antacids, kaolin-pectin: decreased absorption of oral digitoxin. Schedule doses as far as possible from oral digitoxin administration.
Cholestyramine, colestipol, metoclopramide: decreased absorption of oral digitoxin. Monitor for decreased effect and low blood levels. Dosage may have to be increased.
Amphotericin B, carbenicillin, ticarcillin, corticosteroids, and diuretics (including chlorthalidone, ethacrynic acid, furosemide, metolazone, and thiazides): hypokalemia, predisposing patient to digitalis toxicity. Monitor serum potassium.
Parenteral calcium, thiazides: hypercalcemia and hypomagnesemia, predisposing patient to digitalis toxicity. Monitor serum calcium and serum magnesium.
Phenylbutazone, phenobarbital, phenytoin, rifampin: faster metabolism and shorter duration of digitoxin. Observe for underdigitalization.
Cimetidine: decreased digitoxin metabolism. Monitor for digitoxin toxicity.

Specific considerations

• I.M. injection is painful; give I.V. if parenteral route is necessary.
• Digitoxin is a long-acting drug; watch for cumulative effects.
• Protect solution from light.
• Instruct patient and responsible family member about drug action, dosage regimen, how to take pulse, reportable signs, and follow-up plans.
• Do not substitute one brand for another.
• Therapeutic blood levels of digitoxin range from 25 to 35 ng/ml.

Comparing Cardiac Glycosides

DRUG	ONSET	PEAK	HALF-LIFE	DURATION
deslanoside	10 to 30 min	1 to 2 hr	1½ days	2 to 5 days
digitalis leaf	15 to 120 min	4 to 12 hr	5 to 7 days	2 to 3 weeks
digitoxin	30 to 120 min	4 to 12 hr	5 to 7 days	2 to 3 weeks
digoxin	15 to 30 min	1½ to 5 hr	1½ days	2 to 3 days
gitalin	30 to 120 min	12 to 20 hr	8 to 12 days	10 to 12 days

---

digoxin
(Lanoxicaps, Lanoxin)

Indications and dosage
CHF, atrial fibrillation and flutter, paroxysmal atrial tachycardia—
Adults: loading dose 0.5 to 1 mg I.V. or P.O. in divided doses over 24 hours; maintenance 0.125 to 0.5 mg I.V. or P.O. daily (average 0.25 mg). Larger doses are often needed for treatment of dysrhythmias, depending on patient response.
Children over 2 years: loading dose 0.04 to 0.06 mg/kg P.O. divided q 8 hours over 24 hours; I.V. loading dose 0.025 to 0.04 mg/kg; maintenance 0.02 mg/kg P.O. daily divided q 12 hours
Children 1 month to 2 years: loading dose 0.06 to 0.075 mg/kg P.O. divided into three doses over 24 hours; I.V. loading dose 0.035 to 0.05 mg/kg; maintenance 0.02 to 0.025 mg/kg P.O. daily divided q 12 hours
Neonates under 1 month: loading dose 0.05 mg/kg P.O. divided q 8 hours over 24 hours; I.V. loading dose 0.015 to 0.04 mg/kg; maintenance 0.0167 mg/kg P.O. daily divided q 12 hours
Premature infants: loading dose 0.04 mg/kg I.V. divided into 3 doses over 24 hours; maintenance 0.0133 mg/kg I.V. daily divided q 12 hours

Interactions
Antacids, kaolin-pectin: decreased absorption of oral digoxin. Schedule doses as far as possible from oral digoxin administration.
Cholestyramine, colestipol, metoclopramide: decreased absorption of oral digoxin. Monitor for decreased effect and low blood levels. Dosage may have to be increased.
Quinidine, nifedipine, and verapamil: increased digoxin blood levels. Monitor for toxicity.
Amphotericin B, carbenicillin, ticarcillin, corticosteroids, and diuretics (including chlorthalidone, ethacrynic acid, furosemide, metolazone, and thiazides): hypokalemia, predisposing patient to digitalis toxicity. Monitor serum potassium.
Parenteral calcium, thiazides: hypercalcemia and hypomagnesemia, predisposing patient to digitalis toxicity. Monitor serum calcium and serum magnesium.
Anticholinergics: may increase digoxin absorption of oral tablets. Monitor blood levels and observe for toxicity.
Amiloride: inhibits and increases digoxin excretion. Monitor for altered digoxin effect.

Specific considerations
• Withhold for 1 to 2 days before elective electrocardioversion. Adjust dose after cardioversion.
• Instruct patient and responsible family member about drug action, dosage regimen, how to take pulse, reportable

signs, and follow-up plans.
- Do not substitute one brand for another.
- Therapeutic blood levels of digoxin range from 0.5 to 2.5 ng/ml.

ANTIARRHYTHMICS

Antiarrhythmics are used to prevent or treat atrial and ventricular dysrhythmias, including those secondary to myocardial infarction (MI) or digitalis toxicity.

Bradycardia can be due to decreased generation of atrial impulses or to conduction of fewer atrial impulses to the ventricles. Similarly, ventricular tachycardia can develop from an increased number of impulses from either atrial or ventricular areas.

As a group, the antiarrhythmics have a narrow therapeutic index (the toxic dose is not much greater than the therapeutic dose). Careful monitoring of therapy is imperative, since side effects of these drugs are usually serious.

Before therapy begins, underlying conditions, such as electrolyte imbalances, should be corrected.

Synchronized cardioversion and electrical pacemakers are effective antiarrhythmic alternatives.

Major uses
Antiarrhythmics are therapeutic for atrial and ventricular dysrhythmias of various causes. They are both prophylactic and therapeutic for post-MI dysrhythmias.

Mechanism of action
- Group I drugs (disopyramide, lidocaine, mexiletine hydrochloride, phenytoin, procainamide, quinidine, and tocainide) decrease sodium transport through cardiac tissues, slowing conduction through the AV node. These drugs also prolong the effective refractory period and decrease automaticity; phenytoin may also combat dysrhythmias due to digitalis toxicity.

- Group II drugs (beta blockers) decrease conduction of impulses through the AV node and increase the effective refractory period. In addition to their beta blockade, Group II drugs also have reentry blocking effects similar to those of Group I. Propranolol, the only beta blocker approved for use as an antiarrhythmic, is effective for supraventricular dysrhythmias and, to a lesser extent, for ventricular dysrhythmias.
- The Group III drug bretylium was originally thought to act as an antiadrenergic agent whose action is mediated through the sympathetic division of the autonomic nervous system. Bretylium initially exerts short-lived adrenergic stimulatory effects (caused by release of norepinephrine) on the cardiovascular system. When norepinephrine is depleted, the adrenergic blocking actions predominate. Recent pharmacologic studies indicate that bretylium's action may be due to its large quaternary ammonium structure. Amiodarone, another Group III drug, prolongs the refractory period and repolarization.
- Among the unclassified drugs in this category, atropine blocks the vagal effects on the SA node, relieving severe nodal or sinus bradycardia, or AV block. Increased conduction through the AV node speeds heart rate.

Absorption, distribution, metabolism, and excretion
After oral administration, most antiarrhythmic drugs are well absorbed from the gastrointestinal tract. Bretylium, however, is poorly absorbed and must be given parenterally.

All antiarrhythmics are widely distributed in body tissues and are metabolized primarily in the liver.
- Procainamide is metabolized to an active metabolite, N-acetylprocainamide, which accumulates in patients with impaired renal function. (The other drugs are excreted partly as inactive metabolites and partly as unchanged drug by the kidneys.)
- Propranolol and lidocaine, although well absorbed when administered by

mouth, enter the hepatic portal circulation immediately and are quickly metabolized. This is known as the "first-pass effect." However, the first-pass effect of propranolol may be nullified by administering large oral doses (relative to parenteral doses). Therefore, propranolol is commonly used both orally and parenterally.

Onset and duration
See chart on page 367.

amiodarone hydrochloride (Cordarone)

Indications and dosage
Ventricular and supraventricular dysrhythmias, including recurrent supraventricular tachycardia (including Wolff-Parkinson-White syndrome), atrial fibrillation and flutter, and ventricular tachycardia—
Adults: loading dose 5 to 10 mg/kg I.V. via central line, followed by 10 mg/kg/day I.V. for 3 to 5 days; maintenance 200 to 600 mg P.O. daily

Side effects
CNS: peripheral neuropathy and extrapyramidal symptoms, headache
CV: bradycardia, hypotension
EENT: corneal microdeposits
Endocrine: hypo- and hyperthyroidism
Hepatic: altered liver enzymes, hepatic dysfunction
Respiratory: pneumonitis
Skin: photosensitivity, blue-gray skin pigmentation
Other: muscle weakness

Interactions
None significant

Specific considerations
• Use cautiously in patients with preexisting bradycardia or sinus node disease, conduction disturbances, severely depressed ventricular function, and marked cardiomegaly.
• Amiodarone is often effective for treatment of dysrhythmias resistant to

other drug therapy. However, frequent incidence of side effects limits its use.
• Most patients treated show corneal microdeposits on slit-lamp ophthalmologic examination. Onset of this effect from 1 to 4 months after beginning amiodarone therapy. However, only 2% to 3% have actual visual disturbances. To minimize this complication, recommend instillation of methylcellulose ophthalmic solution during amiodarone therapy.
• Monitor blood pressure, and heart rate and rhythm frequently. Notify doctor of any significant change.
• Monitor hepatic function tests; thyroid function tests.
• Monitor for symptoms of pneumonitis—exertional dyspnea, nonproductive cough, and pleuritic chest pain. Monitor pulmonary function tests and chest X-ray. Pulmonary complications more prevalent in patients taking more than 600 mg daily.
• Advise patient to use a sunscreen to prevent photosensitivity. Monitor for burn or tingling skin followed by erythema and possible skin blistering.
• Amiodarone's side effects are more prevalent at high doses but are generally reversible when drug therapy is stopped. Resolution of side effects may take up to 4 months.

atropine sulfate

Indications and dosage
Symptomatic bradycardia, bradyarrhythmia (junctional or escape rhythm)—
Adults: usually 0.5 to 1 mg I.V. push; repeat q 5 minutes, to maximum 2 mg. Lower doses (less than 0.5 mg) can cause bradycardia.
Children: 0.01 mg/kg dose up to maximum 0.4 mg; or 0.3 mg/m^2 dose; may repeat q 4 to 6 hours

Side effects
Blood: leukocytosis
CNS: with doses greater than 5 mg—headache, restlessness, ataxia, disori-

entation, hallucinations, delirium, coma, *insomnia, dizziness*
CV: 1 to 2 mg—tachycardia, palpitations; greater than 2 mg—extreme tachycardia, angina
EENT: 1 mg—slight mydriasis, photophobia; *2 mg—blurred vision, mydriasis*
GI: dry mouth (common even at low doses), thirst, *constipation,* nausea, vomiting
GU: urinary retention
Skin: 2 mg—flushed, dry skin; 5 mg or more—hot, dry, reddened skin

Interactions
Methotrimeprazine: may produce extrapyramidal symptoms. Monitor patient carefully.

Nursing considerations
• Side effects vary considerably with dose. Most common are dry mouth (which can be treated with pilocarpine syrup) and thirst. Recommend sucking sour hard candy.
• Watch for tachycardia in cardiac patients; report to doctor.
• Antidote for atropine overdose is physostigmine salicylate.
• Other anticholinergic drugs may increase vagal blockage.
• Monitor closely for urinary retention in elderly males with benign prostatic hypertrophy, who are at high risk for this effect.

---

bretylium tosylate (Bretylol)

Indications and dosage
Ventricular fibrillation—
Adults: 5 mg/kg by rapid I.V. injection. If necessary, increase dose to 10 mg/kg and repeat q 15 to 30 minutes until 30 mg/kg have been given.
Other ventricular dysrhythmias—
Adults: initially, 500 mg diluted to 50 ml with dextrose 5% in water or normal saline solution and infused I.V. over more than 8 minutes at 5 to 10 mg/kg. Dose may be repeated in 1 to 2 hours. Thereafter, dose q 6 to 8 hours.

I.V. maintenance—
Adults: infused in diluted solution of 500 ml dextrose 5% in water or normal saline solution at 1 to 2 mg/minute.
I.M. injection—
Adults: 5 to 10 mg/kg undiluted. Repeat in 1 to 2 hours if needed. Thereafter, repeat q 6 to 8 hours.
Not recommended for children

Side effects
CNS: vertigo, dizziness, lightheadedness, syncope (usually secondary to hypotension)
CV: severe hypotension (especially orthostatic), bradycardia, anginal pain
GI: severe nausea, vomiting (with rapid infusion)

Interactions
All antihypertensives: may potentiate hypotension. Monitor blood pressure.

Nursing considerations
• Contraindicated in digitalis-induced dysrhythmias. Use cautiously in patients with fixed cardiac output, aortic stenosis, and pulmonary hypertension to avoid severe and sudden drop in blood pressure.
• Monitor blood pressure, and heart rate and rhythm frequently. Notify doctor immediately of any significant change. If supine systolic blood pressure falls below 75 mm Hg, notify doctor; he may order norepinephrine, dopamine, or volume expansion to raise blood pressure.
• Keep patient in the supine position until tolerance to hypotension develops.
• Avoid sudden postural changes due to postural hypotension.
• Follow dosage directions carefully to avoid nausea and vomiting.
• Give I.V. injections for ventricular fibrillation as rapidly as possible. Do not dilute.
• Rotate I.M. injection sites to prevent tissue damage, and do not exceed 5-ml volume in any one site.
• To be used with other cardiopulmonary-resuscitative measures such as cardiopulmonary resuscitation (CPR), countershock, epinephrine, sodium bi-

carbonate, and lidocaine.
• Avoid subtherapeutic doses (less than 5 mg/kg), since such doses may cause hypotension.
• Ventricular tachycardia and other ventricular dysrhythmias respond less rapidly to treatment than ventricular fibrillation.
• Dosage should be decreased in renal impairment.
• Monitor carefully if pressor amines (sympathomimetics) are given to correct hypotension, as bretylium potentiates pressor amines.
• Ineffective treatment for atrial dysrhythmias
• Has been used investigationally to treat hypertension
• Observe for increased anginal pain in susceptible patients.
• Observe patient for side effects and notify doctor if any occur.

---

disopyramide
(Norpace, Norpace CR)

Indications and dosage
Premature ventricular contractions (unifocal, multifocal, or coupled); ventricular tachycardia not severe enough to require electrocardioversion—
Adults: usual maintenance dose 150 to 200 mg P.O. q 6 hours; for patients who weigh less than 50 kg or those with renal, hepatic, or cardiac impairment— 100 mg P.O. q 6 hours. May give sustained-release capsule q 12 hours. Recommended doses in advanced renal insufficiency: creatinine clearance 15 to 40 ml/minute: 100 mg q 10 hours; creatinine clearance 5 to 15 ml/minute: 100 mg q 20 hours; creatinine clearance 1 to 5 ml/minute: 100 mg q 30 hours
Children 12 to 18 years: 6 to 15 mg/kg daily
Children 4 to 12 years: 10 to 15 mg/kg daily
Children 1 to 4 years: 10 to 20 mg/kg daily
Children less than 1 year: 10 to 30 mg/kg daily

All children's doses should be divided into equal amounts and given every 6 hours.

Side effects
CNS: dizziness, agitation, depression, fatigue, muscle weakness, syncope
CV: hypotension, CHF, heart block
EENT: blurred vision, dry eyes, dry nose
GI: nausea, vomiting, anorexia, bloating, abdominal pain, *constipation, dry mouth*
GU: urinary retention and hesitancy
Hepatic: cholestatic jaundice
Metabolic: hypoglycemia
Skin: rash in 1% to 3% of patients

Interactions
Phenytoin: increases disopyramide's metabolism. Monitor for decreased antiarrhythmic effect.

Nursing considerations
• Contraindicated in cardiogenic shock or second- or third-degree heart block with no pacemaker. Use very cautiously or avoid, if possible, in CHF. Use cautiously in underlying conduction abnormalities, urinary tract diseases (especially prostatic hypertrophy), hepatic or renal impairment, myasthenia gravis, narrow-angle glaucoma. Adjust dosage in renal insufficiency.
• Do not give sustained-release capsule for rapid control of ventricular dysrhythmias; when therapeutic blood levels must be rapidly attained; in patients with cardiomyopathy or possible cardiac decompensation; or in patients with severe renal impairment.
• When transferring your patient from immediate-release to sustained-release capsules, advise him to take a sustained-release capsule 6 hours after the last immediate-release capsule.
• Discontinue drug if heart block develops, if QRS complex widens by more than 25%, or if QT interval lengthens by more than 25% above baseline.
• Correct any underlying electrolyte abnormalities before use.

• Watch for recurrence of dysrhythmias; check for side effects; notify doctor.

• Check apical pulse before administering drug. Notify doctor if pulse rate is slower than 60 beats/minute or faster than 120 beats/minute.

• Teach patient the importance of taking drug on time, exactly as prescribed. To do this, he may have to use an alarm clock for night doses.

• Relieve discomfort of dry mouth with chewing gum or hard candy.

• Manage constipation with proper diet or bulk laxatives.

• Use of disopyramide with other antiarrhythmics may cause further myocardial depression.

• Most doctors prefer to prescribe disopyramide for patients not in heart failure who cannot tolerate quinidine or procainamide.

---

lidocaine
(Xylocaine)

Indications and dosage

Ventricular dysrhythmias from MI, cardiac manipulation, or cardiac glycosides; ventricular tachycardia—
Adults: 50 to 100 mg (1 to 1.5 mg/kg) I.V. bolus at 25 to 50 mg/minute. Give half this amount to elderly or lightweight patients and those with CHF or hepatic disease. Repeat bolus q 3 to 5 minutes until dysrhythmias subside or side effects develop. Do not exceed 300-mg total bolus during a 1-hour period. Simultaneously, begin constant infusion: 1 to 4 mg/minute. Use lower dose in elderly patients, those with CHF or hepatic disease, or patients who weigh less than 50 kg. If single bolus has been given, repeat smaller bolus 15 to 20 minutes after start of infusion to maintain therapeutic serum level. After 24 hours of continuous infusion, decrease rate by half.
I.M. administration: 200 to 300 mg in deltoid muscle only.

Side effects

CNS: confusion, tremors, lethargy, somnolence, *stupor, restlessness,* slurred speech, euphoria, depression, *lightheadedness,* paresthesias, muscle twitching, *convulsions*
CV: hypotension, bradycardia, further dysrhythmias
EENT: tinnitus, blurred or double vision
Other: anaphylaxis, soreness at injection site, sensations of cold, diaphoresis

Interactions

Barbiturates: may decrease patient's response to lidocaine. Adjust dose.
Cimetidine, beta blockers: decreased metabolism of lidocaine. Monitor for toxicity.
Phenytoin: additive cardiac depressant effects. Monitor carefully.
Procainamide: may increase neurologic side effects. Monitor carefully.

Nursing considerations

• Contraindicated in complete or second-degree heart block. Use with epinephrine (for local anesthesia) to treat dysrhythmias contraindicated. Use with caution in elderly patients, those with CHF or renal or hepatic disease, or patients who weigh less than 50 kg. Such patients will need a reduced dose.

• In many severely ill patients, convulsions may be the first clinically apparent sign of toxicity. However, severe reactions usually are preceded by somnolence, confusion, and paresthesias.

• If toxic signs (dizziness) occur, stop drug at once and notify doctor. Continued infusion could lead to convulsions and coma. Give oxygen via nasal cannula, if not contraindicated. Keep oxygen and CPR equipment handy.

• Patients receiving infusions must be *attended at all times* and be on a cardiac monitor. Use an infusion pump or a microdrip system and timer for monitoring infusion precisely. Never exceed an infusion rate of 4 mg/minute, if possible. A faster rate greatly increases risk of toxicity.

• Monitor patient's response, especially blood pressure, serum electrolytes, blood urea nitrogen, and creatinine. Notify doctor promptly if abnormalities develop.
• A bolus dose not followed by infusion will have a short-lived effect.
• A patient who has received lidocaine I.M. will show a sevenfold increase in serum creatine phosphokinase (CPK) levels. Such CPK originates in the skeletal muscle, not the heart. Test isoenzymes if using I.M. route.

mexiletine hydrochloride (Mexitil)

Indications and dosage
Treatment of refractory ventricular dysrhythmias, including ventricular tachycardia—
Adults: 200 to 250 mg I.V. bolus over 3 to 5 minutes followed by 0.5 to 1.5 mg/minute I.V. Maintenance dose 200 to 400 mg P.O. q 8 hours

Side effects
CNS: tremor, dizziness, blurred vision, ataxia, diplopia, confusion, nystagmus
CV: hypotension, bradycardia, widened QRS complex
GI: nausea, vomiting
Skin: rash

Interactions
Phenytoin: decreased mexiletine blood levels. Monitor carefully.

Specific considerations
• Use cautiously in patients with CHF or sinus node disease.
• Early sign of mexiletine toxicity is tremor, usually a fine tremor of the hands. This progresses to dizziness and later to ataxia and nystagmus as the drug's blood level increases. Question patient about these symptoms.
• May administer oral maintenance dose with meals.
• Therapeutic levels range from 0.75 to 2 mcg/ml.

• Oral mexiletine has been found to be as effective as procainamide in reduction of premature ventricular contractions (PVCs) but with fewer side effects.
• Monitor blood pressure, and heart rate and rhythm frequently. Notify doctor of any significant change.

phenytoin (Dilantin)

Indications and dosage
Ventricular dysrhythmias unresponsive to lidocaine or procainamide; supraventricular and ventricular dysrhythmias induced by cardiac glycosides—
Adults: loading dose 1 g P.O. divided over first 24 hours, followed by 500 mg daily for 2 days, then maintenance dose 300 mg P.O. daily; 250 mg I.V. over 5 minutes until dysrhythmias subside, side effects develop, or 1 g has been given. Infusion rate should never exceed 50 mg/minute (slow I.V. push).
Alternate method: 100 mg I.V. q 15 minutes until side effects develop, dysrhythmias are controlled, or 1 g has been given. May also administer entire loading dose of 1 g I.V. slowly at 25 mg/minute. Can be diluted in normal saline solution. I.M. dose not recommended because of pain and erratic absorption.
Children: 3 to 8 mg/kg P.O. or slow I.V. daily or 250 mg/m² daily given as single dose or divided in 2 doses.

Side effects
Blood: thrombocytopenia, leukopenia, *agranulocytosis, pancytopenia, lymphadenopathy,* megaloblastic anemia
CNS: ataxia, slurred speech, insomnia, headache, muscle twitching, *lethargy*
CV: severe hypotension, vascular collapse (with rapid I.V. infusions greater than 50 mg/minute), vasodilation, asystole, ventricular fibrillation, AV block
EENT: nystagmus, diplopia, blurred vision
GI: gingival hyperplasia, nausea, vomiting, constipation
Metabolic: hyperglycemia

Skin: rash (*morbilliform* most common), dermatitis (bullous, *exfoliative,* purpuric), lupus erythematosus, Stevens-Johnson syndrome

Interactions
Alcohol, barbiturates, folic acid, loxapine succinate: monitor for decreased phenytoin activity.
Oral anticoagulants, antihistamines, chloramphenicol, diazepam, diazoxide, disulfiram, isoniazid, phenylbutazone, phenyramidol, salicylates, sulfamethizole, valproate: monitor for increased phenytoin activity.

Nursing considerations
• Contraindicated in heart block, sinus bradycardia, Stokes-Adams attacks. Use cautiously in CHF, hepatic or renal dysfunction, elderly or debilitated patients, hypotension, myocardial insufficiency, respiratory depression. Cardiac patients on thyroid replacement therapy should be given I.V. phenytoin cautiously to prevent supraventricular tachycardia.
• Administer drug slow I.V. push, not to exceed 50 mg/minute in adults.
• Monitor blood pressure and EKG. Notify doctor if side effects occur.
• Do not mix with dextrose 5% I.V. fluids, as crystallization will occur. Flush I.V. line with saline solution before and after administration.
• Watch patients on phenytoin and other antiarrhythmics (disopyramide, quinidine, procainamide, propranolol) closely for signs of additive cardiac depression.
• Phenytoin can be diluted in normal saline solution and infused without precipitation. Such infusions should not take longer than 1 hour.
• Shake oral suspensions well to make dosage uniform. After giving suspension by nasogastric tube, flush tube with water to facilitate passage to stomach.
• Give drug with food or large glass of water to minimize gastric irritation.
• Avoid I.M. route of administration.
• Teach patient importance of taking drug on time, exactly as prescribed.
• Dose should be decreased in hepatic dysfunction.

• Blood levels greater than 20 mcg/ml may be toxic. The difference between therapeutic and toxic levels of phenytoin in the blood is very slight. If toxic symptoms occur, draw blood to determine drug level.
• Stress need for good oral hygiene to minimize gingival hyperplasia.
• Patients with uremia may require dose adjustment for stabilization.
• Patients concurrently on phenytoin and barbiturates, prednisone, or isoniazid should have phenytoin blood levels checked frequently. Observe for phenytoin toxicity and for failure to respond adequately to phenytoin.
• Warn patient not to drink alcohol as he may lose control of previously stable antiarrhythmic effects.

procainamide (Procan, Pronestyl)

Indications and dosage
PVC, ventricular tachycardia, atrial dysrhythmias unresponsive to quinidine, paroxysmal atrial tachycardia—
Adults: 100 mg q 5 minutes slow I.V. push, no faster than 25 to 50 mg/minute until dysrhythmias disappear, side effects develop, or 1 g has been given. When dysrhythmias disappear, give continuous infusion of 2 to 6 mg/minute. Usual effective dose 500 to 600 mg. If dysrhythmias recur, repeat bolus as above and increase infusion rate; 0.5 to 1 g I.M. q 4 to 8 hours until oral therapy begins.
Loading dose for atrial fibrillation or paroxysmal atrial tachycardia—
Adults: 1 to 1.25 g P.O. If dysrhythmias persist after 1 hour, give additional 750 mg. If no change occurs, give 500 mg to 1 g q 2 hours until dysrhythmias disappear or side effects occur.
Loading dose for ventricular tachycardia—
Adults: 1 g P.O. Maintenance 50 mg/kg daily given at 3-hour intervals; average 250 to 500 mg q 3 hours.
Note: Sustained-release tablet may be used for maintenance dosing when treat-

Comparing Antiarrhythmics

DRUG	ROUTE OF ADMIN- ISTRA- TION	ONSET	PEAK	DURA- TION	THERA- PEUTIC BLOOD LEVELS
atropine	I.V.	immedi- ate	within minutes	4 to 6 hr	†
bretylium	I.M.	up to 2 hr	6 to 9 hr	up to 10 hr	†
	I.V.	within minutes	within 20 min	up to 10 hr	†
disopyramide	P.O.	30 min	2 hr	6 to 8 hr	3 to 8 mcg/ml
lidocaine	I.M.	5 to 15 min	20 to 30 min	60 to 90 min	2 to 5 mcg/ml
	I.V.	immedi- ate	immediate (after I.V. bolus)	10 to 20 min	2 to 5 mcg/ml
phenytoin	I.V.	immedi- ate	immediate	up to 24 hr	10 to 20 mcg/ml
	P.O.	2 hr	6 hr	up to 24 hr	10 to 20 mcg/ml
procainamide	I.V.	immedi- ate	25 to 60 min	3 to 4 hr	4 to 8 mcg/ml*
	P.O.	30 min	1 hr	3 to 4 hr	4 to 8 mcg/ml*
propranolol	I.V.	immedi- ate	2 to 4 hr	3 to 6 hr	†
	P.O.	30 min	60 to 90 min	3 to 6 hr	†
quinidine	I.M.	30 min	30 to 90 min	6 to 8 hr	2 to 5 mcg/ml
	I.V.	30 min	immediate	6 to 8 hr	2 to 5 mcg/ml
	P.O.	30 min	1 to 3 hr	6 to 8 hr	2 to 5 mcg/ml

*N-acetylprocainamide (active metabolite of procainamide): 2 to 8 mcg/ml
† Not established

ing ventricular tachycardia, atrial fibrillation, and paroxysmal atrial tachycardia. Dose is 500 mg to 1 g q 6 hours.

Side effects
Blood: thrombocytopenia, *agranulocytosis,* hemolytic anemia, *increased antinuclear antibodies titer*
CNS: hallucinations, confusion, convulsions, depression
CV: severe hypotension, bradycardia, AV block, ventricular fibrillation (after parenteral use)
GI: nausea, vomiting, anorexia, diarrhea, bitter taste
Skin: maculopapular rash
Other: fever, lupus erythematosus syndrome (especially after prolonged administration), myalgia

Interactions
None significant

Nursing considerations
• Contraindicated in patients with hypersensitivity to procaine and related drugs; complete, second-degree, or third-degree heart block unassisted by electrical pacemaker; or myasthenia gravis. Use with caution in CHF or other conduction disturbances, such as bundle branch block or cardiac glycoside intoxication, or with hepatic or renal insufficiency.
• Patients receiving infusions must be *attended at all times.* Use an infusion pump or a microdrip system and timer to monitor the infusion precisely.
• Monitor blood pressure and EKG continuously during I.V. administration. Watch for prolonged QT and QRS intervals, heart block, or increased dysrhythmias. If these occur, withhold drug, obtain rhythm strip, and notify doctor immediately.
• Keep patient in supine position for I.V. administration.
• If procainamide is administered too rapidly, I.V. hypotension can occur.
• Watch closely for side effects and notify doctor if they occur. Instruct patient to report fever, rash, muscle pain, diarrhea, or pleuritic chest pain.

• Decrease dose in hepatic and renal dysfunction, and give over 6 hours. Half-life of procainamide is increased as much as threefold in these states.
• N-acetylprocainamide, an active metabolite, may accumulate when renal function is decreased. This may add to toxicity.
• Patients with CHF have lower volume of distribution and can be treated with lower doses.
• Positive antinuclear antibody titer common in about 60% of patients who do not have symptoms of lupus erythematosus syndrome. This response seems related to prolonged use, not dosage.
• After long-standing atrial fibrillation, restoration of normal rhythm may result in thromboembolism due to dislodging of thrombi from atrial wall. Anticoagulation usually advised before restoration of normal sinus rhythm.
• Stress importance of taking drug exactly as prescribed. Patient may have to set an alarm clock for night doses.

propranolol hydrochloride (Inderal)

Indications and dosage
Supraventricular, ventricular, and atrial dysrhythmias; tachyarrhythmias due to excessive catecholamine action during anesthesia, hyperthyroidism, and pheochromocytoma; angina—
Adults: 1 to 3 mg I.V. diluted in 50 ml dextrose 5% in water or normal saline solution infused slowly, not to exceed 1 mg/minute. After 3 mg have been infused, another dose may be given in 2 minutes; subsequent doses no sooner than q 4 hours. Usual maintenance 10 to 80 mg P.O. t.i.d. or q.i.d.

Side effects
CNS: fatigue, lethargy, vivid dreams, hallucinations
CV: bradycardia, hypotension, CHF, peripheral vascular disease
GI: nausea, vomiting, diarrhea

Metabolic: hypoglycemia without tachycardia
Skin: rash
Other: increased airway resistance, fever

Interactions

Insulin, hypoglycemic drugs (oral): can alter requirements for these drugs in previously stabilized diabetics. Monitor for hypoglycemia.
Cardiac glycosides: cause excessive bradycardia and increased depressant effect on myocardium. Use together cautiously.
Aminophylline: antagonizes beta-blocking effects of propranolol. Use together cautiously.
Isoproterenol, glucagon: antagonizes propranolol effect. May be used therapeutically and in emergencies.
Cimetidine: inhibits propranolol's metabolism. Monitor for greater beta-blocking effect.
Epinephrine: severe vasoconstriction. Monitor blood pressure and observe patient carefully.

Nursing considerations

• Contraindicated in asthma or allergic rhinitis; during ethyl ether anesthesia; in sinus bradycardia and in heart block greater than first-degree; in cardiogenic shock; in right ventricular failure secondary to pulmonary hypertension. Use with caution in patients with CHF, diabetes mellitus, or respiratory disease.
• Always withdraw drug slowly. Abrupt withdrawal might precipitate MI or aggravate angina, thyrotoxicosis, or pheochromocytoma. Abrupt withdrawal in thyrotoxicosis may exacerbate hyperthyroidism or precipitate thyroid storm. In thyrotoxicosis, propranolol may mask clinical signs of hyperthyroidism.
• *Do not discontinue before surgery for pheochromocytoma.* Before any surgical procedure, notify anesthesiologist that patient is receiving propranolol.
• Double-check dose and route. I.V. doses much smaller than P.O.
• Check apical pulse rate and blood pressure before giving drug. If you de-

tect extremes in pulse rate, withhold drug and notify doctor at once. Severe bradycardia may be treated with atropine 0.25 to 1 mg I.V.
• After long-standing atrial fibrillation, restoration of normal sinus rhythm may result in thromboembolism due to dislodging of thrombi from atrial wall. Anticoagulation often advised before restoration of normal atrial rhythm.
• Monitor blood pressure, EKG, and heart rate and rhythm frequently, especially during I.V. administration. When propranolol is used with other antihypertensives, monitor blood pressure while patient is sitting and standing.
• Monitor patient daily for weight gain and development of peripheral edema.
• Auscultate patient's lungs for rales and his heart for gallop rhythm or for third or fourth heart sounds. If these develop, notify doctor at once.

quinidine
(Quinidex, Quinora)

Indications and dosage
Atrial flutter or fibrillation—
Adults: 200 mg quinidine sulfate or equivalent base P.O. q 2 to 3 hours for 5 to 8 doses with subsequent daily increases until sinus rhythm is restored or toxic effects develop. Administer quinidine only after digitalization to avoid increasing AV conduction. Maximum 3 to 4 g daily.
Paroxysmal supraventricular tachycardia—
Adults: 400 to 600 mg I.M. gluconate q 2 to 3 hours until toxic side effects develop or dysrhythmia subsides
Premature atrial and ventricular contractions; paroxysmal atrioventricular junctional rhythm; paroxysmal atrial tachycardia; paroxysmal ventricular tachycardia; maintenance after cardioversion of atrial fibrillation or flutter—
Adults: test dose 50 to 200 mg P.O., then monitor vital signs before beginning therapy. Quinidine sulfate or equivalent base 200 to 400 mg P.O. q 4 to 6 hours; or initially, quinidine gluco-

nate 600 mg I.M., then up to 400 mg q 2 hours, p.r.n.; or quinidine gluconate 800 mg I.V. diluted in 40 ml dextrose 5% in water, infused at 1 mg/minute
Children: test dose 2 mg/kg; 3 to 6 mg/ kg q 2 to 3 hours for 5 doses P.O. daily

Side effects
Blood: hemolytic anemia, thrombocytopenia, agranulocytosis
CNS: vertigo, headache, lightheadedness, confusion, restlessness, cold sweat, pallor, fainting
CV: PVC; *severe hypotension; SA and AV block; ventricular fibrillation, tachycardia; aggravated CHF; EKG changes (particularly widening of QRS complex, notched P waves, widened QT interval, ST-segment depression)*
EENT: tinnitus, excessive salivation, blurred vision
GI: diarrhea, nausea, vomiting, anorexia, abdominal pains
Skin: rash, petechial hemorrhage of buccal mucosa, pruritus
Other: angioedema, acute asthmatic attack, respiratory arrest, *fever, cinchonism*

Interactions
Acetazolamide, antacids, sodium bicarbonate: may increase quinidine blood levels due to alkaline urine. Monitor for increased effect.
Barbiturates, phenytoin, rifampin: may antagonize quinidine activity. Monitor for decreased quinidine effect.
Verapamil: do not use together in patients with cardiomyopathy. May result in hypotension.

Nursing considerations
• Contraindicated in cardiac glycoside toxicity when AV conduction is grossly impaired; complete AV block with AV nodal or idioventricular pacemaker. Use with caution in myasthenia gravis. Anticholinergic drug doses may have to be increased.
• May increase toxicity of digitalis derivatives. Use with caution in patients previously digitalized. Monitor digoxin levels.

• The I.V. route should only be used to treat acute dysrhythmias. For maintenance, give only by oral or I.M. route.
• Dosage varies—some patients may require drug q 4 hours, others q 6 hours. Titrate dose by both clinical response and blood levels.
• When changing route of administration, alter dosage to compensate for variations in quinidine base content.
• Dose should be decreased in CHF and hepatic disease.
• Check apical pulse rate and blood pressure before starting therapy. If you detect extremes in pulse rate, withhold drug and notify doctor at once.
• Lidocaine may be effective in treating quinidine-induced dysrhythmias, since it increases AV conduction.
• GI side effects, especially diarrhea, are signs of toxicity. Notify doctor. Check quinidine blood levels, which are toxic when greater than 8 mcg/ml. GI symptoms may be decreased by giving with meals. Monitor drug response carefully.
• Instruct patient to notify doctor if skin rash, fever, unusual bleeding, bruising, ringing in ears, or visual disturbance occurs.
• After long-standing atrial fibrillation, restoration of normal sinus rhythm may result in thromboembolism due to dislodging of thrombi from atrial wall. Anticoagulation often advised before restoration of normal atrial rhythm.
• Never use discolored (brownish) quinidine solution.

tocainide hydrochloride (Tonocard)

Indications and dosage
Treatment of refractory ventricular dysrhythmias, including ventricular tachycardia—
Adults: 750 mg I.V. over 15 minutes as a bolus loading dose. Then give maintenance dose of 400 to 800 mg P.O. q 8 hours.

Side effects
CNS: tremor, dizziness, paresthesias, anxiety, agitation, memory loss, confusion, headache, convulsions
CV: worsening of CHF
GI: anorexia, nausea, vomiting, abdominal pain, constipation
Skin: rash, lupuslike syndrome

Interactions
None significant

Specific considerations
• Use cautiously in patients with CHF.
• May administer oral maintenance dose with meals.
• Therapeutic levels range from 4 to 10 mcg/ml.
• Tocainide has little or no adverse effect on EKG, heart rate, or blood pressure.
• Although side effects occur in up to 70% of all patients, they are usually mild or transient.
• Some patients may need to take the drug as infrequently as every 12 hours, as tocainide has prolonged duration of action.
• Monitor patient for rare lupuslike rash, which requires discontinuation of drug.

verapamil
(Calan, Isoptin)

Indications and dosage
Treatment of atrial dysrhythmias—
Adults: 0.075 to 0.15 mg/kg (5 to 10 mg) I.V. push over 2 minutes with EKG and blood pressure monitoring. Repeat dose in 30 minutes if no response. Follow bolus injection with maintenance infusion of 0.005 mg/kg/minute.
Children 1 to 15 years: 0.1 to 0.3 mg/kg and I.V. bolus over 2 minutes
Children less than 1 year: 0.1 to 0.2 mg/kg as I.V. bolus over 2 minutes under continuous EKG monitoring. Dose can be repeated in 30 minutes if no response.

Side effects
CNS: dizziness, headache, fatigue
CV: transient hypotension, heart failure, bradycardia, AV block, ventricular asystole, peripheral edema
GI: constipation, nausea (primarily from oral form)
Hepatic: elevated liver enzymes

Interactions
Propranolol (and other beta blockers), *disopyramide:* may cause heart failure. Use together cautiously.
Quinidine: do not use together in patients with cardiomyopathy. May result in hypotension.

Specific considerations
• Contraindicated in patients with advanced heart failure, AV block, severe left ventricular dysfunction, cardiogenic shock, sinus node disease, and severe hypotension.
• Use cautiously in patients with MI followed by coronary occlusion, sick sinus syndrome, impaired AV conduction, and heart failure with atrial tachyarrhythmia.
• Liver function tests should be done periodically.
• Patients with severely compromised cardiac function or those receiving beta blockers should receive lower doses of verapamil. Monitor these patients very closely.
• In older patients, I.V. doses should be administered over at least 3 minutes to minimize the risk of adverse effects.
• Notify doctor if such signs of CHF as swelling of hands and feet or shortness of breath occur.
• A new and very effective drug for treatment of supraventricular dysrhythmias. Not very effective for ventricular dysrhythmias.

ANTIANGINALS

Antianginal drugs are used to treat pain produced by an imbalance between myocardial oxygen demand and supply. These drugs are effective in the treatment of classic effort-induced angina or angina that occurs at rest (Prinzmetal's variant angina).

Drugs used to prevent and treat angina consist chiefly of nitrates, beta-adrenergic blockers, and calcium antagonists.

Treatment with antianginal drugs should be part of a general program designed to alleviate symptoms and reduce risk factors predisposing the patient to coronary artery disease (CAD).

Major uses

• Sublingual nitroglycerin and sublingual or chewable isosorbide dinitrate are indicated for relief of acute anginal episodes.

• Long-acting nitrates and topical, transdermal, transmucosal, and oral extended-release nitroglycerin products are used in prophylaxis and long-term management of patients with recurrent angina.

• Intravenous nitroglycerin is used to treat unstable angina and CHF associated with MI.

• Nitrates are also used to reduce cardiac work load in patients with CHF.

• Nadolol and propranolol, the two beta blockers, are indicated for patients with moderate-to-severe angina.

• Calcium antagonists are used to treat both classic, effort-induced angina and Prinzmetal's angina.

Mechanism of action

• Nitrates (isosorbide dinitrate, nitroglycerin, pentaerythritol tetranitrate) produce relief of angina by reducing the heart's oxygen demand. This reduction occurs because nitrates decrease left ventricular end-diastolic pressure (preload) and systemic vascular resistance (afterload). In addition, nitrates increase blood flow through collateral coronary vessels.

• Beta blockers (nadolol and propranolol hydrochloride) reduce the heart's oxygen demand by blocking catecholamine-induced increases in heart rate, blood pressure, and force of myocardial contraction.

• Calcium antagonists (diltiazem, nifedipine, and verapamil) reduce oxygen demand by inhibiting influx of calcium through the muscle cell. This dilates the coronary arteries and decreases systemic vascular resistance (afterload).

Absorption, distribution, metabolism, and excretion

• Nitrates are well absorbed by their intended routes of administration, metabolized in the liver, and excreted mainly in the urine.

• Beta blockers are absorbed in the gastrointestinal tract. Propranolol is metabolized by the liver and excreted in the urine. Nadolol is excreted unchanged in the urine.

• Calcium antagonists are well absorbed in the gastrointestinal tract, metabolized mainly in the liver, and excreted in the urine.

Onset and duration

• Onset and duration of the nitrates depends on the drug used and the form and route of administration selected. The accompanying chart on page 375 shows the range of onset and duration for these drugs.

• Propranolol's onset of action is 30 minutes; duration of action is about 6 hours.

• Nadolol's onset of action is about 2 hours; duration is from 17 to 24 hours.

• Nifedipine begins to act in 10 minutes; duration of action is approximately 4 hours.

• Verapamil, when administered intravenously, has an onset of action of less than 5 minutes. The oral form begins to act within 1 to 2 hours; duration of action is several hours.

---

diltiazem
(Cardizem)

Indications and dosage

Management of vasospastic (also called Prinzmetal's or variant angina) and classic chronic stable angina pectoris—

Adults: 30 mg P.O. q.i.d., before meals and at bedtime. Dosage may be gradually increased to 240 mg/day, in divided doses.

Side effects
CNS: headache, fatigue, drowsiness, dizziness, nervousness, depression, insomnia, confusion
CV: edema, dysrhythmia, flushing, bradycardia, hypotension, conduction abnormalities
GI: nausea, vomiting, diarrhea
GU: nocturia, polyuria
Hepatic: transient elevation of liver enzymes
Skin: rash, pruritus
Other: photosensitivity

Interactions
Propranolol (and other beta blockers): may prolong cardiac conduction time. Use together cautiously.

Specific considerations
• Contraindicated in sick sinus syndrome, unless a functioning ventricular pacemaker is present; in hypotension when systolic blood pressure is less than 90 mm Hg; and in second- or third-degree AV block.
• Use cautiously in patients with impaired ventricular function or conduction abnormalities.
• Use cautiously in patients with impaired liver or kidney function.
• If nitrate therapy is prescribed during titration of diltiazem dosage, urge patient to continue compliance. Sublingual nitroglycerin, especially, may be taken concomitantly as needed when anginal symptoms are acute.
• Of the available calcium antagonists, diltiazem may offer the lowest risk of side effects.
• Used investigationally to treat supraventricular tachycardia.

---

isosorbide dinitrate
(Isordil, Sorbitrate)

Indications and dosage
Treatment of acute anginal attacks (sublingual and chewable only); prophylaxis in situations likely to cause attacks; treatment of chronic ischemic heart disease (by preload reduction); adjunct with other vasodilators, such as hydralazine and prazosin, in treatment of severe chronic CHF—
Adults:
Sublingual form—2.5 to 10 mg under the tongue for prompt relief of anginal pain, repeated q 2 to 3 hours during acute phase, or q 4 to 6 hours for prophylaxis
Chewable form—5 to 10 mg p.r.n., for acute attack or q 2 to 3 hours for prophylaxis but only after initial test dose of 5 mg to determine risk of severe hypotension
Oral form—5 to 30 mg P.O. q.i.d. for prophylaxis only (use smallest effective dose); sustained-release forms 40 mg P.O. q 6 to 12 hours

Side effects
CNS: headache, sometimes with throbbing; dizziness; weakness
CV: orthostatic hypotension, tachycardia, palpitations, ankle edema, fainting
GI: nausea, vomiting
Local: sublingual burning
Skin: cutaneous vasodilation, *flushing*
Other: hypersensitivity reactions

Interactions
None significant

Nursing considerations
• Contraindicated in hypersensitivity to nitrites, head trauma, cerebral hemorrhage, severe anemia. Use with caution in hypotension.
• Monitor blood pressure and intensity and duration of response to drug.
• May cause headaches, especially at first. Treat headache with aspirin or acetaminophen. Dosage may need to be

reduced temporarily, but tolerance usually develops.

• Tell patient to take medication regularly, even long-term, if ordered, and to keep it easily accessible at all times. Drug is physiologically necessary but not habit-forming.

• Additional dose may be taken before anticipated stress or at bedtime if angina is nocturnal.

• Advise patient to avoid alcoholic beverages; they may produce unpleasant disulfiram-like side effects.

• May cause orthostatic hypotension. To minimize it, patient should change to upright position slowly, go up and down stairs carefully, and lie down at first sign of dizziness.

• Teach patient to take sublingual tablet at first sign of attack. He should wet the tablet with saliva, place it under the tongue until completely absorbed, and sit down and rest. Burning sensation indicates potency. Dose may be repeated every 10 to 15 minutes for a maximum of three doses. If no relief, patient should call doctor or go to hospital emergency room. If patient complains of tingling sensation with drug placed sublingually, he may try holding tablet in buccal pouch.

• Warn patient not to confuse sublingual with oral form.

• Teach patient to take oral tablet on empty stomach, either ½ hour before or 1 to 2 hours after meals, to swallow oral tablets whole, and to chew chewable tablets thoroughly before swallowing.

• Drug should not be discontinued abruptly—coronary vasospasm may occur.

• Store in cool place, in tightly closed container, away from light.

• Has been used investigationally in treatment of CHF.

---

nadolol
(Corgard)

Indications and dosage
Management of angina pectoris—

Adults: 40 mg P.O. once daily, initially. Dosage may be increased in 40- to 80-mg increments until optimum response occurs. Usual maintenance dosage range: 80 to 240 mg once daily

Side effects
CNS: fatigue, lethargy
CV: bradycardia, hypotension, CHF, peripheral vascular disease
GI: nausea, vomiting, diarrhea
Metabolic: hypoglycemia without tachycardia
Skin: rash
Other: increased airway resistance, fever

Interactions
Insulin, hypoglycemic drugs (oral): can alter dosage requirements in previously stabilized diabetics. Observe patient carefully.
Cardiac glycosides: excessive bradycardia and increased depressant effect on myocardium. Use together cautiously.
Epinephrine: severe vasoconstriction. Monitor blood pressure and observe patient carefully.

Nursing considerations
• Contraindicated in patients with bronchial asthma, sinus bradycardia and greater than first-degree conduction block, and cardiogenic shock.

• Use cautiously in patients with heart failure, chronic bronchitis, and emphysema.

• Always check patient's apical pulse before giving drug. If slower than 60 beats/minute, hold drug and call doctor.

• Monitor blood pressure frequently. If patient develops severe hypotension, administer a vasopressor as ordered.

• Do not discontinue abruptly: can exacerbate angina and MI.

• Teach patient about his disease and therapy. Explain importance of taking drug, even when he is feeling well. Tell outpatient not to discontinue drug suddenly, but to call doctor if unpleasant side effects develop.

• Drug masks common signs of shock and hypoglycemia.

Comparing Nitrates

DRUG	FORM	ONSET	DURATION
erythrityl tetranitrate	chewable and sublingual	5 min	2 hr
	oral	30 min	3 to 4 hr
isosorbide dinitrate	chewable and sublingual	2 to 5 min	1 to 2 hr
	oral	15 to 30 min	4 to 6 hr
	oral, extended-release	1 hr	12 hr
nitroglycerin	intravenous	instantaneous	transient
	sublingual	3 min	10 to 30 min
	transmucosal	3 min	6 hr
	oral, extended-release	1 hr	8 to 12 hr
	topical ointment	30 to 60 min	4 to 6 hr
	transdermal	30 to 60 min	24 hr
penta-erythritol tetranitrate	oral	30 min	4 to 5 hr
	oral, extended-release	1 hr	12 hr

• May be given without regard to meals.

---

nifedipine
(Adalat, Procardia)

Indications and dosage

Management of vasospastic (also called Prinzmetal's or variant angina) and classic chronic stable angina pectoris—
Adults: Starting dose is 10 mg P.O. t.i.d. Usual effective dose range is 10 to 20 mg t.i.d. Some patients may require up to 30 mg q.i.d. Maximum daily dose is 180 mg.

Side effects

CNS: dizziness, light-headedness, flushing, headache, weakness, syncope
CV: peripheral edema, hypotension, palpitations
EENT: nasal congestion
GI: nausea, heartburn, diarrhea
Other: muscle cramps, dyspnea

Interactions

Propranolol (and other beta blockers): may cause heart failure. Use together cautiously.

Nursing considerations

• Use cautiously in patients with CHF or hypotension.
• Monitor blood pressure regularly, especially in patients also taking beta blockers or antihypertensives.
• Patient may briefly develop anginal exacerbation when beginning drug therapy or at times of dosage increase. Reassure him that this symptom is temporary.
• Although rebound effect has not been observed when drug is stopped, dosage should still be reduced slowly under doctor's supervision.
• If patient is kept on nitrate therapy while drug dosage is being titrated, urge him to continue compliance. Sublingual nitroglycerin, especially, may be taken

as needed when anginal symptoms are acute.
• Instruct patient to swallow capsule whole without breaking, crushing, or chewing.
• No sublingual form of nifedipine is available. However, the liquid in oral capsule can be withdrawn by puncturing capsule with a needle. Instill drug into buccal pouch.
• Has been used investigationally in treatment of hypertension and Raynaud's phenomenon.

nitroglycerin (Nitrostat, Nitro-Dur)

Indications and dosage
Prophylaxis against chronic anginal attacks—
Adults: 1 sustained-release capsule q 8 to 12 hours; or 2% ointment: Start with ½" ointment, increasing with ½" increments until headache occurs, then decreasing to previous dose. Range of dosage with ointment 2" to 5"; usual dose 1" to 2". Alternatively, transdermal disc or pad (Nitro-Dur) may be applied to hairless site once daily.
Relief of acute angina pectoris, prophylaxis to prevent or minimize anginal attacks when taken immediately prior to stressful events—
Adults: 1 sublingual tablet (gr ¼₀₀, ¼₀₀, ¼₅₀, ¼₀₀) dissolved under tongue or in buccal pouch immediately on indication of anginal attack. May repeat q 5 minutes for 15 minutes.
To control hypertension associated with surgery; to treat CHF associated with MI; to relieve angina pectoris in acute situations; to produce controlled hypotension during surgery (by I.V. infusion)—
Adults: Initial infusion rate is 5 mcg/minute. May be increased by 5 mcg/minute q 3 to 5 minutes until response is noted. If a 20 mcg/minute rate does not produce a response, dosage may be increased by as much as 20 mcg/minute q 3 to 5 minutes.

Side effects
CNS: headache, sometimes with throbbing; dizziness; weakness
CV: orthostatic hypotension, tachycardia, flushing, palpitations, fainting
GI: nausea, vomiting
Skin: cutaneous vasodilation
Local: sublingual burning
Other: hypersensitivity reactions

Interactions
None significant

Nursing considerations
• Contraindicated in hypersensitivity to nitrites, head trauma, cerebral hemorrhage, severe anemia. Use with caution in hypotension.
• Monitor blood pressure and intensity and duration of response to drug.
• May cause headaches, especially at first. Treat headache with aspirin or acetaminophen. Dosage may need to be reduced temporarily, but tolerance usually develops.
• Tell patient to take medication regularly, even long-term, if ordered, and to keep it easily accessible at all times. Drug is physiologically necessary but not habit-forming.
• Additional dose may be taken before anticipated stress or at bedtime if angina is nocturnal.
• Advise patient to avoid alcoholic beverages; they may produce unpleasant disulfiram-like side effects.
• May cause orthostatic hypotension. To minimize it, patient should change to upright position slowly, go up and down stairs carefully, and lie down at first sign of dizziness.
• Only the sublingual form should be used to relieve acute attack.
• Teach patient to take sublingual tablet at first sign of attack. He should wet the tablet with saliva, place it under the tongue until completely absorbed, and sit down and rest. If no relief, he should call doctor or go to hospital emergency room. If patient complains of tingling sensation with drug placed sublingually, he may try holding tablet in buccal pouch.

• Although burning sensation used to be an indication of tablet potency, today many brands do not produce this sensation.

• Teach patient to take oral tablet on empty stomach, either ½ hour before or 1 to 2 hours after meals, to swallow oral tablets whole, and to chew chewable tablets thoroughly before swallowing.

• Store in cool, dark place in tightly closed container. To assure freshness, replace supply every 3 months. Remove cotton from container, since it absorbs drug.

• Buccal sustained-release tablet should be allowed to dissolve between cheek and gum. Dissolves within 3 to 5 minutes.

• To apply ointment, spread in uniform, thin layer on any nonhairy area. Do not rub in. Cover with plastic film to aid absorption and protect clothing.

• Transdermal dosage forms can be applied to any hairless part of the skin except distal parts of the arms or legs, because absorption will not be maximal at these sites.

• Various brands of transdermal nitroglycerin products have different total content and surface-area specifications. Do not interchange brands on same patient without first consulting doctor or pharmacist.

• Doctor may prescribe nitroglycerin by its chemical name, glyceryl trinitrate.

• When administering as an intravenous infusion, be sure to use special nonabsorbing tubing supplied by manufacturer, because up to 80% of drug can be absorbed by regular plastic tubing. Also, be sure to prepare in a glass bottle or container.

---

pentaerythritol tetranitrate (Peritrate)

Indications and dosage
Prophylaxis against angina pectoris—
Adults: 10 to 20 mg P.O. q.i.d.; may be titrated upward to 40 mg P.O. q.i.d. ½ hour before or 1 hour after meals and h.s.; 80 mg sustained-release preparations P.O. b.i.d.

Side effects
CNS: headache, sometimes with throbbing; dizziness; weakness
CV: orthostatic hypotension, tachycardia, flushing, palpitations, fainting
GI: nausea, vomiting
Skin: cutaneous vasodilation
Other: hypersensitivity reactions

Interactions
None significant

Nursing considerations
• Contraindicated in head trauma, cerebral hemorrhage, severe anemia. Use with caution in hypotension and glaucoma.

• Monitor blood pressure and intensity and duration of response to drug.

• Medication may cause headaches, especially at first. Treat with aspirin or acetaminophen. Dosage may need to be reduced temporarily, but tolerance usually develops.

• Medication should be taken regularly, even long-term, if ordered. Drug is physiologically necessary but not habit-forming.

• Additional doses may be taken before anticipated stress or at bedtime for nocturnal angina.

• Not to be used for relief of acute anginal attacks.

• May cause orthostatic hypotension. To minimize it, patient should change to upright position slowly, go up and down stairs carefully, and lie down at first sign of dizziness.

• Drug should not be discontinued abruptly—coronary vasospasm may occur.

• Store medication in cool place in tightly covered, light-resistant container.

---

propranolol hydrochloride (Inderal, Inderal LA)

Indications and dosage
Management of angina pectoris—

Adults: 10 to 20 mg t.i.d. or q.i.d. Or one 80-mg sustained-release capsule daily. Dosage may be increased at 7- to 10-day intervals. The average optimum dose is 160 mg daily.

Side effects
CNS: fatigue, lethargy, vivid dreams, hallucinations
CV: bradycardia, hypotension, CHF, peripheral vascular disease
GI: nausea, vomiting, diarrhea
Metabolic: hypoglycemia without tachycardia
Skin: rash
Other: increased airway resistance, fever

Interactions
Insulin, hypoglycemic drugs (oral): can alter requirements for these drugs in previously stabilized diabetics. Monitor for hypoglycemia.
Cardiac glycosides: excessive bradycardia and increased depressant effect on myocardium. Use together cautiously.
Aminophylline: antagonizes beta-blocking effects of propranolol. Use together cautiously.
Isoproterenol, glucagon: antagonizes propranolol effect. May be used therapeutically and in emergencies.
Cimetidine: inhibits propranolol's metabolism. Monitor for greater beta-blocking effect.
Epinephrine: severe vasoconstriction. Monitor blood pressure and observe patient carefully.

Nursing considerations
• Contraindicated in diabetes mellitus, asthma, allergic rhinitis; during ethyl ether anesthesia; in sinus bradycardia and heart block greater than first-degree; in cardiogenic shock; in right ventricular failure secondary to pulmonary hypertension. Use with caution in patients with CHF or respiratory disease and in patients taking other antihypertensive drugs.
• Always check patient's apical pulse rate before giving drug. If you detect extremes in pulse rates, hold medication

and call doctor immediately.
• Monitor blood pressure frequently. If patient develops severe hypotension, notify doctor. He may prescribe a vasopressor.
• Teach patient about his disease and therapy. Explain importance of taking drug exactly as prescribed, even when he is feeling well. Tell outpatient not to discontinue drug suddenly; abrupt discontinuation can exacerbate angina and MI. Tell patient to call doctor if unpleasant side effects develop.
• Drug masks common signs of shock and hypoglycemia.
• Food may increase absorption of propranolol. Give drug consistently with meals.
• Compliance may be improved by administering drug twice daily or by sustained-release capsule. Check with doctor.
• Propranolol, as well as other beta blockers, is being prescribed to decrease mortality following MI.

---

verapamil
(Calan, Isoptin)

Indications and dosage
Management of vasospastic (also called Prinzmetal's or variant) angina and classic chronic, stable angina pectoris—

Adults: starting dose is 80 mg P.O. t.i.d. or q.i.d. Dosage may be increased at weekly intervals. Some patients may require up to 480 mg daily.

Side effects
CNS: dizziness, headache, fatigue
CV: transient hypotension, heart failure, bradycardia, AV block, ventricular asystole, peripheral edema
GI: constipation, nausea (primarily from oral form)
Hepatic: elevated liver enzymes

Interactions
Propranolol (and other beta blockers), *disopyramide:* may cause heart failure. Use together cautiously.

Quinidine: do not use together in patients with cardiomyopathy. May result in hypotension.

Nursing considerations
• Contraindicated in patients with advanced heart failure, AV block, severe left ventricular dysfunction, cardiogenic shock, sinus node disease, and severe hypotension.
• Use cautiously in patients with MI followed by coronary occlusion, sick sinus syndrome, impaired AV conduction, and heart failure with atrial tachyarrhythmia.
• Liver function tests should be done periodically.
• Patients with severely compromised cardiac function or those receiving beta blockers should receive lower doses of verapamil. Monitor these patients very closely.
• In older patients, I.V. doses should be administered over at least 3 minutes to minimize risk of adverse effects.
• Notify doctor if such signs of CHF as swelling of hands and feet or shortness of breath occur.
• If patient is kept on nitrate therapy while drug dosage of oral verapamil is being titrated, urge him to continue compliance. Sublingual nitroglycerin, especially, may be taken as needed when anginal symptoms are acute.
• Oral verapamil is also used investigationally as a treatment for hypertension.
• A new and very effective drug for treatment of supraventricular dysrhythmias. Not very effective for ventricular dysrhythmias.

ANTIHYPERTENSIVES

Antihypertensives are used to lower blood pressure in patients whose diastolic blood pressure averages 90 to 95 mm Hg or more. To control blood pressure effectively with minimal side effects, two or more antihypertensive agents—with different modes of action—may be needed.

About half these people do not realize they are ill because they remain asymptomatic until complications occur. Untreated hypertension can lead to stroke and cardiac or renal disease.

Hypertension is one of the few chronic diseases for which effective therapy exists. However, treatment depends on accurate diagnosis.

Compliance with prescribed drug regimens is one of the biggest problems in the treatment of this disorder because, to the patient, the side effects from the drugs may seem worse than the disease.

Major uses
Antihypertensives are used primarily to treat mild-to-severe essential hypertension (about 90% of all cases). Virtually all parenteral drugs are reserved for treatment of hypertensive emergencies such as hypertensive encephalopathy or malignant hypertension.

Antihypertensives can also be used to control hypertension in the 10% of patients who have secondary hypertension, until a surgical cure can be obtained.

Some vasodilating antihypertensives can also be used in chronic refractory CHF to decrease the arterial resistance (afterload) that the heart must pump against. This decrease in arterial impedance causes an increase in cardiac output. Minoxidil and hydralazine affect mainly the arterial bed, whereas prazosin and nitroprusside affect both the arterial and venous sides.

A vasodilator affecting the arterial bed (afterload) may be used alone or in combination with a nitrate affecting the venous bed (preload) to treat refractory CHF. Preload and afterload agents are used in combination with standard therapy for CHF (salt reduction, diuretics, and digoxin) to achieve maximal results.

Mechanism of action
The chart on pages 380 to 381 summarizes the neuromuscular and enzymatic mechanisms of the major classes of antihypertensive agents.

Comparing Antihypertensives

DRUG	ROUTE	ONSET	DURATION	SITE AND MECHANISM OF ACTION
Sympatholytics				
reserpine	I.M.	2 hr	10 to 12 hr	Peripherally acting antihypertensive; depletes stores of norepinephrine by inhibiting uptake
	I.V. P.O.	4 to 60 min days to weeks	6 to 8 hr days	
clonidine	P.O.	30 to 60 min	8 hr	Centrally acting drug; decreases central sympathetic outflow
guanadrel	P.O.	2 hr	12 hr	Peripherally acting drug; directly inhibits release of norepinephrine and depletes stores of norepinephrine in adrenergic nerve endings
guanethi- dine	P.O.	1 to 3 weeks	1 to 3 weeks	
trimetha- phan	I.V.	immediate	10 min after infusion is stopped	Ganglionic blocker; stabilizes postsynaptic membranes
methyldopa	I.V.	4 to 6 hr	24 to 48 hr	Centrally acting drug; activates inhibitory alpha-adrenergic receptors, reducing central sympathetic output
	P.O.	12 to 24 hr	24 to 48 hr	
atenolol	P.O.	variable	24 to 36 hr	Beta blockers; drugs block response to beta stimulation; also depress renin output
metoprolol	P.O.	variable	12 to 24 hr	

DRUG	ROUTE	ONSET	DURATION	SITE AND MECHANISM OF ACTION
nadolol	P.O.	variable	24 to 36 hr	Beta blockers; drugs block response to beta stimulation; also depress renin output
pindolol	P.O.	variable	12 to 24 hr	
propranolol	I.V. P.O.	1 to 5 min variable	4 to 6 hr 12 to 24 hr	
timolol	P.O.	variable	12 to 24 hr	
Vasodilators				
diazoxide	I.V.	5 min	3 to 12 hr	
hydralazine	I.M.	10 to 30 min	2 to 6 hr	Directly relaxes arteriolar smooth muscle
	I.V. P.O.	5 to 20 min 20 to 30 min	2 to 6 hr 3 to 8 hr†	
nitroprus-side	I.V.	immediate	1 to 10 min after infusion is stopped (effect dissipates rapidly)	Relax both arteriolar and venous smooth muscle
prazosin	P.O.	2 hr	less than 24 hr	
Enzyme inhibitors				
captopril	P.O.	1 hr	6 to 12 hr	Inhibits angiotensin-converting enzyme and prevents conversion of angiotensin I to angiotensin II in the lungs. Inhibits tyrosine hydroxylase.
metyrosine	P.O.	1 to 2 days	3 to 4 days	

†Depending on acetylator status
*Depending on dosage

Absorption, distribution, metabolism, and excretion

Given orally, most antihypertensives are rapidly absorbed from the GI tract. Methyldopa, however, is erratically absorbed.

All antihypertensives are widely distributed in body tissues, and most are excreted predominantly through the kidneys. Prazosin, however, is eliminated through bile and feces.

• Captopril: This drug is well absorbed from the GI tract, distributed to most body tissues, and partially metabolized in the liver. Both metabolite and unchanged drug are excreted in the urine.

• Hydralazine: Some patients acetylate (metabolize) hydralazine at a faster rate than others (see chart). Since acetylation inactivates the drug, rapid acetylators may require doses up to 60% larger than the usual dose to control their blood pressure.

• Methyldopa: The extent of methyldopa absorption varies in patients from day to day but averages 50% of the administered dose. The drug's onset is delayed about 12 to 24 hours after an oral dose because methyldopa is biotransformed in the liver to the metabolite alpha-methylnorepinephrine, which produces the antihypertensive effect.

Onset and duration

The chart on pages 380 and 381 describes the onset and duration of antihypertensives.

---

atenolol (Tenormin)

Indications and dosage

Treatment of hypertension—
Adults: initially 50 mg P.O. daily single dose. Dosage may be increased to 100 mg once daily after 7 to 14 days. Dosages greater than 100 mg are unlikely to produce further benefit.

Side effects

CNS: fatigue, lethargy

CV: *bradycardia, hypotension, CHF,* peripheral vascular disease
GI: nausea, vomiting, diarrhea
Skin: rash
Other: fever

Interactions

Insulin, hypoglycemic drugs (oral): can alter dosage requirements in previously stabilized diabetics. Observe patient carefully.
Cardiac glycosides: excessive bradycardia and increased depressant effect on myocardium. Use together cautiously.
Indomethacin: decrease in antihypertensive effect. Monitor blood pressure and adjust dosage.

Nursing considerations

• Contraindicated in sinus bradycardia and greater-than-first-degree conduction block and cardiogenic shock.

• Use cautiously in patients with cardiac failure.

• Similar to metoprolol, atenolol is a cardioselective beta blocker. Although atenolol can be used in patients with bronchospastic diseases such as asthma and emphysema, it should be used cautiously in such patients–especially when 100 mg are given.

• Dosage should be reduced if patient has renal insufficiency.

• Once-a-day dosage encourages patient compliance. Counsel patient to take the drug at a regular time every day. Drug can be dispensed in a 28-day calendar pack.

• Always check patient's apical pulse before giving drug; if slower than 60 beats/minute, hold drug and call doctor.

• Monitor blood pressure frequently. If patient develops severe hypotension, administer a vasopressor.

• Do not discontinue abruptly; can exacerbate angina and MI.

• Teach patient about his disease and therapy. Explain importance of taking drug, even when he is feeling well. Tell patient not to discontinue drug suddenly, but to call doctor if unpleasant side effects develop.

• Drug masks common signs of shock and hypoglycemia. However, atenolol does not potentiate insulin-induced hypoglycemia or delay recovery of blood glucose to normal levels.
• Atenolol, as well as other beta blockers, is being prescribed to decrease mortality following MI.

captopril
(Capoten)

Indications and dosage
Treatment of severe hypertension—
Adults: 25 mg t.i.d. initially. If blood pressure is not satisfactorily controlled in 1 to 2 weeks, dose may be increased to 50 mg t.i.d. If not satisfactorily controlled after another 1 to 2 weeks, a diuretic should be added to regimen. If further blood pressure reduction is necessary, dose may be raised to as high as 150 mg t.i.d. while continuing the diuretic. Maximum dose is 450 mg daily.
Heart failure inadequately controlled by digitalis and diuretics—
Adults: 25 mg t.i.d. in addition to the usual diuretic and digitalis regimen. Dosage may be increased to 50 mg t.i.d. If necessary, after 2 weeks, dose may be increased to as much as 150 mg t.i.d.

Side effects
Blood: leukopenia, agranulocytosis, pancytopenia
CNS: dizziness, fainting
CV: tachycardia, hypotension, angina pectoris, CHF
EENT: loss of taste (dysgeusia)
GU: proteinuria, nephrotic syndrome, membranous glomerulopathy, renal failure, urinary frequency
GI: anorexia
Metabolic: hyperkalemia
Skin: urticarial rash, maculopapular rash, pruritus
Other: fever, angioedema of face and extremities, transient increases in liver enzymes

Interactions
None significant

Nursing considerations
• Use cautiously in patients with impaired renal function or serious autoimmune disease (particularly systemic lupus erythematosus) or those who have been exposed to other drugs known to affect white cell counts or immune response.
• Proteinuria and nephrotic syndrome may occur in patients on captopril therapy. Those who develop persistent proteinuria or proteinuria that exceeds 1 g daily should have their captopril therapy reevaluated.
• Monitor patient's blood pressure and pulse rate frequently.
• Perform white blood cell count and differential counts before starting treatment, every 2 weeks for the first 3 months of therapy and periodically thereafter.
• Advise patients to report any sign of infection (sore throat, fever).
• Because captopril may cause serious side effects, it should be reserved for patients who have developed undesirable side effects from or failed to respond to other antihypertensive drugs. Commonly used in patients who fail to respond to "triple-drug therapy" (a diuretic, a beta blocker, and a vasodilator).
• Although captopril can be used alone, its beneficial effects are increased when a thiazide diuretic is added.
• May cause dizziness or fainting; advise patient to avoid sudden postural changes.
• Question patient about impaired taste sensation.
• Should be taken 1 hour before meals since food in the GI tract may reduce absorption.

clonidine hydrochloride
(Catapres)

Indications and dosage
Essential, renal, and malignant hypertension—
Adults: initially, 0.1 mg P.O. b.i.d. Then increase by 0.1 to 0.2 mg daily on a weekly basis. Usual dose range: 0.2 to

0.8 mg daily in divided doses. Infrequently, doses as high as 2.4 mg daily. No dosing recommendations for children.

Side effects
CNS: drowsiness, dizziness, fatigue, sedation, nervousness, headache
CV: orthostatic hypotension, bradycardia
EENT: mouth dryness
GI: constipation
GU: urinary retention
Metabolic: glucose intolerance
Other: impotence

Interactions
Tricyclic antidepressants and monoamine oxidase (MAO) inhibitors: may decrease antihypertensive effect. Use together cautiously.
Propranolol and other beta blockers: paradoxical hypertensive response. Monitor carefully.

Nursing considerations
• Use cautiously in patients with severe coronary insufficiency, diabetes, MI, cerebral vascular disease, chronic renal failure, or history of depression, or in those taking other antihypertensives.
• Monitor blood pressure and pulse rate frequently. Dosage is usually adjusted to patient's blood pressure and tolerance.
• May be given to rapidly lower blood pressure in some hypertensive emergency situations.
• Reduce dose gradually over 2 to 4 days. If discontinued abruptly, this drug may cause severe hypertension.
• Teach patient about his disease and therapy. Explain importance of taking drug exactly as prescribed, even when he is feeling well. Tell outpatient not to discontinue drug suddenly, but to call doctor if unpleasant side effects develop. Warn that drug can cause drowsiness, but that tolerance to this side effect will develop.
• Inform patient that orthostatic hypotension can be minimized by rising slowly and avoiding sudden position changes. Mouth dryness can be relieved with sugarless chewing gum, sour hard candy, or ice chips.
• Last dose should be taken immediately before retiring.

diazoxide
(Hyperstat—I.V. only)

Indications and dosage
Hypertensive crisis—
Adults: 300 mg I.V. bolus push, administered in 30 seconds or less into peripheral vein. Repeat at intervals of 4 to 24 hours p.r.n. Mini-boluses of 1 to 3 mg/kg repeated at intervals of 5 to 15 minutes or infusions of 15 mg/minute are equally effective. Switch to therapy with oral antihypertensives as soon as possible.
Children: 5 mg/kg I.V. rapid bolus push

Side effects
CNS: headaches, dizziness, light-headedness, euphoria
CV: sodium and water retention, orthostatic hypotension, sweating, flushing, warmth, angina, myocardial ischemia, dysrhythmias, EKG changes
GI: nausea, vomiting, abdominal discomfort
Metabolic: hyperglycemia, hyperuricemia
Local: inflammation and pain from extravasation

Interactions
Hydralazine: may cause severe hypotension. Use together cautiously.
Thiazide diuretics: may increase the effects of diazoxide. Use together cautiously.

Nursing considerations
• Use cautiously in patients with impaired cerebral or cardiac function, diabetes, or uremia, or in those taking other antihypertensives.
• Monitor blood pressure frequently. Notify doctor immediately if severe hypotension develops. Keep norepinephrine available.

• Monitor intake and output carefully. If fluid or sodium retention develops, doctor may want to order diuretics.
• Avoid extravasation.
• Drug may alter requirements for insulin, diet, or oral hypoglycemic drugs in previously controlled diabetics. Monitor blood glucose daily.
• Weigh patient daily. Notify doctor of any weight increase.
• Watch diabetics closely for signs of severe hyperglycemia or hyperosmolar nonketotic coma. Insulin may be needed.
• Check uric acid levels frequently. Report abnormalities to doctor.
• Inform patient that orthostatic hypotension can be minimized by rising slowly and avoiding sudden position changes. Instruct him to remain supine for 30 minutes after injection.
• Infusion of diazoxide has been shown to be as effective as a bolus in some patients.

guanabenz acetate
(Wytensin)

Indications and dosage
Treatment of hypertension—
Adults: initially, 4 mg P.O. b.i.d. Dosage may be increased in increments of 4 to 8 mg/day every 1 to 2 weeks. Maximum dose is 32 mg b.i.d.

Side effects
CNS: *drowsiness, sedation, dizziness, weakness,* headache, ataxia, depression
EENT: dry mouth
GU: sexual dysfunction

Interactions
CNS depressants: may cause increased sedation. Use together cautiously.

Nursing considerations
• Use cautiously in patients with vascular insufficiency, coronary insufficiency, recent MI, cerebrovascular disease, or severe hepatic or renal failure.
• Do not stop guanabenz therapy abruptly. Rebound hypertension may

occur.
• Advise patient to drive a car or operate machinery very cautiously until the CNS effects of the drug are determined.
• Warn patient that tolerance to alcohol or other CNS depressants may be diminished.
• Guanabenz can be used alone or in combination with a thiazide diuretic.
• Teach patient about his disease and therapy. Explain importance of taking drug exactly as prescribed, even when he is feeling well.
• To relieve dry mouth, tell patient to chew sugarless gum or dissolve ice chips in the mouth.

guanadrel sulfate
(Hylorel)

Indications and dosage
Treatment of hypertension—
Adults: initially, 5 mg P.O. b.i.d. Dosage can be adjusted until blood pressure is controlled. Most patients require doses of 20 to 75 mg/day, usually given b.i.d.

Side effects
CNS: *fatigue, dizziness,* drowsiness, faintness
CV: *orthostatic hypotension,* edema
Other: impotence, ejaculation disturbances

Interactions
MAO inhibitors, ephedrine, levarterenol, methylphenidate, tricyclic antidepressants, amphetamines, phenothiazines: may inhibit antihypertensive effect of guanadrel. Adjust dose accordingly.

Nursing considerations
• Contraindicated in patients with known or suspected pheochromocytoma or frank CHF.
• Use cautiously in asthmatic patients and in patients with known regional vascular disease or history of peptic ulcer disease.

• Guanadrel should be discontinued 48 to 72 hours before surgery to minimize risk of vascular collapse during anesthesia.

• Do not give concurrently or within 1 week of therapy with an MAO inhibitor.

• Patient response varies widely, and dosage must be individualized. Monitor both supine and standing blood pressure, especially during period of dosage adjustment.

• Teach patient about his disease and therapy. Explain importance of taking drug exactly as prescribed, even when he is feeling well. Tell patient not to discontinue drug suddenly but to call doctor if unpleasant side effects develop.

• Tell outpatient to avoid strenuous exercise, and warn that hot showers may cause hypotensive reaction.

• Inform patient that orthostatic hypotension can be minimized by rising slowly from a supine position and avoiding sudden position changes.

---

guanethidine sulfate (Ismelin)

Indications and dosage

For moderate-to-severe hypertension; usually used in combination with other antihypertensives—
Adults: initially, 10 mg P.O. daily. Increase by 10 mg at weekly to monthly intervals p.r.n. Usual dose is 25 to 50 mg daily. Some patients may require up to 300 mg.
Children: initially, 200 mcg/kg P.O. daily. Increase gradually every 1 to 3 weeks to maximum of 8 times initial dose.

Side effects

CNS: dizziness, weakness, syncope
CV: orthostatic hypotension, bradycardia, CHF, dysrhythmias
EENT: nasal stuffiness, mouth dryness
GI: diarrhea
Other: edema, weight gain, inhibition of ejaculation

Interactions

Levodopa, alcohol: may increase hypotensive effect of guanethidine. Use together cautiously.
MAO inhibitors, ephedrine, levarterenol, methylphenidate, tricyclic antidepressants, amphetamines, phenothiazines: may inhibit the antihypertensive effect of guanethidine. Adjust dose accordingly.

Nursing considerations

• Contraindicated in patients with pheochromocytoma. Use cautiously in patients with severe cardiac disease, recent MI, cerebrovascular disease, peptic ulcer, impaired renal function, or bronchial asthma, or in those taking other antihypertensives.

• Discontinue drug 2 to 3 weeks before elective surgery to reduce possibility of vascular collapse and cardiac arrest during anesthesia.

• Teach patient about his disease and therapy. Explain importance of taking drug exactly as prescribed, even when he is feeling well. Tell patient not to discontinue drug suddenly, but to call doctor if unpleasant side effects develop.

• Tell outpatient to avoid strenuous exercise, and warn that hot showers may cause hypotensive reaction.

• Inform patient that orthostatic hypotension can be minimized by rising slowly and avoiding sudden position changes. Mouth dryness can be relieved with sugarless chewing gum, sour hard candy, or ice chips.

• Give drug with meals to increase absorption.

• If patient develops diarrhea, doctor may prescribe atropine or paregoric.

---

hydralazine (Apresoline)

Indications and dosage

Essential hypertension (oral, alone or in combination with other antihypertensives); to reduce afterload in severe CHF (with nitrates); and severe essential hy-

pertension *(parenteral to lower blood pressure quickly)*—
Adults: initially, 10 mg P.O. q.i.d.; gradually increased to 50 mg q.i.d. Maximum recommended dosage is 200 mg daily, but some patients may require 300 to 400 mg daily.
I.V.—20 to 40 mg given slowly and repeated as necessary, generally q 4 to 6 hours. Switch to oral antihypertensives as soon as possible.
I.M.—20 to 40 mg repeated as necessary, generally q 4 to 6 hours. Switch to oral antihypertensives as soon as possible.
Children: initially, 0.75 mg/kg P.O. daily in 4 divided doses (25 mg/m^2 daily). May increase gradually to 10 times this dose, if necessary.
I.V.—give slowly 1.7 to 3.5 mg/kg daily or 50 to 100 mg/m^2 daily in 4 to 6 divided doses.
I.M.—1.7 to 3.5 mg/kg daily or 50 to 100 mg/m^2 daily in 4 to 6 divided doses.

Side effects

CNS: peripheral neuritis, *headache*, dizziness
CV: orthostatic hypotension, *tachycardia*, dysrhythmias, *angina, palpitations, sodium retention*
GI: nausea, vomiting, diarrhea, anorexia
Skin: rash
Other: lupus erythematosus-like syndrome, weight gain

Interactions

Diazoxide: may cause severe hypotension. Use together cautiously.

Nursing considerations

• Use cautiously in patients with cardiac disease or in those taking other antihypertensives.
• Monitor patient's blood pressure and pulse rate frequently.
• Watch patient closely for signs of lupus erythematosus-like syndrome (sore throat, fever, muscle and joint aches, skin rash). Call doctor immediately if any of these develop.

• Teach patient about his disease and therapy. Explain importance of taking drug exactly as prescribed, even when he is feeling well. Tell outpatient not to discontinue drug suddenly, but to call doctor if unpleasant side effects develop.
• Inform patient that orthostatic hypotension can be minimized by rising slowly and avoiding sudden position changes.
• Give drug with meals to increase absorption.
• Compliance may be improved by administering drug b.i.d. Check with doctor.
• Complete blood count (CBC), LE cell preparation, and antinuclear antibody titer determinations should be done before therapy and periodically during long-term therapy.

labetalol
(Trandate, Normodyne)

Indications and dosage

Treatment of hypertension—
Adults: 100 mg P.O. b.i.d. with or without a diuretic. Dose may be increased to 200 mg b.i.d. after 2 days. Further dose increases may be made every 1 to 3 days until optimum response is reached. Usual maintenance dose is 200 to 400 mg b.i.d.
For severe hypertension and hypertensive emergencies—
Adults: Dilute 200 mg to 200 ml with 5% dextrose in water. Infuse at 2 mg per minute until satisfactory response is obtained. Then stop the infusion. May repeat q 6 to 8 hours.

Side effects

CNS: vivid dreams, fatigue, headache
CV: orthostatic hypotension and dizziness, peripheral vascular disease
EENT: nasal stuffiness
Endocrine: hypoglycemia without tachycardia
GI: nausea, vomiting, diarrhea
GU: sexual dysfunction, urinary retention

Skin: rash
Other: increased airway resistance

Interactions
Insulin, hypoglycemic drugs (oral): can alter dosage requirements in previously stabilized diabetics. Observe patient carefully.

Specific considerations
• Contraindicated in patients with bronchial asthma.
• Use cautiously in CHF, chronic bronchitis, emphysema, and preexisting peripheral vascular disease.
• Monitor blood pressure frequently. If patient develops severe hypotension, notify doctor. He may prescribe a vasopressor.
• Teach patient about his disease and therapy. Explain importance of taking drug exactly as prescribed, even when he is feeling well. Tell outpatient not to discontinue drug suddenly; abrupt discontinuation can exacerbate angina and MI. Tell patient to call doctor if unpleasant side effects develop.
• Drug masks common signs of shock and hypoglycemia.
• Labetalol is a beta-adrenergic blocker that also has unique alpha-adrenergic blocking effects.
• Unlike other beta blockers, labetalol does not decrease heart rate or cardiac output.
• Dizziness is the most troublesome side effect and tends to occur in early stages of treatment, in patients also receiving diuretics, and in patients receiving higher dosages. Inform patient that this can be minimized by rising slowly and avoiding sudden position changes.
• Studies show that labetalol side effects seem less common and more transient than those of other beta blockers.

---

mecamylamine hydrochloride (Inversine)

Indications and dosage
For moderate-to-severe essential hypertension and uncomplicated malignant hypertension—
Adults: initially, 2.5 mg P.O. b.i.d. Increase by 2.5 mg daily every 2 days. Average daily dose 25 mg given in 3 divided doses. No dosing recommendations for children.

Side effects
CNS: paresthesias, sedation, *fatigue, tremor, choreiform movements,* convulsions, psychic changes, dizziness, *weakness, headaches*
CV: orthostatic hypotension
EENT: mouth dryness, glossitis, dilated pupils, *blurred vision*
GI: anorexia, nausea, vomiting, constipation, adynamic ileus, diarrhea
GU: urinary retention
Other: decreased libido, impotence

Interactions
Sodium bicarbonate and acetazolamide: may increase effect of mecamylamine. Use together cautiously. Watch for increased hypotensive effects and toxicity.

Nursing considerations
• Contraindicated in patients with recent MI, uremia, or chronic pyelonephritis. Use cautiously in patients with lower urinary tract pathology, renal insufficiency, glaucoma, pyloric stenosis, coronary insufficiency, or cerebrovascular insufficiency, or in those taking other antihypertensives.
• Effects of drug are increased by high environmental temperature, fever, stress, or severe illness.
• Do not withdraw drug suddenly; rebound hypertension may occur. Tell outpatient to call doctor if unpleasant side effects develop.
• Monitor patient's blood pressure frequently while he is standing.

• Give with meals for better absorption. Do not restrict sodium intake.
• If patient develops constipation from drug, doctor may want him to take milk of magnesia. Instruct patient to avoid bulk laxatives.
• Teach patient about his disease and therapy. Explain importance of taking drug exactly as prescribed, even when he is feeling well.
• Inform patient that orthostatic hypotension can be minimized by rising slowly and avoiding sudden position changes. Mouth dryness can be relieved with sugarless chewing gum, sour hard candy, or ice chips.

---

methyldopa
(Aldomet)

Indications and dosage

For sustained mild-to-severe hypertension; should not be used for acute treatment of hypertensive emergencies—
Adults: initially 250 mg P.O. b.i.d. to t.i.d. in first 48 hours. Then increase as needed every 2 days. May give entire daily dose in the evening or at bedtime. Dosages may need adjustment if other antihypertensive drugs are added to or deleted from therapy.
Maintenance dosages—500 mg to 2 g daily in 2 to 4 divided doses. Maximum recommended daily dose is 3 g.
I.V.—500 mg to 1 g q 6 hours, diluted in dextrose 5% in water and administered over 30 to 60 minutes. Switch to oral antihypertensives as soon as possible.
Children: initially 10 mg/kg daily P.O. in 2 to 3 divided doses; or 20 to 40 mg/kg daily I.V. in 4 divided doses. Increase dose daily until desired response occurs. Maximum daily dose 65 mg/kg.

Side effects

Blood: hemolytic anemia, reversible granulocytopenia, thrombocytopenia
CNS: sedation, headache, asthenia, weakness, dizziness, *decreased mental acuity,* involuntary choreoathetotic movements, psychic disturbances, depression, nightmares
CV: bradycardia, *orthostatic hypotension,* aggravated angina, myocarditis, *edema and weight gain*
EENT: dry mouth, nasal stuffiness
GI: diarrhea, pancreatitis
Hepatic: hepatic necrosis
Other: gynecomastia, lactation, skin rash, drug-induced fever, impotence

Interactions

Norepinephrine, phenothiazines, tricyclic antidepressants, amphetamines: possible hypertensive effects. Monitor carefully.

Nursing considerations

• Use cautiously in patients receiving other antihypertensives or MAO inhibitors and in patients with impaired hepatic function. Monitor blood pressure and pulse rate frequently.
• Observe for involuntary choreoathetoid movements. Report to doctor; he may discontinue drug.
• Observe patient for side effects, particularly unexplained fever. Report side effects to doctor.
• After dialysis, monitor patient for hypertension. Patient may need an extra dose of methyldopa.
• If patient requires blood transfusion, make sure he gets direct and indirect Coombs' tests to avoid cross-matching problems.
• Monitor blood studies (CBC) before and during therapy.
• If patient has been on this drug for several months, positive reaction to direct Coombs' test indicates hemolytic anemia.
• Weigh patient daily. Notify doctor of any weight increase. Salt and water retention may occur but can be relieved with diuretics.
• Tell patient that urine may turn dark in toilet bowls treated with bleach.
• Teach patient about his disease and therapy. Explain importance of taking drug exactly as prescribed, even when he is feeling well. Tell outpatient not to stop drug suddenly, but to call doctor if unpleasant side effects develop. Once-

daily dosage administered at bedtime will minimize drowsiness during daytime. Check with doctor.
• Inform patient that orthostatic hypotension can be minimized by rising slowly and avoiding sudden position changes. Mouth dryness can be relieved with sugarless chewing gum, sour hard candy, or ice chips.

metoprolol tartrate (Lopresor, Lopressor)

Indications and dosage
For hypertension; may be used alone or in combination with other antihypertensives—
Adults— 50 mg b.i.d. or 100 mg once daily P.O. initially. Up to 200 to 400 mg daily in 2 to 3 divided doses. No dosage recommendations for children.

Side effects
CNS: fatigue, lethargy
CV: bradycardia, hypotension, CHF, peripheral vascular disease
GI: nausea, vomiting, diarrhea
Skin: rash
Other: fever

Interactions
Insulin, hypoglycemic drugs (oral): can alter dosage requirements in previously stabilized diabetics. Observe patient carefully.
Cardiac glycosides: excessive bradycardia and increased depressant effect on myocardium. Use together cautiously.
Barbiturates, rifampin: increased metabolism of metoprolol. Monitor for decreased effect.
Chlorpromazine, cimetidine: inhibits metoprolol's metabolism. Monitor for greater beta-blocking effect.
Indomethacin: decrease in antihypertensive effect. Monitor blood pressure and adjust dosage.

Nursing considerations
• Use cautiously in patients with heart block, CHF, diabetes, or respiratory disease, or in those taking other antihyper-

tensives. Always check patient's apical pulse rate before giving drug. If it is slower than 60 beats/minute, hold drug and call doctor immediately.
• Although most patients with asthma and bronchitis can take drug without fear of worsening their condition, higher dosages should be used cautiously in these patients.
• Monitor blood pressure frequently. If patient develops severe hypotension, administer a vasopressor as ordered.
• Teach patient about his disease and therapy. Explain importance of taking drug, even when he is feeling well. Tell outpatient not to discontinue drug suddenly; abrupt discontinuation can exacerbate angina and MI. Instruct patient to call doctor if unpleasant side effects develop.
• Drug masks common signs of shock and hypoglycemia. However, metoprolol does not potentiate insulin-induced hypoglycemia or delay recovery of blood glucose to normal levels.
• Food may increase absorption of metoprolol. Give consistently with meals.
• Metoprolol, as well as other beta blockers, is prescribed to decrease mortality following MI.

metyrosine (Demser)

Indications and dosage
Preoperative preparation of patients with pheochromocytoma; management of such patients when surgery is contraindicated; to control or prevent hypertension before or during pheochromocytomectomy—
Adults and children over 12 years: 250 mg P.O. q.i.d. May be increased by 250 to 500 mg q day to a maximum of 4 g daily in divided doses. When used for preoperative preparation, optimally effective dosage should be given for at least 5 to 7 days.

Side effects
CNS: sedation, extrapyramidal symptoms, such as speech difficulty and

tremors, disorientation
GI: diarrhea, nausea, vomiting, abdominal pain
GU: crystalluria, hematuria
Other: impotence, hypersensitivity

Interactions
Phenothiazines and haloperidol: increased inhibition of catecholamine synthesis may result in extrapyramidal symptoms. Use cautiously.

Nursing considerations
• During surgery, monitor blood pressure and EKG continuously. If a serious dysrhythmia occurs during anesthesia and surgery, treatment with a beta-blocking drug or lidocaine may be necessary.
• Warn patient that sedation almost always occurs with metyrosine. It usually subsides after several days' treatment.
• Instruct patient to increase daily fluid intake to prevent crystalluria. Daily urine volume should be 2,000 ml or more.
• Tell patient to notify doctor if any listed side effects occur.
• Insomnia may occur when metyrosine is stopped.
• If patient's hypertension is not adequately controlled by metyrosine, an alpha-adrenergic blocking agent, such as phenoxybenzamine, should be added to the regimen.

minoxidil
(Loniten)

Indications and dosage
Treatment of severe hypertension—
Adults: 5 mg P.O. initially as a single dose. Effective dosage range is usually 10 to 40 mg daily. Maximum dose is 100 mg daily.
Children under 12 years: 0.2 mg/kg as a single daily dose. Effective dosage range usually 0.25 to 1.0 mg/kg daily. Maximum dose is 50 mg.

Side effects
CV: edema, tachycardia, pericardial effusion and tamponade, CHF, EKG changes
Skin: rash, *Stevens-Johnson syndrome*
Other: hypertrichosis (elongation, thickening, and enhanced pigmentation of fine body hair), breast tenderness

Interactions
Guanethidine: severe orthostatic hypotension. Advise patient to stand up slowly.

Nursing considerations
• Contraindicated in patients with pheochromocytoma.
• A potent vasodilator: Use only when other antihypertensives have failed.
• About 8 out of 10 patients will experience hypertrichosis within 3 to 6 weeks of beginning treatment. Unwanted hair can be controlled with a depilatory or shaving. Assure patient that extra hair will disappear within 1 to 6 months of stopping minoxidil. Advise patient, however, not to discontinue drug without doctor's consent.
• Drug is usually prescribed with a beta-blocking drug to control tachycardia and a diuretic to counteract fluid retention. Make sure patient complies with total treatment regimen.
• A patient package insert has been prepared by the manufacturer of minoxidil, describing in layman's terms the drug and its side effects. Be sure patient receives this insert and reads it thoroughly. Provide an oral explanation also.

nadolol
(Corgard)

Indications and dosage
Treatment of hypertension—
Adults: 40 mg P.O. once daily initially. Dosage may be increased in 40- to 80-mg increments until optimum response occurs. Usual maintenance dosage range: 80 to 320 mg once daily. Doses of 640 mg may be necessary in rare cases.

Long-term management of angina pectoris—
Adults: 40 mg P.O. once daily initially. Dosage may be increased in 40- to 80-mg increments until optimum response occurs. Usual maintenance dosage range: 80 to 240 mg once daily.

Side effects
CNS: fatigue, lethargy
CV: bradycardia, hypotension, CHF, peripheral vascular disease
GI: nausea, vomiting, diarrhea
Metabolic: hypoglycemia without tachycardia
Skin: rash
Other: increased airway resistance, fever

Interactions
Insulin, hypoglycemic drugs (oral): can alter dosage requirements in previously stabilized diabetics. Observe patient carefully.
Cardiac glycosides: excessive bradycardia and increased depressant effect on myocardium. Use together cautiously.
Epinephrine: severe vasoconstriction. Monitor blood pressure and observe patient carefully.
Indomethacin: decrease in antihypertensive effect. Monitor blood pressure and adjust dosage.

Nursing considerations
• Contraindicated in patients with bronchial asthma, sinus bradycardia and greater-than-first-degree conduction block, and cardiogenic shock.
• Use cautiously in patients with heart failure, chronic bronchitis, and emphysema.
• Always check patient's apical pulse before giving drug. If slower than 60 beats/minute, hold drug and call doctor.
• Monitor blood pressure frequently. If patient develops severe hypotension, administer a vasopressor as ordered.
• Do not discontinue abruptly: can exacerbate angina and MI.
• Teach patient about his disease and therapy. Explain importance of taking drug, even when he is feeling well. Tell outpatient not to discontinue drug suddenly, but to call doctor if unpleasant side effects develop.
• Drug masks common signs of shock and hypoglycemia.
• May be given without regard to meals.

nitroprusside sodium (Nipride, Nitropress)

Indications and dosage
To lower blood pressure quickly in hypertensive emergencies; to control hypotension during anesthesia; to reduce preload and afterload in cardiac pump failure or cardiogenic shock; may be used with or without dopamine—
Adults: 50-mg vial diluted with 2 to 3 ml of dextrose 5% in water I.V. and then added to 250, 500, or 1,000 ml dextrose 5% in water. Infuse at 0.5 to 10 mcg/kg/minute.
Average dose: 3 mcg/kg/minute. Maximum infusion rate: 10 mcg/kg/minute.
Patients taking other antihypertensive drugs along with nitroprusside are very sensitive to this drug. Adjust dosage accordingly.

Side effects
The following side effects generally indicate overdosage:
CNS: headache, dizziness, ataxia, loss of consciousness, coma, weak pulse, absent reflexes, widely dilated pupils, *restlessness, muscle twitching, diaphoresis*
CV: distant heart sounds, palpitations, dyspnea, shallow breathing
GI: vomiting, nausea, abdominal pain
Metabolic: acidosis
Skin: pink color

Interactions
None significant

Nursing considerations
• Use cautiously in patients with hypothyroidism or hepatic or renal disease, or in those receiving other antihypertensives.
• Due to light sensitivity, wrap I.V. solution in foil. It is not necessary to wrap

the tubing in foil. Fresh solution should have faint brownish tint. Discard after 24 hours.
• Obtain baseline vital signs before giving drug, and find out what parameters doctor wants to achieve.
• Check blood pressure every 5 minutes at start of infusion and every 15 minutes thereafter. If severe hypotension occurs, turn off I.V. nitroprusside—effects of drug quickly reverse. Notify doctor. If possible, an arterial pressure line should be started. Regulate drug flow to specified level.
• Do not use bacteriostatic water for injection or sterile saline solution for reconstitution.
• Infuse with automatic infusion pump.
• Drug is best run piggybacked through a peripheral line with no other medication. Do not adjust rate of main I.V. line while drug is running. Even small bolus of nitroprusside can cause severe hypotension.
• Drug can cause cyanide toxicity, so check serum thiocyanate levels every 72 hours. Levels greater than 10 mcg/dl are associated with toxicity. Watch for signs of thiocyanate toxicity: profound hypotension, metabolic acidosis, dyspnea, headache, loss of consciousness, ataxia, vomiting. If these occur, discontinue drug immediately and notify doctor.

pindolol
(Visken)

Indications and dosage
Treatment of hypertension—
Adults: initially, 10 mg P.O. b.i.d. Dosage may be increased by 10 mg/day every 2 to 3 weeks up to a maximum of 60 mg/day.

Side effects
CNS: insomnia, fatigue, dizziness, nervousness, vivid dreams, hallucinations, lethargy
CV: edema, bradycardia, CHF, peripheral vascular disease, hypotension
EENT: visual disturbances
GI: nausea, vomiting, diarrhea

Metabolic: hypoglycemia without tachycardia
Skin: rash
Other: increased airway resistance, muscle pain, joint pain, chest pain

Interactions
Insulin, hypoglycemic drugs (oral): can alter requirements for these drugs in previously stabilized diabetics. Monitor for hypoglycemia.
Cardiac glycosides: excessive bradycardia and increased depressant effect on myocardium. Use together cautiously.
Cimetidine: inhibits pindolol metabolism. Monitor for greater beta-blocking effect.
Epinephrine: severe vasoconstriction. Monitor blood pressure and observe patient carefully.
Indomethacin: decreased antihypertensive effect. Monitor blood pressure and adjust dosage.

Nursing considerations
• Contraindicated in diabetes mellitus, asthma, allergic rhinitis, sinus bradycardia and heart block greater than first-degree, cardiogenic shock, right ventricular failure secondary to pulmonary hypertension, and during ethyl ether anesthesia. Use with caution in patients with CHF or respiratory disease and in patients taking other antihypertensive drugs.
• Always check patient's apical pulse rate before giving drug. If you detect extremes in pulse rates, hold medication and call doctor immediately.
• Monitor blood pressure frequently. If patient develops severe hypotension, notify doctor. He may prescribe a vasopressor.
• Teach patient about his disease and therapy. Explain importance of taking drug exactly as prescribed, even when he is feeling well. Tell outpatient not to discontinue drug suddenly; abrupt discontinuation can exacerbate angina and MI. Tell patient to call doctor if unpleasant side effects develop.
• This drug masks common signs of shock and hypoglycemia.

• Pindolol may be taken without any special regard for meals.
• Many patients respond favorably to a dose of 5 mg t.i.d.
• First commercially available beta-blocker with partial beta-*agonist* activity. In other words, pindolol *stimulates* beta-adrenergic receptors as well as blocks them. Therefore, it decreases cardiac output less than other beta-adrenergic blockers.
• May be advantageous for patients who develop bradycardia with other beta blockers.

prazosin hydrochloride (Minipress)

Indications and dosage

For mild-to-moderate hypertension; used alone or in combination with a diuretic or other antihypertensive drugs; also used to decrease afterload in severe chronic CHF—
Adults: P.O. test dose: 1 mg before bedtime to prevent "first-dose syncope." Initial dose: 1 mg t.i.d. Increase dosage slowly. Maximum daily dose 20 mg. Maintenance dose: 3 to 20 mg daily in 3 divided doses. A few patients have required dosages larger than this (up to 40 mg daily). If other antihypertensive drugs or diuretics are added to this drug, decrease prazosin dosage to 1 to 2 mg t.i.d. and retitrate.

Side effects

CNS: dizziness, headache, drowsiness, weakness, *"first-dose syncope,"* depression
CV: orthostatic hypotension, *palpitations*
EENT: blurred vision, dry mouth
GI: vomiting, diarrhea, abdominal cramps, constipation, *nausea*
GU: priapism

Interactions

Propranolol and other beta blockers: syncope with loss of consciousness may occur more frequently. Advise patient to sit or lie down if he feels dizzy.

Nursing considerations

• Use cautiously in patients receiving other antihypertensive drugs.
• Monitor patient's blood pressure and pulse rate frequently.
• If initial dose is greater than 1 mg, patient may develop severe syncope with loss of consciousness (first-dose syncope). Increase dosage slowly. Instruct patient to sit or lie down if dizzy.
• Teach patient about his disease and therapy. Explain importance of taking drug exactly as prescribed, even when he is feeling well. Tell outpatient not to discontinue drug suddenly, but to call doctor if unpleasant side effects develop.
• Inform patient that orthostatic hypotension can be minimized by rising slowly and avoiding sudden position changes. Mouth dryness can be relieved with sugarless chewing gum, sour hard candy, or ice chips.
• Compliance *may* be improved by giving drug once a day. Check with doctor.

propranolol hydrochloride (Inderal, Inderal LA)

Indications and dosage

Hypertension (usually used with thiazide diuretics)—
Adults: initial treatment of hypertension: 80 mg P.O. daily in 2 to 4 divided doses or the sustained-release form once daily. Increase at 3- to 7-day intervals to maximum daily dose of 640 mg. Usual maintenance dose for hypertension: 160 to 480 mg daily. No dosing recommendations for children.

Side effects

CNS: fatigue, lethargy, vivid dreams, hallucinations
CV: bradycardia, hypotension, CHF, peripheral vascular disease
GI: nausea, vomiting, diarrhea
Metabolic: hypoglycemia without tachycardia
Skin: rash
Other: increased airway resistance, fever

Interactions

Insulin, hypoglycemic drugs (oral): can alter requirements for these drugs in previously stabilized diabetics. Monitor for hypoglycemia.

Cardiac glycosides: excessive bradycardia and increased depressant effect on myocardium. Use together cautiously.

Chlorpromazine, cimetidine: inhibit propranolol's metabolism. Monitor for greater beta-blocking effect.

Epinephrine: severe vasoconstriction. Monitor blood pressure and observe patient carefully.

Barbiturates, rifampin: increased metabolism of propranolol. Monitor for decreased effect.

Indomethacin: decrease in antihypertensive effect. Monitor blood pressure and adjust dosage.

Nursing considerations

• Contraindicated in diabetes mellitus, asthma, allergic rhinitis, sinus bradycardia and heart block greater than first-degree, cardiogenic shock, right ventricular failure secondary to pulmonary hypertension, and during ethyl ether anesthesia. Use with caution in patients with CHF or respiratory disease, and in patients taking other antihypertensive drugs.

• Always check patient's apical pulse rate before giving drug. If you detect extremes in pulse rates, hold medication and call doctor immediately.

• Monitor blood pressure frequently. If patient develops severe hypotension, notify doctor. He may prescribe a vasopressor.

• Teach patient about his disease and therapy. Explain importance of taking drug exactly as prescribed, even when he is feeling well. Tell outpatient not to discontinue drug suddenly; abrupt discontinuation can exacerbate angina and MI. Tell patient to call doctor if unpleasant side effects develop.

• Drug masks common signs of shock and hypoglycemia.

• Food may increase absorption of propranolol. Give consistently with meals.

• Compliance may be improved by administering drug on a twice-daily basis. Check with doctor.

• Propranolol, as well as other beta blockers, is prescribed to decrease mortality following MI.

reserpine (Serpasil)

Indications and dosage

Mild-to-moderate essential hypertension (oral); hypertensive emergencies (parenteral)—

Adults: initially, 0.5 mg P.O. daily for 1 to 2 weeks. Maintenance dose: 0.1 to 0.5 mg daily

I.M.—initially 0.5 to 1 mg, followed by doses of 2 to 4 mg at 2-hour intervals. Maximum recommended dose 4 mg.

Children: 0.07 mg/kg or 2 mg/m^2 with hydralazine I.M. every 12 to 24 hours.

Side effects

CNS: mental confusion, *depression, drowsiness, nervousness, anxiety, nightmares,* sedation

CV: orthostatic hypotension, bradycardia, syncope

EENT: mouth dryness, nasal stuffiness, glaucoma

GI: hyperacidity, nausea, vomiting, GI bleeding

Skin: pruritus, rash

Other: impotence, weight gain

Interactions

MAO inhibitors: may cause excitability and hypertension. Use together cautiously.

Nursing considerations

• Contraindicated in patients with depression. Use cautiously in patients with severe cardiac or cerebrovascular disease, peptic ulcer, ulcerative colitis, gallstones, mental depressive disorders; in those undergoing surgery; and in those taking other antihypertensive drugs.

• Monitor patient's blood pressure and pulse rate frequently.

• Teach patient about his disease and therapy. Explain importance of taking drug exactly as prescribed, even when he is feeling well. Tell outpatient not to discontinue drug suddenly, but to call doctor if unpleasant side effects develop. Warn that this drug can cause drowsiness.

• Warn female patient to notify doctor if she becomes pregnant.

• Watch patient closely for signs of mental depression. Warn him to notify doctor promptly if he starts having nightmares.

• Inform patient that orthostatic hypotension can be minimized by rising slowly and avoiding sudden position changes. Mouth dryness can be relieved with sugarless chewing gum, sour hard candy, or ice chips. Tell patient to contact doctor if relief is needed for nasal stuffiness.

• Give drug with meals.

• Patient should weigh himself daily and notify doctor of any weight gain.

• Effects of drug may last for 10 days after it is discontinued.

• Parenteral form erratically absorbed; commonly replaced by other antihypertensives for hypertensive emergencies.

timolol maleate
(Blocadren)

Indications and dosage

Hypertension—
Adults: Initial dosage is 10 mg P.O. b.i.d. Usual daily maintenance dosage is 20 to 40 mg. Maximum daily dosage is 60 mg. Drug is used either alone or in combination with diuretics.
MI (long-term prophylaxis in patients who have survived acute phase)—
Adults: Recommended dosage for long-term prophylaxis in survivors of acute MI is 10 mg P.O. b.i.d.

Side effects

CNS: fatigue, lethargy, vivid dreams
CV: bradycardia, hypotension, CHF, peripheral vascular disease
GI: nausea, vomiting, diarrhea

Metabolic: hypoglycemia without tachycardia
Skin: rash
Other: increased airway resistance, fever

Interactions

Insulin, hypoglycemic drugs (oral): can alter requirements for these drugs in previously stabilized diabetics. Monitor for hypoglycemia.
Cardiac glycosides: excessive bradycardia and increased depressant effect on myocardium. Use together cautiously.
Indomethacin: decrease in antihypertensive effect. Monitor blood pressure and adjust dosage.

Nursing considerations

• Contraindicated in diabetes mellitus, asthma, allergic rhinitis, sinus bradycardia and heart block greater than first-degree, cardiogenic shock, right ventricular failure secondary to pulmonary hypertension, and during ethyl ether anesthesia. Use with caution in CHF, respiratory disease, and in patients taking other antihypertensives.

• Always check patient's apical pulse rate before giving drug. If you detect extremes in pulse rates, withhold medication and call doctor immediately.

• Monitor blood pressure frequently. If patient develops severe hypotension, notify doctor. He may prescribe a vasopressor.

• Instruct patient about the disease and therapy. Explain the importance of taking drug exactly as prescribed, even when he is feeling well. Tell patient not to discontinue drug suddenly; abrupt discontinuation can exacerbate angina and MI. Tell patient to call doctor if unpleasant side effects develop.

• Drug masks common signs of shock and hypoglycemia.

• If patient is taking the drug for hypertension, warn him not to increase dosage without first consulting doctor. At least 7 days should intervene between increases in dosage.

• Timolol is the first beta blocker approved for use in post-MI patients. Like other beta blockers, it prolongs survival of MI patients.

trimethaphan camsylate (Arfonad)

Indications and dosage
To lower blood pressure quickly in hypertensive emergencies; for controlled hypotension during surgery—
Adults: 500 mg (10 ml) diluted in 500 ml dextrose 5% in water to yield concentration of 1 mg/ml I.V. Start I.V. drip at 1 to 2 mg/minute and titrate to achieve desired hypotensive response. Range: 0.3 mg to 6 mg/minute

Side effects
CNS: dilated pupils, *extreme weakness*
CV: severe orthostatic hypotension, tachycardia
GI: anorexia, *nausea, vomiting, dry mouth*
GU: urinary retention
Other: respiratory depression

Interactions
None significant

Nursing considerations
• Contraindicated in patients with anemia, respiratory insufficiency. Use cautiously in patients with arteriosclerosis, cardiac, hepatic, or renal disease, degenerative CNS disorders, Addison's disease, or diabetes. Also use cautiously in patients receiving glucocorticoids or those receiving other antihypertensives.
• Monitor patient's blood pressure and vital signs frequently.
• May require elevation of head of bed for maximal effect.
• If extreme hypotension occurs, discontinue drug and call doctor. Use phenylephrine or mephentermine to counteract hypotension.
• Watch closely for respiratory distress, especially if large doses are used.
• Use infusion pump to administer drug slowly and precisely.
• Discontinue drug before wound closure in surgery to allow blood pressure

to return to normal.
• Position patient to avoid cerebral anoxia.
• Patient should receive oxygen therapy during use of this agent.

VASODILATORS

Peripheral vasodilators have limited clinical value in patients with obstructive vascular disease, although they may be useful in patients with minimal organic involvement. Studies in healthy persons indicate that peripheral vasodilators increase blood flow to vascular areas. Although we lack evidence of their vasodilating effect in diseased vascular areas, these drugs are still widely used.

Major uses
Peripheral vasodilators are used to treat symptoms of peripheral vascular and vasospastic conditions as well as cerebrovascular disease.
• Dipyridamole (in combination with aspirin or warfarin) inhibits platelet aggregation to reduce risk of thrombus formation.

Mechanism of action
• Some peripheral vasodilators directly relax smooth muscle. This effect may be due to inhibition of phosphodiesterase, resulting in increased concentrations of cyclic adenosine monophosphate, which causes vasodilation.
• Other peripheral vasodilators have a different mechanism of action. Tolazoline blocks alpha receptors; isoxsuprine and nylidrin stimulate beta receptors. Although isoxsuprine originally was thought only to stimulate beta receptors, newer evidence indicates that it may also be a direct-acting peripheral vasodilator.
• Dipyridamole, originally classified as a coronary vasodilator, has no value in treating acute attacks of angina. In fact, evidence is lacking that its long-term use is beneficial in preventing chronic angina. It does, however, inhibit platelet

adhesion in patients with prosthetic heart valves.

Absorption, distribution, metabolism, and excretion

Vasodilators are well absorbed, widely distributed in body tissues, metabolized in the liver, and excreted mainly in the urine.

Onset and duration

Onset and duration of vasodilators depend on the drug used, form selected, and route of administration.

amyl nitrite

Indications and dosage

Relief of angina pectoris, bronchospasm, biliary spasm—
Adults and children: 0.2 to 0.3 ml by inhalation (one glass ampul inhaler), p.r.n.

Side effects

Blood: methemoglobinemia
CNS: headache, sometimes with throbbing; dizziness; weakness
CV: orthostatic hypotension, tachycardia, flushing, palpitations, fainting
GI: nausea, vomiting
Skin: cutaneous vasodilation
Other: hypersensitivity reactions

Interactions

None significant

Nursing considerations

• Contraindicated in hypersensitivity to nitrites. Use with caution in cerebral hemorrhage, hypotension, head injury, and glaucoma.
• Watch for orthostatic hypotension. Have patient sit down and avoid rapid position changes while inhaling drug.
• Extinguish all cigarettes before use, or ampul may ignite.
• Wrap ampul in cloth and crush. Hold near patient's nose and mouth so vapor is inhaled.
• Effective within 30 seconds but with a short duration of action (4 to 8 min-

utes).
• Keeping the head low, deep breathing, and movement of extremities may help relieve dizziness, syncope, or weakness from postural hypotension.

cyclandelate (Cyclanfor, Cyclospasmol)

Indications and dosage

Adjunct in intermittent claudication, arteriosclerosis obliterans, vasospasm and muscular ischemia associated with thrombophlebitis, nocturnal leg cramps, Raynaud's phenomenon, selected cases of ischemic cerebral vascular disease—
Adults: initially 200 mg P.O. q.i.d. (before meals and h.s.); maximum 400 mg P.O. q.i.d. When clinical response is noted, decrease dosage gradually until maintenance dosage is reached. Maintenance dose 400 to 800 mg daily in divided doses.

Side effects

CNS: headache, tingling of the extremities, dizziness
CV: mild flushing, tachycardia
GI: pyrosis, eructation, nausea.
Other: sweating

Interactions

None significant

Nursing considerations

• Use with extreme caution in severe obliterative coronary artery or cerebrovascular disease, since circulation to these diseased areas may be compromised by vasodilatory effects of drug elsewhere (coronary steal syndrome). Use with caution in patients with glaucoma, hypotension.
• Give with food or antacids to lessen GI distress.
• Use in conjunction with, not as a substitute for, appropriate medical or surgical therapy for peripheral or cerebrovascular disease.
• Short-term therapy of little benefit. Instruct patient to expect long-term treatment and to continue taking medi-

cation.
• Side effects usually disappear after several weeks of therapy.

dipyridamole
(Persantine)

Indications and dosage
Long-term therapy for chronic angina pectoris, prevention of recurrent transient ischemic attack—
Adults: 50 mg P.O. t.i.d. at least 1 hour before meals, to maximum of 400 mg daily
Inhibition of platelet adhesion in patients with prosthetic heart valves, in combination with warfarin—
Adults: 100 to 400 mg P.O. daily
Transient ischemic attack—
Adults: 100 mg P.O. daily as a single dose

Side effects
CNS: headache, dizziness, weakness
CV: flushing, fainting, *hypotension*
GI: nausea, vomiting, diarrhea
Skin: rash

Interactions
None significant

Nursing considerations
• Use with caution in hypotension, anticoagulant therapy.
• Observe for side effects, especially with large doses. Monitor blood pressure.
• Administer 1 hour before meals.
• Watch for signs of bleeding, prolonged bleeding time (large doses, long-term).
• Clinical response to antianginal therapy may not be evident before second or third month. Tell patient to continue drug despite lack of observable response.

ethaverine hydrochloride
(Cebral)

Indications and dosage
Long-term treatment of peripheral and cerebrovascular insufficiency associated with arterial spasm; spastic conditions of GI and genitourinary tracts—
Adults: 100 to 200 mg P.O. t.i.d. or 150 mg of sustained-release preparation P.O. q 12 hours

Side effects
CNS: headache, drowsiness
CV: hypotension, flushing, sweating, vertigo, cardiac depression, dysrhythmias
GI: nausea, anorexia, abdominal distress, throat dryness, constipation, diarrhea
Hepatic: jaundice, altered liver function tests
Skin: rash
Other: respiratory depression, malaise, lassitude

Interactions
None significant

Nursing considerations
• Contraindicated in complete AV dissociation and in severe hepatic disease. Use with caution in women who are pregnant or of childbearing age and in patients with glaucoma or pulmonary embolus; may precipitate dysrhythmias.
• Hold dose and call doctor if signs of hepatic hypersensitivity develop (GI symptoms, altered liver function tests, jaundice, eosinophilia).
• Monitor and record vital signs during therapy.

isoxsuprine hydrochloride
(Vasodilan)

Indications and dosage
Adjunct for relief of symptoms associated with cerebrovascular insufficiency, peripheral vascular diseases (such as ar-

teriosclerosis obliterans, thromboangiitis obliterans, Raynaud's disease)—
Adults: 10 to 20 mg P.O. t.i.d. or q.i.d.; initially 5 to 10 mg I.M. b.i.d. or t.i.d. in severe or acute conditions, to maximum of 10 mg. Intramuscular doses greater than 10 mg may be associated with hypotension and tachycardia and are not recommended.

Side effects
CNS: dizziness, nervousness, weakness, trembling, *light-headedness*
CV: hypotension, tachycardia, transient palpitations
GI: vomiting, abdominal distress, intestinal distention
Skin: severe rash

Interactions
None significant

Nursing considerations
• Contraindicated in immediate postpartum period and with arterial bleeding; I.M. contraindicated in hypotension or tachycardia.
• Safe use in pregnancy and lactation not established, although drug has been used to inhibit contractions in premature labor.
• Do not give intravenously.
• Observe for hypotension and tachycardia with parenteral use. Monitor blood pressure and pulse rate.
• Discontinue if rash develops.

nylidrin hydrochloride (Arlidin, Pervadil, Rolidrin)

Indications and dosage
To increase blood supply in vasospastic disorders (arteriosclerosis obliterans, thromboangiitis obliterans, diabetic vascular disease, night leg cramps, Raynaud's phenomenon and disease, ischemic ulcer, frostbite, acrocyanosis, acroparesthesia, sequelae of thrombophlebitis)—
Adults: 3 to 12 mg P.O. t.i.d. or q.i.d.

Side effects
CNS: trembling, *nervousness,* weakness, *dizziness (not associated with labyrinth artery insufficiency)*
CV: palpitations, hypotension, flushing
GI: nausea, vomiting

Interactions
None significant

Nursing considerations
• Contraindicated in acute MI, paroxysmal tachycardia, angina pectoris, thyrotoxicosis. Use with caution in uncompensated heart disease or peptic ulcer.

papaverine hydrochloride (Cerespan, Pavabid)

Indications and dosage
Relief of cerebral and peripheral ischemia associated with arterial spasm and myocardial ischemia; treatment of smooth-muscle spasm (coronary occlusion, angina pectoris, sequelae of peripheral and pulmonary embolism, certain cerebral angiospastic states) and visceral spasms (biliary, ureteral, or GI colic)—
Adults: 60 to 300 mg P.O. 1 to 5 times daily, or 150 to 300 mg sustained-release preparations q 8 to 12 hours; 30 to 120 mg I.M. or I.V. q 3 hours, as indicated

Side effects
CNS: headache
CV: *increased heart rate, increased blood pressure* (with parenteral use), depressed AV and intraventricular conduction, dysrhythmias
GI: constipation, *nausea*
Other: sweating, flushing, malaise, increased depth of respiration

Interactions
None significant

Nursing considerations
• Contraindicated for I.V. use in complete AV block. Use with caution in glaucoma.

- Monitor blood pressure, and heart rate and rhythm, especially in cardiac disease. Hold dose and notify doctor immediately if changes occur.
- Not often used parenterally, except when immediate effect is desired.
- Give I.V. slowly (over 1 to 2 minutes) to avoid side effects.
- Most effective when given early in the course of a disorder.
- Tell patient to take medication regularly; long-term therapy is required.
- Do not add lactated Ringer's injection to the injectable form; will precipitate.

tolazoline hydrochloride (Tazol, Toloxan, Tolzol)

Indications and dosage

Spastic peripheral vascular disorders associated with acrocyanosis, acroparesthesia, arteriosclerosis obliterans, Buerger's disease, causalgia, diabetic arteriosclerosis, gangrene, endarteritis, post-thrombotic conditions, Raynaud's disease—

Adults:

Oral—25 mg 4 to 6 times daily, gradually increasing to maximum of 50 mg 6 times daily

Parenteral—10 to 50 mg S.C., I.V., or I.M. q.i.d. Start with low dose, increasing gradually until optimal response (as determined by appearance of flushing) is reached

Intra-arterial—50 to 75 mg/injection, depending on response; 1 or 2 injections may be required initially, then dose of 2 or 3 injections weekly to maintain circulation, possibly coupled with oral tolazoline between injections.

Side effects

CV: dysrhythmias, anginal pain, hypertension, flushing, transient postural vertigo, palpitations
GI: nausea, vomiting, diarrhea, epigastric discomfort, exacerbation of peptic ulcer
Local: burning at injection site
Other: weakness, paradoxical response in seriously damaged limbs, increased

pilomotor activity, tingling, chilliness, apprehension

Interactions

Ethyl alcohol: possible disulfiram reaction from accumulation of acetaldehyde. Use together cautiously.

Nursing considerations

- Contraindicated in CAD, active peptic ulcer, or following cerebrovascular accident. Use with caution in patients with history of peptic ulcer disease, gastritis, or known or suspected mitral stenosis.
- Keep patient warm during parenteral administration to increase response.
- Appearance of flushing usually indicates maximum tolerable dose.
- Monitor vital signs. Watch especially for blood pressure changes, dysrhythmias.
- Instruct patient to avoid alcohol; chills and flushing may occur.
- Due to risks, technique, and precautions, intra-arterial injection should be done only by experienced personnel, in selected cases, and only after maximum benefit has been achieved with oral and parenteral therapy.
- Warn patient against exposure to cold, which can aggravate tissue damage.
- Often used to distinguish between functional (vasospastic) and organic (obstructive) forms of peripheral vascular disease.

ANTILIPEMICS

Antilipemics can retard, and even arrest, atherosclerosis and its resultant complications. Atherosclerosis is associated with increased levels of certain blood lipids. Research thus far, however, has not been able to show a direct clinical relationship between lowered blood lipid levels and reduced incidence of atherosclerosis since other risk factors are reduced as well during the treatment period.

Dietary restriction and physical exercise are essential in treating all hyperlipidemias. If strict dietary therapy does not effectively lower lipid levels after 2 or 3 months, drug therapy may be started.

Hyperlipidemias may be primary or secondary to conditions such as hypothyroidism, hepatic disorders, renal failure, nephrosis, pancreatic insufficiency, malabsorption syndromes, and diabetes mellitus.

Major uses
Antilipemics counteract high concentrations of lipids in the blood. They do this by lowering levels of cholesterol or triglycerides or both, to different degrees.

Mechanism of action
• Both cholestyramine and colestipol combine with bile acid to form an insoluble compound that is excreted.
• Clofibrate—used when triglycerides are high and cholesterol levels are only moderately elevated—seems to inhibit biosynthesis of cholesterol at an early stage, but the exact mechanism is unknown.
• Dextrothyroxine accelerates hepatic catabolism of cholesterol and increases bile secretion to lower cholesterol levels. The drug's serious cardiovascular side effects restrict its use to young patients with no history of CAD.
• Gemfibrozil inhibits peripheral lipolysis and also reduces triglyceride synthesis in the liver.
• Niacin, by an unknown mechanism, decreases synthesis of low-density lipoproteins and inhibits lipolysis in adipose tissue.
• Probucol inhibits cholesterol transport from the intestine and may also decrease cholesterol synthesis. The drug appears to be more effective in patients with mild cholesterol elevations than in those with severe hypercholesterolemia. (See *Effects of Antilipemics on Blood Lipids*, page 405).

Absorption, distribution, metabolism, and excretion
• Cholestyramine, colestipol, and the sitosterols are not appreciably absorbed from the GI tract. They are eliminated in the feces.
• Clofibrate and niacin are well absorbed from the GI tract.
• Dextrothyroxine is poorly absorbed from the GI tract.
• Probucol is very poorly absorbed from the GI tract. It is passed into the bile for elimination in the feces.

Onset and duration
Response to antilipemic therapy varies with adherence to drug and dietary regimens. Drug treatment is effective only when combined with an adequate dietary plan. For maximum benefit, blood cholesterol and triglyceride levels should be tested several times during the first few months of therapy and periodically thereafter.

After administration of dietary or drug therapy, a new lipid steady-state level is reached in 4 weeks. Lipid levels should be rechecked at this time and the regimen changed, if necessary.
• Clofibrate and probucol take up to 2 months to achieve maximum effect.
• Niacin's effect is transient; therefore, free fatty acid levels rebound between meals and at night. The bedtime dose is especially important to counteract the striking rise of free fatty acid levels during the nocturnal fast.

---

cholestyramine (Questran)

Indications and dosage
Primary hyperlipidemia, pruritus, and diarrhea due to excess bile acid—
Adults: 4 g before meals and h.s., not to exceed 32 g daily. Each scoop or packet of Questran contains 4 g cholestyramine.
Children: 240 mg/kg daily P.O. in 3 divided doses with beverage or food. Safe dosage not established for children under 6 years.

Side effects
GI: *constipation,* fecal impaction, hemorrhoids, *abdominal discomfort,* flatulence, *nausea,* vomiting, steatorrhea
Skin: *rash,* irritation of skin, tongue, and perianal area
Other: *vitamin A, D, and K deficiency from decreased absorption;* hyperchloremic acidosis with long-term use or very high dosage

Interactions
None significant

Nursing considerations
• To mix, sprinkle powder on surface of preferred beverage or wet food. Let stand a few minutes, then stir to obtain uniform suspension.
• Mixing with carbonated beverages may result in excess foaming. To avoid, use large glass, and mix slowly.
• Administer all other medications at least 1 hour before or 4 to 6 hours after cholestyramine to avoid blocking their absorption.
• Observe bowel habits; treat constipation as needed. Encourage a diet high in roughage and fluids. If severe constipation develops, decrease dosage, add a stool softener, or discontinue drug.
• Monitor cardiac glycoside levels in patients receiving both medications concurrently. Should cholestyramine therapy be discontinued, cardiac glycoside toxicity may result unless dosage is adjusted.
• Watch for signs of vitamin A, D, and K deficiency.
• May cause decreased absorption of many drugs due to binding. Check drug interaction list of individual drugs.

clofibrate
(Atromid-S)

Indications and dosage
Hyperlipidemia and xanthoma tuberosum—
Adults: 2 g P.O. daily in 4 divided doses. Some patients may respond to lower doses as assessed by serum lipid moni-

toring.
Should not be used in children.

Side effects
Blood: leukopenia
CNS: fatigue, weakness
GI: nausea, diarrhea, vomiting, stomatitis, *dyspepsia,* flatulence
GU: decreased libido
Hepatic: gallstones, *transient and reversible elevations of liver function tests*
Skin: rash, urticaria, pruritus, dry skin and hair
Other: myalgias and arthralgias, resembling a flulike syndrome; *weight gain; polyphagia;* fever

Interactions
Oral contraceptives: may antagonize clofibrate's lipid-lowering effect. Monitor blood lipid level.

Nursing considerations
• Contraindicated in patients with severe renal or hepatic disease.
• Warn patient to report flulike symptoms to doctor immediately.
• Monitor renal and hepatic function, blood counts, serum electrolyte and blood sugar levels. If liver function tests show steady rise, clofibrate should be discontinued.
• Should not be used indiscriminately. May pose increased risk of gallstones, heart disease, and cancer.
• If significant lipid lowering is not achieved within 3 months, drug should be discontinued.

colestipol hydrochloride
(Colestid)

Indications and dosage
Primary hypercholesterolemia and xanthomas—
Adults: 15 to 30 g P.O. daily in 2 to 4 divided doses

Side effects
GI: constipation (common, may require decreasing the dosage), fecal impaction, hemorrhoids, abdominal discomfort,

flatulence, nausea, vomiting, steatorrhea
Skin: rash, irritation of skin, tongue,
and perianal area
Other: vitamin A, D, and K deficiency
from decreased absorption; hyperchloremic acidosis with long-term use or
very high dosage

Interactions
Oral hypoglycemics: may antagonize response to colestipol. Monitor blood lipid
level.

Nursing considerations
• Administer all other medications at
least 1 hour before or 4 to 6 hours after
colestipol to avoid blocking their absorption.
• Monitor cardiac glycoside levels in
patients receiving both medications
concurrently. Should colestipol therapy
be discontinued, cardiac glycoside toxicity may result unless dosage is adjusted.
• Watch for signs of vitamin A, D, and
K deficiency.
• Lowering dosage or adding stool softener may relieve constipation.
• May cause decreased absorption of
many drugs due to binding. Check drug
interaction list of individual drugs.

dextrothyroxine sodium
(Choloxin)

Indications and dosage
*Hyperlipidemia in euthyroid patients,
especially when cholesterol and triglyceride levels are elevated—*
Adults: initial dose 1 to 2 mg daily,
increased by 1 to 2 mg daily at monthly
intervals to a total of 4 to 8 mg daily
Children: initial dose 0.05 mg/kg daily,
increased by 0.05 mg/kg daily at
monthly intervals to a total of 4 mg daily

Side effects
CV: palpitations, angina pectoris, dysrhythmias, ischemic myocardial changes
on EKG, MI.
EENT: visual disturbances, ptosis

GI: nausea, vomiting, diarrhea, constipation, decreased appetite
*Metabolic: insomnia, weight loss,
sweating,* flushing, hyperthermia, hair
loss, menstrual irregularities

Interactions
None significant

Nursing considerations
• Contraindicated in patients with hepatic or renal disease, or iodism. Patients with history of cardiac disease,
including dysrhythmias, hypertension,
or angina pectoris, should receive very
small doses.
• May increase need for insulin, diet
therapy, or oral hypoglycemics in diabetics.
• If use of anticoagulants is being considered, discontinue drug 2 weeks before surgery to avoid possible potentia-
tion of anticoagulant effect.
• Observe patient for signs of hyperthyroidism, such as nervousness, insomnia,
weight loss. If these occur, dosage
should be decreased or drug discontinued.

gemfibrozil
(Lopid)

Indications and dosage
*Treatment of Type IV hyperlipidemia (hy-
pertriglyceridemia) and severe hypercholesterolemia unresponsive to diet and
other drugs—*
Adults: 1,200 mg P.O. administered in
two divided doses. Usual dosage range
is 900 to 1,500 mg daily.

Side effects
Blood: anemia, leukopenia
CNS: blurred vision, headache, dizzi-
ness
*GI: abdominal and epigastric pain,
diarrhea, nausea,* vomiting, flatulence
Hepatic: elevated enzymes
Skin: rash, dermatitis, pruritus
Other: painful extremities

Effects of Antilipemics on Blood Lipids

DRUG	EFFECT ON CHOLESTEROL	EFFECT ON TRIGLYCERIDES
cholestyramine	⬇ (marked decrease)	◯ or ⬆ (no change or mild increase)
clofibrate	⬇ (mild decrease)	⬇ (marked decrease)
colestipol	⬇ (marked decrease)	◯ or ⬆ (no change or mild increase)
dextrothyroxine	⬇ (moderate decrease)	⬇ or ⬆ (mild decrease or mild increase)
gemfibrozil	⬇ (mild decrease)	⬇ (marked decrease)
niacin	⬇ (marked decrease)	⬇ (moderate decrease)
probucol	⬇ (moderate decrease)	◯ or ⬆ (no change or mild increase)

KEY: ⬇ = Mild decrease ⬇ = Moderate decrease ⬇ = Marked decrease ⬆ = Mild increase ◯ = No change

Interactions
None significant

Nursing considerations
• Contraindicated in hepatic or severe renal dysfunction—including primary biliary cirrhosis—and in preexisting gallbladder disease.
• CBC and liver function tests should be done periodically during first 12 months of therapy.
• Gemfibrozil is very closely related to clofibrate both chemically and pharmacologically.
• Instruct patient to take drugs ½ hour before breakfast and dinner.
• Should not be used indiscriminately. May pose risk of gallstones, heart disease, and cancer.
• Patient should adhere strictly to prescribed diet, avoiding saturated fats,

cholesterol, sugars.
• Because of possible dizziness and blurred vision, patient should avoid driving or operating machinery until CNS response to drug is determined.

niacin
(Nicobid)

Indications and dosage
Adjunctive treatment of hyperlipidemias, especially associated with hypercholesterolemia—
Adults: 1.5 to 3 g daily in 3 divided doses with or after meals, increased at intervals to 6 g daily

Side effects
CV: flushing (usually subsides in a few weeks)

GI: nausea, dyspepsia, vomiting, diarrhea, anorexia, flatulence, epigastric pain
Hepatic: liver function test abnormalities
Metabolic: glucose intolerance resulting in hyperglycemia in previously well-controlled diabetics, hyperuricemia
Skin: pruritus, sensation of burning or stinging

Interactions
None significant

Nursing considerations
• Use cautiously in patients with gout, diabetes, gallbladder or hepatic disease, peptic ulcer.
• Advise patient that pruritus and flushing noted in first few weeks of therapy usually lessen with continued use.
• Begin therapy with small doses; then increase gradually.
• Give with meals to minimize GI irritation. Cold water eases swallowing.
• Blood glucose and liver function tests should be performed routinely during early therapy.

probucol
(Lorelco)

Indications and dosage
Primary hypercholesterolemia—
Adults: 2 tablets (500 mg total) P.O. b.i.d. with morning and evening meals. Not recommended for children.

Side effects
GI: diarrhea, flatulence, abdominal pain, nausea, vomiting
Other: hyperhidrosis, fetid sweat, angioneurotic edema

Interactions
None significant

Nursing considerations
• Drug's effect is enhanced when taken with food.
• Contraindicated in patients with dysrhythmias. Drug should be stopped in any patient whose EKG shows prolonged QT interval.

18
ADJUNCTIVE DRUG THERAPY

Certain drug classes—analgesics, adrenergics, adrenergic blockers, diuretics, anticoagulants and their antagonists, and thrombolytic enzymes—are often used as adjunctive therapy in many cardiovascular disorders. These drugs are discussed below.

ANALGESICS

Aspirin and most salicylate derivatives are available without a doctor's prescription.

Narcotic and opioid analgesics are defined by the Comprehensive Drug Abuse Prevention and Control Act of 1970 as controlled substances. They can change a patient's perception of pain so that it is qualitatively less disturbing and can result in physical and psychological dependence. They should be reserved for treatment of severe pain unrelieved by nonnarcotic analgesics.

Major uses
• Salicylates relieve mild-to-moderate pain; alleviate inflammation of rheumatoid arthritis, osteoarthritis, gout, and other conditions; and reduce fever.
• Aspirin also inhibits platelet aggregation, hindering coagulation.
• Narcotic and opioid analgesics relieve moderate-to-severe pain and furnish preoperative sedation, alone or in combination with tranquilizers (such as chlorpromazine, diazepam, and hydroxyzine).

Mechanism of action
• Salicylates produce analgesia by an ill-defined effect on the hypothalamus (central action) and by blocking generation of pain impulses (peripheral action). The peripheral action may involve inhibition of prostaglandin synthesis.

Salicylates probably exert their anti-inflammatory effect by inhibiting prostaglandin synthesis; they may also inhibit the synthesis or action of other mediators of the inflammatory response.

They relieve fever by acting on the hypothalamic heat-regulating center to produce peripheral vasodilation. This increases peripheral blood supply and promotes sweating, which leads to loss of heat and cooling by evaporation.

Aspirin also appears to impede clotting by blocking prostaglandin synthetase action, which prevents formation of the platelet-aggregating substance thromboxane A_2.
• Narcotic and opioid analgesics bind with opiate receptors at many sites in the central nervous system (brain, brain stem, and spinal cord), altering both perception of and emotional response to pain. The precise mechanism of action, however, is unknown.

Absorption, distribution, metabolism, and excretion
All oral and I.M. forms of the analgesics and antipyretics are well absorbed. The drugs are distributed in most body tissues and fluids, largely metabolized in the liver, and eliminated as inactive metabolites in urine and—through the bile—in feces.

Absorption of most narcotic and opioid analgesics is more effective after parenteral than after oral administration.

All narcotic and opioid analgesics are well distributed in body tissues, metabolized in the liver, and excreted in the urine.

Onset and duration
All the nonnarcotic analgesics and antipyretics begin to act 30 to 60 minutes after oral administration and 15 to 30 minutes after I.M. injection. Peak blood levels are reached in 2 to 3 hours. Duration of action of these drugs is generally 4 to 6 hours.

Meperidine begins to act 10 to 15 minutes after parenteral administration. Peak blood levels are reached in 30 to 60 minutes. Duration of action is 2 to 4 hours.

Morphine's action begins within 20 minutes of parenteral administration. Peak blood levels are reached within 30 to 90 minutes. Duration of action is 4 to 7 hours.

---

aspirin

Indications and dosage
Adults:
Mild pain or fever—325 to 650 mg P.O. or rectally q 4 hours p.r.n.
  Thromboembolic disorders—325 to 650 mg P.O. daily or b.i.d.
  Transient ischemic attacks in men— 650 mg P.O. b.i.d. or 325 mg q.i.d.
Children:
Fever—40 to 80 mg/kg P.O. or rectally daily divided q 6 hours p.r.n.
  Mild pain—65 to 100 mg/kg P.O. or rectally daily divided q 4 to 6 hours p.r.n.

Side effects
Blood: prolonged bleeding time
EENT: tinnitus and hearing loss (first signs of toxicity)
GI: nausea, vomiting, GI distress, occult bleeding

Hepatic: abnormal liver function studies, hepatitis
Skin: rash, bruising
Other: hypersensitivity manifested by anaphylaxis or asthma

Interactions
Ammonium chloride (and other urine acidifiers): increases blood levels of aspirin products. Monitor for aspirin toxicity.
Antacids in high doses (and other urine alkalinizers): decrease levels of aspirin products. Monitor for decreased aspirin effect.
Carbonic anhydrase inhibitors, cimetidine: may elevate salicylate levels. Monitor for toxicity.
Corticosteroids: enhance salicylate elimination. Monitor for decreased salicylate effect.
Oral anticoagulants and heparin: increase risk of bleeding. Avoid using together if possible.

Nursing considerations
• Contraindicated in GI ulcer, GI bleeding, aspirin hypersensitivity. Use cautiously in patients with hypoprothrombinemia, vitamin K deficiency, bleeding disorders, Hodgkin's disease (may cause profound hypothermia); and in asthmatics with nasal polyps (may cause severe bronchospasm).
• Because of epidemiologic association with Reye's syndrome, the Centers for Disease Control recommend that children with chicken pox or influenza-like illness should not be given salicylates.
• Febrile, dehydrated children can develop toxicity rapidly.
• Give with food, milk, antacid, or large glass of water to reduce GI side effects.
• Warn patients to check with doctor or pharmacist before taking over-the-counter combinations containing aspirin.
• Alcohol may increase GI blood loss.
• May cause increase in serum levels of serum glutamic-oxaloacetic transaminase (SGOT), serum glutamic-pyruvic transaminase (SGPT), alkaline phosphatase, and bilirubin.

How Narcotics Affect Body Functions

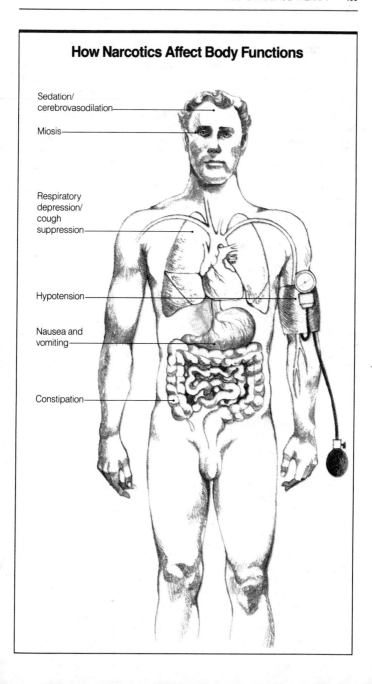

Sedation/
cerebrovasodilation

Miosis

Respiratory
depression/
cough
suppression

Hypotension

Nausea and
vomiting

Constipation

meperidine hydrochloride (Demer-Idine, Demerol)

Controlled Substance Schedule II

Indications and dosage

Moderate-to-severe pain—
Adults: 50 to 150 mg P.O., I.M., or S.C. q 3 to 4 hours p.r.n.
Children: 1 mg/kg P.O., I.M., or S.C. q 4 to 6 hours. Maximum—100 mg q 4 hours p.r.n.
Preoperatively—
Adults: 50 to 100 mg I.M. or S.C. 30 to 90 minutes before surgery
Children: 1 to 2.2 mg/kg I.M. or S.C. 30 to 90 minutes before surgery

Side effects

CNS: sedation, somnolence, clouded sensorium, euphoria, convulsions with large doses
CV: hypotension, bradycardia
GI: nausea, vomiting, constipation, ileus
GU: urinary retention
Local: pain at injection site, local tissue irritation and induration after S.C. injection; phlebitis after I.V. injection
Other: respiratory depression, physical dependence

Interactions

MAO inhibitors, barbiturates, isoniazid: increased CNS excitation or depression can be severe or fatal. Do not use together.
Alcohol, CNS depressants: additive effects. Use together cautiously.
Phenytoin: decreased blood levels of meperidine. Monitor for decreased analgesia.

Nursing considerations

• Contraindicated if patient has used MAO inhibitors within 14 days. Use with extreme caution in patients with increased intracranial pressure, increased cerebrospinal fluid pressure, shock, CNS depression, head injury, asthma, chronic obstructive pulmonary disease (COPD), respiratory depression, supraventricular tachycardias, seizures, acute abdominal conditions, hepatic or renal disease, hypothyroidism, Addison's disease, urethral stricture, prostatic hypertrophy, alcoholism, in children under 12 years, and in elderly or debilitated patients.
• May be used in patients allergic to morphine.
• Meperidine and active metabolite normeperidine accumulate in renal failure. Monitor for increased toxic effect in patients with poor renal function.
• Meperidine may be given slow I.V., preferably as a diluted solution. S.C. injection very painful.
• Keep narcotic antagonist (naloxone) available when giving this drug I.V.
• P.O. dose less than half as effective as parenteral dose. Give I.M. if possible. When changing from parenteral to P.O. route, dose should be increased.
• Chemically incompatible with barbiturates. Do not mix together.
• Monitor respiratory and cardiovascular status carefully. Do not give if respirations are below 12/minute or if change in pupils is noted.
• If used with other narcotic analgesics, general anesthetics, phenothiazines, sedatives, hypnotics, tricyclic antidepressants, or alcohol, respiratory depression, hypotension, profound sedation, or coma may occur. Reduce meperidine dose. Use together with extreme caution.
• For better analgesic effect, give before patient has intense pain. (See *How Narcotics Affect Body Functions,* page 409).

morphine sulfate

Controlled Substance Schedule II RMS

Indications and dosage

Severe pain—
Adults: 5 to 15 mg S.C. or I.M., or 30 to 60 mg P.O. or by rectum q 4 hours p.r.n. or around the clock. May be injected slow I.V. (over 4 to 5 minutes) diluted in 4 to 5 ml water.

Children: 0.1 to 0.2 mg/kg dose S.C.
Maximum 15 mg

Side effects
CNS: sedation, somnolence, clouded sensorium, euphoria, convulsions with large doses
CV: nausea, vomiting, constipation, ileus
GU: urinary retention
Other: respiratory depression, physical dependence

Interactions
Alcohol, CNS depressants: additional effects. Use together cautiously.

Nursing considerations
• Use with extreme caution in patients with head injury, increased intracranial pressure, seizures, asthma, COPD, alcoholism, prostatic hypertrophy, severe hepatic or renal disease, acute abdominal conditions, hypothyroidism, Addison's disease.
• Monitor circulatory and respiratory status and bowel function. Do not give if respirations are below 12/minute.
• Drug of choice in relieving pain of myocardial infarction (MI). May cause transient decrease in blood pressure.
• Keep narcotic antagonist (naloxone) and resuscitative equipment available.
• Constipation often severe with maintenance. Make sure stool softener or other laxative is ordered.
• Respiratory depression, hypotension, profound sedation, or coma may occur if used with general anesthetics, tranquilizers, sedatives, hypnotics, alcohol, tricyclic antidepressants, or monoamine oxidase (MAO) inhibitors. Reduce morphine dose. Use together with extreme caution. Monitor patient's response.
• When used postoperatively, encourage turning, coughing, and deep breathing to avoid atelectasis.
• Patients with very severe pain may receive up to 150 mg of morphine sulfate every 3 hours in some situations.

ADRENERGICS (SYMPATHOMIMETICS)

Adrenergics produce their effect by either mimicking the actions of epinephrine or norepinephrine at receptor sites in the sympathetic nervous system, or displacing natural norepinephrine from neural storage sites. Because these drugs do not simulate all classes of adrenergic receptors equally, their effects and indications for use differ.

As with most drugs, the actions of adrenergics are not organ- or site-specific; they may occur at other than the desired sites.

The sympathetic nervous system innervates numerous organs (for example, the heart, blood vessels, respiratory tract, liver, urinary bladder, and intestines) and significantly affects the regulation of many body functions. When stimulated, sympathetic nerves release norepinephrine (except for sympathetic nerves that innervate sweat glands, which release acetylcholine). Norepinephrine combines with receptor sites on the innervated organ to elicit a response.

The three major types of receptors within the sympathetic system are alpha, beta, and dopaminergic. Stimulation of alpha receptors causes vasoconstriction and uterine and sphincter contraction. Beta receptors are divided into two subgroups, beta$_1$ and beta$_2$. Beta$_1$ receptors are largely in the heart; when stimulated, they increase the rate and force of myocardial contraction and the rate of atrioventricular node conduction. Beta$_2$ receptors are primarily in the bronchi, blood vessels, and uterus; stimulation produces bronchodilation, vasodilation, and uterine relaxation, respectively. Dopaminergic receptors are primarily in splanchnic blood vessels; stimulation dilates these vessels.

The adrenal medulla is a major part of the sympathetic nervous system. During times of danger or acute stress, it releases large amounts of epinephrine into the systemic circulation. Epinephrine activates alpha and beta receptors, ultimately producing physiologic and metabolic effects that prepare the person to cope with the stress (as in the fight-or-flight response).

Major uses
• Dobutamine, dopamine, mephentermine, metaraminol, and norepinephrine raise blood pressure and cardiac output in severely decompensated states, such as cardiogenic shock and heart failure.
• Epinephrine and isoproterenol are used to treat heart block and certain dysrhythmias, and to restore cardiac rhythm in cardiac arrest.

Mechanism of action
Adrenergics simulate or increase the effect of epinephrine and norepinephrine on alpha- and beta-adrenergic receptors within the sympathetic nervous system. Effects vary and include bronchodilation, release of glucose from the liver, increase in heart rate and ventricular contractility, central nervous system excitation, dilation (beta effect) of blood vessels in skeletal muscles, and constriction (alpha effect) of blood vessels in cutaneous areas.

Absorption, distribution, metabolism, and excretion
• Dobutamine and dopamine are not absorbed from the GI tract and must be given parenterally. They are metabolized by the liver to inactive compounds and excreted in urine.
• Ephedrine is rapidly absorbed after oral, I.M., or subcutaneous administration. Some of the drug is metabolized by the liver; both unchanged compound and metabolites are excreted in the urine.
• Epinephrine is not well absorbed from the GI tract after oral administration. Absorption is efficient, however, after I.M. or S.C. injection. The drugs are extensively metabolized in the liver and excreted in the urine.
• Isoproterenol is irregularly absorbed after oral or sublingual administration, but is well absorbed following parenteral administration or oral inhalation. It is metabolized in the liver and other tissues and excreted in the urine.
• Mephentermine is not absorbed from the GI tract and must be given parenterally. It is metabolized in the liver and excreted in the urine; excretion is increased in an acidic urine.
• Metaraminol is erratically absorbed from the GI tract after being given orally, so it must be given parenterally. Distribution, metabolism, and route of excretion are not completely known. Its pharmacologic effects are stopped by its uptake into body tissues.
• Norepinephrine is not absorbed after oral administration and is poorly absorbed after S.C. injection. The drug is taken up by nerve endings where it is metabolized; it is also metabolized by the liver and other tissues. Metabolites are excreted in urine.

Onset and duration
Most adrenergics, when given I.V., have an immediate onset. Their duration is as long as the infusion is continued. However, when the route of administration is I.M. or S.C., the onset is delayed 3 to 5 minutes and lasts about 15 to 30 minutes after injection. Oral medications take the longest to act, with their action lasting up to 4 hours. (See *Comparing Adrenergics,* page 413).

dobutamine hydrochloride (Dobutrex)

Indications and dosage
Refractory heart failure and as adjunct in cardiac surgery—
Adults: 2.5 to 10 mcg/kg/minute as an I.V. infusion. Rarely, infusion rates up to 40 mcg/kg/minute have been required. May be reconstituted with dextrose 5% in water, normal saline solution, or lactated Ringer's solution.

Side effects
CNS: headache
CV: increased heart rate, hypertension, premature ventricular beats, angina,

Comparing Adrenergics

DRUG	ROUTE	ONSET	DURATION
albuterol	inhalation	within 15 min; peaks in 1 hr	3 to 4 hr
	P.O.	within 30 min	4 to 6 hr
dobutamine	I.V.	within 2 min	until shortly after infusion is stopped
dopamine	I.V.	within 5 min	less than 10 min, or as long as infusion is continued
ephedrine	P.O.	less than 1 hr	4 to 12 hr, depending on form of P.O. dosage
epinephrine	I.M. S.C.	3 to 5 min	20 to 30 min
isoproterenol	I.V.	immediate	as long as infusion is continued
	P.O.	20 min	1 hr
mephentermine	I.M.	5 to 15 min	1 to 4 hr
	I.V.	immediate	15 to 30 min after injection
metaraminol	I.M.	within 10 min	1 hr
	I.V.	1 to 2 min	5 to 15 min
	S.C.	5 to 20 min	1 hr
norepinephrine	I.V.	immediate	until shortly after infusion is stopped
phenylephrine	S.C.	10-15 minutes	15 minutes-1 hr
hydrochloride	I.M.		30 minutes-2 hr
	I.V.	immediate	15-20 minutes

nonspecific chest pain
GI: nausea, vomiting
Other: shortness of breath

Interactions

Propranolol, metoprolol: These beta blockers may make dobutamine ineffective. Do not use together.

Nursing considerations

• Contraindicated in idiopathic hypertrophic subaortic stenosis.
• A unique agent. Increases contractility of failing heart without inducing marked tachycardia, except at high doses.
• Dobutamine is chemical modification of isoproterenol.
• Often used with nitroprusside for additive effects.
• Electrocardiogram (EKG), blood pressure, pulmonary wedge pressure, and cardiac output should be monitored continuously. Also monitor urinary output.
• Incompatible with alkaline solutions. Do not mix with sodium bicarbonate injection.
• Infusions of up to 72 hours produce no more adverse effects than shorter infusions.
• Oxidation of drug may slightly discolor admixtures containing dobutamine. This does not indicate a significant loss of potency.
• Intravenous solutions remain stable for 24 hours.

---

dopamine hydrochloride (Dopastat)

Indications and dosage

To treat shock and correct hemodynamic imbalances; to improve perfusion to vital organs, increase cardiac output; to correct hypotension—
Adults: 2 to 5 mcg/kg/minute I.V. infusion, up to 50 mcg/kg/minute
Titrate the dosage to the desired hemodynamic or renal response.

Side effects

CNS: headache
CV: ectopic beats, tachycardia, anginal pain, palpitations, *hypotension,* bradycardia, widening of QRS complex, conduction disturbances, vasoconstriction
GI: nausea, vomiting
Local: necrosis and tissue sloughing with extravasation
Other: piloerection, dyspnea

Interactions

Ergot alkaloids: extreme elevations in blood pressure. Do not use together.
Phenytoin: may lower blood pressure of dopamine-stabilized patients. Monitor carefully.

Nursing considerations

• Contraindicated in uncorrected tachyarrhythmias, pheochromocytoma, ventricular fibrillation. Use cautiously in patients with occlusive vascular disease, cold injuries, diabetic endarteritis, arterial embolism, and in pregnant patients and those taking MAO inhibitors.
• Not a substitute for blood or fluid volume deficit. If volume deficit exists, it should be replaced before vasopressors are administered.
• Use large vein, as in antecubital fossa, to minimize risk of extravasation. Watch site carefully for signs of extravasation. If it occurs, stop infusion immediately and call doctor. He may want to counteract effect by infiltrating the area with 5 to 10 mg phentolamine and 10 to 15 ml normal saline solution.
• Check blood pressure, pulse rate, urinary output, and extremity color and temperature often during infusion. Titrate infusion rate according to findings, using doctor's guidelines. Use a microdrip or infusion pump to regulate flow rate.
• Observe patient closely for side effects. If adverse effects develop, dosage may need to be adjusted or discontinued.
• If a disproportionate rise in the diastolic pressure (a marked decrease in pulse pressure) is observed in patients receiving dopamine, decrease infusion

rate and observe carefully for further evidence of predominant vasoconstrictor activity, unless such an effect is desired.

• Most patients satisfactorily maintained on less than 20 mcg/kg/minute.

• If doses exceed 50 mcg/kg/minute, check urinary output often. If urine flow decreases without hypotension, consider reducing dose.

• If drug is stopped, watch closely for sudden drop in blood pressure.

• Do not mix with alkaline solutions. Use dextrose 5% in water, normal saline solution, or combination of dextrose 5% in water and saline solution. Mix just before use.

• Dopamine solutions deteriorate after 24 hours. Discard at that time or earlier if solution is discolored.

• Do not mix other drugs in bottle containing dopamine.

• Do not give alkaline drugs (sodium bicarbonate, phenytoin sodium) through I.V. line containing dopamine.

ephedrine sulfate

Indications and dosage

To correct hypotensive states; to support ventricular rate in Adams-Stokes syndrome—
Adults: 25 to 50 mg I.M. or S.C., or 10 to 25 mg I.V. p.r.n. to maximum 150 mg/24 hours
Children: 3 mg/kg S.C. or I.V. daily, divided into 4 to 6 doses

Side effects

CNS: *insomnia, nervousness,* dizziness, headache, muscle weakness, sweating, euphoria, confusion, delirium
CV: *palpitations,* tachycardia, hypertension
EENT: dryness of nose and throat
GI: nausea, vomiting, anorexia
GU: urinary retention, painful urination due to visceral sphincter spasm

Interactions

MAO inhibitors and tricyclic antidepressants: when given with sympathomimetics, may cause severe hypertension (hypertensive crisis). Do not use together.
Methyldopa: may inhibit effect of ephedrine. Give together cautiously.

Nursing considerations

• Contraindicated in patients with porphyria, severe coronary artery disease, cardiac dysrhythmias, narrow-angle glaucoma, psychoneurosis, and in patients on MAO-inhibitor therapy. Use with caution in elderly patients and those with hypertension, hyperthyroidism, nervous or excitable states, cardiovascular disease, or prostatic hypertrophy.

• Not a substitute for blood or fluid volume deficit. Volume deficit should be replaced before vasopressors are administered.

• Give I.V. injection slowly.

• Hypoxia, hypercapnia, and acidosis, which may reduce effectiveness or increase incidence of adverse effects, must be identified and corrected before or during ephedrine administration.

• Effectiveness decreases after 2 to 3 weeks. Then increased dosage may be needed. Tolerance develops, but drug is not known to cause addiction.

• To prevent insomnia, avoid giving within 2 hours before bedtime.

• Warn patient not to take over-the-counter drugs that contain ephedrine without informing doctor.

epinephrine hydrochloride (Adrenalin Chloride, Sus-Phrine)

Indications and dosage

To restore cardiac rhythm in cardiac arrest—
Adults: 0.5 to 1 mg I.V. or into endotracheal tube. May be given intracardiac if no I.V. route or intratracheal route available
Children: 10 mcg/kg I.V. or 5 to 10 mcg (0.05 to 0.1 ml of 1:10,000)/kg intracardiac
Note: 1 mg = 1 ml of 1:1,000 or 10 ml of 1:10,000.

Side effects

CNS: nervousness, tremor, euphoria, anxiety, coldness of extremities, vertigo, *headache,* sweating, cerebral hemorrhage, disorientation, agitation. In patients with Parkinson's disease, drug increases rigidity and tremor.

CV: palpitations, widened pulse pressure, hypertension, *tachycardia, ventricular fibrillation, cerebrovascular accident (CVA),* anginal pain, EKG changes, including a decrease in T-wave amplitude

Metabolic: hyperglycemia, glycosuria

Other: pulmonary edema, dyspnea, *pallor*

Interactions

Tricyclic antidepressants: when given with sympathomimetics, may cause severe hypertension (hypertensive crisis). Do not give together.

Propranolol: vasoconstriction and reflex bradycardia. Monitor patient carefully.

Nursing considerations

• Contraindicated in narrow-angle glaucoma, shock (other than anaphylactic shock), organic brain damage, cardiac dilatation, and coronary insufficiency; also during general anesthesia with halogenated hydrocarbons or cyclopropane and in labor (may delay second stage). Use with extreme caution in patients with long-standing bronchial asthma and emphysema who have developed degenerative heart disease. Use with caution in elderly patients and those with hyperthyroidism, angina, hypertension, psychoneurosis, diabetes.

• Do not mix with alkaline solutions. Use dextrose 5% in water, normal saline solution, or a combination of dextrose 5% in water and saline solution. Mix just before use.

• Epinephrine is rapidly destroyed by oxidizing agents, such as iodine, chromates, nitrates, nitrites, oxygen, and salts of easily reducible metals such as iron.

• Epinephrine solutions deteriorate after 24 hours. Discard after that time or

before if solution is discolored or contains precipitate. Keep solution in light-resistant container, and do not remove before use.

• Massage site after injection to counteract possible vasoconstriction. Repeated local injection can cause necrosis at site due to vasoconstriction.

• Avoid intramuscular administration of oil injection into buttocks. Gas gangrene may occur because epinephrine reduces oxygen tension of the tissues, encouraging the growth of contaminating organisms.

• Drug may widen patient's pulse pressure.

• In the event of a sharp blood pressure rise, rapid-acting vasodilators, such as nitrites or alpha-adrenergic blocking agents, can be given to counteract the marked pressor effect of large doses of epinephrine.

• Observe patient closely for side effects. If they develop, dosage may need to be adjusted or discontinued.

isoproterenol hydrochloride (Isuprel, Proternol—tabs)

Indications and dosage

Heart block and ventricular dysrhythmias—

Adults: initially, 0.02 to 0.06 mg I.V. Subsequent doses 0.01 to 0.2 mg I.V. or 5 mcg/minute I.V.; or 0.2 mg I.M. initially, then 0.02 to 1 mg p.r.n.

Children: may give ½ of initial adult dose

Maintenance for Stokes-Adams disease or AV block—

Adults: 30- to 180-mg timed-release tablets P.O. daily swallowed whole

Shock—

Adults and children: 0.5 to 5 mcg/ minute by continuous I.V. infusion. Usual concentration: 1 mg (5 ml) in 500 ml dextrose 5% in water. Adjust rate according to heart rate, central venous pressure (CVP), blood pressure, and urine flow.

Side effects
CNS: headache, mild tremor, weakness, dizziness, nervousness, insomnia
CV: palpitations, tachycardia, anginal pain; blood pressure may be elevated and then fall
GI: nausea, vomiting
Metabolic: hyperglycemia
Other: sweating, flushing of face, bronchial edema and inflammation

Interactions
Propranolol and other beta blockers: blocked bronchodilating effect of isoproterenol. Monitor patient carefully if used together.

Nursing considerations
• Contraindicated in tachycardia caused by digitalis intoxication and in patients with preexisting dysrhythmias, especially tachycardia, because chronotropic effect on heart may aggravate such disorders. Contraindicated in recent MI. Use cautiously in coronary insufficiency, diabetes, hyperthyroidism.
• Not a substitute for blood or fluid volume deficit. If deficit exists, it should be replaced before vasopressors are administered.
• If heart rate exceeds 110 beats/minute, it may be advisable to decrease infusion rate or temporarily stop infusion. Doses sufficient to increase heart rate to more than 130 beats/minute may induce ventricular dysrhythmias.
• If precordial distress or anginal pain occurs, stop drug immediately.
• When administering I.V. isoproterenol for shock, closely monitor blood pressure, CVP, EKG, arterial blood gas measurements, and urinary output. Carefully adjust infusion rate according to these measurements.
• Oral and sublingual tablets are poorly and erratically absorbed.
• Teach patient how to take sublingual tablet properly. Tell him to hold tablet under tongue until it dissolves and is absorbed and not to swallow saliva until that time. Prolonged use of sublingual tablets can cause tooth decay. Instruct patient to rinse mouth with water between doses, which will also help prevent dryness of oropharynx.
• If possible, do not give at bedtime because it interrupts sleep patterns.
• Oral tablets not for sublingual use; must be swallowed whole, not broken. Store in cool, dry place in airtight, light-resistant container. Keep bottle tightly capped after opening.
• Drug may cause slight rise in systolic blood pressure and slight-to-marked drop in diastolic blood pressure.
• Use a microdrip or infusion pump to regulate infusion flow rate.
• Observe patient closely for side effects. Dosage may need to be adjusted or discontinued.

mephentermine sulfate (Wyamine)

Indications and dosage
Treatment of shock and hypotension—
Adults: 0.5 mg/kg I.V.
Children: 0.4 mg/kg I.V.

Side effects
CNS: euphoria, nervousness, anxiety, tremor, incoherence, drowsiness, convulsions
CV: dysrhythmias, marked elevation of blood pressure (with large doses)

Interactions
Propranolol and other beta blockers: blocked bronchodilating effect of metaproterenol. Monitor patient carefully if used together.

Nursing considerations
• Contraindicated in concealed hemorrhage or hypotension from hemorrhage, except in emergencies; also in patients receiving phenothiazines, or who have received MAO inhibitors within 2 weeks. Use cautiously in arteriosclerosis, cardiovascular disease, hyperthyroidism, hypertension, chronic illness.
• Not a substitute for blood or fluid volume deficit. If deficit exists, it should be replaced before vasopressors are administered.

• During infusion, check blood pressure every 5 minutes until stabilized; then every 15 minutes.
• Observe patient closely for side effects. If adverse effects develop, dosage may need to be adjusted or discontinued.
• Monitor blood pressure even after stopping drug.
• I.M. route may be used since drug is not irritating to tissue.
• I.V. drug is not irritating to tissue, and extravasation is not dangerous. To prepare 0.1% I.V. solution, add 16.6 ml mephentermine (30 mg/ml) to 500 ml dextrose 5% in water.
• Can be given I.V. undiluted
• May increase uterine contractions during third trimester of pregnancy
• Hypercapnia, hypoxia, and acidosis may reduce effectiveness or increase adverse effects. Identify and correct before and during administration.

metaraminol bitartrate (Aramine)

Indications and dosage
Prevention of hypotension—
Adults: 2 to 10 mg I.M. or S.C.
Severe shock—
Adults: 0.5 to 5 mg direct I.V. followed by I.V. infusion
Treatment of hypotension due to shock—
Adults: 15 to 100 mg in 500 ml normal saline solution or dextrose 5% in water I.V. infusion. Adjust rate to maintain blood pressure.
All indications—
Children: 0.01 mg/kg as single I.V. injection; 1 mg/25 ml dextrose 5% in water as I.V. infusion. Adjust rate to maintain blood pressure in normal range. 0.1 mg/kg I.M. as single dose p.r.n. Allow at least 10 minutes to elapse before increasing dose because maximum effect is not immediately apparent.

Side effects
CNS: apprehension, restlessness, dizziness, headache, tremor, weakness; with excessive use, convulsions

CV: hypertension, hypotension, precordial pain, palpitations, dysrhythmias, including sinus or ventricular tachycardia, bradycardia, premature supraventricular beats, atrioventricular dissociation
GI: nausea, vomiting
GU: decreased urinary output
Metabolic: hyperglycemia
Skin: flushing, pallor, sweating
Local: irritation on extravasation
Other: metabolic acidosis in hypovolemia, increased body temperature, respiratory distress

Interactions
MAO inhibitors: may cause severe hypertension (hypertensive crisis). Do not use together.

Nursing considerations
• Contraindicated in peripheral or mesenteric thrombosis, pulmonary edema, hypercarbia, and acidosis; also during anesthesia with cyclopropane and halogenated hydrocarbon anesthetics. Use cautiously in patients with hypertension, thyroid disease, diabetes, cirrhosis, or malaria, and those receiving digitalis.
• Not a substitute for blood or fluid volume deficit. Fluid deficit should be replaced before vasopressors are administered.
• Keep solution in light-resistant container, away from heat.
• Use large veins, as in antecubital fossa, to minimize risk of extravasation. Watch infusion site carefully for signs of extravasation. If it occurs, stop infusion immediately and call doctor.
• During infusion, check blood pressure every 5 minutes until stabilized; then every 15 minutes. Check pulse rates, urinary output, and color and temperature of extremities. Titrate infusion rate according to findings, using doctor's guidelines.
• Use a microdrip or infusion pump to regulate infusion flow rate.
• Observe the patient closely for side effects. If adverse effects develop, dosage may need to be adjusted or discon-

tinued.
• For I.V. therapy, use two-bottle setup so I.V. can continue if drug is stopped.
• Blood pressure should be raised to slightly less than patient's normal level. Be careful to avoid excessive blood pressure response. Rapidly induced hypertensive response can cause acute pulmonary edema, dysrhythmias, and cardiac arrest.
• Because of prolonged action, a cumulative effect is possible. With an excessive vasopressor response, elevated blood pressure may persist after drug is stopped.
• Urinary output may decrease initially, then increase as blood pressure reaches normal level. Report persistent decreased urinary output.
• When discontinuing therapy, slow infusion rate gradually. Continue monitoring vital signs, watching for possible severe drop in blood pressure. Keep equipment nearby to start drug again, if necessary. Pressor therapy should not be reinstated until systolic blood pressure falls below 70 to 80 mm Hg.
• Keep emergency drugs on hand to reverse effects of metaraminol: atropine for reflex bradycardia; phentolamine to decrease vasopressor effects; propranolol for dysrhythmias.
• Closely monitor patients with diabetes. Adjustment in insulin dose may be needed.
• Metaraminol should not be mixed with other drugs.

---

norepinephrine
(Levophed)

Indications and dosage

To restore blood pressure in acute hypotensive states—
Adults: initially, 8 to 12 mcg/minute I.V. infusion, then adjust to maintain normal blood pressure. Average maintenance dose 2 to 4 mcg/minute

Side effects

CNS: headache, anxiety, weakness, dizziness, tremor, restlessness, insomnia
CV: bradycardia, severe hypertension, marked increase in peripheral resistance, decreased cardiac output, dysrhythmias, *ventricular tachycardia, fibrillation,* bigeminal rhythm, atrioventricular dissociation, precordial pain
GU: decreased urinary output
Metabolic: metabolic acidosis, hyperglycemia, increased glycogenolysis
Local: irritation with extravasation
Other: fever, respiratory difficulty

Interactions

Tricyclic antidepressants: when given with sympathomimetics, may cause severe hypertension (hypertensive crisis). Do not give together.

Nursing considerations

• Contraindicated in mesenteric or peripheral vascular thrombosis, pregnancy, profound hypoxia, hypercarbia, hypotension from blood volume deficits, or during cyclopropane and halothane anesthesia. Use cautiously in hypertension, hyperthyroidism, severe cardiac disease. Use with extreme caution in patients receiving MAO inhibitors or tricyclic antidepressants.
• Not a substitute for blood or fluid volume deficit. If deficit exists, it should be replaced before vasopressors are administered.
• Norepinephrine solutions deteriorate after 24 hours. Discard after that time.
• Use large vein, as in antecubital fossa, to minimize risk of extravasation. Check site frequently for signs of extravasation. If it occurs, stop infusion immediately and call doctor. He may counteract effect by infiltrating area with 5 to 10 mg phentolamine and 10 to 15 ml normal saline solution. Also check for blanching along course of infused vein; may progress to superficial slough. During infusion, check blood pressure every 2 minutes until stabilized; then every 5 minutes. Also check pulse rates, urinary output, and color and temperature of extremities. Titrate infusion rate according to findings, using doctor's guide-

lines. In previously hypertensive patients, blood pressure should be raised no more than 40 mm Hg below preexisting systolic pressure.
• Never leave patient unattended during infusion.
• Use a microdrip or infusion pump to regulate infusion flow rate.
• For I.V. therapy, use two-bottle setup with Y-port so I.V. can continue if norepinephrine is stopped.
• Report decreased urinary output to doctor immediately.
• If prolonged I.V. therapy is necessary, change injection site frequently.
• When stopping drug, slow infusion rate gradually. Monitor vital signs, even after drug is stopped. Watch for possible severe drop in blood pressure.
• Keep emergency drugs on hand to reverse effects of norepinephrine: atropine for reflex bradycardia, propranolol for dysrhythmias, phentolamine for increased vasopressor effects.
• Administer in dextrose and saline solution; saline solution alone is not recommended.

phenylephrine hydrochloride (Neo-Synephrine)

Indications and dosage
Mild-to-moderate hypotension—
Adults: 2 to 5 mg S.C. or I.M.; 0.1 to 0.5 mg I.V. Not to be repeated more often than 10 to 15 minutes
Paroxysmal supraventricular tachycardia—Adults: initially, 0.5 mg rapid I.V.; subsequent doses should not exceed the preceding dose by more than 0.1 to 0.2 mg and should not exceed 1 mg.
Severe hypotension and shock (including drug-induced)—
Adults: 10 mg in 500 ml dextrose 5% in water. Start 100 to 180 drops per minute I.V. infusion, then 40 to 60 drops per minute. Adjust to patient response.

Side effects
CNS: trembling, sweating, pallor, sense of fullness in head, *tingling in extremities,* sleeplessness, dizziness, *paresthe-*

sia in extremities from injection, lightheadedness, weakness
CV: palpitations, tachycardia, extrasystoles, short paroxysms of ventricular tachycardia, hypertension, anginal pain
EENT: blurred vision
Skin: gooseflesh, feeling of coolness
Other: tachyphylaxis with continued use

Interactions
MAO inhibitors: may cause severe hypertension (hypertensive crisis). Do not use together.
Tricyclic antidepressants: increased pressor response. Observe patient carefully.

Nursing considerations
• Contraindicated in narrow-angle glaucoma and with MAO inhibitors, tricyclic antidepressants, hypotension, ventricular tachycardia, severe coronary disease, or cardiovascular disease (including MI). Use with extreme caution in heart disease, hyperthyroidism, diabetes, severe atherosclerosis, bradycardia, partial heart block, myocardial disease, and the elderly.
• Longer acting than ephedrine and epinephrine
• Causes little or no central nervous system (CNS) stimulation.
• Monitor blood pressure frequently. Avoid excessive rise in blood pressure. Maintain blood pressure at slightly below patient's normal level. In previously normotensive patients, maintain systolic blood pressure at 80 to 100 mm Hg; in previously hypertensive patients, maintain systolic blood pressure at 30 to 40 mm Hg below their usual level.
• May reverse severe increase in blood pressure with phentolamine.
• With I.V. infusions, avoid abrupt withdrawal. Monitor blood pressure throughout. Reverse therapy if blood pressure falls too rapidly.

ADRENERGIC BLOCKERS (SYMPATHOLYTICS)

Adrenergic blockers inhibit the effects of epinephrine and norepinephrine released from sympathetic nerve endings, as well as the effects of other sympathomimetic amines.

The sympathetic nervous system has two types of receptors: alpha and beta. Stimulation of alpha receptors—located in smooth muscle—causes smooth-muscle contraction, such as vasoconstriction and sphincteric and uterine contraction.

Beta receptors are classified as $beta_1$ and $beta_2$. $Beta_1$ receptors—located mainly in the heart—increase heart rate, cardiac contraction, and atrioventricular conduction. $Beta_2$ receptors—in bronchi, blood vessels, and uterus—are responsible for smooth-muscle relaxation, such as vasodilation, bronchodilation, and uterine relaxation.

Major uses
● Propranolol is effective in prophylaxis and treatment of vascular headaches as well as in treatment of atrial dysrhythmias. (See Chapter 18, Antiarrhythmics.)
● Phenoxybenzamine is used to treat symptoms of spastic peripheral vascular disease.

Mechanism of action
● Alpha blockers inhibit the effects of epinephrine, norepinephrine, and other sympathomimetic amines on both smooth muscle and exocrine glands, preventing sympathetic stimulation.
● Propranolol's beta-blocking action prevents vasodilation of cerebral arteries.

Absorption, distribution, metabolism, and excretion
Although absorption varies with the specific drug, all adrenergic blockers are widely distributed to organs innervated by the sympathetic nervous system.

● Propranolol is well absorbed orally, metabolized in the liver, and excreted in urine.
● Phenoxybenzamine is variably absorbed when given orally; it is excreted by the kidneys as both the parent compound and inactive metabolites.

Onset and duration
● Onset of adrenergic blockers after oral administration varies from 30 minutes for ergot alkaloids to several hours for phenoxybenzamine. Duration of action varies from 3 to 4 hours for ergot alkaloids, methysergide, and propranolol to 3 to 4 days for phenoxybenzamine.
● Onset after I.M. or S.C. injection of ergot alkaloids is 15 to 30 minutes. Onset after I.V. administration (recommended for acute symptomatic episodes) is immediate.

phenoxybenzamine hydrochloride (Dibenzyline)

Indications and dosage
To control Raynaud's syndrome, frostbite, acrocyanosis—
Adults: initially 10 mg P.O., then increase by 10 mg q 4 days to a maximum of 60 mg daily

Side effects
CNS: sedation, fatigue, lassitude
CV: tachycardia, *postural hypotension with dizziness*
EENT: miosis, nasal congestion
GI: irritation
GU: inhibition of ejaculation

Interactions
None significant

Nursing considerations
● Contraindicated when fall in blood pressure is undesirable. Use cautiously in cerebral or coronary arteriosclerosis, renal damage, or respiratory disease.
● May aggravate symptoms of respiratory infections.

• Reduce gastric irritation by giving with milk or in divided doses.
• Instruct patient to change position slowly to prevent possible hypotension. Advise him to dangle legs for a few minutes before standing if he has been lying down.
• Place overdosed patient in Trendelenburg position. Treat hypotension with I.V. infusion of norepinephrine.
• Full therapeutic effect may not be seen for several weeks.
• Store drug in airtight containers, protected from light.

propranolol hydrochloride (Inderal, Inderal LA)

Indications and dosage
Prevention of frequent, severe, uncontrollable, or disabling migraine or vascular headache—
Adults: initially, 80 mg daily in divided doses or one sustained-release capsule once daily. Usual maintenance dose: 160 to 240 mg daily, divided t.i.d. or q.i.d.

Side effects
CNS: fatigue, lethargy, vivid dreams, hallucinations
CV: bradycardia, hypotension, congestive heart failure (CHF), peripheral vascular disease
GI: nausea, vomiting, diarrhea
Metabolic: hypoglycemia without symptoms
Skin: rash
Other: increased airway resistance, fever

Interactions
Insulin, hypoglycemic drugs (oral): can alter requirements for these drugs in previously stabilized diabetics. Monitor for hypoglycemia.
Cardiotonic glycosides: excessive bradycardia and increased depressant effect on myocardium. Monitor pulse.
Chlorpromazine, cimetidine: inhibit propranolol's metabolism. Monitor for greater beta-blocking effect.

Epinephrine: severe vasoconstriction. Monitor blood pressure.
Barbiturates, rifampin: increased metabolism of propranolol. Monitor for decreased effect.
Indomethacin: antihypertensive effect. Monitor blood pressure.

Nursing considerations
• Contraindicated in diabetes mellitus, asthma, allergic rhinitis, sinus bradycardia and heart block greater than first degree, cardiogenic shock, right ventricular failure secondary to pulmonary hypertension, and during ethyl ether anesthesia. Use with caution in CHF respiratory disease.
• Withdraw drug slowly in patients with CAD. Abrupt withdrawal might precipitate MI or aggravate angina or pheochromocytoma. Abrupt withdrawal in thyrotoxicosis may exacerbate hyperthyroidism or precipitate thyroid storm. In thyrotoxicosis, propranolol may mask clinical signs of hyperthyroidism.
• Do not stop drug before surgery for pheochromocytoma. Before any surgical procedure, notify anesthesiologist that patient is receiving propranolol.
• Monitor blood pressure frequently. If patient develops excessive hypotension, notify doctor. Tell patient that orthostatic hypotension can be minimized by rising slowly and avoiding sudden position changes.
• Compliance may be improved by administering drug twice daily or giving sustained-release form once daily.
• Drug masks common signs of shock and hypoglycemia.

Diuretics

Thiazide diuretics
Thiazide-like diuretics
Loop diuretics
Miscellaneous diuretics

Diuretics reduce the body's total volume of water and salt by increasing their urinary excretion. This occurs mainly because diuretics impair sodium chloride reabsorption in the renal tubules.

Major Uses of Diuretics

	THIAZIDE DIURETICS	THIAZIDE-LIKE DIURETICS	LOOP DIURETICS	AMILORIDE	MANNITOL	SPIRONOLACTONE	TRIAMTERENE	UREA
Treatment of essential hypertension	•	•	•	•		•	•	
Treatment of edema associated with CHF, cirrhosis of the liver, and renal disease	•	•	•	•		•	•	
Treatment of pulmonary edema			•					
Reduction of intracranial pressure in hydrocephalus					•			•
Reduction of intraocular pressure					•			•
Treatment of primary aldosteronism						•		

Diuretics can be classified according to chemical structure (thiazide and thiazide-like drugs), location of salt- and water-depleting effect on the kidney's nephrons (loop diuretics), and pharmacologic activity (miscellaneous drugs with other mechanisms).

Major uses

The matrix above indicates the major uses of diuretics.

Mechanism of action

• The thiazide and thiazide-like diuretics increase urinary excretion of sodium and water by inhibiting sodium reabsorption in the cortical diluting site of the ascending loop of Henle. They also increase urinary excretion of chloride, potassium, and—to a lesser extent—bicarbonate ions.

• Loop diuretics inhibit reabsorption of sodium and chloride at the proximal portion of the ascending loop of Henle, enhancing water excretion. These very potent diuretics can be effective in patients with markedly reduced glomerular filtration rates (in whom other diuretics usually fail).

• Among miscellaneous diuretics, mannitol increases the osmotic pressure of glomerular filtrate, inhibiting tubular reabsorption of water and electrolytes.

Spironolactone antagonizes the hormone aldosterone in the distal tubule, increasing excretion of sodium and water but sparing potassium.

Triamterene and amiloride depress sodium reabsorption and potassium secretion by direct action on the distal segment of the uriniferous tubule. This reduces potassium excretion.

Urea rapidly increases blood tonicity, which results in passage of fluid from the tissue (including the brain) to the blood.

Absorption, distribution, metabolism, and excretion

• Thiazides and thiazide-like diuretics are all well absorbed from the GI tract, well distributed to the body tissues, and excreted primarily unchanged in urine.

• Among loop diuretics ethacrynic acid is rapidly absorbed after oral administration, metabolized in the liver, and excreted by the kidneys. Ethacrynate sodium is administered parenterally. Its metabolism and excretion are the same as ethacrynic acid's.

Bumetanide is well absorbed from the GI tract; both metabolite and unchanged drug are excreted in urine.

Furosemide is partially (about 60%) absorbed from the GI tract; a small amount is metabolized. Both metabolite and unchanged drug are excreted in urine.

• Among miscellaneous diuretics, mannitol remains in the extracellular fluid, is filtered by the glomeruli, and is excreted unchanged in urine.

Spironolactone is absorbed from the GI tract, distributed to body tissues, metabolized in the liver, and eliminated in both urine and feces.

Amiloride and triamterene are absorbed from the GI tract, partially bound to plasma proteins, distributed to body tissues, and rapidly excreted unchanged in urine.

Urea is well absorbed after oral administration, but it is seldom given orally because of its unpleasant taste. After I.V. administration, it is distributed to intracellular and extracellular fluids, including cerebrospinal fluid (CSF). It is hydrolyzed in the GI tract by bacterial ureases and excreted by the kidneys.

Onset and duration

• Thiazides and thiazide-like diuretics begin to act 1 to 2 hours after oral administration. Most of them have a duration of action of 12 to 24 hours, but several act as long as 36 to 72 hours. I.V. chlorothiazide takes effect within 15 minutes after administration and has a duration of 2 hours.

• Among loop diuretics, ethacrynic acid begins to act 30 minutes after oral administration and has a duration of up to 12 hours. Ethacrynate sodium, after I.V. administration, begins to act within 5 minutes. Its duration is 2 hours.

Bumetanide and furosemide, after oral administration, begin to act in 30 to 60 minutes and have a duration of 6 to 8 hours. After I.V. administration, onset occurs within 5 minutes, with a duration of 2 hours. After I.M. injection, they begin to act within 30 minutes and have a duration of 6 to 8 hours.

• Among the miscellaneous diuretics, mannitol begins to act 15 to 30 minutes after I.V. administration; diuresis occurs in 1 to 3 hours. Duration is 4 to 6 hours, but it may reduce CSF pressure for up to 8 hours.

Spironolactone's onset occurs gradually over 2 to 3 days, but a loading dose may be used for faster effect. The drug continues to act for 2 to 3 days.

Triamterene begins to act in 2 to 4 hours and has a duration of up to 24 hours. Maximal therapeutic effect may not occur during the first few days of therapy.

Amiloride begins to act within 2 hours, reaches a peak effect between 6 to 10 hours, and has a duration of 24 hours.

Urea begins to act 1 to 2 hours after I.V. administration and has a duration of 3 to 10 hours.

---

amiloride hydrochloride (Midamor)

Indications and dosage

Hypertension; or edema associated with CHF, usually in patients who are also taking thiazide or other potassium-wasting diuretics—
Adults: Usual dosage is 5 mg P.O. daily. May be increased to 10 mg daily, if necessary. As much as 20 mg daily can be given.

Side effects

CNS: headache, weakness, dizziness

CV: orthostatic hypotension
GI: nausea, anorexia, diarrhea, vomiting, abdominal pain, constipation
GU: impotence
Metabolic: hyperkalemia

Interactions
None significant

Nursing considerations
• Contraindicated with elevated serum potassium levels (greater than 5.5 mEq/liter). Do not administer to patients receiving other potassium-sparing diuretics, such as spironolactone and triamterene. Also contraindicated in anuria.
• Use cautiously in patients with renal impairment, because potassium retention is increased.
• Risk of hyperkalemia is greater when a potassium-wasting drug is not taken concurrently. When amiloride is taken this way, be sure to monitor daily potassium levels.
• Discontinue immediately if potassium level exceeds 6.5 mEq/liter.
• Warn patient to avoid excessive ingestion of potassium-rich foods or potassium-containing salt substitutes. Concomitant potassium supplement can lead to serious hyperkalemia.
• Administer with meals to prevent nausea.

bumetanide
(Bumex)

Indications and dosage
Edema (CHF, hepatic and renal disease)—
Adults: 0.5 to 2 mg P.O. once daily. If diuretic response not adequate, second or third dose may be given at 4- to 5-hour intervals. Maximum dose is 10 mg/day. May be administered parenterally when P.O. not feasible. Usual initial dose is 0.5 to 1 mg I.V. or I.M. If response is not adequate, second or third dose may be given at intervals of 2 to 3 hours. Maximum dose is 10 mg/day.

Side effects
CNS: dizziness, headache
CV: volume depletion and dehydration, orthostatic hypotension, EKG changes
EENT: transient deafness
GI: nausea
Metabolic: hypokalemia, hypochloremic alkalosis, asymptomatic hyperuricemia, fluid and electrolyte imbalances, including dilutional hyponatremia, hypocalcemia, hypomagnesemia, hyperglycemia and impairment of glucose tolerance
Skin: rash
Other: muscle pain and tenderness

Interactions
Aminoglycoside antibiotics: potentiated ototoxicity. Use together cautiously.
Probenecid, indomethacin: inhibited diuretic response. Use cautiously.

Nursing considerations
• Contraindicated in anuria, hepatic coma, and states of severe electrolyte depletion
• Use cautiously in patients with hepatic cirrhosis and ascites. Supplemental potassium or potassium-sparing diuretics may be used to prevent hypokalemia and metabolic alkalosis in these patients. Use cautiously in patients with depressed renal function.
• Use cautiously in patients allergic to sulfonamides. They may show hypersensitivity to bumetanide.
• Potent loop diuretic; can lead to profound water and electrolyte depletion. Monitor blood pressure and pulse rate during rapid diuresis.
• If oliguria or azotemia develop or increase, may require stopping drug.
• Monitor serum electrolytes, blood urea nitrogen (BUN), and CO_2 frequently.
• Monitor serum potassium levels. Watch for signs of hypokalemia (for example, muscle weakness, cramps). Patients also receiving digitalis have an increased risk of digitalis toxicity due to potassium-depleting effect of diuretic.
• Consult with doctor and dietitian to provide high-potassium diet.

• Foods rich in potassium include citrus fruits, tomatoes, bananas, dates, and apricots.

• Monitor blood sugar levels in patients with diabetes. May treat severe hyperglycemia with oral antidiabetic agents.

• Monitor blood uric acid levels, especially in patients with history of gout.

• Give I.V. doses over 1 to 2 minutes.

• Advise patients taking bumetanide to stand up slowly to prevent dizziness and to limit alcohol intake and strenuous exercise in hot weather since these exacerbate orthostatic hypotension.

• Bumetanide can be safely prescribed in patients allergic to furosemide.

• 1 mg of bumetanide is equal to 40 mg of furosemide.

• May be less ototoxic than furosemide, but the clinical relevance of this has not been determined.

• Intermittent dosage given on alternate days, or for 3 to 4 days with 1 or 2 days intervening, is recommended as safest and most effective dosage schedule for control of edema.

---

chlorothiazide
(Diuril)

Indications and dosage
Diuresis—
Children over 6 months: 20 mg/kg P.O. or I.V. daily in divided doses
Children under 6 months: may require 30 mg/kg P.O. or I.V. daily in two divided doses
Edema, hypertension—
Adults: 500 mg to 2 g P.O. or I.V. daily or in two divided doses

Side effects
Blood: *aplastic anemia, agranulocytosis,* leukopenia, thrombocytopenia
CV: *volume depletion and dehydration,* orthostatic hypotension
GI: anorexia, nausea, pancreatitis
Hepatic: hepatic encephalopathy
Metabolic: *hypokalemia, asymptomatic hyperuricemia, hyperglycemia and impairment of glucose tolerance,* fluid and electrolyte imbalances including dilu-

tional hyponatremia and hypochloremia, metabolic alkalosis, hypercalcemia, gout
Skin: dermatitis, photosensitivity, rash
Other: hypersensitivity reactions such as pneumonitis and vasculitis

Interactions
Cholestyramine, colestipol: intestinal absorption of thiazides decreased. Keep doses as separate as possible.
Diazoxide: increased antihypertensive, hyperglycemic, hyperuricemic effects. Use together cautiously.

Nursing considerations
• Contraindicated in anuria, hypersensitivity to other thiazides or other sulfonamide-derived drugs, impaired hepatic function, progressive hepatic disease. Use cautiously in severe renal disease.

• Monitor intake/output, weight, and serum electrolytes regularly.

• Monitor potassium levels; consult with doctor and dietitian to provide high-potassium diet. Watch for signs of hypokalemia (for example, muscle weakness, cramps). Patients on digitalis have increased risk of digitalis toxicity due to potassium-depleting effect of diuretic. May use with potassium-sparing diuretic to prevent potassium loss.

• Foods rich in potassium include citrus fruits, tomatoes, bananas, dates, and apricots.

• Monitor blood sugar. Check insulin requirements in patients with diabetes. May treat severe hyperglycemia with oral antidiabetic agents.

• Monitor serum creatinine and BUN levels regularly. Not as effective if these levels are more than twice normal.

• Monitor blood uric acid levels, especially in patients with history of gout.

• Watch for decreased calcium excretion, progressive renal impairment.

• Only injectable thiazide. For I.V. use only—not I.M. or subcutaneous. Reconstitute with 18 ml sterile water for injection/500 mg vial. May store reconstituted solutions at room temperature up to 24 hours. Compatible with intra-

venous dextrose or sodium chloride solutions.
• Avoid I.V. infiltration; can be very painful.
• Give in the morning to prevent nocturia.
• In hypertension, therapeutic response may be delayed several days.
• Elderly patients are especially susceptible to excessive diuresis.
• Only thiazide available in liquid form.
• Thiazides and thiazide-like diuretics should be stopped before tests for parathyroid function are performed.

---

chlorthalidone
(Hygroton, Novothalidone)

Indications and dosage
Edema, hypertension—
Adults: 25 to 100 mg P.O. daily or 100 mg three times weekly or on alternate days
Children: 2 mg/kg P.O. three times weekly

Side effects
Blood: *aplastic anemia, agranulocytosis,* leukopenia, thrombocytopenia
CV: *volume depletion and dehydration,* orthostatic hypotension
GI: anorexia, nausea, pancreatitis
GU: impotence
Hepatic: hepatic encephalopathy
Metabolic: *hypokalemia, asymptomatic hyperuricemia, hyperglycemia and impairment of glucose tolerance,* fluid and electrolyte imbalances including dilutional hyponatremia and hypochloremia, metabolic alkalosis, hypercalcemia, gout
Skin: dermatitis, photosensitivity, rash
Other: hypersensitivity reactions, such as pneumonitis and vasculitis

Interactions
Cholestyramine, colestipol: intestinal absorption of thiazides decreased. Keep doses as separate as possible.
Diazoxide: increased antihypertensive, hyperglycemic, hyperuricemic effects. Use together cautiously.

Nursing considerations
• Contraindicated in anuria; hypersensitivity to thiazides or other sulfonamide-derived drugs. Use cautiously in severe renal disease, progressive hepatic disease, impaired hepatic function.
• Monitor intake/output, weight, and serum electrolytes regularly.
• Monitor serum potassium levels; consult with doctor and dietitian to provide high-potassium diet. Watch for signs of hypokalemia (for example, muscle weakness, cramps). Patients on digitalis have increased risk of digitalis toxicity due to potassium-depleting effect of diuretic. May use with potassium-sparing diuretic to prevent potassium loss.
• Foods rich in potassium include citrus fruits, tomatoes, bananas, dates, and apricots.
• Monitor serum creatinine and BUN levels regularly. Not as effective if levels are more than twice normal.
• Monitor blood uric acid levels, especially in patients with history of gout.
• Monitor blood sugar. Check insulin requirements in diabetics. May treat severe hyperglycemia with oral antidiabetic agents.
• In hypertension, therapeutic response may be delayed several days.
• Give in the morning to prevent nocturia.
• Elderly patients are especially susceptible to excessive diuresis.
• Thiazides and thiazide-like diuretics should be stopped before tests for parathyroid function are performed.

---

ethacrynic acid
(Edecrin)

Indications and dosage
Acute pulmonary edema—
Adults: 50 to 100 mg of ethacrynate sodium I.V. slowly over several minutes
Edema—
Adults: 50 to 200 mg P.O. daily. Refractory cases may require up to 200 mg b.i.d.
Children: initial dose 25 mg P.O. cautiously, increased in 25-mg increments

daily until desired effect is obtained

Side effects

Blood: *agranulocytosis,* neutropenia, thrombocytopenia
CV: volume depletion and dehydration, orthostatic hypotension
EENT: transient deafness with too-rapid I.V. injection
GI: abdominal discomfort and pain, diarrhea
Metabolic: *hypokalemia, hypochloremic alkalosis, asymptomatic hyperuricemia, fluid and electrolyte imbalances including dilutional hyponatremia, hypocalcemia, and hypomagnesemia,* hyperglycemia and impairment of glucose tolerance
Skin: dermatitis

Interactions

Aminoglycoside antibiotics: potentiated ototoxic side effects of both ethacrynic acid and aminoglycosides. Use together cautiously.

Nursing considerations

• Contraindicated in patients with anuria and in infants. Use cautiously in electrolyte abnormalities. If electrolyte imbalance, azotemia, or oliguria develop, may require discontinuing drug.
• Drug is a very potent diuretic.
• Monitor intake/output, weight, and serum electrolytes regularly.
• Monitor serum potassium levels; consult with doctor and dietitian to provide high-potassium diet. Watch for signs of hypokalemia (e.g., muscle weakness, cramps).
• Foods rich in potassium include citrus fruits, tomatoes, bananas, dates, and apricots.
• Patients also on digitalis have increased risk of digitalis toxicity due to potassium-depleting effect of diuretic.
• I.V. injection painful; may cause thrombophlebitis. Do not give subcutaneously or I.M. Give slowly through tubing of running infusion over several minutes.
• Salt and potassium chloride supplement may be needed during therapy.

• Reconstitute vacuum vial with 50 ml of dextrose 5% injection or NaCl injection. Discard unused solution after 24 hours. Do not use cloudy or opalescent solutions.
• Elderly patients are especially susceptible to excessive diuresis.
• Give P.O. doses in the morning to prevent nocturia.
• Severe diarrhea may necessitate discontinuing drug.
• Monitor blood uric acid levels, especially in patients with history of gout.
• May potentiate effects of the anticoagulant warfarin; carefully monitor patients receiving both drugs.

furosemide
(Lasix)

Indications and dosage

Acute pulmonary edema—
Adults: 40 mg I.V. injected slowly; then 40 mg I.V. in 1 to 1½ hours if needed
Edema—
Adults: 20 to 80 mg P.O. daily in the morning, second dose can be given in 6 to 8 hours; carefully titrated up to 600 mg daily if needed; or 20 to 40 mg I.M. or I.V. Increase by 20 mg q 2 hours until desired response is achieved. I.V. dose should be given slowly over 1 to 2 minutes.
Infants and children: 2 mg/kg daily; dose increased by 1 to 2 mg/kg in 6 to 8 hours if needed; carefully titrated up to 6 mg/kg daily if needed
Hypertensive crisis, acute renal failure—
Adults: 100 to 200 mg I.V. over 1 to 2 minutes
Chronic renal failure—
Adults: initially 80 mg P.O. daily. Increase by 80 to 120 mg daily until desired response is achieved.

Side effects

Blood: *agranulocytosis,* leukopenia, thrombocytopenia
CV: volume depletion and dehydration, orthostatic hypotension
EENT: transient deafness with too rapid I.V. injection

GI: abdominal discomfort and pain, diarrhea (with oral solution)
Metabolic: hypokalemia, hypochloremic alkalosis, asymptomatic hyperuricemia, fluid and electrolyte imbalances including dilutional hyponatremia, hypocalcemia, and hypomagnesemia, hyperglycemia and impairment of glucose tolerance
Skin: dermatitis

Interactions
Aminoglycoside antibiotics: potentiated ototoxicity. Use together cautiously.
Chloral hydrate: sweating, flushing with I.V. furosemide. Observe patient.
Clofibrate: enhanced furosemide effects. Use cautiously.
Indomethacin: inhibited diuretic response. Use cautiously.

Nursing considerations
• Use cautiously in cardiogenic shock complicated by pulmonary edema, anuria, hepatic coma, or electrolyte imbalances. Drug is not routinely administered to women of childbearing age because its safety in pregnancy has not been established.
• Potent loop diuretic; can lead to profound water and electrolyte depletion. Monitor blood pressure and pulse rate during rapid diuresis.
• Sulfonamide-sensitive patients may have allergic reactions to furosemide.
• If oliguria or azotemia develops or increases, may require stopping drug.
• Monitor serum electrolytes, BUN, and CO_2 frequently.
• Monitor serum potassium levels. Watch for signs of hypokalemia (for example, muscle weakness, cramps). Patients also on digitalis have increased risk of digitalis toxicity due to potassium-depleting effect of diuretic.
• Consult with doctor and dietitian to provide high-potassium diet.
• Foods rich in potassium include citrus fruits, tomatoes, bananas, dates, and apricots.
• Monitor blood sugar levels in patients with diabetes. May treat severe hyperglycemia with oral antidiabetic agents.

• Monitor blood uric acid levels, especially in patients with history of gout.
• Give I.V. doses over 1 to 2 minutes.
• Do not use parenteral route in infants and children unless oral dosage form is not practical.
• I.M. injection causes transient pain; moderate by using "Z" track to limit leakage into subcutaneous tissues.
• Give P.O. and I.M. preparations in the morning to prevent nocturia. Give second doses in early afternoon.
• Elderly patients are especially susceptible to excessive diuresis, with potential for circulatory collapse and thromboembolic complications.
• Store tablets in light-resistant container to prevent discoloration (does not affect potency). Do not use discolored (yellow) injectable preparation. Oral furosemide solution should be stored in refrigerator to ensure stability of drug.
• Promotes calcium excretion. I.V. furosemide often used to treat hypercalcemia.
• Advise patients taking furosemide to stand slowly to prevent dizziness and to limit alcohol intake and strenuous exercise in hot weather, since these exacerbate orthostatic hypotension.
• Advise patients to report immediately ringing in ears, severe abdominal pain, or sore throat and fever; may indicate furosemide toxicity.
• Discourage patients receiving furosemide therapy at home from storing different types of medication in the same container. This increases risk of drug errors, especially for patients taking both furosemide and digoxin, since most popular strengths of these drugs are white tablets approximately equal in size.
• To prepare parenteral furosemide for I.V. infusion, mix drug with dextrose 5% in water, 0.9% sodium chloride solution, or lactated Ringer's solution. Use prepared infusion solution within 24 hours.

hydrochlorothiazide
(Esidrix, Hydro Diuril)

Indications and dosage
Edema—
Adults: initially 25 to 100 mg P.O. daily or intermittently for maintenance to minimize electrolyte imbalance
Children over 6 months: 2.2 mg/kg P.O. daily divided b.i.d.
Children under 6 months: up to 3.3 mg/kg P.O. daily divided b.i.d.
Hypertension—
Adults: 25 to 100 mg P.O. daily or divided dosage. Daily dosage increased or decreased according to blood pressure

Side effects
Blood: aplastic anemia, agranulocytosis, leukopenia, thrombocytopenia
CV: volume depletion and dehydration, orthostatic hypotension
GI: anorexia, nausea, pancreatitis
Hepatic: hepatic encephalopathy
Metabolic: hypokalemia, asymptomatic hyperuricemia, hyperglycemia and impairment of glucose tolerance, fluid and electrolyte imbalances including dilutional hyponatremia and hypochloremia, metabolic alkalosis, hypercalcemia, gout
Skin: dermatitis, photosensitivity, rash
Other: hypersensitivity reactions, such as pneumonitis and vasculitis

Interactions
Cholestyramine, colestipol: intestinal absorption of thiazides decreased. Keep doses as separate as possible.
Diazoxide: increased antihypertensive, hyperglycemic, hyperuricemic effects. Use together cautiously.

Nursing considerations
• Contraindicated in anuria and hypersensitivity to other thiazides or sulfonamide derivatives. Use cautiously in severe renal disease, impaired hepatic function, progressive hepatic disease.
• Monitor intake/output, weight, and serum electrolytes regularly.
• Monitor serum potassium levels; consult with doctor and dietitian to provide high-potassium diet. Watch for hypokalemia (for example, muscle weakness, cramps). Patients also on digitalis have increased risk of digitalis toxicity due to potassium-depleting effect of diuretic. May use with potassium-sparing diuretic to prevent potassium loss.
• Foods rich in potassium include citrus fruits, tomatoes, bananas, dates, and apricots.
• Monitor serum creatinine and BUN levels regularly. Not as effective if levels are more than twice normal.
• Monitor blood uric acid levels, especially in patients with history of gout.
• Check insulin requirements in patients with diabetes. May treat severe hyperglycemia with oral antidiabetic agents.
• In hypertension, therapeutic response may be delayed several days.
• Give in the morning to prevent nocturia. Studies have shown that drug is as effective when administered once daily as when given more frequently.
• Elderly patients are especially susceptible to excessive diuresis.
• Thiazides and thiazide-like diuretics should be stopped before tests for parathyroid function are performed.

mannitol
(Osmitrol)

Indications and dosage
Adults and children over 12 years: To reduce intraocular pressure or intracranial pressure—
1.5 to 2 g/kg as a 15% to 25% solution I.V. over 30 to 60 minutes
To promote diuresis in drug intoxication—
5% to 10% solution continuously up to 200 g I.V., while maintaining 100 to 500 ml urinary output/hour and a positive fluid balance

Side effects
CNS: rebound increase in intracranial pressure 8 to 12 hours after diuresis,

headache, confusion
CV: transient expansion of plasma volume during infusion causing circulatory overload and pulmonary edema, tachycardia, angina-like chest pain
EENT: blurred vision, rhinitis
GI: thirst, nausea, vomiting
GU: urinary retention
Metabolic: fluid and electrolyte imbalance, water intoxication, cellular dehydration

Interactions
None significant

Nursing considerations
• Contraindicated in anuria, severe pulmonary congestion, frank pulmonary edema, severe congestive heart disease, severe dehydration, metabolic edema, progressive renal disease or dysfunction, progressive heart failure during administration, active intracranial bleeding except during craniotomy.
• Monitor vital signs (including CVP) at least hourly; intake/output hourly (report increasing oliguria). Monitor daily: weight, renal function, fluid balance, serum and urine sodium and potassium levels.
• Solution often crystallizes, especially at low temperatures. To redissolve, warm bottle in hot water bath, shake vigorously. Cool to body temperature before giving. Concentrations greater than 15% have greater tendency to crystallize. Do not use solution with undissolved crystals.
• Infusions should always be given I.V. via in-line filter.
• Avoid infiltration; observe for inflammation, edema, potential necrosis.
• For maximum pressure reduction before surgery, give 1 to 1½ hours preoperatively.
• Give frequent mouth care or fluids as permitted to relieve thirst.
• Urethral catheter is inserted in comatose or incontinent patients because therapy is based on strict evaluation of intake and output. In patients with urethral catheters, use an hourly urometer collection bag to facilitate accurate evaluation of output.
• An osmotic diuretic

---

metolazone
(Diulo, Zaroxolyn)

Indications and dosage
Edema (heart failure)—
Adults: 5 to 10 mg P.O. daily
Edema (renal disease)—
Adults: 5 to 20 mg P.O. daily
Hypertension—
Adults: 2.5 to 5 mg P.O. daily. Maintenance dose determined by patient's blood pressure

Side effects
Blood: aplastic anemia, agranulocytosis, leukopenia, thrombocytopenia
CV: volume depletion and dehydration, orthostatic hypotension
GI: anorexia, nausea, pancreatitis
Hepatic: hepatic encephalopathy
Metabolic: hypokalemia, asymptomatic hyperuricemia, hyperglycemia and impairment of glucose tolerance, fluid and electrolyte imbalances including dilutional hyponatremia and hypochloremia, metabolic alkalosis, hypercalcemia, gout
Skin: dermatitis, photosensitivity, rash
Other: hypersensitivity reactions, such as pneumonitis and vasculitis

Interactions
Cholestyramine, colestipol: intestinal absorption of thiazides decreased. Keep doses as separate as possible.
Diazoxide: increased antihypertensive, hyperglycemic, hyperuricemic effects. Use together cautiously.

Nursing considerations
• Contraindicated in anuria, hepatic coma or precoma, hypersensitivity to thiazides or other sulfonamide-derived drugs. Use cautiously in hyperuricemia or gout and severely impaired renal function.
• Monitor intake/output, weight, and serum electrolytes regularly.

• Monitor serum potassium levels; consult with doctor and dietitian to provide high-potassium diet. Foods rich in potassium include citrus fruits, tomatoes, bananas, dates, and apricots. Watch for hypokalemia (for example, muscle weakness, cramps). Patients also on digitalis may have increased risk of digitalis toxicity due to potassium-depleting effect of diuretic. May use with potassium-sparing diuretic to prevent potassium loss.

• Check insulin requirements in diabetics. May treat severe hyperglycemia with oral antidiabetic agents.

• Monitor blood uric acid levels, especially in patients with history of gout.

• In hypertension, therapeutic response may be delayed several days.

• Give in morning to prevent nocturia.

• Elderly patients are especially susceptible to excessive diuresis.

• A thiazide-related diuretic. However, unlike thiazide diuretics, metolazone is effective in patients with decreased renal function.

• Used as an adjunct in furosemide-resistant edema.

• Thiazides and thiazide-like diuretics should be stopped before tests for parathyroid function are performed.

polythiazide (Renese)

Indications and dosage
Hypertension—
Adults: 2 to 4 mg P.O. daily
Edema (heart failure, renal failure)—
Adults: 1 to 4 mg P.O. daily

Side effects
Blood: aplastic anemia, agranulocytosis, leukopenia, thrombocytopenia
CV: volume depletion and dehydration, orthostatic hypotension
GI: anorexia, nausea, pancreatitis
Hepatic: hepatic encephalopathy
Metabolic: hypokalemia, asymptomatic hyperuricemia, hyperglycemia and impairment of glucose tolerance, fluid and electrolyte imbalances including dilu-
tional hyponatremia and hypochloremia, metabolic alkalosis, hypercalcemia, gout
Skin: dermatitis, photosensitivity, rash
Other: hypersensitivity reactions, such as pneumonitis and vasculitis

Interactions
Cholestyramine, colestipol: intestinal absorption of thiazides decreased. Keep doses as separate as possible.
Diazoxide: increased antihypertensive, hyperglycemic, hyperuricemic effects. Use together cautiously.

Nursing considerations
• Contraindicated in anuria, hypersensitivity to other thiazides or other sulfonamide-derived drugs. Use cautiously in severe renal disease, impaired hepatic function, allergies.

• Monitor intake/output, weight, and serum electrolytes regularly.

• Monitor serum potassium levels; consult with doctor and dietitian to provide high-potassium diet. Foods rich in potassium include citrus fruits, tomatoes, bananas, dates, and apricots. Watch for hypokalemia (for example, muscle weakness, cramps). Patients also on digitalis may have increased risk of digitalis toxicity due to potassium-depleting effect of diuretic. May use with potassium-sparing diuretic to prevent potassium loss.

• Monitor serum creatinine and BUN levels regularly. Not as effective if levels are more than twice normal.

• Monitor blood uric acid levels, especially in patients with history of gout.

• Check insulin requirements in diabetics. May treat severe hyperglycemia with oral antidiabetic agents.

• In hypertension, therapeutic response may be delayed several days.

• Give in the morning to prevent nocturia.

• Elderly patients are especially susceptible to excessive diuresis.

• Thiazides and thiazide-like diuretics should be stopped before tests for parathyroid function are performed.

spironolactone
(Aldactone)

Indications and dosage
Edema—
Adults: 25 to 200 mg P.O. daily in divided doses
Children: initially 3.3 mg/kg P.O. daily in divided doses
Hypertension—
Adults: 50 to 100 mg P.O. daily in divided doses
Treatment of diuretic-induced hypokalemia—
Adults: 25 to 100 mg P.O. daily when oral potassium supplements are considered inappropriate
Detection of primary hyperaldosteronism—
Adults: 400 mg P.O. daily for 4 days (short test) or for 3 to 4 weeks (long test). If hypokalemia and hypertension are corrected, a presumptive diagnosis of primary hyperaldosteronism is made.

Side effects
CNS: headache
GI: anorexia, nausea, diarrhea
Metabolic: hyperkalemia, dehydration, hyponatremia, transient rise in BUN, acidosis
Skin: urticaria
Other: gynecomastia in males, breast soreness and menstrual disturbances in females

Interactions
Aspirin: possible blocked spironolactone effect. Watch for diminished spironolactone response.

Nursing considerations
• Contraindicated in anuria, acute or progressive renal insufficiency, hyperkalemia. Use cautiously in fluid or electrolyte imbalances, impaired renal function, and hepatic disease.
• A mild acidosis may occur during therapy. This may be dangerous in patients with hepatic cirrhosis.
• Monitor serum potassium levels, electrolytes, intake/output, weight, and blood pressure regularly.
• Potassium-sparing diuretic; useful as an adjunct to other diuretic therapy. Less potent diuretic than thiazide and loop types. Diuretic effect delayed 2 to 3 days when used alone.
• Maximum antihypertensive response may be delayed up to 2 weeks.
• Warn patient to avoid excessive ingestion of potassium-rich foods or potassium-containing salt substitutes. Concomitant potassium supplement can lead to serious hyperkalemia.
• Elderly patients are more susceptible to excessive diuresis.
• Protect drug from light.
• Breast cancer reported in some patients taking spironolactone, but cause-and-effect relationship not confirmed. Warn against taking drug indiscriminately.
• Give with meals to enhance absorption.

triamterene
(Dyrenium)

Indications and dosage
Diuresis—
Adults: initially 100 mg P.O. b.i.d. after meals. Total daily dosage should not exceed 300 mg.

Side effects
Blood: megaloblastic anemia related to low folic acid levels
CNS: dizziness
CV: hypotension
EENT: sore throat
GI: dry mouth, nausea, vomiting
Metabolic: hyperkalemia, dehydration, hyponatremia, transient rise in BUN, acidosis
Skin: photosensitivity, rash
Other: anaphylaxis, muscle cramps

Interactions
None significant

Nursing considerations

• Contraindicated in anuria, severe or progressive renal disease or dysfunction, severe hepatic disease, hyperkalemia. Use cautiously in impaired hepatic function, diabetes mellitus, pregnancy, or lactation.

• Watch for blood dyscrasias.

• Monitor BUN and serum potassium, electrolytes.

• A potassium-sparing diuretic, useful as an adjunct to other diuretic therapy. Less potent than thiazides and loop diuretics. Full diuretic effect delayed 2 to 3 days.

• Warn patients to avoid excessive ingestion of potassium-rich foods or potassium-containing salt substitutes. Concomitant potassium supplement can lead to serious hyperkalemia.

• Give medication after meals to prevent nausea.

• Should be withdrawn gradually to prevent excessive rebound potassium excretion.

• Concomitant use of spironolactone is not recommended.

---

urea—carbamide (Ureaphil)

Indications and dosage

Intracranial or intraocular pressure—
Adults: 1 to 1.5 g/kg as a 30% solution by slow I.V. infusion over 1 to 2.5 hours
Children over 2 years: 0.5 to 1.5 g/kg slow I.V. infusion
Children under 2 years: as little as 0.1 g/kg slow I.V. infusion. Maximum 4 ml/minute

Maximum adult daily dose 120 g. To prepare 135 ml 30% solution, mix contents of 40-g vial of urea with 105 ml dextrose 5% or 10% in water or 10% invert sugar in water. Each ml of 30% solution provides 300 mg urea.

Side effects

CNS: headache
CV: tachycardia, volume expansion
GI: nausea, vomiting

Metabolic: sodium and potassium depletion
Local: irritation or necrotic sloughing may occur with extravasation.

Interactions

None significant

Nursing considerations

• Contraindicated in severely impaired renal function, marked dehydration, frank hepatic failure, active intracranial bleeding. Use cautiously in pregnancy, lactation, cardiac disease, hepatic impairment, or sickle cell damage with CNS involvement.

• Avoid rapid I.V. infusion; may cause hemolysis or increased capillary bleeding. Avoid extravasation; may cause reactions ranging from mild irritation to necrosis.

• Do not administer through the same infusion as blood.

• Do not infuse into leg veins; may cause phlebitis or thrombosis, especially in the elderly.

• Watch for hyponatremia or hypokalemia (muscle weakness, lethargy); may indicate electrolyte depletion before serum levels are reduced.

• Maintain adequate hydration; monitor fluid and electrolyte balance.

• In renal disease, monitor BUN frequently.

• Indwelling urethral catheter should be used in comatose patients to assure bladder emptying. Use an hourly urometer collection bag to facilitate accurate evaluation of diuresis.

• If satisfactory diuresis does not occur in 6 to 12 hours, urea should be discontinued and renal function reevaluated.

• Use freshly reconstituted urea only for I.V. infusion; solution becomes ammonia upon oxidation when standing.

• Use within minutes of reconstitution.

ANTICOAGULANTS AND ANTAGONISTS

Anticoagulants are given to patients at risk of developing clots (thromboses).

Understanding Anticoagulant Action

A fibrin clot is the final step of the coagulation process. The schematic diagram illustrates the steps that lead up to this.

Coagulation results from the activation of a series of *factors*—a sequence known as a cascade. The process occurs by the intrinsic (intravascular) pathway and the extrinsic (extravascular) pathway. Both pathways are shown here.

The intrinsic pathway is started when Factor XII is disturbed (by coming in contact with collagen). This produces Factor XII$_a$ (activated Factor XII) and the activation of Factor XI and Factor IX. Factor IX$_a$—with Factor VIII (as a cofactor) and phospholipids—then activates Factor X.

Factor X is also activated by the extrinsic pathway. As blood reaches the tissues, tissue factors or thromboplastin activate Factor VII. Factor VII$_a$ then activates Factor X. As you can see, Factor X occupies a key position at the junction of the extrinsic and intrinsic pathways.

Coagulation then proceeds along a common pathway of more clotting factor activation. Factor X$_a$—with cofactor Factor V and

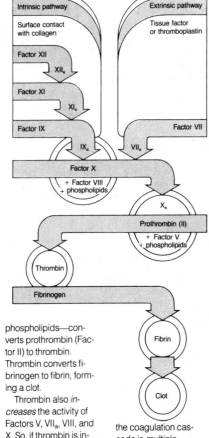

phospholipids—converts prothrombin (Factor II) to thrombin. Thrombin converts fibrinogen to fibrin, forming a clot.

Thrombin also *increases* the activity of Factors V, VII$_a$, VIII, and X. So, if thrombin is inhibited, coagulation will be significantly affected. A naturally occurring protein, antithrombin III, neutralizes thrombin. Heparin acts by potentiating (increasing) the thrombin-neutralizing action of antithrombin III. Therefore, heparin's effect on

the coagulation cascade is *multiple*.

Oral anticoagulants antagonize vitamin K, which is responsible for the formation of Factors II, VII, IX, and X from the liver.

Diagram adapted from the figure "The Coagulation System," in "Clinical Uses of Warfarin," *Drug Therapy*, January 1981. Used with permission of the publisher.

These drugs are also used to prevent clot enlargement or fragmentation (thromboembolism).

Oral anticoagulants include the coumarin derivatives (dicumarol, phenprocoumon, warfarin potassium, and warfarin sodium) and the indandione derivative phenindione. Heparin sodium, a parenteral anticoagulant, is antagonized by protamine sulfate.

Phytonadione is the antagonist for the coumarin derivatives.

Heparin, the coumarin derivatives, and the indandione derivatives impede clotting by preventing fibrin formation.

Major uses

All anticoagulants are used to treat pulmonary emboli and deep vein thrombosis (DVT) and to reduce thrombus formation after MI.

• Heparin is administered subcutaneously in low doses (minidoses) to prevent DVT and pulmonary embolism as well.

• Oral anticoagulants are also used in rheumatic heart disease with valvular damage and in atrial dysrhythmias that obstruct hemodynamics.

• Protamine sulfate neutralizes the effects of heparin.

• Phytonadione neutralizes the effects of coumadin.

Mechanism of action

• Heparin accelerates formation of an antithrombin III-thrombin complex. It inactivates thrombin and prevents conversion of fibrinogen to fibrin.

• The oral anticoagulants inhibit vitamin K–dependent activation of clotting factors II, VII, IX, and X, which are formed in the liver.

• Protamine sulfate, a strong base, forms a physiologically inert complex with heparin sodium, a strong acid. (See *Understanding Anticoagulant Action*, page 435).

Absorption, distribution, metabolism, and excretion

• Heparin is not absorbed from the GI tract and must be administered parenter-

ally. Although absorption after S.C. injection varies greatly among patients, heparin is generally well absorbed and is usually administered by this route.

Heparin is distributed widely in the blood.

Although heparin's metabolism is not completely clear, most of the drug seems to be removed from circulation by the reticuloendothelial cells. However, some heparin is probably metabolized by the liver. A small fraction of the drug is excreted unchanged in urine.

• The oral anticoagulants, phenindione, phenprocoumon, and warfarin salts are well absorbed from the GI tract; dicumarol is incompletely absorbed.

Oral anticoagulants are 98% bound to plasma proteins, primarily albumin, and are widely distributed in body tissues.

They are largely metabolized in the liver, secreted into the bile as inactive metabolites, reabsorbed, and excreted in the urine.

• Protamine's metabolism and excretion are unclear.

Phytonadione is absorbed through the GI tract and requires the presence of bile salts.

Onset and duration

• Heparin sodium begins to act immediately, with peak effects occurring within minutes. Clotting time returns to normal within 2 to 6 hours.

• Oral anticoagulants are detectable in the blood within 1 hour after administration, and blood levels usually peak within 12 hours. However, oral anticoagulants require 1 to 3 days to produce therapeutic anticoagulation, even though they alter prothrombin time the first day of therapy. The average course of therapy is 3 to 6 months, but the anticoagulants should be used for the shortest period necessary. Durations vary from 1 to 14 days.

• Protamine sulfate neutralizes heparin within 5 minutes after I.V. administration.

• Phytonadione's onset of action depends on the route of administration—

Oral: 6-12 hours; I.M. or I.V.: 1-2 hours

dicumarol
(Dicumarol Pulvules)

Indications and dosage
Treatment of pulmonary emboli; prevention and treatment of deep vein thrombosis, MI, rheumatic heart disease with heart valve damage, atrial dysrhythmias—
Adults: 200 to 300 mg P.O. on first day, 25 to 200 mg P.O. daily thereafter, based on prothrombin times

Side effects
Blood: hemorrhage with excessive dosage, leukopenia, *agranulocytosis*
GI: anorexia, nausea, vomiting, cramps, *diarrhea,* mouth ulcers
GU: hematuria
Skin: dermatitis, urticaria, alopecia, rash
Other: fever

Interactions
Allopurinol, chloramphenicol, danazol, clofibrate, diflunisal, dextrothyroxine, thyroid drugs, heparin, anabolic steroids, cimetidine, disulfiram, glucagon, inhalation anesthetics, metronidazole, quinidine, influenza vaccine, sulindac, sulfonamides: increased prothrombin time. Monitor patient carefully for bleeding. Consider anticoagulant dose reduction.
Ethacrynic acid, indomethacin, mefenamic acid, oxyphenbutazone, phenylbutazone, salicylates: increased prothrombin time; ulcerogenic effects. Do not use together.
Acetaminophen: increased bleeding possible with chronic (greater than 2 weeks) therapy with acetaminophen. Monitor very carefully.
Griseofulvin, haloperidol, carbamazepine, paraldehyde, rifampin: decreased prothrombin time with reduced anticoagulant effect. Monitor patient carefully.
Glutethimide, chloral hydrate, sulfinpyrazone, triclofos sodium: increased or

decreased prothrombin time. Avoid use if possible, or monitor patient carefully.
Barbiturates: inhibition of hypoprothrombinemic effect of anticoagulants. If barbiturates are withdrawn, reduce anticoagulant dose; inhibition may last weeks after barbiturate is withdrawn, but fatal hemorrhage can occur when inhibiting effect disappears.
Cholestyramine: decreased response when administered too close together. Administer 6 hours after oral anticoagulants.

Nursing considerations
• Contraindicated in hemophilia, thrombocytopenic purpura, leukemia with pronounced bleeding tendency, open wounds or ulcers, impaired hepatic or renal function, severe hypertension, acute nephritis, subacute bacterial endocarditis. Use cautiously in pregnancy or lactation, during menses, during use of any drainage tube, and in any patient in whom slight bleeding is dangerous. Use with extreme caution (if at all) in psychiatric, debilitated, or cachectic patients.
• Use caution when adding or stopping any drug for patient receiving anticoagulants. May change clotting status and result in hemorrhage.
• Fever and skin rash signal severe complications.
• Give drug at same time daily. Stress importance of complying with recommended dosage and keeping follow-up appointments. Patient should carry a card that identifies him as a potential bleeder.
• Regularly inspect patient for bleeding gums, bruises on arms or legs, petechiae, nosebleeds, melena, tarry stools, hematuria, hematemesis. Tell patient and family to watch for these signs and notify doctor immediately.
• Warn patient to avoid over-the-counter products containing aspirin, other salicylates, or drugs that may interact with dicumarol.
• Because onset of action is delayed, heparin sodium is often given during first few days of treatment. When hepa-

rin is being given simultaneously, do not draw blood for prothrombin time within 5 hours after I.V. heparin administration.

• Dose given depends on prothrombin time (PT). Doctors usually try to maintain PT at 1.5 to 2 times normal. PT values depend on procedure and reagents used in individual laboratory.

• Tell patient to notify doctor if menses is heavier than usual. May require adjusting dose.

• Tell patient to use electric razor when shaving to avoid scratching skin and to brush teeth with soft toothbrush.

• May turn alkaline urine red-orange.

• Duration of action 2 to 6 days

• Formerly known as bishydroxycoumarin.

• Light-to-moderate alcohol intake does not significantly affect prothrombin times.

• Tell patient to eat a consistent amount of leafy green vegetables every day. These contain vitamin K, and eating different amounts daily will alter anticoagulant effect.

---

heparin
(Hepalean, Liquaemin Sodium)

Indications and dosage
Treatment of deep vein thrombosis, MI—

Adults: initially 5,000 to 7,500 units I.V. push, then adjust dose according to partial thromboplastin time (PTT) results and give dose I.V. q 4 hours (usually 4,000 to 5,000 units); or 5,000 to 7,500 units I.V. bolus, then 1,000 units/ hour by I.V. infusion pump. Wait 8 hours following bolus dose, and adjust hourly rate according to PTT.
Treatment of pulmonary embolism—
Adults: initially 7,500 to 10,000 units I.V. push, then adjust dose according to PTT results and give dose I.V. q 4 hours (usually 4,000 to 5,000 units); or 7,500 to 10,000 units I.V. bolus, then 1,000 units hourly by I.V. infusion pump. Wait 8 hours following bolus dose, and adjust

hourly rate according to PTT.
Prophylaxis of embolism—
Adults: 5,000 units S.C. q 12 hours
Open heart surgery—
Adults: (total body perfusion) 150 to 300 units/kg continuous I.V infusion
Treatment of pulmonary emboli; prevention and treatment of deep vein thrombosis—
Children: initially 50 units/kg I.V. drip. Maintenance dose 100 units/kg I.V. drip q 4 hours. Constant infusion: 20,000 units/m^2 daily. Dosages adjusted according to PTT.

Heparin dosing is highly individualized, depending on disease state, age, renal and hepatic status.

Side effects
Blood: hemorrhage with excessive dosage, overly prolonged clotting time, thrombocytopenia
Local: irritation, mild pain
Other: hypersensitivity reactions including chills, fever, pruritus, rhinitis, burning of feet, conjunctivitis, lacrimation, arthralgia, urticaria

Interactions
Salicylates: increased anticoagulant effect. Do not use together.
Anticoagulants, oral: additive anticoagulation. Monitor prothrombin time and partial thromboplastin time.

Nursing considerations
• Conditionally contraindicated in active bleeding, blood dyscrasias, or bleeding tendencies such as hemophilia, thrombocytopenia, or hepatic disease with hypoprothrombinemia; suspected intracranial hemorrhage; suppurative thrombophlebitis; inaccessible ulcerative lesions (especially of GI tract); open ulcerative wounds; extensive denudation of skin; ascorbic acid deficiency and other conditions causing increased capillary permeability; during or after brain, eye, or spinal cord surgery; during continuous tube drainage of stomach or small intestine; in subacute bacterial endocarditis; shock; advanced renal disease; threatened abor-

tion; severe hypertension. Although use of heparin is clearly hazardous in these conditions, decision to use it depends on comparative risk in failure to treat coexisting thromboembolic disorder.

• Use cautiously during menses; in mild hepatic or renal disease, alcoholism, patients in occupations with risk of physical injury; immediately postpartum; and in patients with history of allergies, asthma, or GI ulcers.

• Monitor platelet counts regularly. Thrombocytopenia caused by heparin may be associated with arterial thrombosis.

• Measure PTT carefully and regularly. Anticoagulation is present when PTT values are 1.5 to 2 times control values.

• Drug requirements are higher in early phases of thrombogenic diseases and febrile states; lower when patient becomes stabilized.

• Regularly inspect patient for bleeding gums, bruises on arms or legs, petechiae, nosebleeds, melena, tarry stools, hematuria, hematemesis. Tell patient and family to watch for these signs and notify doctor immediately.

• Tell patient to avoid over-the-counter medications containing aspirin, other salicylates, or drugs that may interact with heparin.

• Heparin comes in various concentrations. Check order and vial carefully.

• Low-dose injections given sequentially between iliac crests in lower abdomen deep into subcutaneous fat. Inject drug slowly S.C. into fat pad. Leave needle in place for 10 seconds after injection; then withdraw. Alternate site every 12 hours—right for morning, left for evening.

• Do not massage after S.C. injection. Watch for signs of bleeding at injection site. Rotate sites and keep accurate record.

• Check constant I.V. infusions regularly, even when pumps are in good working order, to prevent overdosage or underdosage.

• I.M. administration is not recommended.

• I.V. administration preferred because of long-term effect and irregular absorption when given S.C. Whenever possible, administer I.V. heparin using infusion pump to provide maximum safety.

• Concentrated heparin solutions (greater than 100 units/ml) can irritate blood vessels.

• Place notice above patient's bed to inform I.V. team or lab personnel to apply pressure dressings after taking blood.

• Avoid excessive I.M. injections of other drugs to prevent or minimize hematomas. If possible, do not give I.M. injections at all.

• Elderly patients should usually start at lower doses.

• When intermittent I.V. therapy is used, always draw blood ½ hour before next scheduled dose to avoid falsely elevated PTT.

• Blood for PTT can be drawn any time after 8 hours of initiation of continuous I.V. heparin therapy. Never draw blood for PTT from the I.V. tubing of the heparin infusion, or from vein of infusion. Falsely elevated PTT will result. Always draw blood from opposite arm.

• Give on time; try not to skip a dose or "catch up" with an I.V. containing heparin. If I.V. is out, get it restarted as soon as possible, and reschedule bolus dose immediately.

• Never piggyback other drugs into an infusion line while heparin is running. Many antibiotics and other drugs inactivate heparin. Never mix any drug with heparin in syringe when bolus therapy is used.

• Abrupt withdrawal may cause increased coagulability. Usually, heparin therapy is followed by oral anticoagulants for prophylaxis.

phenindione
(Danilone, Eridione, Hedulin)

Indications and dosage

Treatment of pulmonary emboli; prevention and treatment of deep vein throm-

bosis, MI, rheumatic heart disease with heart valve damage, atrial dysrhythmias—
Adults: 300 mg P.O. first day; 200 mg P.O. second day. Maintenance dose: 50 to 150 mg daily, based on PT.

Side effects

Blood: *hemorrhage with excessive dosage, agranulocytosis,* leukopenia, leukocytosis, eosinophilia
CNS: headache
CV: myocarditis, tachycardia
EENT: conjunctivitis, blurred vision, paralysis of ocular accommodation
GI: diarrhea, sore mouth and throat
GU: *nephropathy with renal tubular necrosis,* albuminuria
Hepatic: jaundice
Skin: rash, severe exfoliative dermatitis
Other: fever

Interactions

Allopurinol, chloramphenicol, danazol, clofibrate, diflunisal, dextrothyroxine, thyroid drugs, heparin, anabolic steroids, cimetidine, disulfiram, glucagon, inhalation anesthetics, metronidazole, quinidine, influenza vaccine, sulindac, sulfonamides: increased prothrombin time. Monitor patient carefully for bleeding. Consider anticoagulant dose reduction.
Ethacrynic acid, indomethacin, mefenamic acid, oxyphenbutazone, phenylbutazone, salicylates: increased PT, ulcerogenic effects. Do not use together.
Griseofulvin, haloperidol, carbamazepine, paraldehyde, rifampin: decreased prothrombin time with reduced anticoagulant effect. Monitor patient carefully.
Glutethimide, chloral hydrate, sulfinpyrazone, triclofos sodium: increased or decreased PT. Avoid use if possible, or monitor patient carefully.
Barbiturates: inhibition of hypoprothrombinemic effect of anticoagulants. If barbiturates are withdrawn, reduce anticoagulant dose; inhibition may last weeks after barbiturate is withdrawn, but fatal hemorrhage can occur when inhibiting effect disappears.

Cholestyramine: decreased response when administered too close together. Administer 6 hours after oral anticoagulants.

Nursing considerations
• Contraindicated in hemophilia, thrombocytopenic purpura, leukemia with pronounced bleeding tendency, open wounds or ulcers, impaired hepatic or renal function, severe hypertension, acute nephritis, and subacute bacterial endocarditis. Use cautiously in pregnancy or lactation, during menses, during use of any drainage tube in any orifice, and in any patient in whom slight bleeding is dangerous. Use with extreme caution (if at all) in psychiatric, debilitated, or cachectic patients.
• Use caution when adding or stopping any drug. May change clotting status and result in hemorrhage.
• Fever and skin rash signal severe complications.
• Give drug at same time daily. Stress importance of complying with recommended dosage and keeping follow-up appointments. Patient should carry a card that identifies him as a potential bleeder.
• Regularly inspect patient for bleeding gums, bruises on arms or legs, petechiae, nosebleeds, melena, tarry stools, hematuria, hematemesis. Tell patient and family to watch for these signs and notify doctor immediately.
• Warn patient to avoid over-the-counter products containing aspirin, salicylates, or other drugs that may interact with phenindione.
• Because onset of action is delayed, heparin sodium is often given during first few days of treatment. When heparin is being given simultaneously, do not draw blood for PT within 5 hours after I.V. heparin administration.
• Dose given depends on PT. Doctors usually try to maintain PT at 1.5 to 2 times normal. Numerical PT values depend on procedure and reagents used in individual laboratory.
• Tell patient to notify doctor if menses is heavier than usual. May require ad-

justing dose.
• Tell patient to use electric razor when shaving to avoid scratching skin and to brush teeth with soft toothbrush.
• Warn patient that alkaline urine may turn red-orange.
• Duration of action is 2 to 4 days.
• Light-to-moderate alcohol intake does not significantly affect PT.
• Tell patient to eat a consistent amount of leafy green vegetables every day. These contain vitamin K, and eating different amounts daily will alter anticoagulant effect.

phenprocoumon (Liquamar)

Indications and dosage
Treatment of pulmonary emboli; prevention and treatment of deep vein thrombosis, MI, rheumatic heart disease with heart valve damage, atrial dysrhythmias—
Adults: initially 24 mg P.O. Maintenance dose: 0.75 to 6 mg daily, based on PT

Side effects
Blood: hemorrhage with excessive dosage, agranulocytosis, leukopenia
GI: paralytic ileus and intestinal obstruction (both resulting from hemorrhage), nausea, vomiting, cramps, diarrhea, mouth ulcers
GU: nephropathy, hematuria
Skin: rash, alopecia, necrosis
Other: fever

Interactions
Allopurinol, chloramphenicol, danazol, clofibrate, diflunisal, dextrothyroxine, thyroid drugs, heparin, anabolic steroids, cimetidine, disulfiram, glucagon, inhalation anesthetics, metronidazole, quinidine, influenza vaccine, sulindac, sulfonamides: increased PT. Monitor patient carefully for bleeding. Consider anticoagulant dose reduction.
Ethacrynic acid, indomethacin, mefenamic acid, oxyphenbutazone, phenylbutazone, salicylates: increased PT, ul-cerogenic effects. Do not use together.
Acetaminophen: increased bleeding possible with chronic (greater than 2 weeks) therapy with acetaminophen. Monitor very carefully.
Griseofulvin, haloperidol, carbamazepine, paraldehyde, rifampin: decreased PT with reduced anticoagulant effect. Monitor patient carefully.
Glutethimide, chloral hydrate, sulfinpyrazone, triclofos sodium: increased or decreased PT. Avoid use if possible, or monitor patient carefully.
Barbiturates: inhibition of hypoprothrombinemic effect of anticoagulants. If barbiturates are withdrawn, reduce anticoagulant dose; inhibition may last weeks after barbiturate is withdrawn, but fatal hemorrhage can occur when inhibiting effect disappears.
Cholestyramine: decreased response when administered too close together. Administer 6 hours after oral anticoagulants.

Nursing considerations
• Contraindicated in hemophilia, thrombocytopenic purpura, leukemia with pronounced bleeding tendency, open wounds or ulcers, impaired hepatic or renal function, severe hypertension, acute nephritis, and subacute bacterial endocarditis. Use cautiously in pregnancy or lactation, during menses, during use of any drainage tube in any orifice, and in any patient in whom slight bleeding is dangerous. Use with extreme caution (if at all) in psychiatric, debilitated, or cachectic patients.
• Use caution when adding or stopping any drug for patient receiving anticoagulants. May change clotting status and result in hemorrhage.
• Fever and skin rash signal severe complications.
• Give drug at same time daily. Stress importance of complying with recommended dosage and keeping follow-up appointments. Patient should carry a card that identifies him as a potential bleeder.
• Regularly inspect patient for bleeding gums, bruises on arms or legs, pete-

chiae, nosebleeds, melena, tarry stools, hematuria, hematemesis. Tell patient and family to watch for these signs and notify doctor immediately.

• Warn patient to avoid over-the-counter products containing aspirin, other salicylates, or drugs that may interact with phenprocoumon.

• Because onset of action is delayed, heparin sodium is often given during first few days of treatment. When heparin is being given simultaneously, do not draw blood for PT within 5 hours of I.V. heparin administration.

• Dose given depends on PT. Doctors usually try to maintain PT at 1.5 to 2 times normal. Numerical PT values depend on procedure and reagents used in individual laboratory.

• Tell patient to notify doctor if menses is heavier than usual. May require adjusting dose.

• Tell patient to use electric razor when shaving to avoid scratching skin and to brush teeth with soft toothbrush.

• Warn patient that alkaline urine may turn orange-red.

• A coumarin derivative

• Duration of action is 7 to 14 days.

• Light-to-moderate alcohol intake does not significantly affect prothrombin times.

• Tell patient to eat a consistent amount of leafy green vegetables every day. These contain vitamin K, and eating different amounts daily will alter anticoagulant effect.

---

phytonadione— vitamin K₁ (AquaMEPHYTON)

Indications and dosage
Hypoprothrombinemia secondary to vitamin K malabsorption, drug therapy, or excess vitamin A—
Adults: 2 to 25 mg, depending on severity, P.O. or parenterally, repeated and increased up to 50 mg, if necessary
Children: 5 to 10 mg P.O. or parenterally

Infants: 2 mg P.O. or parenterally. I.V. injection rate for children and infants should not exceed 3 mg/m²/minute or a total of 5 mg.
Hypoprothrombinemia secondary to effect of oral anticoagulants—
Adults: 2.5 to 10 mg P.O., S.C., or I.M., based on PT, repeated, if necessary, 12 to 48 hours after oral dose or 6 to 8 hours after parenteral dose. In emergency, give 10 to 50 mg slow I.V., rate not to exceed 1 mg/minute, repeated q 4 hours, as needed.

Side effects
CNS: dizziness, convulsive movement
CV: transient hypotension after I.V. administration, rapid, weak pulse, cardiac irregularities
GI: nausea, vomiting
Skin: sweating, flushing, erythema
Local: pain, swelling, and hematoma at injection site
Other: bronchospasms, dyspnea, cramp-like pain, *anaphylaxis and anaphylactoid reactions (usually after rapid I.V. administration)*

Interactions
Mineral oil, cholestyramine resin: inhibited GI absorption of oral vitamin K. Use together cautiously.

Nursing considerations
• Contraindicated in hereditary hypoprothrombinemia, bleeding secondary to heparin therapy or overdose, hepatocellular disease, unless caused by biliary obstruction (vitamin K can paradoxically worsen hypoprothrombinemia). Oral administration contraindicated if bile secretion inadequate, unless supplemented with bile salts. Use cautiously, if at all, during last weeks of pregnancy to avoid toxic reactions in newborns; in G-6-PD deficiency to avoid hemolysis. Use large doses cautiously in severe hepatic disease.

• Failure to respond to vitamin K may indicate coagulation defects.

• In severe bleeding, do not delay other measures such as fresh frozen plasma or whole blood.

- Protect parenteral products from light. Wrap infusion container with aluminum foil.
- Effects of I.V. injections more rapid but shorter lived than S.C. or I.M. injections.
- Monitor PT to determine dosage effectiveness.
- Observe for signs of side effects and report them to doctor.
- Phytonadione therapy for hemorrhagic disease in infants causes fewer adverse reactions than do other vitamin K analogs.
- Check brand name labels for administration route restrictions.
- Administer I.V. by slow infusion (over 2 to 3 hours). Mix in normal saline solution, dextrose 5% in water, or dextrose 5% in normal saline solution. Observe patient closely for signs of flushing, weakness, tachycardia, and hypotension; may progress to shock.
- Leafy vegetables are high in vitamin K and may alter warfarin needs.
- Vitamin is fat soluble.

protamine sulfate

Indications and dosage
Heparin overdose—
Adults: dosage based on venous blood coagulation studies, generally 1 mg for each 78 to 95 units of heparin. Give diluted to 1% (10 mg/ml) slow I.V. injection over 1 to 3 minutes. Maximum 50 mg/10 minutes

Side effects
CV: fall in blood pressure, bradycardia
Other: transitory flushing, feeling of warmth, dyspnea

Interactions
None significant

Nursing considerations
- Use cautiously after cardiac surgery.
- Doctor gives drug. Should be given slowly to reduce side effects. Have equipment available to treat shock.

- Monitor patient continually. Check vital signs frequently.
- Watch for spontaneous bleeding (heparin "rebound"), especially in patients undergoing dialysis or who have had cardiac surgery.
- Protamine sulfate may act as anticoagulant in very high doses.
- 1 mg of protamine neutralizes 78 to 95 units of heparin.
- Heparin antagonist.

warfarin (Coumadin)

Indications and dosage
Treatment of pulmonary emboli; prevention and treatment of deep vein thrombosis, MI, rheumatic heart disease with heart valve damage, atrial arrhythmias—
Adults: 10 to 15 mg P.O. for 3 days, then dosage based on daily PT. Usual maintenance dose 2 to 10 mg P.O. daily. Alternate regimen: initially, 40 to 60 mg P.O. daily; then 2 to 10 mg daily based on PT determinations
Warfarin sodium also available for I.V. use (50 mg/vial). Reconstitute with sterile water for injection. I.V. form rarely used and may be in periodic short supply.

Side effects
Blood: *hemorrhage with excessive dosage,* leukopenia
GI: paralytic ileus, intestinal obstruction (both resulting from hemorrhage), diarrhea, vomiting, cramps, nausea
GU: excessive uterine bleeding
Skin: dermatitis, urticaria, *rash,* necrosis, alopecia
Other: fever

Interactions
Allopurinol, chloramphenicol, danazol, clofibrate, diflunisal, dextrothyraxine, thyroid drugs, heparin, anabolic steroids, cimetidine, disulfiram, glucagon, inhalation anesthetics, metronidazole, quinidine, influenza vaccine, sulindac, sulfonamides: increased PT. Monitor

patient carefully for bleeding. Consider anticoagulant dose reduction.

Ethacrynic acid, indomethacin, mefenamic acid, oxyphenbutazone, phenylbutazone, salicylates: increased prothrombin time, ulcerogenic effects. Do not use together.

Acetaminophen: increased bleeding possible with chronic (greater than 2 weeks) therapy with acetaminophen. Monitor very carefully.

Griseofulvin, haloperidol, carbamazepine, paraldehyde, rifampin: decreased PT with reduced anticoagulant effect. Monitor patient carefully.

Glutethimide, chloral hydrate, sulfinpyrazone, triclofos sodium: increased or decreased PT. Avoid use if possible, or monitor patient carefully.

Barbiturates: inhibition of hypoprothrombinemic effect of anticoagulants. If barbiturates are withdrawn, reduce anticoagulant dose. Inhibition may last weeks after barbiturate is withdrawn, but fatal hemorrhage can occur when inhibiting effect disappears.

Cholestyramine: decreased response when administered too close together. Administer 6 hours after oral anticoagulants.

Nursing considerations

• Contraindicated in bleeding or hemorrhagic tendencies resulting from open wounds, visceral cancer, GI ulcers, severe hepatic or renal disease, severe uncontrolled hypertension, subacute bacterial endocarditis, vitamin K deficiency, and after recent eye, brain, or spinal cord surgery. Use cautiously in diverticulitis, colitis, lactation, mild or moderate hypertension, hepatic or renal disease, lactation; in presence of drainage tubes in any orifice, with regional or lumbar block anesthesia, or in any condition increasing risk of hemorrhage.

• Observe nursing infants of mothers on drug for unexpected bleeding.

• PT determinations essential for proper control. High incidence of bleeding when PT exceeds 2.5 times control values. Doctors usually try to maintain PT at 1.5 to 2 times normal.

• Give at same time daily. Stress importance of complying with recommended dosage and keeping follow-up appointments. Patient should carry a card that identifies him as a potential bleeder.

• Elderly patients and patients with renal or hepatic failure are especially sensitive to warfarin effect.

• Half-life of warfarin is 36 to 44 hours.

• Warfarin effect can be neutralized by vitamin K injections.

• Regularly inspect patient for bleeding gums, bruises on arms or legs, petechiae, nosebleeds, melena, tarry stools, hematuria, hematemesis. Tell patient and family to watch for these signs and notify doctor immediately.

• Warn patient to avoid over-the-counter products containing aspirin, other salicylates, or drugs that may interact with warfarin potassium or warfarin sodium.

• Food and enteral feedings that contain vitamin K may cause inadequate anticoagulation. Warn patient to read labels.

• Because onset of action is delayed, heparin sodium is often given during first few days of treatment. When heparin is being given simultaneously, do not draw blood for prothrombin time within 5 hours of I.V. heparin administration.

• Fever and skin rash signal severe complications.

• Tell patient to notify doctor if menses is heavier than usual. May require adjusting dose.

• Tell patient to use electric razor when shaving to avoid scratching skin and to brush teeth with soft toothbrush.

• Best oral anticoagulant when patient must receive antacids or phenytoin

• Light-to-moderate alcohol intake does not significantly affect prothrombin time.

• Possibly effective in treatment of transient cerebral ischemic attacks

• Tell patient to eat a consistent amount of leafy green vegetables every day. These contain vitamin K, and eating different amounts daily will alter anticoagulant effects.

Thrombolytic enzymes

Thrombolytic enzymes are effective in treating acute and extensive episodes of thrombotic disorders. Before administering these enzymes, however, be aware of the increased risk of hemorrhage that attends their use. Although major bleeding is a possible complication, bruising and oozing of blood at the incision site and surgical trauma are more likely. Because of the inherent risk of hemorrhage, thrombolytic enzyme therapy should be initiated only by doctors skilled in its use and under close laboratory monitoring.

Major uses
Streptokinase and urokinase are used to treat acute, massive pulmonary emboli. Streptokinase is also used to dissolve acute, extensive deep-vein thrombi and acute arterial thromboemboli.

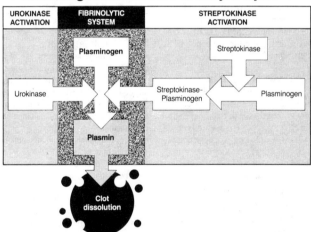

How Drugs Activate the Fibrinolytic System

When blood begins to form a clot, the natural mechanism for dissolving this clot is also initiated.

The mechanism for dissolving clotted blood when it is no longer needed is called the fibrinolytic system. Its physiologic stimuli are kinases, activated Factor XII, and certain tissue activators. They activate plasminogen to form plasmin, the proteolytic enzyme that dissolves a clot's fibrin threads.

When undesirable clots form, the fibrinolytic system's anticoagulant action can be hastened with the thrombolytic drugs streptokinase and urokinase.

These drugs imitate the system's natural activators. Urokinase reacts directly with plasminogen to create the lysing agent plasmin; streptokinase joins plasminogen in a complex that then reacts with plasminogen to form plasmin. This activated plasmin then dissolves the clot.

Adapted with permission from Philip P. Gerbino and Sanford J. Shattil, "Prevention and Treatment of Pulmonary Embolism," *U.S. Pharmacist*, 5:5:H-1, May 1980.

Mechanism of action

Both streptokinase and urokinase activate plasminogen and convert it to plasmin, which degrades fibrin clots, fibrinogen, and other plasma proteins.

• Streptokinase activates plasminogen in a two-step process. Plasminogen and streptokinase form a complex that exposes the plasminogen-activating site. Plasminogen is converted to plasmin by cleavage of the peptide bond.

• Urokinase activates plasminogen by directly cleaving peptide bonds at two different sites (See *How Drugs Activate the Fibrinolytic System,* page 445.)

Absorption, distribution, metabolism, and excretion

Streptokinase and urokinase are administered only by I.V. infusion and are distributed throughout the body. Their metabolism and excretion have not been fully elucidated.

Onset and duration

Streptokinase and urokinase begin to act immediately. They must be infused at a constant dosage level to maintain therapeutic effectiveness. Their action ceases when the I.V. infusion is discontinued, but residual effects on coagulation may last as long as 12 hours.

---

streptokinase
(Kabikinase, Streptase)

Indications and dosage

Arteriovenous cannula occlusion—
Adults: 250,000 IU in 2 ml I.V. solution by I.V. pump infusion into each occluded limb of the cannula over 25 to 35 minutes. Clamp off cannula for 2 hours. Then aspirate contents of cannula, flush with saline solution, and reconnect.
Venous thrombosis, pulmonary embolism, and arterial thrombosis and embolism—
Adults: loading dose: 250,000 IU I.V. infusion over 30 minutes. Sustaining dose: 100,000 IU/hour I.V. infusion for 72 hours for deep vein thrombosis and 100,000 IU/hour over 24 to 72 hours by

I.V. infusion pump for pulmonary embolism
Lysis of coronary artery thrombi following acute MI—
Adults: loading dose: 20,000 IU via coronary catheter, followed by a maintenance dose. Maintenance dose: 2,000 IU/minute for 60 minutes as an infusion

Side effects

Blood: *bleeding, decreased hematocrit*
CV: *transient lowering or elevation of blood pressure*
EENT: *periorbital edema*
Local: *phlebitis at injection site*
Skin: urticaria
Other: *hypersensitivity to drug, fever, anaphylaxis,* musculoskeletal pain, minor breathing difficulty, bronchospasms, angioneurotic edema

Interactions

Anticoagulants: concurrent use of anticoagulants with streptokinase is not recommended. Reversing the effects of oral anticoagulants must be considered before beginning therapy, and heparin must be stopped and its effect allowed to diminish.
Aspirin, indomethacin, phenylbutazone, drugs affecting platelet activity: increased risk of bleeding. Do not use together.

Nursing considerations

• Contraindicated in ulcerative wounds, active internal bleeding, recent CVA, recent trauma with possible internal injuries, visceral or intracranial malignancy, ulcerative colitis, diverticulitis, severe hypertension, acute or chronic hepatic or renal insufficiency, uncontrolled hypocoagulation, chronic pulmonary disease with cavitation, subacute bacterial endocarditis or rheumatic valvular disease, recent cerebral embolism, thrombosis, or hemorrhage. Also contraindicated within 10 days after intraarterial diagnostic procedure or any surgery, including liver or kidney biopsy, lumbar puncture, thoracentesis, paracentesis, or extensive or multiple cutdowns.

• Use cautiously when treating arterial emboli that originate from left side of heart because of danger of cerebral infarction.

• I.M. injections contraindicated during streptokinase therapy

• Before initiating therapy, draw blood to determine PTT and PT. Rate of I.V. infusion depends on thrombin time and streptokinase resistance.

• If patient has had either recent streptococcal infection or recent treatment with streptokinase, higher loading dose may be necessary.

• Preparation of I.V. solution: reconstitute each vial with 5 ml sodium chloride for injection. Further dilute to 45 ml. Do not shake; roll gently to mix. Use within 24 hours. Store at room temperature in powder form; refrigerate after reconstitution.

• Monitor patient for excessive bleeding every 15 minutes for the first hour; every 30 minutes for the second through eighth hours; then once every shift. If bleeding is evident, stop therapy. Pretreatment with heparin or drugs affecting platelets causes high risk of bleeding.

• Monitor pulses, color, and sensitivities of extremities every hour.

• Have typed and crossmatched packed red cells and whole blood available to treat possible hemorrhage.

• Keep aminocaproic acid available to treat bleeding. Corticosteroids are used to treat allergic reactions.

• Before using streptokinase to clear an occluded arteriovenous cannula, try flushing with heparinized saline solution.

• Bruising more likely during therapy; avoid unnecessary handling of patient. Side rails should be padded.

• Maintain the involved extremity in straight alignment to prevent bleeding from infusion site.

• Keep venipuncture sites to a minimum; use pressure dressing on puncture sites for at least 15 minutes.

• Keep a laboratory flow sheet on patient's chart so you can monitor PPT, PT, hemoglobin, and hematocrit.

• Monitor vital signs frequently.

• Watch for signs of hypersensitivity. Notify doctor immediately.

• Heparin by continuous infusion is usually started within an hour after stopping streptokinase. Use infusion pump to administer heparin.

• Should be used only by doctors with wide experience in thrombotic disease management where clinical and laboratory monitoring can be performed.

• In treatment of acute MI, streptokinase prevents primary or secondary thrombus formation in microcirculation surrounding necrotic area.

urokinase
(Abbokinase)

Indications and dosage
Lysis of acute massive pulmonary emboli and pulmonary emboli accompanied by unstable hemodynamics—
Adults: for I.V. infusion only by constant infusion pump that will deliver a total volume of 195 ml
Priming dose: 4,400 IU/kg hourly of urokinase-normal saline solution admixture given over 10 minutes

Follow with 4,400 IU/kg hourly for 12 to 24 hours. Total volume should not exceed 200 ml.

Follow therapy with continuous I.V. infusion of heparin, then oral anticoagulants.

Side effects
Blood: bleeding, decreased hematocrit
Local: phlebitis at injection site
Other: hypersensitivity (not as frequent as streptokinase), musculoskeletal pain, bronchospasm, *anaphylaxis*

Interactions
Anticoagulants: concurrent use of anticoagulants with urokinase is not recommended. Reversing effects of oral anticoagulants must be considered before beginning therapy, and heparin must be stopped and its effect allowed to diminish.

Aspirin, indomethacin, phenylbutazone, other drugs affecting platelet activity: increased risk of bleeding. Do not use together.

Nursing considerations
• Contraindicated in ulcerative wounds, active internal bleeding, CVA, recent trauma with possible internal injuries, visceral or intracranial malignancy, pregnancy and first 10 days postpartum, ulcerative colitis, diverticulitis, severe hypertension, acute or chronic hepatic or renal insufficiency, uncontrolled hypocoagulation, chronic pulmonary disease with cavitation, subacute bacterial endocarditis or rheumatic valvular disease, and recent cerebral embolism, thrombosis, or hemorrhage. Also contraindicated within 10 days after intraarterial diagnostic procedure or any surgery, including liver or kidney biopsy, lumbar puncture, thoracentesis, paracentesis, or extensive or multiple cutdowns.
• I.M. injections are contraindicated during urokinase therapy.
• Maintain the involved extremity in straight alignment to prevent bleeding from infusion site.
• Preparation of I.V. solution: add 5.2 ml sterile water for injection to vial. Dilute further with 0.9% saline solution before infusion. Do not use bacteriostatic water for injection to reconstitute; it contains preservatives.

• Monitor patient for bleeding every 15 minutes for the first hour; every 30 minutes for the second through eighth hours; then once every shift. Pretreatment with drugs affecting platelets places patient at high risk of bleeding.
• Monitor pulses, color, and sensitivities of extremities every hour.
• Have typed and crossmatched red cells and whole blood available to treat possible hemorrhage.
• Keep a laboratory flow sheet on patient's chart so you can monitor PTT, PT, hemoglobin, and hematocrit.
• Keep aminocaproic acid available to treat bleeding. Corticosteroids are used to treat allergic reactions.
• Watch for signs of hypersensitivity. Notify doctor immediately.
• Monitor vital signs.
• Keep venipuncture sites to a minimum; use pressure dressing on puncture sites for at least 15 minutes.
• Heparin by continuous infusion usually started within an hour after urokinase has been stopped. Use infusion pump to administer heparin.
• Bruising more likely during therapy; avoid unnecessary handling of patient. Side rails should be padded.
• Should be used only by doctors with wide experience in thrombotic disease management where clinical and laboratory monitoring can be performed.
• Also used to clear I.V. catheters obstructed by clotted blood or fibrin deposits.

19
CARDIAC REHABILITATION

I n the past decade, cardiac rehabilitation has become recognized as a crucial stage of care for the cardiac patient and a challenging assignment for the nurse.

Nurses involved in cardiac rehabilitation deliver physical, educational, and psychosocial care to the cardiac patient and his family and help bring patients who might have been "cardiac cripples" back into the mainstream of life. To meet this challenge, the nurse must be committed to the nursing philosophy and objectives of the program.

INPATIENT PROGRAM

A comprehensive cardiac rehabilitation program should meet the patient's educational, psychosocial, and physical activity needs as they relate to his cardiovascular functioning. The cardiac rehabilitation nurse coordinates care in both inpatient and outpatient settings and works with other health professionals, including doctors, physical therapists, social workers, and dietitians.

Ideally, cardiac rehabilitation should begin before overt signs and symptoms of heart disease develop, so nurses should also promote and assist with community educational programs to increase public awareness of cardiac risk factors.

Patient teaching and discharge planning

Cardiac rehabilitation can be divided into four phases. (See *The Four Phases of Cardiac Rehabilitation,* page 450.)

If the patient is a good candidate for rehabilitation, the program is started during the acute phase of illness and continued through the posthospitalization phase.

Patients may enter the program as either inpatients or outpatients. (See *Cardiac Rehabilitation Program,* page 451.) Typically, they enter as inpatients following an acute myocardial infarction (MI) and progress through both inpatient and outpatient programs.

All three program components—education, psychosocial support, and physical activity—should be offered in both inpatient and outpatient settings.

A patient hospitalized with a cardiac condition often feels overwhelmed with despair. He may think that his best years are over and that he will never be able to resume the activities he once enjoyed. In short, he feels that he has lost all control over his life.

Usually, he is wrong. But he will need your help to understand why.

How can you help him? By implementing a comprehensive cardiac rehabilitation program that includes:
• providing emotional and social support for the patient and his family
• supervising a physical activity program
• teaching the patient about his condition and necessary life-style changes.

Remember, cardiac rehabilitation is a continuous process from diagnosis through long-term maintenance: The needs of the patient and family will naturally change as they progress through each phase. Keep in mind that the specific programs presented here are only

The Four Phases of Cardiac Rehabilitation

Phase I Acute illness phase
Begins in the cardiac care unit almost immediately following admission
Phase II Remainder of hospitalization
Takes place on step-down unit or medical unit
Phase III Convalescence
Begins after discharge from hospital
Phase IV Conditioning for long-term maintenance of optimum cardiac health
Takes place at home, with periodic visits to outpatient clinic or doctor's office

examples—your hospital's program may be different in many ways. However, the goals are the same: to give the patient a sense of control over his life and health and to encourage a positive approach to living with a heart condition.

Providing emotional support

Nearly every patient with a serious cardiac condition initially experiences some emotional upset: panic, depression, sleeplessness, anxiety, anger. In fact, a cardiac patient probably feels *all* of these emotions sooner or later.

He is not alone. Almost certainly, his spouse and family feel upset too, although they may be reluctant to share their feelings with the patient.

To help the patient and his family understand these powerful emotions, try planning several discussion sessions for the entire family. Your support and guidance can encourage them to cope realistically with their problems.

What you discuss in each session will vary. Be flexible—let the patient and family direct the discussions, according to their biggest concerns. But use these suggestions as a guide:
• Explain common emotional responses evoked by an MI (and other acute cardiac events).
• Discuss the patient's personal reaction to his MI, and reassure him that his feelings are normal.
• Encourage the patient and his family to share their emotional reactions with each other.

• Discuss practical problems (medical expenses, for example), and refer the family to appropriate agencies for help, if needed.
• Explain life-style changes the patient faces after discharge, and suggest ways the family can adapt to them.
• Prepare the patient for feelings of depression and fatigue, which he may experience after he returns home.
• Recommend that the patient and his family join a support group, which can provide continuing support throughout the recovery period.

Why exercise?

When the patient is recovering from an acute cardiac event, the doctor will prescribe a progressive activity and exercise program that involves progression in activities of daily living and exercise. As well as combating anxiety, fatigue, and depression, physical activity helps prevent or lessen these debilitating effects of prolonged bed rest:
• muscle atrophy
• orthostatic hypotension
• decreased lung volume
• decreased circulating blood volume
• moderate tachycardia in response to exercise
• negative nitrogen balance
• increased risk of thromboembolism.

Managing a seven-step rehabilitation program

"When can I get out of bed? Feed myself? Walk down the hall? Go home?"

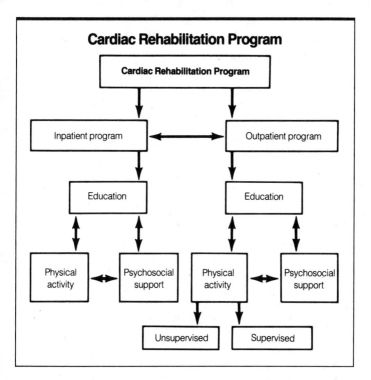

Cardiac Rehabilitation Program

These are commonly asked questions by a usually active person who is confined to bed rest because of a cardiovascular problem.

Your answers will depend on two things: The extent of damage to the patient's heart (the doctor determines this), and your hospital's inpatient physical rehabilitation program. But one thing is certain. A gradual but progressive return to activity is what the patient needs to strengthen his heart and reassure him that he can eventually return to an active life-style.

On the following pages, you will see an inpatient rehabilitation program developed at Grady Memorial Hospital, Atlanta. (See *Seven-Step Program of Physical Activity,* pages 452 and 453.) Your hospital's program may differ. For example, the exercises may not be the same or the program itself may be longer, to accommodate different lengths of stay.

What are your responsibilities in carrying out such a program? Once again, that depends on your hospital's policy. A physical therapist may supervise exercise activities while you supervise ordinary daily activities. Or you may share responsibilities for both. (The doctor will determine how quickly the patient progresses from one step to the next.) Make sure you know exactly how your hospital's policy assigns responsibility.

Important: When you supervise a patient's physical rehabilitation, make sure he gets at least 1 hour's rest between daily activities or sets of exercises, unless the doctor directs otherwise. Remember, your goal is to exercise his heart without overworking it.

Seven-Step Program of Physical Activity

Daily Activities

CCU

Step #1
- Partial bath in bed (hands, feet, teeth)
- Feed self
- Use bedside commode
- Sit in chair 1 or 2 times/day (maximum of 15 minutes each)
- Insure 1-hour rest between activities

Step #2
- Bathe entire body (in bed) with assistance for back and legs
- Feed self
- Use bedside commode
- Sit in chair 15 to 30 minutes, 2 or 3 times/day

Medical floor

Step #3
- Complete self-care, sitting on side of bed
- May eat out of bed
- Sitting out of bed (OOB) as tolerated
- Walk in room at will

Step #4
- Wash self at sink in bathroom
- OOB in room as tolerated
- Walk in hall (50' at 2 mph) with nurse supervision

Step #5
- Continue with room activity as above
- Sitting shower with supervision (warm, not hot water)
- Walk in hall 100'

Step #6
- Standing shower with supervision (warm water)
- May walk in hallway up to 200'
- Continue all previous activities

Step #7
- Standing shower without supervision
- May walk in hallway as desired
- Continue all other activities from before

Exercises

While in bed, *passive/active range of motion (ROM)* to all extremities 3 times/day,
5 times each
- Shoulder and elbow flexion and extension
- Hip and knee flexion and extension
- Hip abduction and adduction
- Teach patient active dorsiflexion and plantar flexion

Active ROM to all extremities 5 times each
- Do same exercises as above, sitting on side of bed

Warm-up exercises—moderate manual resistance (while sitting on edge of bed)
5 times each
- For shoulder, elbow, and hip flexion to knee extension (unilaterally)
- Ambulate in hall 50′ at 2 mph (15 paces/15 seconds)

Warm-up exercises—standing-shoulder circles 10 times each; stand on toes 10
times each
- Hip abduction/adduction 5 times each
- Trunk twists 5 times each
- Ambulate in hallway 100′ at 2 mph with rest stop if needed

Warm-up exercises—same as above
- Stair climbing—up and down 2 to 4 steps
- Ambulate—hallway walk 150′ to 200′ at 2 mph

Warm-up exercises—same as above, plus add lateral side bends 5 times each
- Ambulate in hallway 300′ at 2 to 2.5 mph (15 to 18 paces/15 seconds)
- Walk down one flight of stairs (12 to 14 steps) and return by elevator

Warm-up exercises—same as above.
- Ambulate in hallway 500′ at 2.5 mph (18 paces/15 seconds)
- Walk up one flight of stairs; rest; down one flight or return by elevator

Adapted from the Grady Memorial Hospital and the Emory University School of Medicine.

Teaching the patient about heart disease

To teach your patient about his heart condition and how to live with it, use either a group program or individual teaching sessions.

Which type of teaching session is better? That depends. Group sessions have two advantages: They use your time efficiently, and they encourage support and sharing among members.

But group sessions have one major disadvantage. They are not as effective as individual sessions for meeting each patient's special needs. As a result, you may prefer to teach some topics (risk-factor modification, for example, or returning to sexual activity) in individual sessions.

Use your judgment. Do not hesitate to teach your patient individually whenever it seems appropriate.

Here is an example of a five-session teaching program.

Teaching the patient how to take his own pulse

When the patient begins an exercise program, his doctor will set maximum rates, called target heart rates, for him to achieve. Because of the linear relationship between heart rate and oxygen intake during exercise, the heart rate can be used to control exercise intensity. The calculated heart rate range that is high enough to have a conditioning effect but within safe limits for the patient is called the *target heart range*. *(See Criteria for Terminating Exercise, page 456.)* As rehabilitation advances, the doctor may want him to achieve progressively higher target heart rates.

To comply, the patient needs to know how to take his own pulse. Begin teaching him by explaining why he needs to monitor his heart rate during exercise. Say something like this: "Your heart is a muscle that needs exercise to stay in shape. That is why the doctor wants you to temporarily raise your heart rate slightly every few days. However, he doesn't want you to overwork your heart while it's still healing.

To make sure you give your heart no more than the correct amount of work, you must know how to take your own pulse. The number of pulse beats you count each minute is the same as the number of times your heart beats every minute."

Next, make sure the patient understands the target heart rates his doctor has set for him. Explain that these rates are based on the results of his exercise electrocardiogram (EKG) or treadmill test. These tests show his maximum attainable heart rate. Taking 70% to 85% of that gives you the target heart rate range. Then, answer the patient's questions.

Now, you are ready to show him the proper technique for taking a pulse. Make sure he has a watch or clock with a second hand. Then, show him how to place his index and middle fingers on his radial pulse. Warn him not to use his thumb, since it has a strong pulse of its own, which may confuse him.

Tell the patient to press firmly until he feels the pulse beat. Ask him to count the beats for exactly 1 minute, while he observes his watch's second hand.

Important: To take his pulse rate during exercise, the patient should count for only 15 seconds, then multiply by 4. He may cool down too quickly if he counts an entire minute.

For safety, do not encourage the patient to take his carotid pulse. Pressure on the carotid artery may produce dysrhythmias or asystole.

If the patient plans to exercise at home, encourage him to write down his pulse rate and the time, date, and what he was doing just before taking his pulse. The doctor will use this information to assess the patient's recovery.

Important: Instruct the patient to call the doctor if his pulse ever seems faint, irregular, too fast, or too slow. (See *Monitoring Your Heart Rate*, page 458.)

Counseling the cardiac patient about sex

What you should know: The cardiac patient is in a dilemma: He would like to

Cardiac Teaching Program: Five Sessions

ONE
• How heart functions (including its anatomy)
• How and why coronary arteries harden
• How heart heals after a heart attack
• How heart is affected by these risk factors: stress, smoking, high blood pressure, high cholesterol and triglyceride levels in blood, obesity, uncontrolled diabetes, lack of exercise, family history

TWO
• What patient's personal risk factors are
• How to reduce risk factors while he is in hospital
• How to minimize risk factors after discharge

THREE
• How blood cholesterol contributes to hardening of coronary arteries
• How patient can reduce level of blood cholesterol by limiting high-cholesterol foods and saturated fats in diet
• How excess sodium contributes to fluid retention
• What foods and seasonings contribute to excess sodium
• How to recognize warning signs of fluid retention

• How excess weight contributes to heart disease
• How to devise a plan for losing excess weight

FOUR
• How a progressive activity program helps the heart heal
• What activities are appropriate for patient after discharge
• When patient may resume sexual activity and what precautions to take
• How to devise a plan for conserving physical energy during usual daily activities
• Why he should continue with an exercise program after discharge
• How he should take his own pulse

FIVE
• How to recognize signs and symptoms of heart attack and distinguish them from those of angina pectoris
• How to devise a plan for responding to a heart attack (or other cardiac emergency)
• What medications doctor has prescribed, and what each one is for
• How and when to take each medication
• What side effects are possible with each medication, and how to deal with them
• What special precautions medications require

know if he can resume sexual activity, but he is too shy to ask anyone about it. So instead of waiting for him to broach the subject, take the initiative yourself. Break the ice by giving him a pamphlet on sexual activity for patients who have had cardiac problems.

After he has done some reading, ask for his comments. If he is reluctant to discuss the subject, respect his wishes. Usually, though, when a patient knows the subject is not taboo, he will eagerly

share his concerns.

What do you need to know to answer his questions? Consider the following:
Q. Is sexual activity dangerous for a cardiac patient?
A. No, provided the doctor has given him an OK. For the heart, sex is just a moderate form of exercise, no more stressful than a brisk walk. However, sexual activity can become dangerous if it is accompanied by great emotional stress. For example, the patient may

---

Criteria for Terminating Exercise

Exercise will be terminated immediately if any of the following responses occur.

• **Blood Pressure:** any decrease in systolic blood pressure increase in systolic blood pressure greater than 20 mm Hg.

• **Heart Rate and Rhythm:** increase of 20 beats above resting heart rate decrease of 10 beats/minute below resting heart rate development of arrhythmias

• **Subjective Complaints:** chest pain, SOB, diaphoresis, fatigue, dizziness

Albert Einstein Medical Center, Mt. Sinai— Daroff Division

---

place an additional burden on his heart if he has extramarital sex.

Q. When can my patient safely resume sexual activity?

A. That is up to the doctor, based on his assessment of the patient's recovery. But most patients can resume sexual activity within 6 weeks of a heart attack.

Q. Should my patient reduce or modify sexual activity?

A. Probably not, unless he suffers from advanced congestive heart failure, unstable dysrhythmias or angina, or severe heart tissue damage. If his sex life must be curtailed for one of these reasons, suggest that he and his partner receive special counseling from a sex therapist, marriage counselor, or psychiatrist.

Q. Should my patient take any special precautions during sexual activity?

A. Yes. For guidelines, review the list of Do's and Don'ts below.

Q. How can I help if the patient loses sexual desire or his ability to perform?

A. Try to find the cause of the problem. Some patients lose their desire for sex because they are depressed; others are afraid sex will trigger another heart attack. (The partners of cardiac patients may be overcome by this fear, too.) If

your patient is fearful or depressed, urge him to discuss his anxieties with his partner. Counseling, education, and support by you or a professional therapist or support group will also help.

Keep in mind that cardiac medications may cause impotence in some patients. If your patient suffers this side effect, tell him to discuss it with his doctor.

What the patient should know: Do not let your patient leave the hospital before you have discussed how he can safely resume sexual activity. If possible, include his partner in the discussion. Use these Do's and Don'ts as a guide:

DON'T be afraid to resume sexual activity with your partner. A satisfying sex life can help speed your recovery.

DO choose a quiet, familiar setting for sex. A strange environment may cause stress. Make sure the room temperature is moderate; excessive heat or cold makes your heart work harder.

DO choose times when you are rested and relaxed. Avoid sex when you are fatigued or emotionally upset. A good time for sex is the morning, after a good night's sleep.

DON'T have sex after drinking a lot of alcohol. Alcohol expands your blood vessels, which makes the heart work harder.

DO choose positions that are relaxing and permit unrestricted breathing. Any position that is comfortable for you is OK. Don't be afraid to experiment. At first, you may be more comfortable if your partner assumes a dominant role.

DO ask your doctor if you should take nitroglycerin before sexual activity. This medication can prevent angina attacks during or after sex.

DO call your doctor at once if you have any of these symptoms after sexual activity:

• sweating or palpitations for 15 minutes or longer

• breathlessness or increased heart rate for 15 minutes or longer

• chest pain or angina that is not relieved by two or three nitroglycerin tab-

lets or a rest period
• sleeplessness after sexual activity or extreme fatigue the following day.

Low-level treadmill test
Before discharge, a low-level treadmill test (LLTT) may be performed. The test has three purposes:
1.) to provide the doctor with quantitative information on the patient's cardiovascular response to exercise
2.) to determine functional exercise capacity that can help in formulating guidelines for activity after discharge (See *Using MET Measurements to Determine Safe Activity Levels,* pages 460 and 461.)
3.) to try to predict the patient's mortality in the year following his MI.

Unlike the maximal strength stress test, the LLTT is done at lower intensity and smaller graduations. Monitoring is done before, during, and after the exercise.

Establishing home exercise guidelines
The patient's physical rehabilitation will continue after he leaves the hospital. Most likely, the doctor will prescribe an exercise routine that includes a daily walk and will also set a target heart rate for the patient to achieve.

Before the patient leaves your care, teach him how to determine his heart rate by taking his pulse. Then, give him these exercise guidelines:
• Do not walk right after a meal. Wait about 2 hours.
• Do not walk in extreme heat or cold. The best temperature range is 40° to 85° F. (4.4° to 29.4° C.). If the weather is unpleasant, try walking in an indoor shopping mall.
• Wear comfortable shoes and loose-fitting clothes.
• Warm up for 3 to 5 minutes before walking (or beginning any other prolonged exercise). Perform the warm-up exercises you learned in the hospital or outpatient facility; for example, arm circles, toe raises, trunk twists, front and side bends, and stretching.

• Walk at an even pace, maintaining the speed your doctor has prescribed. As you walk, rhythmically swing your arms at your sides.
• After your walk, cool down slowly. Walk in place while you take your pulse. Then, walk slowly for about 5 more minutes before stopping. This maintains good circulation while your heart rate returns to normal.
• Do not exceed your target heart rate. If your pulse rate rises above your target heart rate, walk more slowly next time.
• Notify your doctor if your pulse is irregular after your walk or if you experience pain in your chest, teeth, ears, jaw, or arms, or extreme breathlessness, fatigue, dizziness, nausea, or vomiting. (See *Learning Walking Speeds,* page 459.)

OUTPATIENT PROGRAM

Continuing rehabilitation after hospital discharge

Outpatient cardiac rehabilitation facilities are usually run by a team that includes nurses, doctors, and physical therapists. Together, they help patients return to active lives.

The nurse is usually responsible for tailoring the program to each patient's needs. To do this, assess the patient before he begins the program, and follow these guidelines:
• Conduct a thorough assessment interview. Explore the patient's cardiac history, and note the medications he is taking. Then, find out how well he understands his condition, and identify his risk factors. Finally, try to determine how well he has adjusted, emotionally and psychologically, to his heart condition. All of this information helps you decide how much teaching and counseling the patient needs.
• Set rehabilitation goals based on the patient's age, condition, and desired activity level. Discuss his plans with him. For example, suppose he plans to return

Monitoring Your Heart Rate

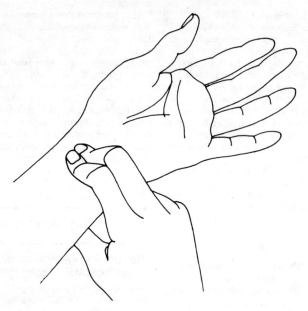

Your doctor has given you exercise guidelines. Follow these special instructions: _____
_____
_____
_____
_____
_____
_____
_____ .

During exercise, monitor your heart rate, as the nurse taught you. Use this teaching aid as a reminder of what you have learned.

Your target heart rate is _____ . beats/minute. Try to maintain this rate when you exercise.

How can you check your heart rate? First, get a watch with a second hand. Then, as soon as you stop exercising, take your pulse.

Place your index and middle fingers on your wrist just below the thumb, as shown below. (Do not use your thumb to feel for a pulse—it has a strong pulse of its own, which may confuse you.)

Count the pulse beats for 15 seconds; then, multiply by 4. This gives you a reliable estimate of your working heart rate for 1 minute. (Do not count your pulse for a whole minute. Because your heart rate slows quickly when you rest, that figure will not be reliable.)

If your working heart rate is 10 beats or more above your target heart rate, do not work so hard the next time. But if your working heart rate is lower than your target rate, work a little *harder* next time. For instance, if you walk, walk faster—or even jog, if the doctor approves.

Learning Walking Speeds

When the doctor or physical therapist designs a patient's exercise program, he will specify walking speeds. For example, he may tell the patient to walk at a speed of 2 miles per hour (0.4 km at 3 km/hr). Can you explain to the patient what this means, in terms he can understand? Tell him how many METs he consumes at each speed, and use this chart as a guide.

Speed							
mph	2	2.5	3	3.5	4	4.5	5
km/hr	3.2	4	4.8	5.6	6.4	7.2	8
Number of paces every 15 seconds	15	18 to 19	22	26	30	34	37 to 38
Number of paces every minute	60	75	88	104	120	135	150
METs	2 to 3	2 to 3	3 to 4	4 to 5	5 to 6	5 to 6	6 to 7

Note: 10 city blocks approximates 1 mile (1.6 km)

to a job that requires lifting and would also like to resume playing golf. To help him reach these goals, design an exercise program that emphasizes arm exercises, using equipment such as a rowing machine and an arm ergometer.

• Obtain the results of a low-level exercise EKG (stress test). Most likely, the patient underwent this test before discharge. If not, the doctor will order one before the patient begins an exercise program. The information provided by an exercise EKG helps you and the doctor devise an appropriate exercise prescription for the patient.

• If ordered, take blood samples for laboratory studies. Once you know the patient's fasting cholesterol, triglyceride, and high-density lipoprotein levels, you can suggest diet modifications, if necessary.

Education

Of course, not all information taught during the inpatient phase of cardiac rehabilitation is learned or retained. Thus, an important part of the outpatient program is providing patients, families, and friends with additional information so they can better learn to live with cardiac illness. This is done in two ways: by incidental teaching that occurs at exercise sessions each day and by formal outpatient education.

Incidental teaching. As participants discuss diet, exercise, and risk factors, they begin to ask many questions. Consequently, individual and informal small-group education occurs during daily exercise sessions.

Group education. These programs can be held before or after exercise sessions or as evening sessions and are planned and implemented according to the needs of the patient, family, and community. The cardiac rehabilitation team speaks or participates with guest speakers, and those attending ask questions and share experiences.

Psychosocial Support

The patient with extensive coronary heart disease sees a tremendous alteration in his life-style. Inability to return to work often causes role changes at home. Inactivity due to the extent of disease, fear, or lack of knowledge can cause overprotection by spouses and loss of autonomy and independence. Restrictions on cigarettes, alcohol, or food can

Using MET Measurements to Determine Safe Activity Levels

Suppose, after the patient's exercise EKG (stress test), or low-level treadmill test, the doctor tells you that the patient can safely tolerate 8 metabolic energy equivalents (METs) of activity. Do you know how this translates into daily activity? More important, can you explain it to the patient in words he will understand? The information on this page can help.

An MET is an amount of metabolic energy consumed at rest. When the patient uses 1 MET of energy, his body consumes about 3.5 ml of oxygen/kilogram of body weight each minute.

What does this mean to the patient? The chart below provides practical guidelines. Refer to it when you discuss safe activity levels with any patient. *Note:* Keep in mind that these are only general guidelines—general fitness, excitement, fatigue, or emotional stress may alter MET levels for any activity.

1 MET
Home activities
- Bed rest
- Sitting
- Eating
- Reading
- Sewing
- Watching television

Occupational activities
- No activity allowed

Exercise or sports activities
- No activity allowed

1 to 2 METs
Home activities
- Dressing
- Shaving
- Brushing teeth
- Washing at sink
- Making bed
- Desk work
- Driving car
- Playing cards
- Knitting

Occupational activities
- Typing (electric typewriter)

Exercise or sports activities
- Walking 1 mph (1.6 km/hr) on level ground

2 to 3 METs
Home activities
- Tub bathing
- Cooking
- Waxing floor
- Riding power lawn mower
- Playing piano

Occupational activities
- Driving small truck
- Using hand tools
- Typing (manual typewriter)
- Repairing car

Exercise or sports activities
- Walking 2 mph (3.2 km/hr) on level ground
- Bicycling 5 mph (8 km/hr) on level ground
- Playing billiards

- Fishing
- Bowling
- Golfing (with motor cart)
- Operating motorboat
- Riding horseback (at walk)

3 to 4 METs
Home activities
- General housework
- Cleaning windows
- Light gardening
- Pushing light power mower
- Sexual intercourse

Occupational activities
- Assembly-line work
- Driving large truck
- Bricklaying
- Plastering

Exercise or sports activities
- Walking 3 mph (4.8 km/hr)
- Bicycling 6 mph (9.7 km/hr)
- Sailing
- Golfing (pulling hand cart)
- Pitching horseshoes

- Archery
- Badminton (doubles)
- Horseback riding (at slow trot)
- Fly-fishing

4 to 5 METs
Home activities
- Heavy housework
- Heavy gardening
- Home repairs, including painting and light carpentry
- Raking leaves
Occupational activities
- Painting
- Masonry
- Paperhanging
Exercise or sports activities
- Calisthenics
- Table tennis
- Golfing (carrying bag)
- Tennis (doubles)
- Dancing
- Slow swimming

5 to 6 METs
Home activities
- Sawing softwood
- Digging garden
- Shoveling light loads
Occupational activities
- Using heavy tools
- Lifting 50 lbs
Exercise or sports activities
- Walking 4 mph (6.4 km/hr)

- Bicycling 10 mph (16.1 km/hr)
- Skating
- Fishing with waders
- Hiking
- Hunting
- Square dancing
- Horseback riding (at brisk trot)

6 to 7 METs
Home activities
- Shoveling snow
- Splitting wood
- Mowing lawn with hand mower
Occupational activities
- All activities listed previously
Exercise or sports activities
- Walking or jogging 5 mph (8.0 km/hr)
- Bicycling 11 mph (17.7 km/hr)
- Tennis (singles)
- Waterskiing
- Light downhill skiing

7 to 8 METs
Home activities
- Sawing hardwood
Occupational activities
- Digging ditches
- Lifting 80 lbs
- Moving heavy furniture
Exercise or sports activities
- Paddleball
- Touch football

- Swimming (backstroke)
- Basketball
- Ice hockey

8 to 9 METs
Home activities
- All activities listed previously
Occupational activities
- Lifting 100 lbs
Exercise or sports activities
- Running 5.5 mph (8.9 km/hr)
- Bicycling 13 mph (20.9 km/hr)
- Swimming (breaststroke)
- Handball (noncompetitive)
- Cross-country skiing
- Fencing

10 or more METs
Home activities
- All activities listed previously
Occupational activities
- All activities listed previously
Exercise or sports activities
- Running 6 mph (9.7 km/hr) or faster
- Handball (competitive)
- Squash (competitive)
- Gymnastics
- Football (contact)

make a patient feel even more deprived. In many instances, these alterations isolate him from his friends and family at the time when he needs companionship most.

Informal supervised exercise sessions and group psychological support sessions can help patients accept their disease, vent frustrations, and find friendship and companionship.

Evaluation

Evaluation is an ongoing process in the outpatient as well as inpatient program. Most evaluation occurs during the physical activity section of the outpatient program, when the patient is observed at exercise sessions and his objective (blood pressure, EKG, and pulse response) and subjective (how he perceives his work load) reactions are monitored. He also is reevaluated for functional work capacity and cardiovascular response at 3-month intervals while he is in the supervised program and at 6-month intervals after he progresses into an unsupervised home-maintenance program.

When the patient completes the supervised outpatient program, his entrance goals are reviewed along with the overall program objectives. He then formulates his revised maintenance goals and makes these plans: to return for follow-up exercise test evaluations, to maintain regular telephone contact with the nurses (1 or 2 times per month) concerning his home exercise, and to try to return for monthly meetings.

Selected References

Andreoli, Kathleen, et al. *Comprehensive Cardiac Care: A Text for Nurses, Physicians, and Other Health Practitioners,* 5th ed. St. Louis: C.V. Mosby Co., 1983.

Cornett, Sandra J., and Watson, Joan E. *Cardiac Rehabilitation: An Interdisciplinary Team Approach.* New York: John Wiley & Sons, 1984.

Fardy, Paul S., et al. *Cardiac Rehabilitation: Implications for the Nurse and Other Health Professionals.* St. Louis: C.V. Mosby Co., 1980.

Fischbach, Frances. *A Manual of Laboratory Diagnostic Tests,* 2nd ed. Philadelphia: J.B. Lippincott Co., 1984.

Fowler, Noble O. *Cardiac Diagnosis and Treatment,* 3rd ed. New York: Harper & Row Publishers, 1980.

Guzzetta, Cathie C., and Dossey, Barbara M. *Cardiovascular Nursing: Bodymind Tapestry.* St. Louis: C.V. Mosby Co., 1984.

Hurst, J. Willis, et al. *The Heart,* 5th ed. New York: McGraw-Hill Book Co., 1982.

Jackle, Mary, and Halligan, Marney. *Cardiovascular Problems: A Critical Care Nursing Focus.* Bowie, Md.: Robert J. Brady Co., 1980.

Kim, Mi J., et al. *Classification of Nursing Diagnoses: Proceedings of the Fifth National Conference.* St. Louis: C.V. Mosby Co., 1984.

Nieminski, K.E., et al. "Current Concepts and Management of the Sick Sinus Syndrome," *Heart & Lung* 13(6):675-81, November 1984.

Nissen, M.B. "Streptokinase Therapy in Acute Myocardial Infarction," *Heart & Lung* 13(3):223-30, May 1984.

Page, G.G. "Patent Ductus Arteriosus in the Premature Neonate," *Heart & Lung* 14(2):156-62, March 1985.

Parker, M.M., and Lemberg, L. "Pacemaker Update 1984, Part IV: DDD Pacemaker—Electrocardiographic Assessment and Problem Solving," *Heart & Lung* 13(6):687-90, November 1984.

Riedinger, M.S., and Shellock, F.G. "Technical Aspects of the Thermodilution Method for Measuring Cardiac Output," *Heart & Lung* 13(3):215-22, May 1984.

Sadler, D. *Nursing for Cardiovascular Health.* East Norwalk, Conn.: Appleton-Century-Crofts, 1983.

Shoemaker, William C., et al. *The Society of Critical Care Medicine: Textbook of Critical Care.* Philadelphia: W.B. Saunders Co., 1984.

Underhill, Sandra L., and Woods, Susan L. *Cardiac Nursing.* Philadelphia: J.B. Lippincott Co., 1982.

Wells, Sara J., et al. *Manual of Cardiovascular Assessment.* Reston, Va.: Reston Publishing Co., 1982.

Wenger, Nanette K., et al. *Cardiology for Nurses.* New York: McGraw-Hill Book Co., 1980.

Nurse's Guide to Cardiovascular Conditions

Angina pectoris

CHIEF COMPLAINT
• *Chest pain:* may be dull or burning, or described as pressure, tightness, heaviness; builds and fades gradually; may be in abdomen; may radiate to jaw, teeth, face, or left arm
• *Dyspnea:* possible, with sense of constriction around larynx or upper trachea
• *Fatigue:* absent
• *Irregular heartbeat:* may be present; patient complains of palpitations or skipped beats
• *Peripheral changes:* none

HISTORY
• Risk factors include family history of coronary artery disease, arteriosclerotic heart disease, cerebrovascular accident (CVA), diabetes, gout, hypertension, renal disease, obesity caused by excessive carbohydrate and saturated fat intake, smoking, lack of exercise, and stress.
• Higher incidence in men over age 40; lower incidence in women prior to menopause
• Precipitating factors include exertion, stress, cold or hot weather, and emotional excitement.

PHYSICAL EXAMINATION
• Inspection reveals patient anxiety and diaphoresis.
• Palpation reveals tachycardia.
• Auscultation reveals change in blood pressure, possibly hypertension, especially during anginal attack; transient rales associated with congestive heart failure (CHF); paradoxical splitting of S_2 possible.

DIAGNOSTIC STUDIES
• Electrocardiogram (EKG) may show depressed ST segments during ischemia attack but may be within normal limits; atrioventricular conduction defect
• Thallium stress imaging or stress EKG may show ischemic areas.

Acute myocardial infarction

CHIEF COMPLAINT
• *Chest pain:* sudden but not instantaneous onset of constricting, crushing, heavy weightlike chest pain occurring at any time—not relieved by nitroglycerin; located centrally and substernally, although not usually in left chest; may build rapidly or in waves to maximum intensity in a few minutes; may be accompanied by nausea and vomiting
• *Dyspnea:* present; may be accompanied by orthopnea, cough, and wheezing
• *Fatigue:* present; indicated by weakness and apprehension
• *Irregular heartbeat:* may be present; patient complains of palpitations or skipped beats
• *Peripheral changes:* peripheral cyanosis, with decreased perfusion

HISTORY
• Risk factors same as in angina pectoris
• Past medical history may include episodes of angina pectoris.

PHYSICAL EXAMINATION
• Fever after 24 hours
• Inspection reveals anxiety, tenseness, sense of impending doom, nausea, vomiting, and possibly distended neck veins, sweating, pallor, cyanosis, and shock.
• Palpation reveals tachycardia or bradycardia and weak pulse.
• Auscultation reveals normal or decreased blood pressure (less than 80 mm Hg), significant murmurs that may preexist or occur with ruptured sep-

tum or ruptured papillary muscle, diminished gallop rhythm, pericardial friction rub and rales.

• In severe attack, shock, decreased urinary output, pulmonary edema.

DIAGNOSTIC STUDIES

• EKG at onset shows elevated ST segment, which then returns to baseline; T waves become symmetrically inverted; abnormal Q waves present; may also show dysrhythmias

• White blood cell (WBC) count shows leukocytosis on second day (lasts 1 week); erythrocyte sedimentation rate normal at first, rises on second or third day

• Enzyme testing shows elevated creatine phosphokinase (CPK) and CPK-MB initially; then increased serum glutamic-oxaloacetic transaminase.

Left ventricular failure

CHIEF COMPLAINT

• *Chest pain:* usually absent
• *Dyspnea:* present on exertion, accompanied by cough, orthopnea, paroxysmal nocturnal dyspnea; in advanced disease, present at rest
• *Fatigue:* present on exertion, accompanied by weakness
• *Irregular heartbeat:* may be present; patient may complain of rapid heart rate and skipped beats

HISTORY

• Patient uses pillow to prop self up for sleep; wakes up gasping for breath; must sit or stand for relief

• History of present illness includes wheezing on inspiration and expiration (cardiac asthma), right upper abdominal pain or discomfort on exertion, daytime oliguria, nighttime polyuria, constipation (uncommon), anorexia, progressive weight gain,

generalized edema, progressive weakness, fatigue, decreased mentation.

• Past medical history includes severe CHF.

PHYSICAL EXAMINATION

• Inspection reveals profuse sweating, pallor or cyanosis, frothy white or pink sputum, heaving apical impulse, hand veins that remain distended when patient puts hands above level of right atrium.

• Palpation reveals enlarged, diffuse, and sustained left ventricular impulse at precordium, displaced to left; pulsus alternans at peripheral pulses.

• Percussion reveals pleural fluid (indicated by dullness at lung bases) and decreased tactile fremitus.

• Auscultation reveals S_3 and S_4 sounds, possibly mitral and tricuspid regurgitation murmurs, accentuated pulmonary component of second sound, decreased or absent breath sounds, rales (basilar) that do not clear on cough.

DIAGNOSTIC STUDIES

• Pulmonary artery and pulmonary capillary wedge pressures elevated
• Central venous pressure elevated if condition has advanced to right ventricular failure, or hypervolemia from increased sodium and water retention
• EKG reflects heart strain or left ventricular enlargement, ischemia, and dysrhythmias.
• X-ray shows left atrial enlargement and pulmonary venous congestion.

Acute right ventricular failure

CHIEF COMPLAINT

• *Chest pain:* usually absent
• *Dyspnea:* respiratory distress secondary to pulmonary disease or advanced left ventricular failure
• *Fatigue:* in severe cases, weakness

(continued)

Nurse's Guide to Cardiovascular Conditions *continued*

and mental aberration
• *Irregular heartbeat:* atrial dysrhythmias common
• *Peripheral changes:* dependent edema: begins in ankles but progresses to legs and genitalia; initially subsides at night, later does not; ascites; weight gain

HISTORY
• History of present illness includes anorexia, right upper abdominal pain or discomfort during exertion, nausea, and vomiting.
• Past medical history includes left ventricular failure, mitral stenosis, pulmonic valve stenosis, tricuspid regurgitation, pulmonary hypertension, chronic obstructive pulmonary disease.

PHYSICAL EXAMINATION
• Inspection reveals lower sternal or left parasternal heave independent of apical impulse.
• Palpation and percussion reveal enlarged, tender, pulsating liver, with tricuspid regurgitation; abdomen fluid wave and shifting dullness; hepatojugular reflux, indicating jugular vein distention; tachycardia.
• Auscultation reveals right ventricular S_3 sound; murmur of tricuspid regurgitation.

DIAGNOSTIC STUDIES
• Central venous pressure readings are elevated.

Cardiomyopathies

CHIEF COMPLAINT
• *Dyspnea:* paroxysmal nocturnal, accompanied by orthopnea
• *Fatigue:* present
• *Irregular heartbeat:* palpitations; Stokes-Adams attacks with conduction defects

• *Peripheral changes:* dry skin, extremity pain, edema and ascites with right-sided failure

HISTORY
• Past medical history includes viral illness, alcoholism, chronic debilitating illnesses.

PHYSICAL EXAMINATION
• Fever
• Signs of right or left heart failure
• Palpation reveals displaced cardiac impulse to left; tachycardia.
• Auscultation reveals systolic murmur, S_3 sound, and postural hypotension.

DIAGNOSTIC STUDIES
• EKG reveals nonspecific ST-T changes, decreased height of R wave; may show dysrhythmias and conduction defects (especially atrial fibrillation).
• Echocardiography and chest X-ray may help determine heart size.

Idiopathic hypertrophic subaortic stenosis (IHSS) or asymmetric septal hypertrophy

CHIEF COMPLAINT
• *Chest pain:* present; similar to angina pectoris, but unrelieved by nitroglycerin
• *Dyspnea:* present on exertion
• *Fatigue:* present; accompanied by dizziness and syncope
• *Irregular heartbeat:* may be present; patient may complain of palpitations or skipped beats
• *Peripheral changes:* peripheral edema (uncommon)

HISTORY
• Symptoms may be induced by high temperatures, pregnancy, exercise, standing suddenly, Valsalva's maneuver.

PHYSICAL EXAMINATION
• Palpation reveals peripheral pulse with characteristic double impulse.

- Auscultation reveals systolic ejection murmur.
- In advanced stage, signs of mitral insufficiency (such as systolic murmur), CHF, and sudden death possible

DIAGNOSTIC STUDIES
- EKG reveals left ventricular hypertrophy, ST segment, and T wave abnormalities.
- Echocardiography shows increased thickness of the interventricular system and abnormal motion of the mitral valve.

Pericarditis

CHIEF COMPLAINT
- *Chest pain:* sudden onset; precordial or substernal, pleuritic, radiating to left neck, shoulder, back, or epigastrium; worsened by lying down or swallowing
- *Dyspnea:* usually absent; breathing may cause pain
- *Fatigue:* usually absent
- *Irregular heartbeat:* absent
- *Peripheral changes:* none

HISTORY
- Past medical history includes viral respiratory infection, recent pericardiotomy or MI, disseminated lupus erythematosus, serum sickness, acute rheumatic fever, trauma, uremia, lymphoma, dissecting aorta.
- Most common in men between ages 20 and 50

PHYSICAL EXAMINATION
- Fever: 100° to 103° F. (37.8° to 39.4° C.)
- Palpation reveals tachycardia.
- Auscultation reveals pericardial friction rub.

DIAGNOSTIC STUDIES
- EKG shows ST-T segment elevation in all leads; returns to baseline in a few days, with T wave inversion.
- Possibly atrial fibrillation

Pericarditis with effusion

CHIEF COMPLAINT
- *Chest pain:* may be present as dull, diffuse oppressive precordial or substernal distress; dysphagia
- *Dyspnea:* present; associated with cough that causes patient to lean forward for relief
- *Fatigue:* usually absent
- *Irregular heartbeat:* absent
- *Peripheral changes:* none

HISTORY
- Past medical history includes uremia, malignancy, connective tissue disorder, viral pericarditis.

PHYSICAL EXAMINATION
- Inspection reveals distended neck veins.
- Palpation and percussion reveal tachycardia, enlarged area of cardiac dullness, apical beat that is within dullness border or not palpable.
- Auscultation reveals abnormal blood pressure and possibly pericardial friction rub, and acute cardiac tamponade (inspiratory distention of neck veins, narrow pulse pressure, paradoxic pulse); may progress to shock.

DIAGNOSTIC STUDIES
- EKG shows flat T waves, low diphasic or inverted leads, QRS voltage uniformly low.

Subacute and acute bacterial endocarditis

CHIEF COMPLAINT
- *Chest pain:* present; also in abdomen and flanks (uncommon)
- *Dyspnea:* present in approximately 50% of cases; depends on severity of

(continued)

Nurse's Guide to Cardiovascular Conditions *continued*

disease or valve involved
- *Fatigue:* present, usually as malaise
- *Irregular heartbeat:* absent
- *Peripheral changes:* weight loss, redness or swelling, heart failure symptoms

HISTORY
- Present or recent history includes acute infection, surgery or instrumentation, dental work, drug abuse, abortion, transurethral prostatectomy.
- Past medical history includes rheumatic, congenital, or artherosclerotic heart disease.

PHYSICAL EXAMINATION
- Daily fever
- Inspection may reveal petechiae on conjunctivae and palate buccal mucosa; long-standing endocarditis, clubbed fingers and toes; splinter hemorrhages beneath nails; tender red nodules on finger and toe pads (Osler nodes); pallor or yellow-brown tint to skin; oval, pale, retinal lesion around optic disk (seen with ophthalmoscope)
- Palpation reveals splenomegaly.
- Auscultation reveals sudden change in present heart murmur or development of new murmur and possibly signs of early heart failure or emboli.

DIAGNOSTIC STUDIES
- Blood cultures determine causative organism.
- Echocardiography—particularly the two-dimensional (2-D) method—looks for vegetation.

Rheumatic fever (acute)

CHIEF COMPLAINT
- *Chest pain:* absent
- *Dyspnea:* may be present
- *Fatigue:* malaise
- *Irregular heartbeat:* absent
- *Peripheral changes:* weight loss

HISTORY
- Recent history includes streptococcal infection of upper respiratory tract (in previous 4 weeks), anorexia.
- Past medical history includes migratory, gradually beginning arthritis; recurrent epistaxis; "growing pains" in joints (arthralgia).
- Increased clumsiness

PHYSICAL EXAMINATION
- Usually low-grade fever, with sinus tachycardia disproportional to fever level
- Inspection reveals erythema marginatum (ring- or crescent-shaped macular rash), subcutaneous nodules (uncommon except in children), swollen joints (arthritis), Sydenham's chorea.
- Palpation reveals enlarged heart.
- Auscultation reveals mitral or aortic diastolic murmurs, varying heart sound quality, and possibly gallop rhythm dysrhythmias and ectopic beats.

DIAGNOSTIC STUDIES
- Erythrocyte sedimentation rate and WBC count elevated
- Throat cultures positive for beta-hemolytic streptococci
- Antistreptolysin titer elevated
- Chest X-ray may show cardiac enlargement.
- EKG shows PR greater than 0.2 seconds; may further define dysrhythmias.

Varicose veins

CHIEF COMPLAINT
- *Chest pain:* absent
- *Peripheral changes:* aching discomfort or pain in legs, pigmentation and ulceration of distal leg, possibly edema

HISTORY
• History of present illness includes leg cramps at night that may be relieved by leg elevation, itching in vein regions, leg fatigue caused by periods of standing.
• Past medical history includes thrombophlebitis and family history of varicosities.
PHYSICAL EXAMINATION
• Inspection reveals dilated tortuous vessels in legs, visible when patient stands; brown pigmentation and thinning of skin above ankles; ulceration of distal leg; positive Trendelenburg's test.
DIAGNOSTIC STUDIES
• None usually performed

Thrombophlebitis

CHIEF COMPLAINT
• *Chest pain:* present with pulmonary embolism
• *Peripheral changes:* pain and swelling of affected extremity; if leg veins affected, pain may increase with walking
HISTORY
• Childbirth 4 to 14 days before onset
• History of present illness includes fracture, trauma, deep vein surgery, cardiac disease, CVA, prolonged bed rest.
• Past medical history includes malignancy, shock, dehydration, anemia, obesity, chronic infection, use of oral contraceptives.
• In superficial vein thrombophlebitis, recent history includes superficial vein I.V. therapy with irritating solutions.
PHYSICAL EXAMINATION
• Slight fever
• In deep vein involvement, inspection

reveals, with severe venous obstruction, cyanotic skin in affected area; with reflex arterial spasm, pale, cool skin.
• Palpation reveals warm affected leg, spasm and pain in calf muscles with dorsiflexion of foot (positive Homans' sign).
• In superficial vein involvement, inspection reveals induration, redness, tenderness along course of vein; possibly no clinical manifestations.
DIAGNOSTIC STUDIES
• Ultrasound blood flow detector, thermography, and phlebography used to confirm diagnosis

---

Dissecting thoracic aortic aneurysms

CHIEF COMPLAINT
• *Chest pain:* present; sudden and severe, radiating to back, abdomen, and hips
• *Peripheral changes:* paralysis of legs possible
HISTORY
• Recent history may include convulsions.
• Past medical history includes hypertension, arteriosclerosis, congenital heart disease, Marfan's syndrome, pregnancy, trauma
PHYSICAL EXAMINATION
• Fever
• Palpation reveals unequal or diminished peripheral pulses.
• Auscultation reveals aortic diastolic murmur and murmurs over arteries.
DIAGNOSTIC STUDIES
• Aortography shows size and extent of aneurysm.

Abdominal aortic aneurysm

CHIEF COMPLAINT
• *Chest pain:* absent
• *Peripheral changes:* none

(continued)

Nurse's Guide to Cardiovascular Conditions *continued*

HISTORY
• Most common in men over age 50
PHYSICAL EXAMINATION
• Inspection reveals subcutaneous ecchymosis in flank or groin.
• Palpation reveals pulsating midabdominal and upper abdominal mass.
DIAGNOSTIC STUDIES
• Aortography shows size of aneurysm.
• EKG, urinalysis, blood urea nitrogen (BUN) evaluate renal and cardiac function.

Raynaud's disease and Raynaud's phenomenon

CHIEF COMPLAINT
• *Chest pain:* absent
• *Peripheral changes:* with Raynaud's disease: attacks of cyanosis, followed by pallor in fingers (rarely in thumbs or toes); redness, swelling, throbbing, and paresthesia during recovery, occurring when areas are warmed; numbness, stiffness, diminished sensation; with Raynaud's phenomenon: usually unilateral cyanosis, which may involve only one or two fingers
HISTORY
• Most common in women between puberty and age 40
• Precipitating factors include emotional upsets or a cold.
• Past history includes immunologic abnormalities.
• Family history of vasospastic diseases
• Raynaud's phenomenon may accompany cervical rib, carpal tunnel syndrome, scleroderma, systemic lupus erythematosus, frostbite, ergot poisoning.
PHYSICAL EXAMINATION
• Inspection reveals atrophy of terminal fat pads of fingers.
DIAGNOSTIC STUDIES
• None usually performed.

Tricuspid stenosis

CHIEF COMPLAINT
• *Chest pain:* usually absent
• *Dyspnea:* present in varying degrees
• *Fatigue:* present; often severe
• *Irregular heartbeat:* usually absent
• *Peripheral changes:* dependent peripheral edema
HISTORY
• Most common in women
• Past medical history includes mitral valve disease.
PHYSICAL EXAMINATION
• Inspection may reveal olive skin.
• Palpation may reveal presystolic liver pulsation if in sinus rhythm; middiastolic thrill between lower left sternal border and apical impulse.
• Auscultation reveals diastolic rumbling murmur heard along lower left sternal border, slow y descent in jugular pulse, normal blood pressure.
DIAGNOSTIC STUDIES
• EKG shows wide, tall, peaked P waves, normal axis.
• Echocardiography may permit stenosis recognition.
• X-ray shows enlarged right atrium.
• Cardiac catheterization may reveal site of stenosis.

Tricuspid regurgitation (incompetence)

CHIEF COMPLAINT
• *Chest pain:* absent
• *Dyspnea:* present
• *Fatigue:* present; tires easily
• *Irregular heartbeat:* atrial fibrillation; usually not noticed by patient
• *Peripheral changes:* none

HISTORY
• Past medical history includes right ventricular failure, rheumatic fever, trauma, endocarditis, pulmonary hypertension.
PHYSICAL EXAMINATION
• Palpation reveals right ventricular pulsation, systolic liver pulsation, and possibly systolic thrill at lower left sternal edge.
• Auscultation reveals blowing, coarse, or harsh systolic murmur heard along lower left sternal border; increases on inspiration.
DIAGNOSTIC STUDIES
• EKG usually shows atrial fibrillation.

Aortic stenosis

CHIEF COMPLAINT
• *Chest pain:* present in severe stenosis
• *Dyspnea:* present, with coughing, on exertion; paroxysmal nocturnal
• *Fatigue:* usually present; syncope
• *Irregular heartbeat:* present, as palpitations occasionally
HISTORY
• More common in men
• Usually asymptomatic unless severe
PHYSICAL EXAMINATION
• Inspection reveals apical impulse localized and heaving, usually not laterally displaced.
• Palpation reveals sustained localized forceful apical impulse; systolic thrill over aortic area and neck vessels; small, slowly rising plateau pulse, best appreciated in carotid pulse.
• Auscultation reveals harsh, rough, systolic ejection murmur in aortic area, radiating to the neck and apex; possibly systolic ejection click at aortic area just before murmur; paradoxical splitting of second sound with significant stenosis; normal or high diastolic blood pressure.

DIAGNOSTIC STUDIES
• EKG shows criteria for left ventricular hypertrophy; possibly complete heart block.
• X-rays and fluoroscopy may show calcified aortic valve, poststenotic dilatation of ascending aorta (hyperactivity evident with fluoroscopy), left ventricular hypertrophy.
• Echocardiography may identify level of obstruction and a bicuspid aortic valve.
• Cardiac catheterization indicates the severity and location of the obstruction as well as left ventricular function.

Aortic regurgitation (incompetence)

CHIEF COMPLAINT
• *Chest pain:* angina pectoris
• *Dyspnea:* on exertion early in disease; paroxysmal nocturnal dyspnea; orthopnea and cough signal beginning of decompensation
• *Fatigue:* present; weakness if left ventricular failure present
• *Irregular heartbeat:* palpitations (signal beginning of decompensation)
• *Peripheral changes:* none
HISTORY
• Past medical history includes Reiter's syndrome, rheumatoid arthritis, psoriasis, rheumatic fever, syphilis, subacute bacterial endocarditis.
PHYSICAL EXAMINATION
• Inspection reveals generalized skin pallor; strong, abrupt carotid pulsations; forceful apical impulse to left of left midclavicular line and downward; capillary pulsations.
• Palpation reveals sustained and forceful apical impulse, displaced to

(continued)

Nurse's Guide to Cardiovascular Conditions *continued*

left and downward; rapidly rising and collapsing pulses.
• Auscultation reveals normal heart sounds; soft, blowing, diastolic murmur (heard over aortic area and apex; usually loudest along left sternal border); in advanced aortic insufficiency, Austin Flint murmur that may be heard at apex; with diastolic pressure less than 60 mm Hg, possibly wide pulse pressure.
DIAGNOSTIC STUDIES
• EKG shows evidence of left ventricular hypertrophy.
• X-ray shows enlarged left ventricle.
• Echocardiography helps establish aortic valve incompetence.
• Cardiac catheterization and angiocardiography performed to exclude complicating lesions and to assess left ventricular function and magnitude of leak.

Mitral stenosis

CHIEF COMPLAINT
• *Chest pain:* usually absent
• *Dyspnea:* present; induced by exertion; may also occur during rest; orthopnea; paroxysmal nocturnal dyspnea; hemoptysis
• *Fatigue:* present; increased with decreased exercise tolerance
• *Irregular heartbeat:* usually absent
• *Peripheral changes:* extremity pain
HISTORY
• Most common in women under age 45
• Recent bronchitis or upper respiratory tract infection may worsen symptoms.
• Past medical history includes rheumatic fever, congenital valve disorder, tumor (myxoma).
PHYSICAL EXAMINATION
• Inspection reveals malar flush; in young patients, precordial bulge and

diffuse pulsation.
• Palpation reveals tapping sensation over area of expected apical impulse, middiastolic or presystolic thrill at apex, small pulse, overactive right ventricle with elevated pulmonary pressure.
• Auscultation reveals localized, delayed, rumbling, low-pitched, diastolic murmur at or near apex (duration of murmur varies depending on severity of stenosis; onset of murmur at opening snap early in diastole); possibly loud S_2 with elevated pulmonary pressure; normal blood pressure.
DIAGNOSTIC STUDIES
• EKG shows notched and broad P waves in standard leads, inverted P in V_1 lead; atrial fibrillation common.
• X-ray and fluoroscopy show left atrial enlargement.
• Echocardiography helps assess severity of stenosis.
• Cardiac catheterization and angiocardiography help determine amount of regurgitation that may also be present.

Mitral regurgitation (incompetence)

CHIEF COMPLAINT
• *Chest pain:* absent
• *Dyspnea:* present, progressive with exertion; orthopnea, paroxysmal dyspnea
• *Fatigue:* present, progressive with exertion
• *Irregular heartbeat:* present as palpitations
• *Peripheral changes:* none
HISTORY
• Past medical history includes rheumatic fever, endocarditis, congenital

mitral valve defect, papillary muscle dysfunction or rupture, chordae tendinae dysfunction or rupture, heart failure associated with left ventricular dilation, blunt injury to the chest.

PHYSICAL EXAMINATION
• Inspection reveals forceful apical impulse to left of left midclavicular line.
• Palpation reveals forceful, brisk apical impulse; systolic thrill over apical impulse; normal, small, or slightly collapsing pulse.
• Auscultation reveals blowing, high-pitched, harsh, or musical pansystolic apical murmur maximal at apex and transmitted to axilla; abnormally wide splitting of S_2; possibly S_3 present; normal blood pressure.

DIAGNOSTIC STUDIES
• EKG shows P waves broad or notched in standard leads; with pulmonary hypertension, tall peaked P waves, right axis deviation, or right ventricular hypertrophy; possibly atrial fibrillation.
• X-ray shows enlargement of left ventricle and moderate aneurysmal dilatation of left atrium.
• Echocardiography shows dilated left ventricle and left atrium; pattern of contraction of left ventricle suggests diastolic overload.
• Cardiac catheterization and ventriculography help determine amount of regurgitation and identify prolapsing cusps.

Pulmonic stenosis

CHIEF COMPLAINT
• *Chest pain:* usually not present
• *Dyspnea:* present on exertion
• *Fatigue:* present
• *Irregular heartbeat:* absent
• *Peripheral changes:* peripheral edema possible

HISTORY
• Congenital stenosis or rheumatic heart disease, associated with other congenital heart defects, such as tetralogy of Fallot.

PHYSICAL EXAMINATION
• Inspection reveals jugular vein distention.
• Palpation reveals hepatomegaly.
• Auscultation reveals systolic murmur at left sternal border and split S_2 sound, with delayed or absent pulmonic component.

DIAGNOSTIC STUDIES
• EKG shows right ventricular hypertrophy, right axis deviation, right atrial hypertrophy.

Pulmonic regurgitation (incompetence)

CHIEF COMPLAINT
• *Chest pain:* absent
• *Dyspnea:* present
• *Fatigue:* present; patient tires easily; weakness
• *Irregular heartbeat:* absent
• *Peripheral changes:* peripheral edema

HISTORY
• Pulmonary hypertension
• Congenital defect

PHYSICAL EXAMINATION
• Inspection reveals jugular vein distention.
• Palpation reveals hepatomegaly.
• Auscultation reveals diastolic murmur in pulmonic area.

DIAGNOSTIC STUDIES
• EKG shows right ventricular or right atrial enlargement.

Cardiac Dysrhythmias

Normal sinus rhythm (NSR) in adults

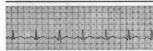

- Ventricular and atrial rates of 60 to 100 beats per minute (bpm)
- QRS complexes and P waves regular and uniform
- PR interval 0.12 to 0.2 second
- QRS duration < 0.12 second
- Identical atrial and ventricular rates, with constant PR interval

Sinus arrhythmia

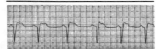

CAUSE
- Usually a normal variation of NSR, associated with sinus bradycardia
DESCRIPTION
- Slight irregularity of heartbeat, usually corresponding to respiratory cycle
- PR interval increases with inspiration and decreases with expiration
TREATMENT
- None

Sinus tachycardia

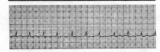

CAUSES
- Normal physiologic response to fever, exercise, anxiety, pain, dehydration; may also accompany shock, left ventricular failure, cardiac tamponade, anemia, hyperthyroidism, hypovolemia, pulmonary embolus
- May result from treatment with va-
golytic and sympathetic stimulating drugs
DESCRIPTION
- Rate > 100 bpm; rarely > 160 bpm
- Every QRS wave follows a P wave
TREATMENT
- Correct underlying cause

Sinus bradycardia

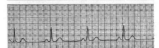

CAUSES
- Increased intracranial pressure: increased vagal tone due to bowel straining, vomiting, intubation, mechanical ventilation, sick sinus syndrome, or hypothyroidism
- Treatment with betablockers and sympatholytic drugs
- May be normal in athletes
DESCRIPTION
- Rate < 60 bpm
- A QRS complex follows each P wave
TREATMENT
- For signs of low cardiac output, dizziness, weakness, altered level of consciousness, or low blood pressure, 0.5 mg atropine every 5 minutes to total 2 mg
- Temporary pacemaker or isoproterenol, if atropine fails

Sinoatrial arrest or block (sinus arrest)

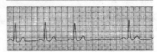

CAUSES
- Vagal stimulation, digitalis or quinidine toxicity
- Often a sign of sick sinus syndrome

DESCRIPTION
- NSR interrupted by unexpectedly prolonged PP interval; often terminated by a junctional escape beat or return to NSR
- QRS complexes uniform but irregular

TREATMENT
- Pacemaker for repeated episodes

Wandering atrial pacemaker

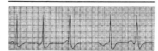

CAUSES
- Seen in rheumatic pancarditis as a result of inflammation involving the SA node; digitalis toxicity; sick sinus syndrome

DESCRIPTION
- Rate varies
- QRS complexes uniform in shape but irregular in rhythm
- P waves irregular with changing configuration, indicating they are not all from sinus node or single atrial focus
- PR interval varies from short to normal

TREATMENT
- Caution with digitalis administration
- No other treatment

Premature atrial contraction (PAC)

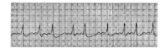

CAUSES
- CHF, ischemic heart disease, acute respiratory failure, or chronic obstructive pulmonary disease
- May result from treatment with digitalis, aminophylline, or adrenergic drugs; or from anxiety, amphetamines, or caffeine ingestion
- Occasional PAC may be normal

DESCRIPTION
- Premature, occasionally abnormal-looking P waves
- QRS complexes follow, except in very early or blocked PACs
- P wave often buried in the preceding T wave or can often be identified in the preceding T wave

TREATMENT
- If more than six times per minute or if frequency is increasing, give digitalis, quinidine, or propranolol; after revascularization surgery, propranolol
- Eliminate known causes, such as caffeine or drugs

Paroxysmal atrial tachycardia or paroxysmal supraventricular tachycardia

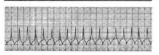

CAUSES
- Intrinsic abnormality of AV conduction system
- Congential accessory atrial conduction pathway
- Physical or psychological stress, hypoxia, hypokalemia, caffeine, marijuana, stimulants, digitalis toxicity

DESCRIPTION
- Heart rate > 140 bpm; rarely exceeds 250 bpm
- P waves regular but aberrant; difficult to differentiate from preceding T wave
- Onset and termination of dysrhythmia occur suddenly
- May cause palpitations and lightheadedness

(continued)

Cardiac Dysrhythmias *continued*

TREATMENT
• Verapamil, a calcium blocker, given first.
• Vagal maneuvers, sympathetic blockers (propranolol, digitalis [when not caused by digitalis toxicity], quinidine), or calcium blockers to alter AV node conduction
• Elective cardioversion, if patient is symptomatic and unresponsive to drugs

Atrial flutter

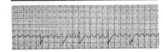

CAUSES
• Heart failure, valvular heart disease, pulmonary embolism, digitalis toxicity, postoperative revascularization
DESCRIPTION
• Ventricular rate depends on degree of AV block (usually 60 to 100 bpm)
• Atrial rate 240 to 400 bpm and regular
• QRS complexes uniform in shape but often irregular in rate
• P waves may have sawtooth configuration
TREATMENT
• Digitalis (unless dysrhythmia is due to digitalis toxicity), propranolol, or quinidine
• May require synchronized cardiovascular atrial pacemaker or vagal stimulation

Atrial fibrillation

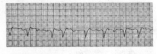

CAUSES
• CHF, chronic obstructive pulmonary disease, hyperthyroidism, sepsis, pulmonary embolus, mitral stenosis, digitalis toxicity (rare), atrial irritation, postcoronary bypass or valve replacement surgery
DESCRIPTION
• Atrial rate > 400 bpm
• Ventricular rate varies
• QRS complexes uniform in shape, but at irregular intervals
• PR interval indiscernible
• No P waves; or P waves appear as erratic, irregular baseline F waves
• Irregular QRS complexes
TREATMENT
• Digitalis and quinidine, to slow ventricular rate, and quinidine to convert rhythm to NSR: diuretics, such as furosemide, for CHF
• May require elective cardioversion for rapid rate

Nodal rhythm
(AV junctional rhythm)

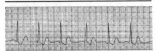

CAUSES
• Digitalis toxicity, inferior wall MI or ischemia, hypoxia, vagal stimulation
• Acute rheumatic fever
• Valve surgery
DESCRIPTION
• Ventricular rate usually 40 to 60 bpm (60 to 100 bpm is accelerated junctional rhythm)
• P waves may precede, be hidden within (absent), or follow QRS; if visible, they are altered
• Normal QRS duration, except in aberrant conduction
• Patient may be asymptomatic, unless ventricular rate is very slow

TREATMENT
- Symptomatic
- Atropine, with slow rate
- If patient is taking digitalis, it is discontinued.

Premature nodal contractions or junctional premature beats

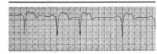

CAUSES
- MI or ischemia, digitalis toxicity, amphetamines, caffeine

DESCRIPTION
- Premature QRS complexes of uniform shape
- P waves irregular, with premature beat; may precede, be hidden within, or follow QRS

TREATMENT
- Correct underlying cause
- Quinidine or disopyramide, as ordered
- If patient is taking digitalis, it may be discontinued.

First-degree AV block

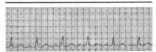

CAUSES
- Inferior myocardial ischemia or infarction, hypothyroidism, digitalis toxicity, potassium imbalance

DESCRIPTION
- PR interval prolonged > 0.2 second
- QRS complex normal

TREATMENT
- Caution, with digitalis administration
- Correct underlying cause; otherwise, be alert for increasing block

Second-degree AV block Mobitz Type I (Wenckebach)

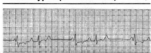

CAUSES
- *Mobitz Type I:* Inferior wall MI, digitalis toxicity, vagal stimulation

DESCRIPTION
- *Mobitz Type I:* PR interval becomes progressively longer with each cycle until QRS disappears (dropped beat). After a dropped beat, PR interval is shorter. Ventricular rate is irregular; atrial rhythm, regular.

TREATMENT
- *Mobitz Type I:* atropine, if patient is symptomatic
- Discontinue digitalis

Second-degree AV block Mobitz Type II

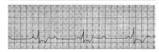

CAUSES
- *Mobitz Type II:* Degenerative disease of conduction system, ischemia of AV node in anterior MI, digitalis toxicity, anteroseptal infarction

DESCRIPTION
- *Mobitz Type II:* PR interval is constant, with QRS complexes dropped
- Ventricular rhythm may be irregular, with varying degree of block
- Atrial rate regular

TREATMENT
- *Mobitz Type II:* temporary pacemaker, sometimes followed by permanent pacemaker
- Atropine, for slow rate
- If patient is taking digitalis, it is discontinued.

(continued)

Cardiac Dysrhythmias *continued*

Third-degree AV block (complete heart block)

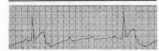

CAUSES
• Ischemic heart disease or infarction; postsurgical complications of mitral valve replacement; digitalis toxicity; hypoxia sometimes causing syncope due to decreased cerebral blood flow, as in Stokes-Adams syndrome

DESCRIPTION
• Atrial rate regular; ventricular rate slow and regular
• No relationship between P waves and QRS complexes
• No constant PR interval
• QRS interval normal (nodal pacemaker); wide and bizarre (ventricular pacemaker)

TREATMENT
• Usually requires temporary pacemaker, followed by permanent pacemaker
• Epinephrine or isoproterenol

Nodal tachycardia (junctional tachycardia)

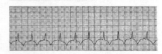

CAUSES
• Digitalis toxicity, myocarditis, cardiomyopathy, myocardial ischemia or infarction

DESCRIPTION
• Onset of rhythm often sudden, occurring in bursts
• Ventricular rate > 100 bpm
• Other characteristics same as junctional rhythm

TREATMENT
• Vagal stimulation
• Propranolol, quinidine, digitalis (if cause is not digitalis toxicity)
• Elective cardioversion

Premature ventricular contraction (PVC)

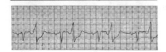

CAUSES
• Heart failure; old or acute MI or contusion with trauma; myocardial irritation by ventricular catheter, such as a pacemaker; hypoxia, as in anemia and acute respiratory failure; drug toxicity (digitalis, aminophylline, tricyclic antidepressants, betaadrenergics [isoproterenol or dopamine]); electrolyte imbalances (especially hypokalemia); psychological stress

DESCRIPTION
• Beat occurs prematurely, usually followed by a complete compensatory pause after PVC; irregular pulse
• QRS complex wide and distorted
• Can occur singly, in pairs, or in threes; can alternate with normal beats
• Focus can be from one or more sites
• PVCs are most ominous when clustered, multifocal, with R wave on T pattern

TREATMENT
• Lidocaine I.V. bolus and drip infusion; procainamide I.V. If induced by digitalis toxicity, stop the digitalis; if induced by hypokalemia, give potassium chloride I.V.
• Inderal (propranolol)

Ventricular tachycardia

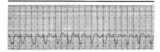

CAUSES
Myocardial ischemia, infarction, or aneurysm; ventricular catheters; digitalis or quinidine toxicity; hypokalemia; hypercalcemia; anxiety; Torsades de Pointes

DESCRIPTION
• Ventricular rate 140 to 220 bpm; may be regular
• QRS complexes are wide, bizarre, and independent of P waves.
• No visible P waves
• Can produce chest pain, anxiety, palpitations, dyspnea, shock, coma, and death

TREATMENT
• Cardiopulmonary resuscitation (CPR) if no pulse, followed by lidocaine I.V. (bolus and drip infusion); synchronized cardioversion with pulse, countershock without pulse
• Bretylium tosylate and procainamide

Ventricular fibrillation

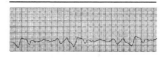

CAUSES
• Myocardial ischemia or infarction, untreated ventricular tachycardia, electrolyte imbalances (hypokalemia and alkalosis; hyperkalemia and hypercalcemia), digitalis or quinidine toxicity, electric shock, hypothermia

DESCRIPTION
• Ventricular rhythm rapid and chaotic
• QRS complexes are wide and irregular; no visible P waves

• Loss of consciousness, with no peripheral pulses, blood pressure, or respirations; possible seizures; sudden death

TREATMENT
• CPR
• Asynchronized counter-shock (200-300 watts/second then 300-400 watts/second). If rhythm does not return, shock again.
• Drugs such as bretylium tosylate I.V., lidocaine, or procainamide (for recurrent episodes)

Ventricular standstill (asystole)

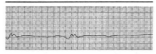

CAUSES
• Acute respiratory failure, myocardial ischemia or infarction, ruptured ventricular aneurysm, aortic valve disease, or hyperkalemia

DESCRIPTION
• Primary ventricular standstill—regular P waves, no QRS complexes
• Secondary ventricular standstill—QRS complexes wide and slurred, occurring at irregular intervals; agonal heart rhythm
• Loss of consciousness, with no peripheral pulses, blood pressure, respirations

TREATMENT
• CPR
• Endotracheal intubation; pacemaker should be available
• Epinephrine, calcium gluconate, sodium bicarbonate, atropine, and isoproterenol

Supportive Cardiovascular Drugs

DRUG, DOSE, ROUTE	INTERACTIONS
Antianxiety Drugs **alprazolam** 0.25 to 0.5 mg t.i.d. Maximum daily dosage 4 mg in divided doses	None significant
chlordiazepoxide hydrochloride 5 to 25 mg t.i.d. or q.i.d. Children over 6 years: 5 mg P.O. b.i.d. to q.i.d. Maximum 10 mg b.i.d. or t.i.d.	*Cimetidine:* increases sedation
diazepam Adults: 2 to 10 mg P.O. b.i.d. to q.i.d. Children: same as above	*Phenobarbital:* increased interactions of both drugs
Electrolytes **calcium salts** Adults and children: initially 500 mg to 1 g elemental calcium I.V., with further dosage based on serum calcium determinants	*Cardiac glycosides:* increased digitalis toxicity
magnesium sulfate Adults: 1 g or 8.12 mEq of 50% solution (2 ml) I.M. q 6 hours for four doses, depending on serum magnesium level	None significant
potassium acetate Adults and children: 20 mEq P.O. daily in divided doses b.i.d. to q.i.d.	None significant

SIDE EFFECTS	SPECIAL CONSIDERATIONS
Drowsiness, light-headedness, headache, confusion, transient hypotension, dry mouth, nausea, vomiting	Reduce dose in elderly or debilitated patients. Do not withdraw drug abruptly. Warn patient not to combine with alcohol or other depressants
Drowsiness, lethargy, hangover, fainting, transient hypotension, nausea, vomiting, abdominal discomfort	Monitor patient carefully. Reduce dosage in the elderly. Warn patient not to combine with alcohol or other depressants. Withdrawal symptoms are similar to barbiturates.
Fatigue, drowsiness, ataxia, dizziness, headache, slurred speech, hypotension, cardiovascular collapse, blurred vision, nausea, urinary retention, rash, respiratory depression	Monitor respirations. Drug should not be withdrawn abruptly. Warn patient not to mix with alcohol or other depressants.
I.V. administration: tingling sensations, syncope, heat waves, vasodilation, bradycardia, cardiac dysrhythmias, cardiac arrest *P.O. administration:* stomach irritation, hemorrhage, constipation, mild fall in blood pressure	Monitor EKG when giving I.V.; patient should remain recumbent for a short while. Monitor blood calcium levels frequently. Solutions should be warmed to body temperature before administration. Make sure doctor specifies which salt he wants administered.
Toxicity: weak or absent deep tendon reflexes, flaccid paralysis, hypothermia, drowsiness, respiratory depression, paralysis, twitching, tetany, seizures, cardiac dysrhythmias, slow, weak pulse, hypotension	I.V. bolus must be injected slowly to avoid respiratory or cardiac arrest. If available, use constant infusion pump. Monitor vital signs every 15 minutes when infusing. Monitor intake and output. Check serum magnesium levels before each dose.
Paresthesias of extremities, listlessness, mental confusion, weakness, flaccid paralysis, peripheral vascular collapse with fall in blood pressure, cardiac dysrhythmias, heart block, possible cardiac arrest, EKG changes, nausea, vomiting, diarrhea, oliguria, gray pallor	During therapy, monitor EKG, serum potassium level, renal function, BUN, serum creatinine, intake and output. Give slowly as diluted solution. Monitor patient carefully.

(continued)

Supportive Cardiovascular Drugs *continued*

DRUG, DOSE, ROUTE	INTERACTIONS
potassium bicarbonate 25 mEq or 50 mEq tablet dissolved in water one to four times a day	None significant
potassium chloride 40 to 100 mEq P.O. divided into three to four doses daily. Give by I.V. route when patient cannot take orally, 40 mEq/liter or less	None significant
potassium gluconate 40 to 100 mEq P.O. divided into three to four doses daily	None significant
sodium bicarbonate Adults and children: as a 7.5% or 8.4% solution, 1 to 3 mEq/kg I.V. initially; may repeat in 10 minutes	None significant
Laxatives **docusate calcium, docusate potassium, docusate sodium.** Adults and older children: 50 to 300 mg (sodium) P.O. daily or 240 mg (calcium and potassium) P.O. daily until bowel movements are normal	None significant
glycerine Adults and children over 6 years: 3 g as a suppository, or 5 to 15 ml as an enema	None significant

SIDE EFFECTS	SPECIAL CONSIDERATIONS
Mental confusion, weakness, cardiac dysrhythmias, EKG changes (prolonged P-R interval, wide QRS, ST-segment depression; tall, tented T waves), nausea, vomiting, abdominal pain, diarrhea, perforation of bowel, ulcerations	Monitor patient carefully. Never switch potassium products without a doctor's order. Have patient take with meals and sip slowly over a 5- to 10-minute period.
Mental confusion, weakness, peripheral vascular collapse with fall in blood pressure, cardiac dysrhythmias, heart block, cardiac arrest, EKG changes, nausea, vomiting, diarrhea, possible ulcerations and hemorrhage, oliguria, gray pallor	Never give I.V. push or I.M.; give slowly as dilute solution. Give P.O. forms after meals, with full glass of water or fruit juice. Monitor patient carefully.
Mental confusion, paresthesias, weakness, flaccid paralysis, cardiac dysrhythmias, EKG changes, nausea, vomiting, diarrhea, abdominal pain, intestinal obstructions, stenosis, hemorrhage, perforation	Monitor patient carefully. Give with or after meals with full glass of water or fruit juice, to lessen GI distress. Monitor EKG, serum potassium, other electrolytes, creatinine, and BUN during therapy.
Gastric distention, renal calculi or crystals, (with overdose) alkalosis, hyperkalemia, hyperosmolarity	May be added to other I.V. fluids. Parenteral solutions will precipitate calcium salts. Do not mix with norepinephrine and dopamine. Monitor patient's blood pH, Pao_2, $Paco_2$, and electrolytes.
Throat irritation, bitter taste, mild abdominal cramping, diarrhea	Use sodium salt preparation cautiously in patients on sodium-restricted diets. Not to be used to treat constipation, but to prevent it.
Cramping pain, rectal discomfort, hyperemia of rectal mucosa	Used mainly to reestablish proper toilet habits in laxative-dependent patients.

(continued)

Supportive Cardiovascular Drugs *continued*

DRUG, DOSE, ROUTE	INTERACTIONS
magnesium salts Adults and children over 6 years: 15 g magnesium sulfate P.O. in glass of water; or 10 to 20 ml concentrated milk of magnesia P.O.; or 15 to 60 ml milk of magnesia P.O.; or 5 to 10 oz magnesium citrate at bedtime	None significant
methylcellulose Adults: 5 to 20 ml liquid P.O. t.i.d. with a glass of water; or 15 ml syrup P.O. morning and evening	None significant
mineral oil Adults: 15 to 30 ml P.O. at bedtime; or 4 oz enema Children: 5 to 15 ml P.O. at bedtime; or 1 to 2 oz enema	None significant
psyllium Adults: 1 to 2 rounded teaspoonfuls P.O. in full glass of liquid daily, b.i.d. or t.i.d., followed by a second glass of liquid Children over 6 years: 1 level teaspoonful P.O. in ½ glass of liquid at bedtime	None significant
Sedatives and hypnotics **chloral hydrate** Adults: 250 mg P.O. or rectally t.i.d. after meals Children: 8 mg/kg P.O. t.i.d.	*Alcohol or other other CNS depressants, including narcotic analgesics:* excessive CNS depression or vasodilation reaction *Furosamide I.V.:* sweating, flushing, variable blood pressure, uneasiness
flurazepam hydrochloride 15 to 30 mg P.O. at bedtime	*Cimetidine:* increased sedation *Alcohol and other CNS depressants:* increased CNS depression
triazolam Adults: 0.125 to 0.5 mg P.O. at bedtime.	*Alcohol and other CNS depressants, including narcotic analgesics:* excessive CNS depression

SIDE EFFECTS	SPECIAL CONSIDERATIONS
Abdominal cramping, nausea, fluid and electrolyte disturbances, laxative dependence	For short-term therapy. Do not give oral drugs 1 to 2 hours before or after. Monitor serum electrolytes during prolonged therapy.
Nausea; vomiting; diarrhea; esophageal, gastric, small intestine, or colonic strictures, abdominal cramps	Use for short-term therapy. Not absorbed systemically; nontoxic.
Nausea, vomiting, diarrhea, abdominal cramps, decreased absorption of nutrients and fat-soluble vitamins	Do not give drug with meals or directly after, as it delays passage of food from stomach. To be taken only at bedtime. Give with fruit juice or carbonated beverage to disguise taste.
Nausea; vomiting; diarrhea; abdominal cramps; esophageal, gastric, small intestinal, or colonic strictures when taken in dry form	Contains significant amount of sodium; should not be given to patients on sodium-restricted diets. Some brands contain sugar; be careful with diabetic patients. For short-term treatment. May reduce appetite if given before meals.
Hangover, drowsiness, nightmares, dizziness, ataxia, nausea, vomiting, diarrhea	Supervise walking and all out-of-bed activities. Raise bed rails, especially with elderly patients. If patient is on anticoagulant therapy, monitor for increased prothrombin time during first several days.
Daytime sedation, dizziness, drowsiness, disturbed coordination, headache	Monitor all out-of-bed activities. Raise bed rails, especially with elderly patients.
Drowsiness, dizziness, headache, rebound insomnia, amnesia, nausea, vomiting	Supervise walking and all out-of-bed activities. Raise bed rails, especially with elderly patients. Dependence is possible with long-term use.

INDEX

D

E

J

K

I

L

W

Notes

Notes

499

Notes

Nursing85 Books™

CLINICAL POCKET MANUAL™ SERIES
Diagnostic Tests
Emergency Care
Fluids and Electrolytes
Signs and Symptoms
Cardiovascular Care
Respiratory Care
Critical Care
Neurologic Care
Surgical Care

NURSING NOW™ SERIES
Shock
Hypertension
Drug Interactions
Cardiac Crises
Respiratory Emergencies
Pain

NURSE'S CLINICAL LIBRARY™
Cardiovascular Disorders
Respiratory Disorders
Endocrine Disorders
Neurologic Disorders
Renal and Urologic Disorders
Gastrointestinal Disorders
Neoplastic Disorders
Immune Disorders

NURSE REVIEW™ SERIES
Cardiac Problems

Nursing85 DRUG HANDBOOK™

NURSING PHOTOBOOK™ SERIES
Providing Respiratory Care
Managing I.V. Therapy
Dealing with Emergencies
Giving Medications
Assessing Your Patients
Using Monitors
Providing Early Mobility
Giving Cardiac Care
Performing GI Procedures
Implementing Urologic Procedures
Controlling Infection
Ensuring Intensive Care
Coping with Neurologic Disorders
Caring for Surgical Patients
Working with Orthopedic Patients
Nursing Pediatric Patients
Helping Geriatric Patients
Attending Ob/Gyn Patients
Aiding Ambulatory Patients
Carrying Out Special Procedures

NURSE'S REFERENCE LIBRARY®
Diseases
Diagnostics
Drugs
Assessment
Procedures
Definitions
Practices
Emergencies
Signs and Symptoms

PROFESSIONAL TRADE BOOKS
Health Assessment Handbook
MediQuik Cards™
Nurse's Legal Handbook
Cardiovascular Care Handbook
Emergency Care Handbook